Stedman's
EMERGENCY
MEDICINE
WORDS

INCLUDES
TRAUMA & CRITICAL CARE

D1166198

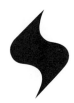

Stedman's

EMERGENCY MEDICINE

WORDS

INCLUDES
TRAUMA & CRITICAL CARE

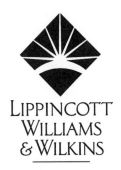

LIPPINCOTT
WILLIAMS
& WILKINS

Publisher: Julie K. Stegman
Series Managing Editor: Trista A. DiPaula
Associate Managing Editor: Steve Lichtenstein
Typesetter: Peirce Graphic Services, LLC.
Printer & Binder: Malloy Litho, Inc.

Copyright © 2004 Lippincott Williams & Wilkins
351 West Camden Street
Baltimore, Maryland 21201-2436

Printed in the United States of America

2004

Library of Congress Cataloging-in-Publication Data

Stedman's emergency medicine words including trauma and critical care.—1st ed.
   p. ; cm.
Includes bibliographical references and index.
ISBN 0-7817-4421-0 (alk. paper)
1. Emergency medicine—Terminology. 2. Critical care medicine—Terminology.
[DNLM: 1. Emergencies—Terminology—English. 2. Emergency Medicine—
Terminology—English. WB 15 S8122 2004] I. Title: Emergency medicine words
including trauma and critical care. II. Stedman, Thomas Lathrop, 1853–1938.
III. Lippincott Williams & Wilkins.

RC86.3.S74 2004
616.02′5′014—dc22
                                               2003019049
                                                      01
1 2 3 4 5 6 7 8 9 10

Contents

Acknowledgments

An important part of our editorial process is the involvement of medical transcriptionists—as advisors, reviewers, and/or editors.

We extend special thanks to Jeanne Bock, CSR, MT, and Nicole Peck, CMT, for editing the manuscript, helping resolve many difficult questions, and contributing material for the appendix sections. We are grateful to our Editorial Advisory Board members, including Barbara Batchelder, RHIT, Quality Assurance Manager; Cheryl J. Blake; R. Jo-Ann Clarke; Judith Lichtenberger, CMT; Beverly S. Oberline, CMT; Cheryl Rittschoff; Anne Thorpe; and Terri L. Unkelhaeuser, who were instrumental in the development of this reference. They recommended sources and shared their valuable judgment, insight, and perspective.

Additional thanks to Helen Littrell for performing the final prepublication review. Other important contributors to this edition include Susan Bartolucci; Marty Cantu, CMT; Shemah Fletcher; Robin Koza; Heather Little, CMT; Judy Moody; and Linda Waugh. Thanks to Roger Stone, MD, for his valuable help with the appendix.

And, as always, Barb Ferretti played an integral role in the process by reviewing the content files for format, updating the content, and providing a final quality check. Special thanks also goes to Lisa Fahnestock for her assistance with this work.

As with all our *Stedman's* word references, this resource incorporates the suggestions and expertise of our many contacts in the medical transcriptionist community. Thanks to all of our advisory board participants, reviewers, and editors; AAMT meeting attendees; and others who have written us with requests and comments—keep talking, and we'll keep listening.

Editor's Preface

It's the sound we hope to never hear coming to our home—the wail of ambulance sirens. That sound is associated with tragedy and pain—someone somewhere has been hurt. However, it is also reassuring to know that help is on the way. It is a sound many take for granted, because it is heard so often and because we know help will come if and when we need it. Once in the ambulance, the work begins. EMTs begin the task of evaluating, stabilizing, resuscitating, and treating the patient to facilitate the best outcome.

Every medical transcriptionist I have ever met who has cable TV has watched, at least once, *Trauma: Life in the ER*. This show reveals the nitty gritty, real-life situations encountered in emergency rooms all over the United States. What is our fascination with this show and others like it? I can't speak for the whole profession, but much of the fascination for me is because every time I turn on a reality medical program like this, all the situations I hear about and transcribe in my work-day world come to life! The intubation maneuver I've transcribed over and over is occurring before my very eyes, as is the treatment of a gunshot wound victim.

Stedman's Emergency Medicine Words, Includes Trauma and Critical Care contains terminology used in dictation, describing situations and conditions encountered from the time a patient is evaluated by the EMTs on the scene to the time the patient is discharged to the medical floor, operating room, or home. The terms here cover a broad range of medical conditions and anatomy, because we understand many causes can bring a person to the ER—anything from a bean in the nose of a young child to the multiple traumas of a plane crash victim. We have also included terminology used for those patients transferred to and treated in the critical care units of a hospital.

You will find the appendix section of this book to be a unique and informative resource in its own right. We have included terminology that is often heard but hard to confirm, specifically slang and abbreviations used nearly exclusively in the environment of emergency medicine. We have also included lists of fractures and sutures, as well as listings of poisons and their antidotes. Because emergency medicine can be focused on any part of a patient's anatomy, we have devised a very inclusive section of anatomical illustrations to cover the complete human body, as well as illustrations of intubation techniques and IV line placement positions.

This preface would not be complete without thanking everyone involved in the process of putting this Word Book together: the reviewers who searched journals, texts, and the Internet to find the terms included in this book; the transcriptionists who requested this book and sent in their own lists of terms; and the entire Stedman's team for listening to transcriptionists everywhere and making this Word Book possible. We also extend special thanks to Trista DiPaula, Steve Lichtenstein, and Barb Ferretti for their valuable assistance.

We hope you find this newest Word Book to be another valuable tool in completing emergency medicine and trauma reports. We also hope you will send in your word lists and suggestions to contribute to the next edition of this book, as each edition is only made better with help from its users—you!

Jeanne Bock, CSR, MT
Nicole G. Peck, CMT

Publisher's Preface

Stedman's Emergency Medicine Words, Includes Trauma and Critical Care, offers an authoritative assurance of quality and exactness to the wordsmiths of the healthcare professions—medical transcriptionists, medical editors and copyeditors, health information management personnel, court reporters, and the many other users and producers of medical documentation.

In this new title, we have included emergency medicine, trauma, and critical care terminology. Users will find protocols, diagnoses, and therapeutic procedures, new techniques, lab tests, clinical research terms, as well as abbreviations with their expansions pertinent to emergency medicine, trauma, and critical care. The appendix sections include anatomical illustrations with useful captions and labels; a table of fracture and sutures; normal lab values; poisons and antidotes; poisonous and hazardous organisms and their antidotes; emergency medicine abbreviations and slang; and drugs by indication.

This new edition, including more than 30,000 entries, includes the *Stedman's Word Book Series'* trademarks: terms fully cross-indexed by first and last word, an A-Z format with main entries and subentries, and appendix material for additional comprehension and application of the terminology.

We at Lippincott Williams & Wilkins strive to provide you with the most up-to-date and accurate word references available. Your use of this Word Book will prompt new editions, which we will publish as often as updates and revisions justify. We welcome your suggestions for improvements, changes, corrections, and additions—whatever will make this *Stedman's* product more useful to you. Please complete the postage-paid card in this book for future suggestions and recommendations, or visit us online at www.stedmans.com.

Explanatory Notes

Medical transcription is an art as well as a science. Both approaches are needed to correctly interpret the dictation of a physician, whose language is a product of education, training, and experience. This variety in medical language means that there are several acceptable ways to express certain terms, including jargon. *Stedman's Emergency Medicine Words, Includes Trauma and Critical Care,* provides variant spellings and phrasings for many terms. These elements, in addition to complete cross-referencing, make *Stedman's Emergency Medicine Words, Includes Trauma and Critical Care* a valuable resource for determining the validity of terms as they are encountered.

Alphabetical Organization

Alphabetization of main entries is letter by letter as spelled, ignoring punctuation, spaces, prefixed numbers, or other characters. In compliance with the *AAMT Book of Style, 2nd Edition,* the numbers 1 through 9 are no longer spelled out in medical transcription, so these terms will be ordered by the first letter in the phrase. For example:

fighter's fracture	**personality**	**head-down position**
figure-of-8 suture	**1-person stretcher**	**4-headed muscle**
filament suture	**pertinent negative**	**headlamp**

Terms beginning or ending with Greek letters show the Greek letters spelled out and listed alphabetically. For example:

alpha, α
   a. phase
   a. radiation

In subentry alphabetization, the abbreviated singular form or the spelled-out plural form of the noun main entry word is ignored.

Format and Style

All main entries are in **boldface** to expedite locating a sought-after term, to enhance distinction between main entries and subentries, and to relieve the textual density of the pages.

Irregular plurals and variant spellings are shown on the same line as the singular or preferred form of the word. For example:

alveolus, pl. alveoli
anular, annular

Hyphenation
As a rule of style, multiple eponyms (e.g., Mears-Rubash approach) are hyphenated. Also, hyphens have been added between a manufacturer and one or more eponyms (e.g., Vital-Metzenbaum dissecting scissors). Please note that in many cases, hyphenation is a question of style, not of accuracy, and thus is a matter of choice.

Possessives
Possessive forms have been dropped in this reference for the sake of consistency and conformance with the guidelines of the American Association for Medical Transcription (AAMT) and other groups. Please note, however, that in many cases, retaining the possessive, like hyphenating, is a question of style, not of accuracy, and thus is a matter of choice. To form the possessive of a word, simply add the apostrophe or apostrophe "s" to the end of the word.

Cross-indexing
The word list is in an index-like main entry-subentry format that contains two combined alphabetical listings:

(1) A *noun* main entry-subentry organization, which is typical of the A-Z section of medical dictionaries like *Stedman's:*

aorta
  abdominal a.
  ascending a.
  coarctation of a.

monitor
  cardiac m.
  Holter m.
  impedance m.

(2) An *adjective* main entry-subentry organization, which lists words and phrases as you hear them. The main entries are the adjectives or modifiers in a multiword term. The subentries are the nouns around which the terms are constructed and to which the adjectives or modifiers pertain:

spinal
    s. column
    s. cord concussion
    s. fracture

ovarian
    o. bursa
    o. cyst
    o. ligament

This format provides the user with more than one way to locate and identify a multiword term. For example:

contrast
    c. esophagram

esophagram
    contrast e.

skull
    s. fracture

fracture
    skull f.

It also allows the user to see together all terms that contain a particular descriptor, as well as all types, kinds, or variations of a noun entity. For example:

material
    bone grafting m.
    hazardous m.
    suture m.

popliteal
    p. aneurysm
    p. muscle
    p. nerve

Wherever possible, abbreviations are separately defined and cross-referenced. For example:

RAP
    right atrial pressure

right
    r. atrial pressure (RAP)

pressure
    right atrial p. (RAP)

References

In addition to the manufacturers' literature we gather at various medical meetings, scientific reports from hospitals, and the lists of our Editorial Advisory Board members (from their daily transcription work), we used the following sources for new terms in *Stedman's Emergency Medicine Words Includes Trauma and Critical Care.*

Books

The AAMT Book of Style, 2nd Edition. Modesto, CA: AAMT, 2002.

Aehlert B. *Aehlert's EMT-Basic Study Guide.* Baltimore: Williams & Wilkins, 1998.

Aghababian RV. *Emergency Medicine: The Core Curriculum.* Philadelphia: Lippincott-Raven, 1998.

Birrer RB. *Management of Adult Urgencies and Emergencies.* Philadelphia: Lippincott Williams & Wilkins, 2001.

Chan ED. *Bedside Critical Care Manual, 2nd Edition.* Philadelphia: Hanley & Belfus, 2002.

Civetta JM, Taylor RW, Kirby RR. *Critical Care, 3rd Edition.* Philadelphia: Lippincott Williams & Wilkins, 1996.

Critical Care Challenges: Disorders, Treatments, and Procedures. Philadelphia: Lippincott Williams & Wilkins, 2003.

Diepenbrock NH. *Quick Reference to Critical Care.* Philadelphia: Lippincott Williams & Wilkins, 1999.

Drake E. *Sloane's Medical Word Book, 4th Edition.* Philadelphia: Saunders, 2001.

Harwood-Nuss A, Wolfson AB, Linden CH, Shepherd SM, Stenklyft PH. *The Clinical Practice of Emergency Medicine, 3rd Edition.* Philadelphia: Lippincott Williams & Wilkins, 2001.

Hogan DE, Burstein JL. *Disaster Medicine.* Philadelphia: Lippincott Williams & Wilkins, 2002.

Hurford WE, Hess D. *Critical Care Handbook of Massachusetts General Hospital, 3rd Edition.* Philadelphia: Lippincott Williams & Wilkins, 2000.

Irwin RS, Rippe RS. *Manual of Intensive Care Medicine: With Annotated Key References, 3rd Edition.* Philadelphia: Lippincott Williams & Wilkins, 2000.

James DM. *Field Guide to Urgent and Ambulatory Care Procedures.* Philadelphia: Lippincott Williams & Wilkins, 2001.

Jenkins JL, Braen GR. *Manual of Emergency Medicine, 4th Edition.* Philadelphia: Lippincott Williams & Wilkins, 2000

Lance LL. *Quick Look Drug Book 2003.* Baltimore: Lippincott Williams & Wilkins, 2003.

Marini JJ. *Critical Care Medicine: The Essentials, 2nd Edition.* Baltimore: Lippincott Williams & Wilkins, 1997.

NMS Clinical Manuals: *Emergency Medicine, 2nd Edition*. Baltimore: Lippincott Williams & Wilkins, 2002.

Olshaker JS, Jackson MC, Smock WS. *Forensic Emergency Medicine*. Philadelphia: Lippincott Williams & Wilkins, 2001.

Peitzman AB. *The Trauma Manual, 2nd Edition*. Philadelphia: Lippincott Williams & Wilkins, 2002.

Rosen P. *5-Minute Emergency Medicine Consult*. Philadelphia: Lippincott Williams & Wilkins, 1999.

Schwartz GR. *Principles and Practice: Emergency Medicine, 4th Edition*. Baltimore: Lippincott Williams & Wilkins, 1999.

Simon RR, Brenner BE. *Emergency Procedures and Techniques, 4th Edition*. Philadelphia: Lippincott Williams & Wilkins, 2001.

Stedman's Concise Medical Dictionary for the Health Professions, 4th Edition. Baltimore: Lippincott Williams & Wilkins, 2001.

Stedman's Medical Dictionary, 27th Edition. Baltimore: Lippincott Williams & Wilkins, 2000.

Sullivan JB Jr, Krieger GR. *Clinical Environmental Health and Toxic Exposures*. Philadelphia: Lippincott Williams & Wilkins, 2001.

Viccellio P. *Emergency Toxicology, 2nd Edition*. Philadelphia: Lippincott-Raven, 1998.

Walls RM, Luten RC, Murphy MF, Schneider RE. *Manual of Emergency Airway Management*. Philadelphia: Lippincott Williams & Wilkins, 2000.

Wilson RF. *Handbook of Trauma: Pitfalls and Pearls*. Philadelphia: Lippincott Williams & Wilkins, 1999.

Images

Agur AMR, Lee MJ. *Grant's Atlas of Anatomy, 10th Edition*. Baltimore: Lippincott Williams & Wilkins, 1999.

Battista K, Baltimore, MD. From Oatis C. *Kinesiology: The Mechanics and Pathomechanics of Human Movement*. Baltimore: Lippincott Williams & Wilkins, 2003.

Caldwell S, Pikesville, MD. From *Stedman's Medical Dictionary, 27th Edition*. Baltimore: Lippincott Williams & Wilkins, 2000.

Hardy NO, Westport, CT. From *Stedman's Medical Dictionary, 27th Edition*. Baltimore: Lippincott Williams & Wilkins, 2000.

LifeART Emergency Collection 2, CD-ROM. Baltimore: Lippincott Williams & Wilkins.

LifeART Emergency Collection 3, CD-ROM. Baltimore: Lippincott Williams & Wilkins.

LifeART Emergency Collection 4, CD-ROM. Baltimore: Lippincott Williams & Wilkins.

LifeART Emergency Collection 5, CD-ROM. Baltimore: Lippincott Williams & Wilkins.

LifeART Nursing Collection 1, CD-ROM. Baltimore: Lippincott Williams & Wilkins.

LifeART Nursing Collection 3, CD-ROM. Baltimore: Lippincott Williams & Wilkins.

LifeART Pediatrics Collection 1, CD-ROM. Baltimore: Lippincott Williams & Wilkins.

LifeART Super Anatomy Collection 1, CD-ROM. Baltimore: Lippincott Williams & Wilkins.

LifeART Super Anatomy Collection 2, CD-ROM. Baltimore: Lippincott Williams & Wilkins.

LifeART Super Anatomy Collection 5, CD-ROM. Baltimore: Lippincott Williams & Wilkins.

LifeART Super Anatomy Collection 7, CD-ROM. Baltimore: Lippincott Williams & Wilkins.

LifeART Super Anatomy Collection 9, CD-ROM. Baltimore: Lippincott Williams & Wilkins.

MediClip Human Anatomy 1–3, CD-ROM. Baltimore: Lippincott Williams & Wilkins.

MediClip Manual Medicine 2, CD-ROM. Baltimore: Lippincott Williams & Wilkins.

Senkarik M, San Antonio, TX. From *Stedman's Medical Dictionary, 27th Edition*. Baltimore: Lippincott Williams & Wilkins.

Senkarik M, San Antonio, TX. Smeltzer SC & Bare BG. *Brunner & Suddarth's Textbook of Medical Surgical-Nursing, 8th Edition*. Philadelphia: JB Lippincott & Wilkins, 1996.

Stedman's Orthopaedic & Rehab Words, 4th Edition. Baltimore: Lippincott Williams & Wilkins, 2003.

Journals

Critical Care Medicine. Baltimore: Lippincott Williams & Wilkins, 2002–2003.

Emergency Medical Services. Sherman Oaks, Ca: Emergency Medical Services, 2002–2003.

Emergency Medicine News. Baltimore: Lippincott Williams & Wilkins, 2002–2003.

Latest Word. Philadelphia: Saunders, 1999–2003.

Pediatric Critical Care Medicine. Baltimore: Lippincott Williams & Wilkins, 2002.

Pediatric Emergency Care. Baltimore: Lippincott Williams & Wilkins, 2002.

Perspectives on the Medical Transcription Profession. Modesto, CA: Health Professions Institute, 2002.

Websites

http://ccforum.com/

http://health.ucsd.edu/poison/marine.asp

http://pedsccm.wustl.edu/All-Net/main.html

http://rnbob.tripod.com/abbreviationsandrespiratoryterms.htm

http://www.calpoison.org/

http://www.calpoison.org/public/mushrooms.html

http://www.ccme.org/EMA/index.html

http://www.ccmjournal.com/

http://www.emedhome.com/

http://www.emedicine.com/emerg/index.shtml

http://www.emedmag.com/

http://www.enw.org/Lexicon.htm

http://www.er365.com/germ%20warfare-nerve%20gas-anthrax-biological%
20warfare%20treat ment.htm#Anthrax

http://www.eurasiahealth.org/english/gloss/results.cfm

http://www.ispub.com/ostia/index.php?xmlFilePath=journals/ijeicm/front.xml

http://www.medscape.com/criticalcarehome

http://www.nbc-med.org/SiteContent/HomePage/WhatsNew/MedAspects/contents.html

http://www.ncemi.org/

http://www.nda.ox.ac.uk/ptc/

http://www.regionshospital.com/Regions/Menu/0,1592,3795,00.html

http://www.sccm.org

http://www.sccm.org/patient/glossary.html

http://www.thrombosis-consult.com/articles/Textbook/118_poison.htm

http://www.trauma.org/

http://www.umm.edu/ency/article/002852.htm

http://www.wwrem.com/

α (*var. of* alpha)
A2
    aortic second sound
AA
    Alcoholics Anonymous
        AA neurotransmitter
AAA
    abdominal aortic aneurysm
AAO3
    awake, alert, and oriented ×3
AAPCC
    American Association of Poison Control
    Centers
Aaron sign
AAS
    acute abdominal series
abandon
        threat to a.
abandonment
Abbreviated Injury Scale
ABC
    airway, breathing, circulation
ABCDE
    airway, breathing, circulation, disability,
    and exposure
        ABCDE of trauma
abciximab
abdomen
        doughy a.
        intrathoracic a.
        patulous a.
        protuberant a.
abdominal
    a. aneurysm
    a. aorta
    a. aortic aneurysm (AAA)
    a. apron
    a. breathing
    a. cavity
    a. circumference
    a. closure
    a. compartment syndrome
    a. crisis
    a. CT
    a. distention
    a. evisceration
    a. gangrene
    a. gunshot wound
    a. hypertension
    a. ischemia
    a. muscle
    a. packing
    a. paracentesis
    a. pressure
    a. reflex

    a. region
    a. tenderness
    a. thrust
    a. trauma
    a. trauma imaging
    a. triangular ligament
    a. ultrasonography
    a. view
    a. visceral organ injury scale
    a. wall pain
abdominis muscle
abdominoanterior
abdominopelvic cavity
abdominoposterior
abducent nerve
abduct
abduction
    a. finger splint
    a. fracture
    a. muscle
    a. thumb splint
abduction-external rotation fracture
abductor
    a. digiti minimi muscle
    a. digiti quinti muscle
    a. digiti quinti tendon
    a. hallucis brevis muscle
    a. hallucis tendon
    a. magnus muscle
    a. pollicis brevis muscle
    a. pollicis brevis tendon
    a. pollicis longus muscle
    a. pollicis longus tendon
aberrancy
aberrant obturator vein
aberration
        coma a.
ABG
    arterial blood gas
ablation
        nerve rootlet a.
able
    a. to ambulate
    a. to maintain hydration
abnormal
    a. breath sound
    a. respiratory rate
abnormality
        acid-base a.
        bone marrow a.
        bony a.
        conduction a.
        electrolyte a.
        joint a.
        metabolic a.

abnormality *(continued)*
    ocular a.
    scalp a.
    spinal cord injury without
      radiographic a. (SCIWORA)
ABO incompatibility
abortion
    complete a.
    criminal a.
    incomplete a.
    induced a.
    inevitable a.
    missed a.
    septic a.
    spontaneous a.
    therapeutic a.
    threatened a. (TAB)
abortive neurofibromatosis
ABP
    arterial blood pressure
ABR
    absolute bedrest
abraded wound
abrasion
    a. collar
    corneal a.
    dicing a.
    facial a.
    marginal a.
abrasive agent
abrupt exacerbation
abruption
    previous a.
    traumatic a.
abruptio placentae
Abrus precatorius
abscess
    amebic hepatic a.
    apical a.
    Bartholin a.
    Bezold a.
    bone a.
    brain a.
    breast a.
    caseous a.
    cerebellar a.
    cheesy a.
    chronic a.
    cutaneous a.
    deep a.
    diffuse a.
    Eikenella corrodens brain a.
    encapsulated a.
    encysted a.
    enteric a.
    epidural a.
    epidural brain a.
    external ear a.
    external ear chondritis a.

    gas a.
    glandular a.
    hematogenous a.
    hemorrhagic a.
    hepatic a.
    hot a.
    idiopathic a.
    intersphincteric a.
    intraabdominal a.
    intracranial a.
    ischiorectal a.
    locus of brain a.
    marginal a.
    migrating a.
    miliary a.
    milk a.
    mural a.
    pancreatic a.
    perianal a.
    periapical a.
    perinephric a.
    periodontal a.
    perirectal a.
    peritoneal a.
    peritonsillar a.
    phlegmonous a.
    pilonidal a.
    primary a.
    puerperal breast a.
    pulmonary a.
    pyemic a.
    pyogenic a.
    recrudescent a.
    renal a.
    residual a.
    retropharyngeal a.
    satellite a.
    secondary a.
    septicemic a.
    serous a.
    simple a.
    skin a.
    soft tissue a.
    stellate a.
    sterile a.
    stitch a.
    subacute a.
    subaponeurotic a.
    subdiaphragmatic a.
    subfascial a.
    subpectoral a.
    subscapular a.
    supralevator a.
    suture a.
    traumatic a.
    tuboovarian a.
    tympanic a.
    verminous a.
    wound a.

abscessed vein
absence
    a. attack
    a. of gag reflex
    muscle a.
    a. of rectal muscle
    a. seizure
absent
    a. bowel sound
    a. bow-tie sign
    a. peripheral vein
    a. pulse
    a. respiration
absolute
    a. bedrest (ABR)
    a. lymphocytic count (ALC)
absorbable suture
absorption
    a. atelectasis denitrogenation
    bone a.
    bone radiation a.
    drug a.
    a. powder
absorptive atelectasis
abuse
    alcohol a.
    amphetamine a.
    anabolic-androgenic steroid a.
    barbiturate a.
    caffeine a.
    calcium laxative a.
    chemical a.
    child a.
    child sexual a.
    chromium picolinate a.
    clenbuterol a.
    creatine monohydrate a.
    drug a.
    elder a.
    emotional a.
    erythropoietin a.
    ethanol a.
    financial a.
    glycerin laxative a.
    inhalant a.
    insulin a.
    intimate partner a. (IPA)
    lactulose a.
    laxative a.
    Metamucil a.
    mixed drug a.

    National Institute on Drug A.
      (NIDA)
    pediatric a.
    physical a.
    polypharmacy a.
    polysubstance a.
    sexual a.
    spousal a.
    spouse a.
    substance a.
    tobacco a.
abuser
    intravenous drug a. (IVDA)
abusive home condition
abut
ACA
    adenocarcinoma
acalculous cholecystitis
ACC
    ambulatory care center
accelerant
accelerated
    a. diagnostic protocol (ADP)
    a. hypertension
    a. idioventricular rhythm
    a. respiration
accelerating angina
acceleration
    defective a.
accelerator
    thromboplastin generation a.
access
    central a.
    complex a.
    hemodialysis vascular a.
    intraosseous venous a.
    intravenous a.
    simple a.
    vascular a.
AccessAED defibrillator
AccessALS defibrillator
accessory
    a. atlantoaxial ligament
    a. cephalic vein
    a. communicating tendon
    a. flexor muscle
    a. gland
    a. hemiazygos vein
    a. hepatic vein
    a. inspiratory muscle
    a. lateral collateral ligament
    a. ligament

NOTES

accessory (continued)
    a. multangular bone
    a. muscle
    a. muscles of respiration
    a. muscle use
    a. navicular bone
    a. navicular fracture
    a. organ
    a. ossicle fracture
    a. pathway
    a. phrenic nerve
    a. plantar ligament
    a. saphenous vein
    a. sesamoid bone
    a. sign
    a. soleus muscle
    a. venous vein
    a. vertebral vein
    a. volar ligament
accident
    bicycle a.
    cardiac a.
    cardiovascular a.
    car versus pedestrian a.
    cerebral vascular a.
    cerebrovascular a. (CVA)
    mass poisoning a.
    motor vehicle a. (MVA)
    multiple casualty a. (MCA)
    scuba diving a.
accidental
    a. hemorrhage
    a. hypothermia
    a. poisoning
acclimate
Accolate
accommodate
    inability to a.
accommodation
    pupils equal and react to light
      and a. (PERLA)
    pupils equal, round, and reactive
      to light and a. (PERRLA)
accompanying vein
accomplice
accreta
    placenta a.
accretion
    bone mass a.
    bone mineral a.
accrual
    bone mineral a.
Accu-Chek
accuracy
ACD-CPR
    active compression-decompression
    cardiopulmonary resuscitation
ACE
    angiotensin-converting enzyme

    ACE inhibitor
    ACE inhibitor overdose
Ace bandage
ACEP
    American College of Emergency
    Physicians
acetabula, pl. acetabulum
acetabular
    a. bone
    a. posterior wall fracture
    a. rim fracture
acetaldehyde
acetaminophen-alcohol interaction
acetaminophen poisoning
acetanilid poisoning
acetate
    aluminum a.
    flecainide a.
    a. kinase
    mafenide a.
acetazolamide
acetone
acetylation
acetylcholine excess
acetylcholinesterase inhibitor
N-acetylcysteine
N-acetyl-p-benzoquinone imine
acetylsalicylic
    a. acid
    a. acid, phenacetin, caffeine (APC)
    a. acid poisoning
ACF
    acute care facility
achalasia
    sphincteral a.
ache
    bone a.
Achilles
    A. tendon
    A. tendon bursa
    A. tendon injury
aching
    a. abdominal wall pain
    a. chest pain
ACI
    asymptomatic cardiac ischemia
acid
    acetylsalicylic a.
    acidic amino a.
    acrylic a.
    aminocaproic a.
    anthranilic a.
    boric a.
    a. burn
    carbolic a.
    citric a.
    clavulanic a.
    dimercaptosuccinic a. (DMSA)
    dimethyl iminodiacetic a. (HIDA)

a. diuresis
epsilon aminocaproic a. (EACA)
ethylenediamine tetraacetic a.
  (EDTA)
folic a.
formic a.
fusidic a.
gamma-aminobutyric a. (GABA)
hydrofluoric a.
indoleacetic a.
a. ingestion
mefenamic a.
muriatic a.
nitric a.
a. rain
salicylic a.
saturated fatty a.
sulfuric a.
tannic a.
titratable a.
tranexamic a.
trichloroacetic a.
unsaturated fatty a.
valproic a.
acid-base
a.-b. abnormality
a.-b. balance
a.-b. disorder
a.-b. disturbance
acidemia
acidic
a. agent
a. amino acid
acidification
acidity
titratable a.
acidosis
anion gap metabolic a.
dilutional a.
elevated a.
a., epilepsy, insulin, overdose,
  uremia, tumor, infection,
  psychosis, and stroke (AEIOU
  TIPS)
lactic a.
metabolic a.
mild lactic a.
paradoxical a.
profound lactic a.
renal tubular a. (RTA)
renal tubule a.
resolving anion gap metabolic a.

respiratory a.
uncompensated metabolic a.
acid-pepsin problem
Acier stainless steel suture
Acinetobacter **infection**
ACI-TIPI
acute cardiac ischemia-time insensitive
  predictive instrument
ACL
anterior cruciate ligament
ACLLA
anticardiolipin lupus anticoagulant
ACLS
advanced cardiac life support
  ACLS protocol
acne
chemical a.
a. vulgaris
acneiform lesion
acolous
aconite
acoustic
a. nerve
a. neuroma
a. reflectometry
a. window
acousticofacial nerve
acquired
a. anemia
a. immunodeficiency syndrome
  (AIDS)
ACR
active core rewarming
acritical
acrodynia
acrolein inhalation injury
acromegaly
acromial bone
acromioclavicular
a. injury
a. joint
a. joint injury
a. ligament
a. separation
acromiocoracoid ligament
acrylamide
acrylate
ethyl a.
acrylic acid
ACS
acute coronary syndrome

NOTES

ACT
activated clotting time
act
Federal Hazardous Substance A.
(FHSA)
Labeling of Art Materials A.
Toxic Substances Control A.
(TOSCA)
ACTH
adrenocorticotropic hormone
ACTH suppression
Actidose activated charcoal
actin
muscle a.
actinomycosis
action
cumulative a.
electrophysiologic a.
mechanism of a.
activated
a. charcoal
a. clotting time (ACT)
a. partial thromboplastin time
(aPTT)
activation
neurohormonal a.
activator
intravenous tissue plasminogen a.
plasminogen a.
tissue plasminogen a. (TPA, t-PA)
active
a. compression-decompression
cardiopulmonary resuscitation
(ACD-CPR)
a. core rewarming (ACR)
a. external rewarming (AER)
a. rewarming
activity
activities of daily living (ADL)
bone morphogenetic a.
delta-aminolevulinate dehydratase a.
muscle a.
muscle sympathetic nerve a.
pulseless electrical a. (PEA)
spinal cord motor a.
strenuous a.
tonic-clonic a.
ACTS
acute cervical traumatic sprain
actuator
mechanical ventilator a.
Acufex bioabsorbable Suretac suture
acuity
visual a.
acuminata
condyloma a.
perianal condyloma a.
acute
a. abdominal series (AAS)

a. adrenal insufficiency
a. airway obstruction
a. alveolar hyperventilation on
chronic ventilatory failure
a. anemia
a. angle closure glaucoma
a. appendicitis
a. avulsion fracture
a. azotemia
a. bronchitis
a. cardiac ischemia-time insensitive
predictive instrument (ACI-TIPI)
a. cardiovascular disease
a. care
a. care facility (ACF)
a. care medicine
a. cervical traumatic sprain (ACTS)
a. cholecystitis
a. compression triad
a. compressive optic neuropathy
a. coronary syndrome (ACS)
a. cystitis
a. delirium
a. digoxin toxicity
a. diverticulosis
a. eosinophilic pneumonia (AEP)
a. fatty liver
a. fracture
a. gas embolism
a. gastritis
a. gingivitis
a. hemorrhagic pancreatitis
a. infective endocarditis
a. intermittent peritoneal dialysis
(AIPD)
a. interstitial nephritis
a. interstitial pneumonia (AIP)
a. intoxication
a. intracerebral hemorrhage
a. intracranial hypertension
a. intracranial injury
a. limb ischemia
a. lung injury (ALI)
a. mesenteric ischemia
a. mitral regurgitation
a. myocardial infarction (AMI)
a. necrotizing ulcerative gingivitis
(ANUG)
a. neurologic impairment
a. on chronic fracture
a. on chronic illness
a. on chronic symptoms
a. onset hepatotoxicity
otitis media, purulent, a. (OMPA)
A. Physiology and Chronic Health
Evaluation (APACHE)
a. psychosis
a. pulmonary edema
a. Q-wave myocardial infarction

a. recurrent rhabdomyolysis
a. renal failure (ARF)
a. respiratory disease (ARD)
a. respiratory distress (ARD)
a. respiratory distress syndrome (ARDS)
a. respiratory failure (ARF)
a. severe asthma
a. spinal cord compression
a. suppurative parotitis
a. tubular interstitial nephritis (ATIN)
a. tubular necrosis (ATN)
a. tumor lysis syndrome
a. vestibular labyrinthitis
a. wound
acuteness of onset
Acutrol suture
ACV
assist control ventilation
ACVD
arteriosclerotic cardiovascular disease
acyanotic
a. congenital heart disease
a. heart disease
a. limb
acyclic compound
acyclovir
AD
admitting diagnosis
advanced directive
Adam's apple
adaptability
adaptation
physiologic a.
sensory a.
Adaptiv biphasic technology
adaptor
portable radio a.
ADCC
antibody-dependent cellular cytotoxicity
addiction
marijuana a.
opioid a.
addictive personality
additive
a. effect
food a.
ADDU
alcohol and drug dependency unit
adduction fracture

adductor
a. brevis muscle
a. hallucis muscle
a. hallucis tendon
a. magnus muscle
a. magnus tendon
a. minimus muscle
a. muscle strain
a. pollicis brevis tendon
a. pollicis longus muscle
adenalgia
adenine
citrate phosphate dextrose a.
adenitis
cervical a.
mesenteric a.
adenocarcinoma (ACA)
Adenocard
adenodynia
adenogenous
adenohypophyseal disorder
adenosine
a. therapy
a. triphosphatase (ATPase)
a. triphosphatase inhibitor
adenous
adenoviral
adenovirus
adequate
a. depth
a. immobilization
a. nutrition
a. ventilation
ADH
antidiuretic hormone
adhere
adherent profundus tendon
adhesion
lysis of a.
tendon a.
adhesive
a. arachnoiditis
cyanoacrylate a.
DERMABOND topical skin a.
surgical a.
adhesiveness
adhesive-type dressing
adiposalgia
adipose
a. ligament
a. tissue
adjacent

NOTES

adjunct
    airway a.
adjunctive
adjustable
    a. external suture
    a. splint
adjusted-dose unfractionated heparin
adjustment
    a. disorder
    suture a.
adjuvant therapy
ADL
    activities of daily living
administration
    bicarbonate a.
    enteral a.
    Food and Drug A. (FDA)
    National Highway Traffic
      Safety A. (NHTSA)
    Occupational Safety and Health A.
      (OSHA)
    parenteral a.
admission
    a. criteria
    emergency a.
    a. for observation
    a. for operative repair
    prior to a.
admitting diagnosis (AD)
adnexal
    a. infection
    a. mass
    a. torsion
adolescence
adolescent
    a. crisis
    a. medicine
ADP
    accelerated diagnostic protocol
ADR
    adverse drug reaction
adrenal
    a. crisis
    a. disease
    a. hyperplasia
    a. insufficiency
    a. shock
    a. vein
adrenalectomy
Adrenalin Chloride
adrenaline
adrenalitis
    autoimmune a.
adrenergic
    a. agent
    a. agonist
    a. blocking agent

adrenocortical
    a. insufficiency
    a. suppression
adrenocorticotropic
    a. hormone (ACTH)
    a. hormone stimulation
adrenogenic
adrenoleukodystrophy
Adriamycin cardiotoxicity
Adson forceps
adsorbent gel
adult
    a. asthma
    a. cerebrospinal injury
    a. congregate living facility
    a. diarrhea
    a. epiglottitis
    fever a.
    a. fever
    a. pneumonia
    a. polycystic kidney disease
    a. respiratory distress syndrome
      (ARDS)
    a. seizure
    a. T-cell leukemia
    a. trauma center
    a. urinary tract infection
    a. vomiting
adult-onset epilepsy
adult-type III TIE fracture
advanced
    a. cardiac life support (ACLS)
    a. cardiovascular life support
    a. directive (AD)
    a. life support (ALS)
    a. lung disease
    a. trauma life support (ATLS)
advancement
    tendon a.
adventitia
adventitial dissection
adventitious
    a. breath sound
    a. bursa
adverse
    a. drug reaction (ADR)
    a. effect
adversive movement
advice
    against medical a. (AMA)
advocate
    patient a.
adynamic
    a. bone
    a. ileus
AECG
    ambulatory electrocardiography
AED
    antiepileptic drug

automated external defibrillation
automated external defibrillator
automatic external defibrillation

AEF
aortoenteric fistula

AEIOU TIPS
acidosis, epilepsy, insulin, overdose, uremia, tumor, infection, psychosis, and stroke
alcohol intoxication, epilepsy, insulin, overdose, uremia, trauma, infection, psychosis, and stroke

aEnaC
amiloride-sensitive sodium channel

AEP
acute eosinophilic pneumonia

AER
active external rewarming

aerate

aerobic culture

aerodigestive tract injury

aeromedical transport

Aeromonas hydrophila

aerophagia

aerosol
Combivent inhalation a.
a. delivery
a. mask
a. therapy

aerosolization

aerosolized medication

aeruginosa
Pneumocystis a.
Pseudomonas a.

AF
Asian female

AFE
amniotic fluid embolism

afebrile

affect
apathetic a.
bland a.
blunted a.
congruent a.
depressed a.
depressive a.
euphoric a.
flat a.
impaired a.
inappropriate a.
labile a.
restricted a.

afferent
a. digital nerve
a. renal nerve
a. vein

AFL
air-fluid level

aflatoxin

aforementioned treatment

African-American
A.-A. female
A.-A. male

aftercare plan

aftercoming
a. fetal head
a. fetal part

afterload
a. reduction
ventricular a.

aftermath

against medical advice (AMA)

aganglionic megacolon

AGE
arterial gas embolism

age
anatomical a.
bone a.
childbearing a.
chronological a.
a. of consent
developmental a.
emotional a.
functional a.
increased maternal a.
mental a.
physical a.
physiological a.
skeletal a.

agency
Drug Enforcement A. (DEA)
Environmental Protection A. (EPA)
Federal Emergency Management A. (FEMA)
welfare a.

agenetic fracture

agent
abrasive a.
acidic a.
adrenergic a.
adrenergic blocking a.
alpha-adrenergic a.
antiarrhythmic a.
antibiotic-steroid a.

NOTES

agent *(continued)*
    anticholinergic a.
    anticonvulsant a.
    antiestrogen a.
    antihistamine a.
    antihyperlipidemic a.
    antiinfective a.
    antiischemic a.
    antilymphocyte a.
    antiplatelet a.
    antipsychotic a.
    antituberculous a.
    antivenin a.
    beta-blocking a.
    biological warfare a.
    blister-causing a.
    bone formation-stimulating a.
    bone marrow a.
    cardioprotective a.
    caustic a.
    chelating a.
    chemical warfare a.
    cholinergic a.
    cholinesterase chemical warfare a.
    Class IA, IB, IC antiarrhythmic a.
    Class II, IV, V antiarrhythmic a.
    corrosive a.
    cytoprotective a.
    emetic a.
    gallstone-solubilizing a.
    inotropic a.
    magnesium and thermite
      incendiary a.
    mixed pressor a.
    muscle relaxing a.
    neuroleptic a.
    neuromuscular blocking a. (NMBA)
    neutralizing a.
    nondepolarizing neuromuscular
      blocking a.
    nonsteroidal antiinflammatory a.
    A. Orange
    paralytic a.
    riot control a.
    Sarin nerve a.
    Soman nerve a.
    Tabun nerve a.
    thrombolytic a.
    vasoconstrictor a.
    vasopressor a.
age-specific pediatric trauma score (ASPTS)
aggregate
    bone a.
aggressive
    a. fluid resuscitation
    a. manner
    a. treatment

aggressiveness
    bone tumor a.
agitated
    a. behavior
    highly a.
agitation
    patient a.
    psychomotor a.
agonal
    a. breathing
    a. respiration
agonist
    adrenergic a.
    beta-adrenergic a.
    cholinergic a.
    dopaminergic a.
    a. muscle
    narcotic a.
    prostaglandin a.
agonist-antagonist
    narcotic a.-a.
agonistic muscle
agoraphobia
agranulocytosis
agrypnotic
AHA
    American Heart Association
AHFS
    American Hospital Formulary Service
aid
    bone conduction hearing a.
    first a.
    pharmaceutic a.
    pharmaceutical a.
aide
    nurse's a.
AIDS
    acquired immunodeficiency syndrome
    AIDS dementia complex
AIIRA
    angiotensin II receptor antagonist
AIIS
    anterior inferior iliac spine
    AIIS avulsion fracture
ailment
    current a.
AIP
    acute interstitial pneumonia
AIPD
    acute intermittent peritoneal dialysis
air
    ambient a.
    a. bag injury
    a. bed
    a. cushion
    a. embolism
    a. entrainment face mask
    a. entrapment mask
    free intraperitoneal a.

high-efficiency particulate a.
(HEPA)
joint space a.
a. leak syndrome
a. medical transport
a. pollutant
a. pressure splint
a. reduction
subcutaneous a.
a. trapping
a. trapping in ventricle
airbag
toxic substance in automobile a.
airborne
a. disease
a. droplet
a. pathogen
a. transmission
air-fluidized bed
air-fluid level (AFL)
airsickness
airway
a. adjunct
anatomical a.
artificial a.
binasal pharyngeal a. (BNPA)
a. and breathing
a., breathing, circulation (ABC)
a., breathing, circulation, disability,
and exposure (ABCDE)
a. burn
a. compromise
a. constriction
a. edema
esophageal gastric tube a. (EGTA)
esophageal obturator a. (EOA)
esophagogastric tube a. (EGTA)
failed a.
Guedel a.
a. injury
laryngeal mask a. (LMA)
lower a.
a. management
nasopharyngeal a. (NPA)
a. obstruction
oropharyngeal a. (OPA)
pharyngeal tracheal lumen a.
(PTLA)
a. pressure release ventilation
(APRV)
a. protection
a. smooth muscle

a. stabilization
a. status assessment
upper a.
**Aitken classification of epiphysial
fracture**
AKA
alcoholic ketoacidosis
akathisia
akinetic mutism
alanine transaminase
alar
a. bone
a. fold
a. ligament
a. muscle
alba
pityriasis a.
Albert-Lembert suture
Albert suture
albicans
Candida a.
Albinus muscle
albumin level
albuminoid
albuminous
albuterol toxicity
ALC
absolute lymphocytic count
alcohol
a. abuse
a. dependency
a. dependent
a. and drug dependency unit
(ADDU)
ethyl a. (EtOH, ETOH)
grain a.
a. intoxication
a. intoxication, epilepsy, insulin,
overdose, uremia, trauma,
infection, psychosis, and stroke
(AEIOU TIPS)
a. on breath (AOB)
a. poisoning
a. withdrawal
a. withdrawal delirium
a. withdrawal syndrome
wood a.
alcoholic
A.'s Anonymous (AA)
a. blackout
a. cardiomyopathy
chronic a.

NOTES

alcoholic *(continued)*
    a. hallucinosis
    a. ketoacidosis (AKA)
    a. paresis
    a. withdrawal seizure
Alcon suture
aldehyde
alert, verbal stimuli, painful stimuli, unresponsive (AVPU)
alfentanil
algorithm
    bone a.
    NAEPP a.
ALI
    acute lung injury
Alice in Wonderland syndrome
alignment
    body a.
alimentation
    parenteral a.
aliphatic
    a. halogenated hydrocarbon
    a. hydrocarbon poisoning
aliquot
alisphenoid bone
alkalemia
    metabolic a.
alkali, pl. **alkalies**
    a. burn
    caustic a.
    a. ingestion
    a. reserve
alkaline
    a. caustic injury
    a. phosphatase
alkalinity
alkalinization therapy
alkalinize
alkaloid
    ergot a.
    a. poisoning
alkalosis
    chloride-resistant a.
    compensatory renal metabolic a.
    metabolic a.
    respiratory a.
Allen
    A. open reduction of calcaneal fracture
    A. test
allergen
    food a.
allergenic extract
allergic
    a. bronchopulmonary aspergillosis
    a. conjunctivitis
    a. coryza
    a. dermatitis
    a. reaction

    a. rhinitis
    a. trigger
allergy
    contact a.
    drug a.
    latex a.
    no known a. (NKA)
Allevyn foam
alliance
    therapeutic a.
    working a.
alligator forceps
allogenic bone
allograft
    bone a.
    cadaver a.
    a. iliac bone
    a. rejection
allografting
    nerve a.
allopurinol
allowance
    recommended daily a. (RDA)
allude
allusion
allylamine
almond
    bitter a.
    a. odor
aloe
alopecia
Aloprim
alpha, α
    interferon a.
    a. phase
    a. radiation
    tumor necrosis factor a.
alpha-1 acid glycoprotein
alpha-2 receptor withdrawal
alpha-adrenergic
    a.-a. agent
    a.-a. blocker
    a.-a. therapy
5-alpha reductase inhibitor
alprazolam
alprostadil
already-threaded suture
ALS
    advanced life support
    amyotrophic lateral sclerosis
ALTE
    apparent life-threatening event
alteration
    bone matrix a.
    pH a.
altered
    a. mental status (AMS)
    a. mentation

A

alternans
    total electrical a.
alternate mode of mechanical ventilation
alternating suture
alternative
    viable a.
alternobaric
    a. facial paralysis
    a. vertigo
altitude illness
altitude-related disorder
Alumafoam splint
aluminum
    a. acetate
    a. hydroxide
    a. nicotinate
    a. phosphate
    a. sulfate
aluminum-bronze wire suture
Alupent
Alvarado appendicitis score
alveolar
    a. bone
    a. bone fracture
    a. duct
    a. effector cell
    a. fracture
    a. nerve
    a. oxygen tension
    a. process fracture
    a. recruitment
    a. socket wall fracture
    a. supporting bone
    a. supporting bone ankle bone
    a. ventilation
alveolar-capillary gas exchange
alveolate
alveoli (*pl. of* alveolus)
alveolitis
    fibrosing a.
alveolodental ligament
alveolus, pl. **alveoli**
AMA
    against medical advice
Amanita
    A. *muscaria* mushroom
    A. *phalloides*
    A. *phalloides* mushroom
amantadine
amatoxin

ambient
    a. air
    a. oxygen pressure
    a. temperature
ambivalent behavior
Ambu bag
ambulance
    a. attendant
    a. call report
    a. service
ambulant edema
ambulate
    able to a.
ambulation
ambulatory
    a. care
    a. care center (ACC)
    a. electrocardiography (AECG)
    a. surgery
amebiasis
amebic hepatic abscess
amebicide
ameliorate
amelioration
amenable
amenorrhea
American
    A. Academy of Emergency Medicine
    A. Association of Poison Control Centers (AAPCC)
    A. College of Emergency Physicians (ACEP)
    A. Heart Association (AHA)
    A. hellebore
    A. Hospital Formulary Service (AHFS)
    A. silk suture
    A. Spinal Injury Association (ASIA)
    A. Spinal Injury Association Impairment Scale
    A. trypanosomiasis
    A. yew ingestion
americana
    Phytolacca a.
amethocaine gel
AMI
    acute myocardial infarction
Amidate
amide
    angiotensin a.

NOTES

13

amikacin sulfate
amiloride
amiloride-sensitive sodium channel
    (aEnaC)
amine
    benzyl a.
aminocaproic
    a. acid
    a. acid therapy
aminoglycoside
    a. antibiotic
    a. nephrotoxicity
    a. therapy
aminoketone
aminopenicillin
aminophylline, phenobarbital, ephedrine
    (APE)
21-aminosteroid
aminotransferase
    aspartate a. (AST)
amiodarone hydrochloride
amitriptyline
ammonia
    a. capsule
    a. compound
    a. gas inhalation
    a. ingestion
    a. liquefaction necrosis
    a. odor
    quaternary a.
amnesia
    posttraumatic a. (PTA)
    traumatic a.
amnestic shellfish poisoning
amniotic
    a. fluid
    a. fluid embolism (AFE)
    a. sac
amobarbital
A-mode ultrasound
amoxapine
amoxicillin
amperage
amphetamine
    a. abuse
    a. aspartate
    crank a.
    a. derivative
    a. poisoning
    a. sulfate
    a. toxicity
    a. withdrawal
amphibian toxin
amphotericin
    a. B
    a. B deoxycholate
    a. therapy
ampicillin
ampicillin-sulbactam

amplitude
    P-wave a.
ampule
ampulla of Vater
amputated part
amputation
    Chopart a.
    guillotine a.
    metacarpal a.
    midfoot a.
    reimplantation a.
    a. reimplantation
    Syme a.
    traumatic a.
amrinone
AMS
    altered mental status
amygdaloid infarct
amylase
    serum a.
amyl nitrate
amyloidosis
amyotrophic lateral sclerosis (ALS)
anabolic
    a. steroid
    a. steroid toxicity
anabolic-androgenic steroid abuse
anabolism
anacatesthesia
anacrotic limb
anaerobic
    a. culture
    a. infection
anagyroides
    Laburnum a.
anal
    a. canal
    a. canal tumor
    a. cryptitis
    a. fissure
    a. fistula
    a. intercourse
    a. nerve
    a. papilla
    a. sphincter laceration
    a. vein
    a. verge
    a. wound
analeptic enema
analgesia
    patient-controlled a. (PCA)
analgesic
    narcotic a.
    a. nephritis
analog, analogue
analogous
analogy
analysis, pl. analyses
    cerebrospinal fluid a.

muscle a.
pleural fluid a.
shunt gas a.

analyzer
Lactate Pro LT-1710 portable
lactate a.
nerve fiber a.
Rapidpoint 400 critical care a.
sequential multiple a. (SMA)
Sonoclot coagulation and platelet
function a.

anaphrodisiac

anaphylactic
a. reaction
a. shock

anaphylactoid

anaphylaxis
bee sting a.
slow-reacting substance of a.
(SRSA)

anasarca
fetoplacental a.

anastomosis, pl. anastomoses
Billroth a.
nerve a.
suture a.
vascular a.

anastomotic
a. suture
a. vein

anatomic
a. dead space
a. fracture
a. information
a. neck fracture

anatomical
a. age
a. airway
a. position

Ancap braided silk suture

anchor
suture a.
a. suture

anchoring
a. suture
a. tendon

anchovy
a. poisoning
a. sauce pus

ancillary
a. measure

a. study
a. therapy

Ancobon

anconeus muscle

ancrod

Andersch nerve

Anderson-Hutchins unstable tibial shaft fracture

androgen

anechoic
a. stripe
a. structure

Anectine

anemia
acquired a.
acute a.
aplastic a.
autoimmune hemolytic a.
borderline a.
chronic a.
chronic disease a.
dilational a.
hemolytic a.
hypochromic a.
hypochromic microcytic a.
inherited a.
iron deficiency a.
macrocytic a.
megaloblastic a.
microcytic a.
normochromic normocytic a.
pernicious a.
physiologic a.
profound a.
sickle cell a.
sideroblastic a.

anemic ponyneuritis

anencephaly

anergy

anesthesia
benzocaine a.
dissociative a.
infiltration a.
inhalational a.
LET a.
lidocaine a.
local a.
nerve block a.
patient-triggered a.
spinal a.
TAC a.
topical a.

NOTES

anesthesiologist
anesthesiology
anesthetic
    ester a.
    eutectic mixture of local a.'s
      (EMLA)
    intraoral a.
    local a.
anesthetist
aneurismal rupture
aneurysm
    abdominal a.
    abdominal aortic a. (AAA)
    aortic a.
    arterial a.
    ballooning a.
    basilar a.
    berry a.
    cerebral a.
    dissecting thoracic a.
    false a.
    giant a.
    hepatic artery a.
    inflammatory abdominal aortic a.
    intracerebral a.
    lower extremity a.
    mycotic a.
    peripheral arterial a.
    popliteal a.
    ruptured abdominal aortic a.
    splenic artery a.
    suprarenal a.
    syphilitic a.
    thoracic aorta a.
    true a.
    ulnar artery a.
    upper extremity a.
    ventricular a.
    visceral a.
aneurysmal vein
aneurysmatic
angel dust
angina
    accelerating a.
    c7E3 Fab Antiplatelet Therapy in
      Unstable Refractory A.
      (CAPTURE)
    Ludwig a.
    new onset a.
    a. pectoris
    Prinzmetal a.
    rest a.
    stable a.
    unstable a.
anginal
    a. attack
    a. pain
angioblastoma
    bone a.

Angiocath catheter
angiocatheter with looped polypropylene
    suture
angiodysplasia
angioedema
    hereditary a.
    recurrent a.
    secondary a.
angiographic embolization
angiography
    cerebral a.
    coronary a.
    digital subtraction a. (DSA)
    gated radionuclide a.
    magnetic resonance a. (MRA)
    pulmonary a.
    radionuclide a.
angioma
    spider a.
angiomatoid
angiomatosis
    bacillary a.
angioneurotic edema
angioplasty
    emergent a.
    percutaneous coronary a.
    percutaneous transluminal
      coronary a. (PTCA)
    rescue a.
    vein patch a.
angiosarcoma
    bone a.
angiotensin
    a. II, III
    a. receptor antagonist (ARA)
    a. II receptor antagonist (AIIRA)
    a. amide
angiotensin-converting
    a.-c. enzyme (ACE)
    a.-c. enzyme inhibitor
angle
    congruence a.
    costovertebral a. (CVA)
    a. fracture
    Louis a.
    a. of repose
    a. suture
angry appearance
angular vein
angulated fracture
angulation fracture
anhidrosis
anhidrotic
ani (*pl. of* anus)
anicteric sclera
aniline gentian violet
animal bite
anion
    a. exchange resin

a. gap
a. gap metabolic acidosis
Aniridia-Wilms tumor
anisocoria
anisoylated plasminogen streptokinase activator complex (APSAC)
ankle
    a. bone
    a. dislocation
    a. fracture
    a. fracture-dislocation
    a. hitch
    a. inferior transverse ligament
    a. mortise fracture
    a. splint
    a. sprain
ankylosing spondylitis
Annelida **envenomation**
annihilation
annular (*var. of* anular)
annulare granuloma
annulus (*var. of* anulus)
ano
    fissure in a.
anococcygeal
    a. ligament
    a. nerve
anodyne
anomalous
    a. muscle
    a. pulmonary vein
anomaly
    developmental a.
    Ebstein a.
anonymous
    Alcoholics A. (AA)
    a. vein
anorectal
    a. fistula
    a. foreign body
    a. hemorrhoid
    a. herpes simplex infection
    a. ring
anorectic drug
anorectoperineal muscle
anorexia nervosa
anorexiant
anoscope
anoscopy
anovular menstruation
anoxemia
anoxic brain injury

ANP
    atrial natriuretic peptide
ansate
anserine bursa
ant
    a. bite
    a. killer toxicity
    a. sting
Antabuse
antacid
    cytoprotective a.
    a. toxicity
antagonist
    angiotensin II receptor a. (AIIRA)
    angiotensin receptor a. (ARA)
    calcium a.
    H1, H2 a.
    histamine a.
    histamine-2 receptor a.
    5-HT a.
    a. muscle
antebrachial vein
antecedent sign
antecubital vein
anteflexion
antegrade flow
anterior
    a. alveolar nerve
    a. antebrachial nerve
    a. anular ligament
    a. auricular muscle
    a. auricular vein
    a. basal vein
    a. blunt neck trauma
    a. calcaneal process fracture
    a. cardiac vein
    a. cardinal vein
    a. cerebral vein
    a. ciliary vein
    a. circumflex humeral vein
    a. collateral ligament
    a. column fracture
    a. commissure ligament
    a. condylar vein
    a. conjunctival vein
    a. costotransverse ligament
    a. cruciate ligament (ACL)
    a. cruciate ligament injury
    a. displacement
    a. drawer sign
    a. epistaxis
    a. ethmoidal nerve

NOTES

anterior *(continued)*
a. facial vein
a. fascicular block
a. femoral cutaneous nerve
a. fibular ligament
a. fontanelle
a. fracture
a. inferior iliac spine (AIIS)
a. inferior tibiofibular ligament
a. intercostal vein
a. internal vertebral vein
a. interosseous nerve
a. interosseous vein
a. jugular vein
a. labial nerve
a. labial vein
a. longitudinal ligament
a. mallear ligament
a. medial ankle ligament
a. meniscofemoral ligament
a. oblique ligament
a. palatine nerve
a. palatine suture
a. papillary muscle
a. pontomesencephalic vein
a. rectus muscle
a. rib fracture
a. sacrococcygeal ligament
a. sacroiliac ligament
a. sacrosciatic ligament
a. scalene muscle
a. scrotal nerve
a. scrotal vein
a. serratus muscle
a. spinal artery syndrome
a. spinal ligament
a. splenis muscle
a. sternoclavicular ligament
a. superficialis muscle
a. supraclavicular nerve
a. suspensory ligament
a. talocalcaneal ligament
a. talofibular ligament
a. talotibial ligament
a. temporal diploic vein
a. terminal vein
a. thoracic nerve
a. tibial bursa
a. tibialis tendon
a. tibial muscle
a. tibial nerve
a. tibial tendon
a. tibial vein
a. tibiofibular ligament
a. uveitis
a. wound
anteroexternal
anterograde

anteroinferior
a. corner fracture
a. myocardial infarction
anterointernal
anterolateral
a. compression fracture
a. intercostal nerve
a. myocardial infarction
a. thoracotomy
anteromedial
a. approach
a. intercostal nerve
anteromedian
anteroposterior
a. position
a. view
anteroposteriorly
anterosuperiorly
anterosuperior position
anteroventral
anteversion
anteverted uterus
anthelmintic
anthracis
    Bacillus a.
anthracycline
anthranilic acid
anthrax
cutaneous a.
gastrointestinal a.
a. infection
inhalational a.
a. meningitis
a. septicemia
a. toxin
anthropometric measurement
antiadrenergic drug
antiandrogen
antianxiety medication
antiarrhythmic
a. agent
a. drug
a. therapy
antibacterial soap
antibiotic
aminoglycoside a.
bactericidal a.
beta lactam a.
broad-spectrum a.
carbapenem a.
cephalosporin a.
empiric use of a.'s
fluoroquinolone a.
glycopeptide a.
intravenous a.
lincosamide a.
macrolide a.
oral a.
polyene a.

A

a. prophylactic
prophylactic a.
sulfonamide a.
tetracycline a.
topical a.
a. treatment
antibiotic-steroid agent
antibody
antinuclear circulating a.
Rh a.
teichoic acid a.
Wassermann a.
antibody-coated suture
antibody-dependent cellular cytotoxicity (ADCC)
antibromic
anticardiolipin lupus anticoagulant (ACLLA)
anticholinergic
a. agent
a. drug
a. poisoning
a. syndrome
a. toxicity
anticholinesterase
anticoagulant
anticardiolipin lupus a. (ACLLA)
a. rodenticide poisoning
a. toxicity
anticonvulsant
a. agent
a. drug ingestion
a. effect
antidepressant
cyclic a.
tricyclic a.
antidiarrheal therapy
anti-digoxin Fab therapy
antidiuretic
a. hormone (ADH)
a. hormone secretion
antidopaminergic
antidote
chemical a.
poison a.
poisoning a.
a. toxicity
antidromic atrioventricular reentrant tachycardia
antidysrhythmic
a. drug poisoning
a. toxicity

antiemetic
antiepileptic drug (AED)
antiestrogen agent
antifibrinolytic drug
antifungal drug
antigen
a. clearance
a. presenting cell (APC)
antigen-extracted allogeneic bone
antigenic
a. drift
a. shift
antigravity muscle
antihistamine agent
antihyperlipidemic agent
antihypertensive therapy
antiinfective agent
antiinflammatory cytokine
antiischemic agent
antilipemic
antilithic
antilymphocyte
a. agent
a. globulin
antimicrobial spectrum
antimuscarinic
urinary a.
antinauseant
antineoplastic
antinuclear circulating antibody
antioxidant therapy
antiparasitic therapy
antiparkinson
antiperiodic
antiphlogistic
antiplatelet
a. agent
a. therapy
antipsychotic
a. agent
atypical a.
a. intoxication
a. poisoning
a. toxicity
antipyretic therapy
antirabies serum
antisense drug
antisepsis
antiseptic
Savlon a.
Zephiran a.

NOTES

19

antiserum
  nerve growth factor a.
antishock pelvic clamp
antisnakebite serum
antisocial personality disorder
antispasmodic
antitetanic serum
antitetanus prophylaxis
antithrombin III deficiency
antithymocyte globulin (ATG)
antithyroid agent toxicity
antitorque suture
antitoxic unit
antitoxin
  Crotalus a.
  diphtheria a. (DAT)
  tetanus a.
antitragicus muscle
antitragus muscle
antituberculous agent
antitussive
antivenin
  a. agent
  a. therapy
antivenom
  snakebite a.
  stone fish a.
antiviral therapy
ANUG
  acute necrotizing ulcerative gingivitis
anular, annular
  a. fracture
  a. ligament
anulus, annulus
anus, pl. **ani**
  imperforate a.
  pruritus ani
Anusol
anvil bone
anxiety
  a. attack
  a. disorder
AOB
  alcohol on breath
AO classification of ankle fracture
AOD
  atlantooccipital dislocation
aorta, pl. **aortae**
  abdominal a.
  ascending a.
  coarctation of a.
  descending a.
  thoracic a.
  traumatic disruption of a.
aortic
  a. aneurysm
  a. arch
  a. bifurcation
  a. coarctation

a. diameter
a. disruption
a. dissection
a. impedance
a. laceration
a. nerve
a. regurgitation
a. root enlargement
a. rupture
a. second sound (A2)
a. transection
a. valve
a. valve disease
a. valve insufficiency
a. valve stenosis
aortocaval compression
aortoenteric fistula (AEF)
aortography
APACHE
  Acute Physiology and Chronic Health
  Evaluation
    APACHE III database
    APACHE II, III
apathetic
  a. affect
  a. hyperthyroidism
apathy
  extreme a.
APC
  acetylsalicylic acid, phenacetin, caffeine
  antigen presenting cell
APC-C
  aspirin, phenacetin, caffeine with codeine
APE
  aminophylline, phenobarbital, ephedrine
aperture
apex, pl. **apices**
  a. fracture
Apgar score
aphagia
aphasia
  expressive a.
aphasic patient
aphthous ulcer
apical
  a. abscess
  a. dental ligament
  a. nerve block
  a. pole
  a. and subcostal four-chambered
  view
  a. suture
  a. vein
apices (*pl. of* apex)
apicoposterior vein
aplasia
  bone marrow a.
  optic nerve a.
aplastic anemia

Apley test
apnea
    sleep a.
    unexplained a.
apneic spell
aponeurosis
    tendon a.
apophysial fracture
apophysis, pl. **apophyses**
    bone lesion a.
apoplexy
    pituitary a.
apoptosis
apparatus
    self-contained breathing a. (SCBA)
    vestibular a.
apparent life-threatening event (ALTE)
appearance
    angry a.
    drumstick a.
    shocklike a.
    shocky a.
    toxic a.
    water-bottle a.
appendices (*pl. of* appendix)
appendicitis
    acute a.
    a. by contiguity
    fulminating a.
    gangrenous a.
    helminthic a.
    myxoglobulosis a.
    nonobstructive a.
    a. obliterans
    perforating a.
    perforative a.
    stercoral a.
    subperitoneal a.
    suppurative a.
    suspicion of a.
    verminous a.
appendicular
    a. skeletal muscle
    a. skeleton
    a. vein
appendix, pl. **appendices**
    hot a.
    vermiform a.
apperception
apperceptive
applanation tonometry

apple
    Adam's a.
applicator
    cotton-tip a.
Appolito suture
apposition
    a. forceps
    fracture in close a.
    a. of skull suture
appraisal
    health risk a.
approach
    anteromedial a.
    lateral a.
    medial a.
    nonoperative a.
    paramedian a.
approximation
    a. suture
    wound a.
approximator
    nerve a.
apron
    abdominal a.
aprotinin
APRV
    airway pressure release ventilation
APSAC
    anisoylated plasminogen streptokinase
    activator complex
AP supine portable view
aPTT
    activated partial thromboplastin time
apyretic
apyrexia
apyrexial
aquarium toxin
aqueous
    a. humor
    a. vein
AR
    artificial respiration
ARA
    angiotensin receptor antagonist
arachnoid
    a. layer
    a. mater
arachnoiditis
    adhesive a.
Arantius ligament
arbovirus infection

NOTES

arch
    aortic a.
    a. bar
    bone a.
    a. fracture
    U-shaped a.
    zygomatic a.
architectural barrier
architecture
    bone a.
arciform vein
arcual
arcuate
    a. popliteal ligament
    a. pubic ligament
    a. vein
ARD
    acute respiratory disease
    acute respiratory distress
ARDS
    acute respiratory distress syndrome
    adult respiratory distress syndrome
Arduan
area
    body surface a. (BSA)
    genital a.
    Kiesselbach a.
    low-oxygen a.
    total body surface a. (TBSA)
    triangular a.
areolar
ARF
    acute renal failure
    acute respiratory failure
arginine
    a. therapy
    a. vasopressin
***Arisaema triphyllum* ingestion**
arm
    a. bone
    a. splint
armamentarium
armboard
    arterial catheter a.
armed conflict
armpit
Arnold nerve
aromatase inhibitor
aromatic halogenated hydrocarbon toxicity
arrest
    cardiac a.
    full cardiopulmonary a.
    respiratory a.
arrhythmia
    cardiac a.
    digoxin-toxic a.
    junctional a.
    wide-complex a.

arrhythmic beat
arrival
    dead on a. (DOA)
    estimated time of a. (ETA)
    prior to a.
Arroyo encircling suture
Arruga encircling suture
arsenic
    a. poisoning
    a. toxicity
    a. tremor
arsenical paralysis
arsine gas inhalation
artefact (*var. of* artifact)
arterial
    a. air embolism
    a. aneurysm
    a. bleeding
    a. blood gas (ABG)
    a. blood gas test
    a. blood pressure (ABP)
    a. catheter
    a. catheter armboard
    a. gas embolism (AGE)
    a. insufficiency
    a. ketone body ratio
    a. ligament
    a. line
    a. occlusion
    a. priapism
    a. puncture
    a. silk suture
    a. vasospasm
    a. vein
    a. venous blood gas
arterialized leptomeningeal vein
arteriography
    pulmonary a.
arteriolar atherosclerosis
arteriole
    pancreatic a.
arteriosclerotic cardiovascular disease (ACVD)
arteriosum
    ligamentum a.
arteriosus
    ductus a.
    patent ductus a.
arteriovenous (AV)
    a. hemodiafiltration
    a. malformation (AVM)
arteritis
    small vessel a.
    Takayasu a.
    temporal a.
artery
    brachial a.
    carotid a.
    circumflex a.

dorsalis pedis a.
femoral a.
hepatic a.
ileal a.
iliac a.
innominate a.
insular a.
median a.
perforation of pulmonary a.
pulmonary a. (PA)

arthritis, pl. **arthritides**
crystal-induced a.
degenerative a.
hemorrhagic a.
infectious a.
juvenile idiopathic a.
juvenile rheumatoid a.
meningococcal a.
monarticular a.
psoriatic a.
reactive a.
rheumatoid a. (RA)
septic a.

arthrocentesis
knee a.
wrist a.

arthroplasty
tendon interposition a.
total hip a. (THA)
total knee a. (TKA)
total shoulder a.

arthropod
a. bite
a. envenomation
a. sting

Arthus reaction
articular
a. mass separation fracture
a. muscle
a. nerve
a. pillar fracture
a. recurrent nerve

articulate
articulation
artifact, artefact
muscle a.

artificial
a. airway
a. fever
a. fingernail remover
a. fracture
a. ligament

a. respiration (AR)
a. respirator
a. tear
a. ventilation

aryepiglottic muscle
arytenoid
a. muscle
a. subluxation-dislocation

asbestos exposure
asbestosis
ascariasis
Ascaris lumbricoides
ascending
a. aorta
a. cholangitis
a. colon
a. lumbar vein
a. pyelonephritis

Ascher vein
Asch forceps
ascites
chylous a.
leaking a.

ASCOT
A Severity Characterization of Trauma

ASD
atrial septal defect

Asendin
asepsis
aseptic
a. fever
a. meningitis
a. necrosis
a. wound

A Severity Characterization of Trauma (ASCOT)
ASH
asymmetric septal hypertrophy

Ashhurst-Bromer ankle fracture classification
Ashman phenomenon
ASIA
American Spinal Injury Association
ASIA Impairment Scale

Asian female (AF)
aspartate
a. aminotransferase (AST)
amphetamine a.

aspect
dorsal a.
ventral a.

NOTES

aspergillosis
    allergic bronchopulmonary a.
    pulmonary a.
Aspergillus
asphyxia
    autoerotic a.
    sexual a.
    traumatic a.
asphyxiant
    chemical a.
asphyxiate
asphyxiation
    near-drowning a.
aspirate
    bone marrow a.
aspirating
aspiration
    bone marrow a.
    bone plate a.
    fine-needle a. (FNA)
    foreign body a.
    a. of gastric contents
    gastric contents a.
    liquid substance a.
    meconium a.
    oropharyngeal flora a.
    a. pneumonia
    risk of a.
    suprapubic bladder a.
    a. syndrome
aspirator
aspirin
    a. intoxication
    a., phenacetin, caffeine with
      codeine (APC-C)
    a. poisoning
    a. therapy
asplenia
ASPTS
    age-specific pediatric trauma score
assault
    criminal sexual a. (CSA)
    felonious a.
    sexual a.
assaultive injury
assay
    D–dimer a.
    enzyme-linked immunosorbent a.
      (ELISA)
    saliva ethanol a.
assessment
    airway status a.
    focused medical a.
    focused trauma a.
    in-flight a.
    initial a.
    ongoing a.
    a. of patency
    primary a.

    rapid medical a.
    rapid trauma a.
    risk-benefit a.
    secondary a.
    sepsis-related organ failure a.
      (SOFA)
    trauma a.
assimilation
assistance
    international relief a.
assist control ventilation (ACV)
assisted coughing
associated
    a. cause of death
    a. orthostatic change
association
    American Heart A. (AHA)
    American Spinal Injury A. (ASIA)
    A. of Emergency Physicians
assumption
    a. of care
    a. of risk
AST
    aspartate aminotransferase
astemizole
asterixis
asteroid
asteroides
    Nocardia a.
asthenia
    muscle a.
asthenic
asthma
    acute severe a.
    adult a.
    a. flare
    GERD-associated a.
    occupational a.
    occupationally induced a.
    pediatric a.
astragalar bone
astragalocrural bone
astragaloid bone
astragaloscaphoid bone
astragalotibial bone
astragalus bone
astringent
astrocytoma
asymmetrical
asymmetric septal hypertrophy (ASH)
asymmetry
    facial a.
asymptomatic cardiac ischemia (ACI)
asynchronism
asynchrony of respiratory muscle
asystole
    atrial a.
    ventricular a.

ataxia
   gait a.
atelectasis
   absorptive a.
   denitrogenation absorption a.
atelectatic
atenolol
ATG
   antithymocyte globulin
atherosclerosis
   arteriolar a.
atherosclerotic
   a. deposit
   a. plaque
athetoid movement
ATIN
   acute tubular interstitial nephritis
Atkin epiphysial fracture
atlantal
   a. fracture
   a. ligament
atlantoaxial
   a. ligament
   a. subluxation
atlantoepistrophic ligament
atlantooccipital
   a. dislocation (AOD)
   a. ligament
atlas-axis combination fracture
atlas burst fracture
ATLS
   advanced trauma life support
atmospheric cooling power
ATN
   acute tubular necrosis
atonia
   muscle a.
atonic
   a. bladder
   a. seizure
atonicity
atony
   gastric a.
atopic dermatitis
atopy
atovaquone
ATPase
   adenosine triphosphatase
atracurium
Atraloc suture
atraumatic
   a. braided silk suture

   a. chromic suture
   a. patient
atresia
   choanal a.
   intestinal a.
atria (*pl. of* atrium)
atrial
   a. asystole
   a. contraction
   a. fibrillation
   a. flutter
   a. myxoma
   a. natriuretic peptide (ANP)
   a. pacemaker
   a. pressure
   a. septal defect (ASD)
   a. stunning
   a. tachycardia
atrioventricular (AV)
   a. block
   a. conduction block
   a. node
   a. septal defect
   a. valve
atrium, pl. atria
Atropa belladonna
atrophic fracture
atrophy
   bone a.
   brain a.
   compensatory a.
   muscle a.
atropine sulfate
atropinization
Atrovent inhaler
attack
   absence a.
   anginal a.
   anxiety a.
   heart a.
   myocardial infarction/heart a.
   panic a.
   transient ischemic a. (TIA)
attendant
   ambulance a.
attending physician
attenuant
attenuate
attenuated ligament
attenuation
   bone ultrasound a.
   tendon a.

NOTES

25

attic temporal bone
ATV
    automatic transport ventilator
atypia
atypical
    a. antipsychotic
    a. migraine
audible
    a. rhonchi
    a. wheezing
auditory
    a. buzz
    a. click
    a. hallucination
    a. tube nerve
    a. vein
augmentation
Augmentin
augmentor nerve
aura
aural stage
Aureomycin suture
aures (*pl. of* auris)
aureus
    methicillin-resistant
        Staphylococcus a. (MRSA)
        Staphylococcus a.
auricular
    a. hematoma
    a. ligament
    a. muscle
    a. nerve
    a. vein
auriculotemporal nerve
auris, pl. **aures**
auscultation
    heart a.
    percussion and a. (P & A)
auscultatory percussion
auto
    a. positive end-expiratory pressure
    A. Suture
autoerotic asphyxia
autogenesis
autogenous
    a. bone
    a. cartilage implantation
    a. iliac bone
    a. vein
autograft
    bone a.
    a. bone
autoimmune
    a. adrenalitis
    a. hemolytic anemia
    a. thrombocytopenia
    a. thrombocytopenia purpura
auto-injector
    epinephrine a.-i.

autologous
    a. blood
    a. blood transfusion
    a. bone
    a. internal jugular vein
automated
    a. external defibrillation (AED)
    a. external defibrillator (AED)
automatic
    a. external defibrillation (AED)
    a. transport ventilator (ATV)
    a. vehicle locator (AVL)
automaticity
    enhanced cardiac a.
autonomic
    a. dysreflexia
    a. hyperreflexia
    a. innervation
    a. nerve
    a. nervous system
autonomy
autoplastic suture
autopsy
AutoPulse CPR device
autosome
autotransfused blood
autotransplantation spleen
autumn
    a. crocus ingestion
    a. crocus toxicity
autumnale
    Colchicum a.
auxiliary
AV
    arteriovenous
    atrioventricular
    AV bypass tract
avalanche
    dry snow a.
avascular necrosis (AVN)
avium
    Mycobacterium a.
AVL
    automatic vehicle locator
AVM
    arteriovenous malformation
AVN
    avascular necrosis
avoidance
    a. of potassium
    a. of trigger
avoid weightbearing
Avon Skin So Soft toxicity
AVPU
    alert, verbal stimuli, painful stimuli, unresponsive
    AVPU scale
avulsed
    a. laceration

a. ligament
a. tooth
a. wound
avulsion
a. chip fracture
degloving a.
dental a.
facial soft tissue a.
a. fracture
ligament a.
nerve root a.
otologic a.
ring a.
scalp a.
a. stress fracture
vocal cord a.
awake, alert, and oriented ×3 (AAO3)
awareness
scene a.
awl
bone a.
axes (*pl. of* axis)
axial
a. compression fracture
a. loading
a. loading fracture
a. load teardrop fracture
a. load three-part, two-plane
fracture
a. muscle
a. skeleton
a. spine
a. tomography
a. view

Axid
axilla, pl. **axillae**
axillary
a. arch muscle
a. nerve
a. temperature
a. vein
axillofemoral bypass
axis, pl. **axes**
a. bone
celiac a.
a. fracture
gut-liver a.
a. ligament
sympathoadrenal a.
axis-atlas combination fracture
axonal injury
axonotmesis
Azactam
azalea ingestion
azathioprine
azidothymidine (AZT)
azithromycin
azlocillin sodium
azole
azotemia
acute a.
postrenal a.
prerenal a.
AZT
azidothymidine
aztreonam
azygos vein

NOTES

β (*var. of* beta)
Babesia
babesiosis
bacillary angiomatosis
Bacillus
    B. anthracis
    B. infection
bacillus
    gram-negative b.
back
    b. blow
    b. disorder
    b. gunshot wound
    b. pain
    b. wall suture
backboard
    half b.
    long b.
    short b.
    short wooden b.
    vest-type b.
backfire fracture
background radiation
backpacker diarrhea
backup
    radiology b.
backward, upward, and rightward
  pressure (BURP)
baclofen
bacteremia
bacteria (*pl. of* bacterium)
bacterial
    b. cholangitis
    b. endocarditis
    b. food poisoning
    b. infection
    b. meningitis
    b. pneumonia
    b. tracheitis
    b. vaginosis
bactericidal, bacteriocidal
    b. antibiotic
    b. drug
bacteriology
bacteriostatic
bacterium, pl. bacteria
bacteriuria
Bacteroides
    B. fragilis
    B. infection
Bactrim DS
BAER
    brainstem auditory evoked response
bag
    Ambu b.

Boardshield disposable backboard b.
breathing b.
Gamow b.
b. and mask
b. ventilation
bag-and-mask ventilation
bag-mask device
bag-valve
    b.-v. device
    b.-v. device to tracheostomy tube
    b.-v. mask
    b.-v. unit
bag-valve-mask (BVM)
    b.-v.-m. device
    b.-v.-m. technique
    b.-v.-m. ventilation
Bair-Hugger convective warming unit
Baker cyst
BAL
    bronchoalveolar lavage
balance
    acid-base b.
    b. sign
balanced
    b. electrolyte solution (BES)
    b. salt solution (BSS)
balanitis
    circinate b.
balanoposthitis
baldness
    male pattern b.
BALF
    bronchoalveolar lavage fluid
Balke-Ware protocol
Ballance sign
ball-and-socket joint
ballistic
    b. injury
    wound b.'s
balloon
    Bard temporary pacing electrode
      catheter with b.
    b. counterpulsation
    Epistat b.
    b. flotation catheterization
      calibration
    intraaortic counterpulsation b.
    intraluminal b.
    b. tamponade
balloon-expandable tracheal stent
ballooning aneurysm
ballotable
balsamic
bamboo spine

banana
    b. fracture
    b.'s, rice cereal, applesauce, toast (BRAT)
    spider b.
    b. spider
band
    creatine kinase-myocardial b. (CK-MB)
    fracture b.
bandage
    Ace b.
    butterfly b.
    elastic b.
    occlusive b.
    pressure b.
    self-adherent b.
    triangular b.
bandaging technique
Band-Aid
banding of muscle
baneberry ingestion
bank
    blood b.
    bone b.
Bankart fracture
banked
    b. blood
    b. bone
    b. freeze-dried bone
bar
    arch b.
    fracture b.
Bárány test
barbiturate
    b. abuse
    b. intoxication
    b. poisoning
Bardinet ligament
Bard temporary pacing electrode catheter with balloon
bariatrics
barium enema
Barkow ligament
barodontalgia
baroreceptor nerve
barosinusitis
barotitis media
barotrauma
    postintubation b.
    pulmonary b.
barracuda bite
Barraquer silk suture
barrel
    b. chest
    b. hoop sign
Barrett esophagus
barrier
    architectural b.

    blood-brain b.
    ligament b.
    mucosal b.
Bartholin
    B. abscess
    B. cyst
    B. gland disease
Barton fracture
Barton-Smith fracture
basal
    b. body temperature
    b. bone
    b. bunching suture
    b. cell carcinoma
    b. epithelial nerve
    b. metabolic rate (BMR)
    b. neck fracture
    b. skull fracture (BSF)
    b. vein
base
    bleeding surface at ulcer b.
    buffer b.
    b. deficit
    b. excess
    b. excess/deficit
    paramedic b.
    skull fracture b.
    b. station
    b. of support
    ulcer b.
baseball
    b. finger
    b. finger fracture
    b. suture
baseline variability
basic
    b. cardiac life support (BCLS)
    b. life support (BLS)
    b. metabolic panel (BMP)
basicervical fracture
basihyal bone
basilad
basilar
    b. aneurysm
    b. bone
    b. crackle
    b. femoral neck fracture
    b. migraine
    b. skull fracture
    b. suture
basilateral
basilic vein
basin
    emesis b.
    kidney b.
basioccipital bone
basisphenoid bone
basivertebral vein

B

basket
>   Stokes b.
>   b. stretcher

basolateral membrane transport system
basophilic stippling
Bassen-Kornzweig disease
bastard suture
basting suture
BAT
>   blunt abdominal trauma

bath pruritus
bathroom privilege (BRP)
battalion
battered
>   b. child syndrome
>   b. spouse syndrome

battering
>   granny b.

battery
>   button b.
>   b. ingestion
>   b. of tests

Battle sign
Baumgarten vein
bayonet
>   b. forceps
>   b. position
>   b. position of fracture

BBC
>   bromobenzylcyanide

BCI
>   blunt cardiac injury

BCLS
>   basic cardiac life support

BCU
>   body cooling unit

beaded lizard envenomation
beak
>   b. fracture
>   b. ligament

beanbag
bearing-down pain
beat
>   arrhythmic b.
>   ectopic b.

beat-to-beat variability
Beck triad
Beckwith-Wiedemann syndrome
beclomethasone
Beclovent
bed
>   air b.

>   air-fluidized b.
>   bone graft b.
>   fracture b.
>   Gatch b.
>   low air loss b.
>   wound b.

bedbug
bedpan
bedrest
>   absolute b. (ABR)
>   endocrine effects of b.
>   b. physiology

bedridden
bedroom fracture
bedside indirect calorimetry
bedsore
bedwetting
bee
>   b. sting
>   b. sting anaphylaxis

beetle
>   blister b.

behavior
>   agitated b.
>   ambivalent b.
>   combative b.
>   controlling b.
>   inappropriate b.

behavioral disturbance
Behçet disease
belching
Bell
>   B. cruciate paralysis
>   B. muscle
>   B. palsy
>   B. respiratory nerve
>   B. suture

belladonna
>   Atropa b.

2-bellied muscle
Bellini ligament
belly
>   b. button
>   muscle b.

bellyache
below-knee cast
Benadryl
bend fracture
bending
>   b. fracture
>   lateral b.

beneficence

NOTES

beneficial
beneficiary
benefit
    indemnity b.
    maximum hospital b.
    maximum medical b.
    service b.
benign
    b. idiopathic neonatal convulsion (BINC)
    b. intracranial hypertension
    b. positional vertigo (BPV)
    b. prostatic hyperplasia (BPH)
    b. prostatic hypertrophy (BPH)
    b. stupor
Bennett
    B. basic hand fracture
    B. comminuted fracture
benoxaprofen
bent-arm drag technique
Bentley autotransfusion system
benzene
    chloroacetophenone, carbon tetrachloride, b. (CNB)
    b. poisoning
benzilate
    3–quinuclidinyl b.
benzisoxazole
benzocaine
    b. anesthesia
    b. ear drops
benzodiazepine poisoning
benztropine
benzyl amine
benzylpenicillin therapy
bepridil
bergamot
    scarlet b.
Berndt-Hardy classification of transchondral fracture
berry
    b. aneurysm
    B. ligament
Bertin ligament
BES
    balanced electrolyte solution
besylate
    cisatracurium b.
beta, β
    b. lactam antibiotic
    b. lactam therapy
    b. radiation
    b. 1, 2 receptor
beta-adrenergic
    b.-a. agonist
    b.-a. blocker
    b.-a. receptor blocker

beta-blocker
    b.-b. poisoning
    b.-b. toxicity
beta-blocking agent
betacardone
Betadine douche
beta-hCG, beta-HCG
    beta-human chorionic gonadotropin
beta-human chorionic gonadotropin (beta-hCG, beta-HCG)
beta-naphthol toxicity
Betapace
bethanechol
Bezafibrate
    B. Infarction Prevention (BIP)
    B. Infarction Prevention study
bezoar
Bezold abscess
bibasilar
    b. dullness
    b. rale
    b. rhonchi
bibulous dressing
bicarbonate
    b. administration
    b. buffer system
    potassium b.
    renal loss of b.
    b. of soda
    sodium b.
    b. therapy
bicaudal
bicephalus
biceps
    b. brachii rupture
    b. brachii tendon
    b. femoris tendon
Bichat ligament
bicipital
    b. muscle
    b. tendinitis
    b. tendon
bicipitoradial bursa
bicolumn fracture
bicondylar
    b. T-shaped fracture
    b. Y-shaped fracture
bicortical iliac bone
bicuspid valve
bicycle
    b. accident
    b. injury
    b. spoke fracture
bifid
    b. biceps tendon
    b. earlobe
    b. uterus
    b. uvula
bifurcated ligament

B

bifurcate ligament
bifurcation
    aortic b.
Bigelow ligament
bigeminal pregnancy
biguanide hypoglycemic
bilateral
    b. burns
    b. condylar fracture
    b. leg edema
    b. maxillary sinus disease
    b. medial orbital ecchymosis
    b. otitis media (BOM)
    b. rhonchi
    b., symmetrical, and equal (BSE)
    b. tonic deviation
bilberry
bile duct
bilevel positive airway pressure (BiPAP)
biliary
    b. colic
    b. duct disruption
    b. fistula
    b. sepsis
    b. tract
    b. tract disease
    b. tract disorder
bilious vomitus
bilirubin
Billroth anastomosis
biloba
    ginkgo b.
biloma
bimalleolar
    b. ankle fracture
    b. fracture
bimanual examination
binasal pharyngeal airway (BNPA)
binaural stethoscope
BINC
    benign idiopathic neonatal convulsion
binge eating disorder
bioabsorbable Dexon suture
bioavailability
Biobrane
    B. dressing
    B. skin substitute
biochemistry
biocidal
Bioclusive dressing
Bio-FASTak suture
bioflavonoid

biohazard
bioimpedance-determined cardiac output
bioimplant
    bone morphogenetic protein b.
biological
    b. diagnosis
    b. dressing
    b. warfare agent
    b. warfare mass casualty
      management
biomechanics
    bone b.
    muscle b.
biomedicine
biophysical profile (BPP)
biophysiology
biopsy
    bone b.
    bone marrow b.
    bone marrow aspiration and b.
    bone marrow trephine b.
    muscle b.
    nerve b.
    open lung b. (OLB)
    transbronchial b. (TBB)
    wound b.
    wound margin b.
biorhythm
BioSorb suture
Biosyn synthetic monofilament suture
biotransformation
    cytochrome P-450 b.
BIP
    Bezafibrate Infarction Prevention
BiPAP
    bilevel positive airway pressure
biparietal
    b. diameter (BPD)
    b. suture
bipartite
    b. fracture
    b. sesamoid bone
bipennate muscle
biperforate
biphasic
    b. airway pressure
    b. fever
bipolar
    b. affective disorder
    b. disorder
    b. electrocautery

NOTES

bipolar *(continued)*
    b. psychosis
    b. traction splint
bird-beak deformity
birth
    b. canal laceration
    date of b. (DB, DOB)
    b. fracture
    b. history
    b. trauma
    b. weight (BW)
    b. weight discordance
birthing center
bisacodyl
bisaxillary
bischloromethyl ether
bismuth
    b. subnitrate
    b. subsalicylate
    b. subsalicylate toxicity
bisoprolol
bisphosphonate
bite
    animal b.
    ant b.
    arthropod b.
    barracuda b.
    black widow spider b.
    brown recluse spider b.
    cat b.
    cobra b.
    cottonmouth b.
    dog b.
    elapid snake b.
    fire ant b.
    human b.
    Hymenoptera b.
    insect b.
    lizard b.
    mammal b.
    marine organism b.
    scorpion b.
    shark b.
    snake b.
    tarantula b.
16-bite nylon suture
bitolterol
bitter
    b. almond
    b. almond odor
black
    b. braided nylon suture
    b. braided silk suture
    b. female
    b. locust tree ingestion
    b. male
    b. silk sling suture
    b. silk suture
    b. twisted suture

    b. widow spider
    b. widow spider bite
blackout
    alcoholic b.
blacksnake
bladder
    atonic b.
    b. carcinoma
    b. function
    b. injury
    kidneys, ureters, b. (KUB)
    b. laceration
    b. neck detrusor muscle
    neurogenic b.
    b. rupture
    b. smooth muscle
    b. tear
    urinary b.
    b. vein
blade
    b. bone
    curved b.
    Flagg b.
    laryngoscope b.
    MacIntosh b.
    Miller b.
    straight b.
    Wisconsin b.
Blakemore-Sengstaken tube
Blalock suture
blanching
    skin b.
bland-aerosol therapy
bland affect
blanket
    b. drag technique
    hypothermic b.
    b. suture
blast
    chest b.
    b. effect
    b. injury
    lung b.
Blastomyces
    B. dermatitidis
    B. dermatitidis infection
blastomycosis
BLB
    Boothby, Lovelace, Bulbulian
    BLB mask
bleach ingestion
bleed
    gastrointestinal b.
    GI b.
    parenchymal b.
bleeder
bleeding
    arterial b.
    b. bone

capillary b.
colonic b.
b. control
control b.
b. disorder
dysfunctional uterine b.
esophageal variceal b.
external b.
gastric b.
gastroesophageal variceal b.
gastrointestinal b.
heavy b.
hemorrhoidal b.
increase in b.
internal b.
lower gastrointestinal b.
occult b.
b. surface at ulcer base
b. time
b. of undetermined origin (BUO)
upper gastrointestinal b.
vaginal b.
variceal b.
venous b.
blepharitis
blind
b. laparotomy
b. nasotracheal intubation (BNTI)
b. procedure
blindness
cortical b.
blister
b. beetle
bone b.
fracture b.
blister-causing agent
bloc
en b.
block
anterior fascicular b.
apical nerve b.
atrioventricular b.
atrioventricular conduction b.
bone b.
bundle branch b.
caudal b.
digital nerve b.
epidural local anesthesia b.
fascicular b.
field b.
first-degree atrioventricular b.
first-degree AV b.

heart b.
intercostal nerve b.
median fascicular b.
median nerve b.
Mobitz atrioventricular b.
Mobitz I, II AV b.
Mobitz I, II second-degree AV b.
b. nerve
nerve root b.
peripheral nerve b.
pudendal b.
radial nerve b.
second-degree atrioventricular b.
second-degree AV b.
sinoatrial conduction b.
supraperiosteal dental nerve b.
sural nerve b.
third-degree atrioventricular b.
third-degree AV b.
tibial nerve b.
ulnar nerve b.
Wenckebach b.
blockade
paravertebral b.
blocker
alpha-adrenergic b.
beta-adrenergic b.
beta-adrenergic receptor b.
calcium channel b.
calcium entry b.
slow channel b.
sodium channel b.
blood
autologous b.
autotransfused b.
b. bank
banked b.
b. chemistry study
crossmatched b.
b. culture
deoxygenated b.
b. dyscrasia
egress of b.
b. flow
b. gas
b. glucose
leukodepleted b.
b. loss
maldistribution of b.
occult b.
oxygenated b.
b. plasma

NOTES

blood *(continued)*
   b. pressure (BP)
   b. pressure cuff
   b. salvage
   b. substitute
   b. sugar (BS)
   b. and thunder
   b. transfusion
   b. transfusion reaction
   b. type
   type and crossmatch b.
   type-specific b.
   b. typing
   b. typing and crossmatching
   b. urea nitrogen (BUN)
   b. viscosity
   b. volume expander
   whole b.
bloodborne
   b. disease
   b. pathogen
blood-brain barrier
bloodroot plant ingestion
bloody
   b. show
   b. sputum
   b. vomitus
blow
   back b.
blow-by oxygen
blow-in fracture
blowing wound
blowout
   bone lesion b.
   b. fracture
BLS
   basic life support
blue
   b. line on gums
   methylene b.
   b. pus
   b. twisted cotton suture
   b. urine
blue-black monofilament suture
Bluetooth remote wireless technology
   microphone
blunt
   b. abdominal trauma (BAT)
   b. anterior neck trauma
   b. cardiac injury (BCI)
   b. chest trauma
   b. head trauma
   b. neck trauma
   b. thoracic trauma
   b. trauma
blunted
   b. affect
   b. perception
   b. perception of dyspnea

blurred vision
BMP
   basic metabolic panel
BMR
   basal metabolic rate
BNPA
   binasal pharyngeal airway
BNTI
   blind nasotracheal intubation
BO
   bronchiolitis obliterans
board
   b. certified
   spine b.
   transfer b.
Boardshield disposable backboard bag
bobbing
   ocular b.
Bochdalek muscle
Bock nerve
body
   b. alignment
   anorectal foreign b.
   cartilaginous loose b.
   b. cooling unit (BCU)
   corneal foreign b.
   Donovan b.
   ear foreign b.
   esophageal foreign b.
   b. fluid exposure
   foreign b. (FB)
   loose b.
   b. mechanics
   metallic foreign b.
   nasal foreign b.
   nerve cell b.
   b. packer
   rectal foreign b.
   retained foreign b.
   b. substance isolation (BSI)
   b. surface area (BSA)
   b. surface area of burn
   b. temperature
   vaginal foreign b.
   b. water
   b. weight
body-weight ratio
Boerhaave syndrome
boggy
   b. mucous membrane
   b. uterus
bolster suture
bolus dose
BOM
   bilateral otitis media
Bondek absorbable suture
bone
   b. abduction instrument
   b. abscess

B

b. absorption
accessory multangular b.
accessory navicular b.
accessory sesamoid b.
acetabular b.
b. ache
acromial b.
adynamic b.
b. age
b. age determination
b. age imaging
b. age ratio
b. aggregate
alar b.
b. algorithm
alisphenoid b.
b. alkaline phosphatase
allogenic b.
b. allograft
allograft iliac b.
alveolar b.
alveolar supporting b.
alveolar supporting bone ankle b.
b. angioblastoma
b. angiosarcoma
ankle b.
antigen-extracted allogeneic b.
anvil b.
b. arch
b. architecture
arm b.
b. aseptic necrosis
astragalar b.
astragalocrural b.
astragaloid b.
astragaloscaphoid b.
astragalotibial b.
astragalus b.
b. atrophy
b. attenuation coefficient
attic temporal b.
autogenous b.
b. autogenous graft
autogenous iliac b.
autograft b.
b. autograft
autologous b.
b. avascular necrosis
b. awl
axis b.
b. bank
banked b.

banked freeze-dried b.
basal b.
basihyal b.
basilar b.
basioccipital b.
basisphenoid b.
bicortical iliac b.
b. biomechanics
b. biopsy
bipartite sesamoid b.
blade b.
bleeding b.
b. blister
b. block
b. block fusion
b. block graft
b. block procedure
bosselated b.
bowed long b.
b. bowing
breast b.
bregmatic b.
bridging b.
brittle b.
b. bruise
b. bruise sign
bundle b.
b. bur
cadaver b.
calcaneal b.
calcaneocuboid b.
calcaneus b.
calf b.
b. callus
calvarial free b.
b. canaliculus
cancellated b.
cancellous cellular b.
cancellous versus cortical b.
b. cancer
cannon b.
b. capillary hemangioma
capitate b.
b. carbonate
b. carcinoma
carpal navicular b.
carpal row b.
b. carpentry
cartilage b.
cavalry b.
b. cell
b. cell receptor

NOTES

37

bone *(continued)*
b. cement
b. center
central b.
cervical vertebral b.
chalky b.
cheek b.
chevron b.
b. chip
b. chip graft
b. chloroma
chondroid b.
clavicle b.
coalition of b.
b. coccidioidomycosis
coccygeal b.
coccyx b.
coffin b.
collar b.
b. collector
compact b.
b. conduction
b. conduction deafness
b. conduction hearing aid
b. conduction level
b. conduction threshold
condyle b.
b. consolidation
b. contusion
convoluted b.
b. core
3-cornered b.
coronary b.
b. corpuscle
b. cortex
cortical b.
corticocancellous b.
costal b.
coxal b.
cranial b.
b. crater
creeping substitution of b.
crestal cortical b.
b. crib
cribriform b.
b. crisis
cubital b.
cuboid b.
b. culture
cuneiform b.
b. cyst
b. cyst excision
b. cyst fracture probability
b. cyst treatment
dancer's b.
dead b.
b. debris
b. decay
b. defect

b. deficiency
b. demineralization
dense b.
b. densitometer
b. densitometry
b. densitometry study
b. density
b. density imaging
b. density measurement
b. density scan
b. density screening
b. density study
b. deposition
b. depression
dermal b.
b. destruction
b. destructive process
detritus b.
b. development
b. disease
disorganized b.
b. dissection
b. dollop
dorsal talonavicular b.
b. dowel
b. dysplasia
b. dystrophy
ear b.
eburnated b.
b. echinococcosis
ectethmoid b.
ectocuneiform b.
ectopic b.
b. effect
elbow b.
b. elevator
b. embedding
embryonic b.
b. end
entocuneiform b.
entrapped plantar sesamoid b.
eosinophilic granuloma of b.
epihyoid b.
epiphysis b.
epipteric b.
episternal b.
b. erosion
ethmoid b.
exercise b.
exoccipital b.
b. expansion
b. exposure
b. extractor
facial b.
b. felon
femoral b.
b. femoral plug
fencer's b.
b. fibrosarcoma

B

fibular sesamoid b.
b. file
first cuneiform b.
flank b.
b. flap
b. flap osteitis
flat frontal b.
flower b.
b. fluid
foot b.
b. forceps
b. formation
b. formation marker
b. formation rate
b. formation-stimulating agent
fourth turbinated b.
fovea centralis b.
fracture running length of b.
fragile b.
b. fragility
b. fragment
frontal b.
fusiform periosteal new b.
b. gouge
gracile b.
b. graft
b. graft bed
b. graft collapse
b. graft decompression
b. graft extrusion
b. graft incorporation
b. grafting
b. grafting material
b. graft placement
b. graft punch
b. graft repair
b. graft shoe horn
b. graft substitute
b. graft substitute graft
great toe sesamoid b.
b. growth
b. growth chamber
b. growth stimulator
hallux sesamoid b.
hamate b.
b. hardening
b. harvesting
haunch b.
haversian b.
heel b.
b. hemangioma
heterologous b.

heterotopic b.
highest turbinated b.
high frontal b.
hip b.
b. histology
b. histomorphometry
b. holder
b. hook
humeral b.
b. hunger
hungry b.
hydroxyapatite b.
hyoid b.
hyperplastic b.
b. hypertrophy
iliac b.
iliac cancellous b.
ilium b.
b. imaging
immature b.
b. implant
b. implantation cyst
b. implant material
incarial b.
incisive b.
incus b.
b. infarct
b. infarction
infected b.
b. infection
inferior maxillary b.
inferior turbinate b.
b. ingrowth
b. injury radiation
innominate b.
intermaxillary b.
intermediate cuneiform b.
interparietal b.
interproximal b.
b. interstice
intracartilaginous b.
intramembranous b.
irradiated b.
irregular b.
ischial b.
b. island
b. isograft
ivory b.
jaw b.
b. and joint tuberculosis
jugal b.
knee b.

NOTES

39

bone (*continued*)

knuckle b.
lacrimal b.
b. lacuna
laminar b.
lateral condyle b.
lateral cuneiform b.
lateral mastoid b.
lateral sesamoid b.
b. lavage
b. length imaging
b. length study
lenticular b.
lentiform b.
b. lesion apophysis
b. lesion blowout
b. lesion epiphysis
b. lesion of rib
lesser trochanter pubic b.
limbus of sphenoid b.
lingual alveolar b.
b. lipoma
b. liquefaction
long b.
b. loss
lunate b.
lunocapitate b.
luxated b.
b. lymphoma
malar b.
b. mallet
mandibular b.
marble b.
b. margin
b. marrow
b. marrow abnormality
b. marrow agent
b. marrow aplasia
b. marrow aspirate
b. marrow aspiration
b. marrow aspiration and biopsy
b. marrow biopsy
b. marrow boundary
b. marrow cell
b. marrow cellularity
b. marrow culture
b. marrow cytogenetics
b. marrow depression
b. marrow-derived B cell
b. marrow-derived cultured mast cell
b. marrow-derived myogenic progenitor
b. marrow-derived stromal cell
b. marrow differential count
b. marrow donor
b. marrow dose
b. marrow dysfunction
b. marrow edema

b. marrow element
b. marrow embolism
b. marrow embolus
b. marrow examination
b. marrow exposure guideline
b. marrow failure
b. marrow failure state
b. marrow fibroblast
b. marrow fibrosis
b. marrow function
b. marrow puncture
b. marrow purging
b. marrow relapse
b. marrow replacement
b. marrow rescue
b. marrow reserve
b. marrow sampling
b. marrow scan
b. marrow scanning
b. marrow scintigraphy
b. marrow staining
b. marrow stem cell
b. marrow stimulating technique
b. marrow stromal cell
b. marrow suppression
b. marrow toxicity
b. marrow transplant
b. marrow transplantation
b. marrow transplant unit
b. marrow trephine biopsy
b. marrow tumor
b. mass accretion
b. mass density
b. mass maintenance
b. mass measurement
masticatory b.
b. mastocytosis
mastoid b.
b. matrix alteration
b. matrix formation
b. maturation
b. maturity
maxillary b.
b. meal
medial cuneiform b.
medial metacarpal b.
medial sesamoid b.
medial turbinate b.
medullary b.
meiopragic b.
meniscal b.
mesocuneiform b.
b. metabolic unit
metacarpal b.
b. metastasis
middle cuneiform b.
middle turbinate b.
b. mineral
b. mineral accretion

B

b. mineral accrual
b. mineral content
b. mineral content imaging
b. mineral content study
b. mineral densitometry
b. mineral density
b. mineral density study
b. mineral immobilization
b. mineralization
b. mineralization isotope
b. mineral mass
b. mineral measurement
b. mineral metabolism
b. mineral uptake
monocortical b.
morcellized b.
b. morphogenetic activity
b. morphogenetic protein
b. morphogenetic protein bioimplant
b. morphogenetic protein receptor
b. morphogenic protein
b. mortise
b. mucormycosis
b. mulch screw
multangular b.
nasal b.
navicular b.
b. neck
necrotic b.
b. neoplasm
newly woven b.
nonlamellar b.
nonlamellated b.
occipital b.
b. occipital malformation
occiput b.
odontoid b.
omovertebral b.
orbicular b.
orbital b.
orbitosphenoidal b.
os calcis b.
osteoclastic b.
osteonal lamellar b.
osteonic b.
osteopenic b.
osteopetrosis-stricken facial b.
osteoporotic b.
b. overdevelopment
b. oxalosis
pagetic b.
pagetoid b.

b. pain
paired skull b.
palatine b.
parietal skull b.
b. particle
b. paste
patella b.
b. pathology
pedal b.
b. peg
b. pegging
b. peg graft
pelvic b.
perichondral b.
periosteal b.
periotic b.
peroneal b.
petrosal b.
petrous temporal b.
phalangeal b.
phantom b.
b. phase image
b. phase imaging
b. pinhole
pisiform b.
pisohamate b.
b. plate
b. plate aspiration
b. plate selection
b. plombage
pneumatic b.
b. pointing
porotic b.
porous b.
postsphenoid b.
postulnar b.
b. powder
prefrontal b.
preinterparietal b.
premaxillary b.
presphenoid b.
primitive b.
b. production
b. prosthesis
pterygoid b.
pubic b.
pyramidal b.
quadrilateral b.
quadripartite b.
b. quantitative CT
b. quantitative ultrasound velocity
b. quantum

NOTES

bone (continued)
rachitic b.
radial b.
b. radiation absorption
ramus b.
b. rarefaction
raw b.
b. reabsorption
b. recession
b. reconstruction
b. reflex
refractured b.
regenerated b.
b. remodeling
replacement b.
b. resection
b. resorption
b. resorption marker
b. resurfacing
resurrection b.
reticulated b.
b. retractor
rider's b.
round iliac b.
rudimentary b.
sacral b.
sacred b.
b. sarcoidosis
b. sarcoma
sarcomatous b.
scaphoid b.
scapular b.
b. scintiscan imaging
sclerosed temporal b.
b. sclerosis
sclerotic b.
scroll b.
second cuneiform b.
semilunar b.
b. sensibility
septal b.
b. sequestrum
sesamoid b.
b. setting
b. shaft
b. shaft fracture
shank b.
shin b.
short metacarpal b.
shoulder b.
b. sialoprotein
sieve b.
b. skid
b. sliver
b. slurry
small maxillary b.
solid b.
b. spacer
sphenoid b.

b. spiculation
b. spicule
splintered b.
spoke b.
spongy b.
spotted b.
b. spur
squamooccipital b.
squamous b.
stapes b.
b. stippling
stirrup b.
b. stock
b. strength
b. strength measurement
b. structural unit
b. strut
stump of b.
styloid b.
subchondral b.
subcoracoid b.
subperiosteal b.
b. substance
substitution b.
superior maxillary b.
supernumerary sesamoid b.
supporting b.
supraoccipital b.
suprapharyngeal b.
suprasternal b.
supreme turbinate b.
b. surface
b. surface lesion
surface of orbital zygomatic b.
b. survey
sutural b.
b. suture fixation
synthetic b.
b. syphilis
tail b.
talonavicular b.
talus b.
target b.
tarsal b.
temporal b.
thigh b.
third cuneiform b.
thoracic b.
thyroid b.
tibia b.
tibial cortical b.
tibial sesamoid b.
b. tissue
toe b.
tongue b.
b. trabecula
trabeculated b.
b. transfer
b. transport technique

B

trapezoid b.
b. trephine
triangular wrist b.
tripartite b.
triquetrum b.
b. trough
b. tuberculoma
tuberculous b.
tubular b.
tumor b.
b. tumor aggressiveness
tumor-bearing b.
b. tumor matrix
b. tumor scalloping
turbinate b.
b. turnover
tympanic b.
ulnar sesamoid b.
ulnar styloid b.
b. ultrasound attenuation
unciform b.
uncinate b.
b. unloading
upper jaw b.
vascular metaphysial b.
vesalian b.
vomer b.
von Recklinghausen disease of b.
b. wax suture
b. weapon
b. wedge
wedge b.
weightbearing b.
whettle b.
b. window
b. wire guide
wormian b.
woven b.
wrist triquetrum b.
b. xanthogranuloma
xenogeneic b.
xiphoid b.
yoke b.
zygomatic b.
Bonine
bony
b. abnormality
b. crepitus
b. injury
b. insertion
b. suture
b. tenderness

boomerang tendon
BOOP
bronchiolitis obliterans organizing
pneumonia
booster
tetanus toxoid b.
boot
fracture b.
IPC b.
Boothby
B., Lovelace, Bulbulian (BLB)
B. mask
boot-top
b.-t. fracture
b.-t. laceration
border
left sternal b. (LSB)
medial b.
borderline
b. anemia
b. diabetes
b. personality disorder
boric
b. acid
b. acid poisoning
b. acid toxicity
Bornholm disease
Borrelia
B. burgdorferi
B. burgdorferi infection
borreliosis
bosselated bone
Boston
B. ivy
B. ivy ingestion
Bosworth fracture
Botallo ligament
both-bone fracture
both-column fracture
both upper extremities (BUE)
botulinum
Clostridium b.
botulism
b. bacterial infection
fish b.
wound b.
boundary
bone marrow b.
bounding pulse
Bourgery ligament
boutonnière deformity
Bovero muscle

NOTES

Bovie cauterization
bowed long bone
bowel
    edematous b.
    eviscerated b.
    b. function
    b. habit
    irritable b.
    b. ischemia
    ischemic b.
    malrotation of b.
    matted b.
    b. movement
    b. obstruction
    b. perforation
    b. sound (BS)
    b. strangulation
bowing
    bone b.
    b. fracture
    tendon b.
Bowman ciliary muscle
bow-tie sign
box
    fracture b.
    b. jellyfish poisoning
boxcar segmentation
boxer's punch fracture
Boyd
    B. communicating perforation vein
    B. perforating vein
    B. type II fracture
Boyer bursa
Bozeman suture
BP
    blood pressure
BPD
    biparietal diameter
    bronchopleural dysplasia
BPF
    bronchopleural fistula
BPH
    benign prostatic hyperplasia
    benign prostatic hypertrophy
BPP
    biophysical profile
BPV
    benign positional vertigo
bracelet identifier
brachial
    b. artery
    b. cutaneous nerve
    b. muscle
    b. plexus injury
    b. plexus nerve
    b. plexus tendon
    b. pulse
    b. vein
brachiocephalic vein

brachioradial
    b. ligament
    b. muscle
bracing
    fracture b.
bradyarrhythmia
bradycardia
    relative b.
    sinus b.
bradydysrhythmia
bradykinesia
bradykinetic
bradypnea
braided
    b. Ethibond suture
    b. Mersilene suture
    b. Nurolon suture
    b. nylon suture
    b. polyamide suture
    b. polyester suture
    b. polyglactin suture
    b. silk suture
    b. Vicryl suture
    b. wire suture
brain
    b. abscess
    b. atrophy
    b. bridging vein
    b. concussion
    b. contusion
    b. death
    b. hematoma
    b. herniation
    b. infarction
    injured b.
    b. injury
    b. laceration
    b. lesion
    b. monitoring
    penetrating injury of b.
    b. resuscitation
    B. Resuscitation Clinical Trial
    (BRCT)
    b. stem
    uninjured b.
brainstem, brain stem
    b. auditory evoked potential
    b. auditory evoked response
    (BAER)
    b. demyelination
    b. function
    b. infarct
    b. infarction
    b. lesion
Bralon suture
branch
    marginal b.
    nerve b.
branchial nerve

branchiomeric muscle
Branham sign
brash
    water b.
BRAT
    bananas, rice cereal, applesauce, toast
Braune muscle
Braunwald unstable angina classification
brawny edema
Braxton-Hicks contraction
brazing toxin
BRCT
    Brain Resuscitation Clinical Trial
breach of duty
breakdown
    muscle b.
    wound b.
breast
    b. abscess
    b. bone
    b. engorgement
    b. fat necrosis
    b. mass
    b. milk
    pendulous b.
breath
    alcohol on b. (AOB)
    foul b.
    shortness of b. (SOB)
    b. sound
    b. test
Breathalyzer test
breath-holding spell
breathing
    abdominal b.
    agonal b.
    airway and b.
    b. bag
    difficulty b.
    effective b.
    effort of b.
    increased work of b.
    intermittent positive-pressure b.
      (IPPB)
    labored b.
    b. management
    mouth-to-mask b.
    mouth-to-mouth b.
    noisy b.
    positive-pressure b. (PPB)
    pursed lip b.
    quiet b.

    rapid b.
    rescue b.
    seesaw b.
    shallow b.
    b. treatment
    work of b. (WOB)
breathlessness
breech presentation
bregmatic bone
bregmatomastoid suture
Breschet vein
bretylium poisoning
brevis
    flexor pollicis b.
    lateral two lumbricals, opponens
      pollicis, abductor pollicis brevis,
      flexor pollicis b. (LOAF)
    b. muscle
brewer's yeast
bridge
    medical b.
    muscle b.
    suture b.
    b. suture
bridging
    b. bone
    b. vein
bridle suture
brittle bone
broad
    b. ligament
    b. uterine ligament
broad-spectrum antibiotic
Broberg-Morrey fracture
Brodie
    B. bursa
    B. ligament
broken
    b. rib
    b. vein
bromate hair neutralizer
bromethalin poisoning
bromide
    emepronium b.
    ipratropium b.
    b. toxicity
bromobenzylcyanide (BBC)
bromocriptine
bronchi (*pl. of* bronchus)
bronchial
    b. artery embolization
    b. fracture

NOTES

bronchial *(continued)*
    b. smooth muscle
    b. tube
    b. vein
bronchiectasis
bronchiolar
bronchiole
bronchiolitic
bronchiolitis
    exudative b.
    b. obliterans (BO)
    b. obliterans organizing pneumonia
    (BOOP)
    proliferative b.
bronchitis
    acute b.
    chronic b.
bronchoalveolar
    b. lavage (BAL)
    b. lavage fluid (BALF)
bronchodilator
bronchoesophageal muscle
bronchographic
bronchography
bronchopleural
    b. dysplasia (BPD)
    b. fistula (BPF)
bronchopneumonia
bronchopulmonary
    b. dysplasia
    b. lavage
bronchorrhea
bronchoscopy
    fiberoptic b.
    rigid b.
bronchospasm
bronchospirometer
bronchospirometry
bronchotracheal
bronchus, pl. bronchi
    left mainstem b.
    right mainstem b.
Bronkometer
Bronkosol
bronze wire suture
Broselow
    B. emergency tape
    B. pediatric resuscitative tape
Broselow-Hinkle pediatric emergency
  system
Broselow-Luten system
brown
    b. recluse spider
    b. recluse spider bite
    b. snake
    B. syndrome
    B. tendon
brown-black urine
Browning vein

brownish-yellow sputum
Brown-Séquard syndrome
Brown-Sharp gauge suture
Broyle ligament
BRP
    bathroom privilege
brucellosis
Brugmansia ingestion
bruise
    bone b.
    multiple b.'s
    patterned b.
    b. in suspicious location
bruising
    evident b.
bruit
    carotid b.
brush
    b. burn
    B. ECG criteria
    protected specimen b.
bruxism
BS
    blood sugar
    bowel sound
BSA
    body surface area
BSE
    bilateral, symmetrical, and equal
BSF
    basal skull fracture
B&S gauge suture
BSI
    body substance isolation
BSS
    balanced salt solution
    buffered saline solution
BU
    burn unit
bubonic plague
buccal
    b. mucosa
    b. muscle
    b. nerve
    b. smear
    b. vein
buccinator
    b. muscle
    b. nerve
bucket-handle fracture
buckle fracture
buckling
buckthorn ingestion
Budd-Chiari syndrome
buddy
    b. splint
    b. tape
    b. taping
budesonide

B

BUE
    both upper extremities
Buerger disease
bufalin ingestion
buffer
    b. base
    b. nerve
    renal b.
buffered saline solution (BSS)
bufo toad
bulb
    b. suture
    b. syringe
bulbar
    b. conjunctiva
    b. polioencephalitis
bulbocavernous muscle
bulboid
bulbourethral gland
bulbous
Bulbulian
    Boothby, Lovelace, B. (BLB)
bulging fontanelle
bulimia nervosa
bulk
    muscle b.
bulk-producing laxative
bulky dressing
bulla, pl. **bullae**
bullet
    b. embolism
    b. wipe
    b. wipe residue
    b. wound
    b. yaw
bullous
    b. emphysema
    b. myringitis
    b. skin lesion
bumetanide
bump
    goose b.'s
bumper fracture
BUN
    blood urea nitrogen
bundle
    b. bone
    b. branch block
    muscle b.
    nerve fiber b.
    b. suture
    tendon b.

bunk bed fracture
Bunnell
    B. crisscross suture
    B. figure-eight suture
    B. wire pull-out suture
BUO
    bleeding of undetermined origin
bupivacaine with epinephrine
buprenorphine
bupropion
bur
    bone b.
burgdorferi
    Borrelia b.
buried
    b. knot
    b. suture
Burkhalter-Reyes
    B.-R. method
    B.-R. method phalangeal fracture
Burkholderia cepacia
burn
    acid b.
    airway b.
    alkali b.
    bilateral b.'s
    body surface area of b.
    brush b.
    caustic b.
    chemical b.
    coal tar b.
    corneal b.
    electrical b.
    entry-exit b.
    first-degree b.
    flash b.
    fourth-degree b.
    friction b.
    full-thickness b.
    glovelike b.
    high-tension b.
    hydrofluoric acid b.
    immersion b.
    kissing b.
    neglectful b.
    nonthermal b.
    ocular b.
    partial-thickness b.
    powder b.
    radiation b.
    respiratory b.
    rug b.

NOTES

burn *(continued)*
    scald b.
    second-degree b.
    stockinglike b.
    superficial b.
    suspicious b.
    thermal b.
    third-degree b.
    unexplained b.
    b. unit (BU)
    b. wound
burned rope odor
burnetii
    Coxiella b.
burning
    b. chest pain
    b. hands syndrome
burnout
Burns ligament
Burow vein
BURP
  backward, upward, and rightward
  pressure
    BURP maneuver
bursa, pl. **bursae**
    Achilles tendon b.
    adventitious b.
    anserine b.
    anterior tibial b.
    bicipitoradial b.
    Boyer b.
    Brodie b.
    calcaneal b.
    Calori b.
    coracobrachial b.
    coracoid b.
    deep infrapatellar b.
    deltoid b.
    diarthrodial joint bursae
    distended b.
    Fleischmann b.
    flexor b.
    gastrocnemius b.
    gastrocnemius-semimembranosus b.
    gluteofemoral b.
    gluteus medius b.
    gluteus minimus b.
    greater trochanteric b.
    hyoid b.
    iliac b.
    iliopectineal b.
    iliopsoas b.
    inferior recess of omental b.
    infracardiac b.
    infrahyoid b.
    infrapatellar b.
    infraspinatus b.
    interligamentous b.
    intermediate b.

    intermetatarsal b.
    intermetatarsophalangeal b.
    intermuscular gluteal b.
    interosseous cubital b.
    intraligamentous b.
    intrapatellar b.
    intratendinous olecranon b.
    ischial b.
    ischiogluteal b.
    laryngeal b.
    lateral epicondylar b.
    lateral malleolar subcutaneous b.
    lateral malleolus b.
    Liponyssus b.
    Luschka b.
    medial epicondylar b.
    medial malleolar subcutaneous b.
    Monro b.
    nasopharyngeal b.
    olecranon b.
    omental b.
    Ornithonyssus b.
    ovarian b.
    patellar b.
    pharyngeal b.
    pisiform b.
    plantar b.
    popliteus b.
    pre-Achilles b.
    premalleolar b.
    prepatellar b.
    quadratus femoris b.
    radial b.
    radiohumeral b.
    retro-Achilles b.
    retrocalcaneal b.
    retrohyoid b.
    retromammary b.
    rider's b.
    sacral b.
    sartorius b.
    scapulohumeral b.
    scapulothoracic b.
    semimembranous b.
    subacromial b.
    subacromial-subdeltoid b.
    subcoracoid b.
    subcutaneous acromial b.
    subcutaneous calcaneal b.
    subcutaneous infrapatellar b.
    subcutaneous olecranon b.
    subcutaneous patellar b.
    subcutaneous prepatellar b.
    subcutaneous synovial b.
    subcutaneous trochanteric b.
    subdeltoid b.
    subfascial prepatellar b.
    subhyoid b.
    sublingual b.

subscapular b.
subtendinous b.
superior recess of omental b.
suprapatellar b.
synovial b.
synovial trochlear b.
tibial collateral ligament b.
tibial intertendinous b.
Tornwaldt b.
triceps b.
trochanteric b.
trochlear synovial b.
ulnar b.
Voshell b.
bursitis
septic b.
burst
b. fracture
b. lung
bursting fracture
burst-type laceration
buspirone
busulfan
butterfly
b. bandage
b. fracture
buttock
button
b. battery

belly b.
feeding b.
ligament b.
peyote b.
suture b.
b. suture
buttonhole fracture
butyl toxicity
butyrophenone
buzz
auditory b.
BVM
bag-valve-mask
BVM resuscitator
BW
birth weight
bypass
axillofemoral b.
cardiopulmonary b. (CPB)
direct coronary artery b.
femorofemoral b.
minimally invasive direct coronary
artery b.
off-pump coronary artery b.
portable cardiopulmonary b.
bystander

B

NOTES

C
Celsius

c7E3 Fab Antiplatelet Therapy in Unstable Refractory Angina (CAPTURE)

CA
cancer
carcinoma
CA irritant

CABG
coronary artery bypass graft

cable wire suture

cachectic

cachexia
muscle c.

CAD
coronary artery disease

cadaver
c. allograft
c. bone

cadaveric renal transplant

cadaverous

cadmium exposure

caduceus

café coronary

Cafergot

caffeinated

caffeine
c. abuse
acetylsalicylic acid, phenacetin, c. (APC)
c., alcohol, pepper, spicy food (CAPS)
c. toxicity

CAGE
cerebral arterial gas embolism

CAHD
coronary arteriosclerotic heart disease
coronary atherosclerotic heart disease

Caladium **ingestion**

Calan

calcaneal
c. avulsion fracture
c. bone
c. bursa
c. displaced fracture
c. nerve
c. stress fracture
c. tendon
c. type I–III fracture

calcaneoastragaloid ligament

calcaneoclavicular ligament

calcaneocuboid
c. bone
c. ligament

calcaneofibular ligament

calcaneonavicular ligament

calcaneotibial ligament

calcaneus
c. bone
c. tongue fracture

calcification
epigastric c.

calcinosis, Raynaud syndrome, esophageal dysmotility, scleroderma, and telangiectasia (CREST)

calcitabine

calcitonin

calcitriol

calcium
c. antagonist
c. carbonate
c. channel blocker
c. channel blocker overdose
c. channel blocker poisoning
c. channel blocker toxicity
c. chloride
c. cyclamate
c. disodium versenate
c. docusate
c. edetate sodium
c. entry blocker
c. gluconate
c. hydroxide paste
c. laxative abuse
c. salt therapy

calculation
serial c.

calculus, pl. calculi
renal c.

Caldani ligament

Caldwell protection

calf bone

calibration
balloon flotation catheterization c.

Callipesis laureola ingestion

callosum
corpus c.

callous formation

callus
bone c.
fracture c.

Calori bursa

caloric stimulation

calorimetry
bedside indirect c.

Caltha
C. palustris
C. palustris ingestion

calvarial
    c. fracture
    c. free bone
Calymmatobacterium granulomatis
CAMEO
    Computer-Aided Management of
    Emergency Operations
Cammann stethoscope
Campbell ligament
Camper ligament
camphor
    c. poisoning
    c. toxicity
Campylobacter
canadensis
    Sanguinaria c.
    Taxus c.
Canadian Cardiovascular Society
    Classification (CCSC)
canal
    anal c.
    external auditory c.
Canale-Kelly talar neck fracture
canalicular laceration
canaliculus
    bone c.
    c. rod and suture
cancellated bone
cancellous
    c. cellular bone
    c. versus cortical bone
cancer (CA)
    bone c.
    occupational c.
    skin c.
    suture line c.
Candida
    C. albicans
    C. endophthalmitis
    C. glabrata
    C. guilliermondii
    C. infection
    C. krusei
    C. lusitaniae
    C. pneumonia
    C. tropicalis
candidal endocarditis
candidiasis
    disseminated c.
    esophageal c.
    oral c.
    oropharyngeal c.
    pulmonary c.
    vaginal c.
canker sore
cannabinoid receptor
cannabis user
cannon bone

cannula
    nasal c.
cannulated central vein
cannulation
    central venous c.
    clavicular venous c.
    infraclavicular c.
    internal jugular vein c.
    jugular vein c.
    penile venous c.
    radial artery c.
    supraclavicular c.
canthal
    c. ligament
    c. tendon
canthus, pl. canthi
    lateral c.
    medial c.
CAP
    community-acquired pneumonia
cap
    nerve c.
capability
    rapid infuser with warming
        capabilities
capacious vein
capacity
    forced vital c. (FVC)
    functional residual c. (FRC)
    total iron-binding c. (TIBC)
    total lung c. (TLC)
    vital c. (VC)
CAPD
    chronic ambulatory peritoneal dialysis
capillary
    c. bleeding
    c. fracture
    c. muscle
    c. refill
    c. vein
capillary-cellular gas exchange
capital ligament
capitate
    c. bone
    c. fracture
capitation
capitellar fracture
capitis
    tinea c.
capitolunate ligament
capitonnage suture
capitulum fracture
Capnocheck II CO$_2$/pulse oximeter
Capnocytophaga
capnography
    Microstream c.
capnometer
    sidestream c.

capnometry
　　esophageal c.
capreomycin
Caprolactam suture
CAPS
　　caffeine, alcohol, pepper, spicy food
capsaicin
CAPS-free diet
capsular ligament
capsulatum
　　Histoplasma c.
capsule
　　ammonia c.
　　garlic c.
captopril
CAPTURE
　　c7E3 Fab Antiplatelet Therapy in
　　Unstable Refractory Angina
　　CAPTURE trial
carbacephem
carbamate
　　c. poisoning
　　c. poisoning extraalveolar gas
　　c. toxicity
carbamazepine poisoning
carbamide peroxide
carbapenem antibiotic
carbidopa
carbolic acid
carbon
　　c. dioxide (CO_2)
　　c. dioxide narcosis
　　c. dioxide retention
　　c. dioxide store
　　c. disulfide
　　c. monoxide (CO)
　　c. monoxide poisoning
　　c. monoxide toxicity
　　c. tetrachloride
carbon-11 hydroxyephedrine
carbonaceous sputum
carbonate
　　bone c.
　　calcium c.
　　sodium c.
carbonic anhydrase inhibitor
carboplatin
carboprost methylamine
carboxyhemoglobin
carbuncle
carbuncular fever
carbunculoid growth

carbunculosis
Carcassonne ligament
carcinogenesis
carcinoid
　　c. meningitis
　　c. syndrome
carcinoma (CA)
　　basal cell c.
　　bladder c.
　　bone c.
　　lobular c.
　　c. in situ (CIS)
　　squamous cell c.
　　suture line c.
carcinomatous
　　c. dermatitis
　　c. neuromyopathy
cardiac
　　c. accident
　　c. allograft vasculopathy
　　c. arrest
　　c. arrhythmia
　　c. assist device
　　c. care technician
　　c. care unit (CCU)
　　c. catheter
　　c. catheterization
　　c. chronotropy
　　c. compromise
　　c. conduction system
　　c. contractility
　　c. contusion
　　c. defibrillator
　　c. depressant
　　c. enzyme
　　c. excitability
　　c. failure
　　c. function
　　c. glycoside
　　c. glycoside ingestion
　　c. herniation
　　c. index (CI)
　　c. insufficiency
　　c. intensive care unit (CICU)
　　c. massage
　　c. monitor
　　c. muscle
　　c. output (CO)
　　c. pacemaker
　　c. pacing
　　c. rate
　　c. rehabilitation

NOTES

cardiac *(continued)*
    c. reperfusion therapy
    c. rescue technician
    c. risk factor (CRF)
    c. sensory nerve
    c. tamponade
    c. testing
    c. toxin
    c. transplantation complication
    c. transportation complication
    c. trauma
    c. vein
cardinal
    c. ligament
    c. suture
    c. symptom
    c. vein
Cardioflon suture
cardiogenic
    c. pulmonary edema
    c. shock
cardiography
    thoracic impedance c.
cardiology intensive care unit (CICU)
cardiomegaly
cardiomyopathy
    alcoholic c.
    dilated c.
    hypertrophic c.
    peripartum c.
    restrictive c.
cardiomyoplasty
Cardionyl suture
cardioprotective agent
cardiopulmonary
    c. bypass (CPB)
    c. resuscitation (CPR)
    c. splanchnic nerve
cardiorespiratory resuscitation
cardiothoracic surgery
cardiotoxicity
    Adriamycin c.
cardiovascular (CV)
    c. accident
    c. collapse
    c. examination
    c. Prolene suture
    c. silk suture
    c. surgery (CVS)
    c. system (CVS)
cardiovascular-respiratory (CVR)
cardioversion
    chemical c.
    urgent synchronized c.
cardioverter-defibrillator
    implantable c.-d. (ICD)
    internal c.-d. (ICD)
care
    acute c.

    ambulatory c.
    assumption of c.
    continuity of c.
    critical c.
    custodial c.
    delay in seeking c.
    durable power of attorney for
      health c.
    emergency c.
    extended c.
    fast-track c.
    followup c.
    home health c.
    intensive c. (IC)
    intensive coronary c. (ICC)
    obstetric level of c.
    prehospital c.
    skilled nursing c.
    standard of c.
    supportive c.
    tertiary c.
    wound c.
caregiver
    c. dependency
    statement of c.
    c. stress
caries
    dental c.
carina, pl. **carinae**
    tracheal c.
carinii
    Pneumocystis c.
carisoprodol
carmustine
Carney syndrome
ʟ-carnitine
carnivorous
Carolina jessamine plant ingestion
caroticoclinoid ligament
caroticotympanic nerve
carotid
    c. artery
    c. artery dissection
    c. bruit
    c. endarterectomy
    c. pulse
    c. sinus nerve
    c. sinus pressure (CSP)
    c. vein
carotidynia
carpal
    c. bone fracture
    c. bone stress fracture
    c. ligament
    c. navicular bone
    c. navicular fracture
    c. row bone
    c. scaphoid bone fracture
    c. tunnel syndrome

carpentry
  bone c.
carpometacarpal
  c. joint fracture
  c. ligament
Carrel suture
carrier
  suture c.
  tendon c.
carrot odor
cart
  crash c.
cartilage
  c. bone
  cricoid c.
  intraarticular c.
  tendon c.
cartilaginous loose body
cartwheel fracture
Carvallo sign
car versus pedestrian accident
cascade
  coagulation c.
cascara sagrada
case
  c. history
  postoperative c.
caseous
  c. abscess
  c. necrosis
caspofungin
Casser
  C. ligament
  C. muscle
casserian
  c. ligament
  c. muscle
cast
  below-knee c.
  c. padding
  c. room
  c. saw
castor
  c. bean ingestion
  c. bean toxicity
casualty
  pediatric c.
CAT
  computed axial tomography
  computerized axial tomography

cat
  c. bite
  c. scratch
catabolism
  muscle c.
catamenial pneumothorax
cataract
  immature c.
  snowflake c.
catarrhalis
  Moraxella c.
catastrophe
  vascular c.
catatonia
  stuporous c.
catatonic stupor
catecholamine level
categorization
caterpillar
  c. envenomation
  venomous c.
catfish
  c. envenomation
  c. poisoning
catgut suture
catharsis
  emotional c.
cathartic
  saline sulfate c.
  c. therapy
catheter
  Angiocath c.
  arterial c.
  cardiac c.
  central venous c. (CVC)
  central venous pressure c.
  c. colonization
  coudé c.
  Epistat nasal c.
  Epistat II nasal c.
  flexible plastic c.
  flexible plastic suction c.
  Fogarty vascular c.
  Foley c.
  French c.
  Heimlich c.
  Introcan Safety IV c.
  large-bore suction c.
  Melker cuffed emergency
    cricothyrotomy c.
  PA c.

NOTES

catheter *(continued)*
    peripherally inserted central c.
     (PICC)
    peripherally inserted central
     venous c.
    c. port
    pulmonary artery c.
    c. replacement
    right ventricular ejection fraction c.
    rigid suction c.
    soft c.
    suprapubic c.
    Swan-Ganz c.
    tonsil-tip c.
    tunneled c.
    venous c.
    Vietnam c.
    whistle-tip c.
    Word c.
    Yankauer tonsil-tip suction c.
catheter-associated urinary tract infection (CAUTI)
catheter-induced venous thrombosis
catheterization
    cardiac c.
    percutaneous internal jugular
     vein c.
catheter-related septicemia
cationic detergent
cat's claw
cat-scratch
    c.-s. disease (CSD)
    c.-s. fever
Caucasian
    C. female
    C. male
cauda
    c. equina compression
    c. equina syndrome
caudad to cranial
caudal
    c. block
    c. direction
    c. ligament
caudalward
caudate
    c. lobe
    c. vein
causation
    legal c.
causative stress
cause
    c. of death (COD)
    definitive c.
    iatrogenic c.
    metabolic c.
    pathologic c.
    underlying c.

caustic
    c. agent
    c. alkali
    c. burn
    c. ingestion
    c. injury
    c. lesion
    c. substance
cauterization
    Bovie c.
CAUTI
    catheter-associated urinary tract infection
cava
    inferior vena c. (IVC)
caval interruption
cavalry bone
Caverject
cavernosal nerve
cavernous
    c. nerve
    c. sinus
    c. sinus fistula
    c. sinus thrombosis
    c. vein
CAVH
    continuous arteriovenous hemofiltration
CAVHD
    continuous arteriovenous hemodialysis
cavity
    abdominal c.
    abdominopelvic c.
    ventral c.
    wound c.
CBC
    complete blood count
CBF
    cerebral blood flow
CC
    chief complaint
    clinical course
    current complaint
C-collar
    cervical collar
CCS
    central cord syndrome
CCSC
    Canadian Cardiovascular Society Classification
CCU
    cardiac care unit
    coronary care unit
    critical care unit
CDC
    Centers for Disease Control and Prevention
CDU
    chemical dependency unit
cecal volvulus
cecum, pl. **ceca**

Cedell fracture
cefazolin
cefepime
cefixime
Cefobid
cefoperazone
cefotaxime
cefotetan
cefoxitin
cefpodoxime
ceftazidime
ceftizoxime
ceftriaxone
cefuroxime
celiac
    c. axis
    c. axis injury
    c. nerve
celiotomy
cell
    alveolar effector c.
    antigen presenting c. (APC)
    bone c.
    bone marrow c.
    bone marrow-derived B c.
    bone marrow-derived cultured
      mast c.
    bone marrow-derived stromal c.
    bone marrow stem c.
    bone marrow stromal c.
    clue c.
    epidermic c.
    nerve c.
    packed red blood c. (PRBC)
    red blood c. (RBC)
    tendon c.
    white blood c. (WBC)
cell-mediated immunity
cellularity
    bone marrow c.
cellulite
cellulitis
    cutaneous c.
    external ear c.
    orbital c.
    pelvic c.
    periorbital c.
    preseptal orbital c.
    synergistic necrotizing c.
celluloid linen suture
Celsius (C)
    C. thermometer

cement
    bone c.
    c. ingestion
cemental ligament
cementum fracture
center
    adult trauma c.
    ambulatory care c. (ACC)
    American Association of Poison
      Control C.'s (AAPCC)
    birthing c.
    bone c.
    Chemical Transportation
      Emergency C. (CHEMTREC)
    crisis resolution c. (CRC)
    C.'s for Disease Control and
      Prevention (CDC)
    level I trauma c.
    nerve c.
    pediatric trauma c.
    poison control c. (PCC)
    regional poison control c.
    specialty referral c.
    trauma c.
centigrade thermometer
centipede envenomation
central
    c. access
    c. anticholinergic effect
    c. bone
    c. cerebral herniation
    c. cord syndrome (CCS)
    c. fracture
    c. hepatic gunshot wound
    c. herniation syndrome
    c. line
    c. nervous system (CNS)
    c. nervous system intoxication
    c. nervous system tumor
    c. neurogenic hyperventilation
    c. perineal tendon
    c. pontine myelinolysis
    c. pulse
    c. reflex hyperpnea
    c. retroperitoneal hematoma
    c. slip
    c. stellate laceration
    c. tendon
    c. vein
    c. venous cannulation
    c. venous catheter (CVC)
    c. venous pressure (CVP)

C

NOTES

central *(continued)*
    c. venous pressure catheter
    c. vertigo
centralization
    tendon c.
centrally acting agent toxicity
centration
centrifugal nerve
centrilobar emphysema
centripetal nerve
cepacia
    Burkholderia c.
cephalad direction
cephalexin
cephalgia
    histamine c.
cephalic
    c. pole
    c. vein
cephalomedullary nail fracture
cephalosporin antibiotic
cephalothin
cephazolin
ceramic glaze toxicity
ceratocricoid
    c. ligament
    c. muscle
ceratopharyngeal muscle
cerebellar
    c. abscess
    c. hemorrhage
    c. herniation
    c. infarct
    c. sign
    c. tumor
    c. vein
cerebellotonsillar herniation
cerebellum
    posterior lobe of c.
cerebral
    c. aneurysm
    c. angiography
    c. arterial gas embolism (CAGE)
    c. blood flow (CBF)
    c. blood volume
    c. compression
    c. concussion
    c. contusion
    c. cytotoxic edema
    c. death
    c. edema
    c. hematoma
    c. hemorrhage
    c. hyperperfusion syndrome
    c. hypoxia
    c. injury
    c. ischemia
    c. laceration
    c. malaria

    c. metabolism
    c. nerve
    c. palsy pathological fracture
    c. perfusion pressure (CPP)
    c. reperfusion
    c. reperfusion therapy
    c. resuscitation
    c. salt-wasting
    c. vascular accident
    c. vascular lesion
    c. vasculitis
    c. vasogenic edema
    c. vasospasm
    c. vein
    c. vomiting
cerebri
    gliomatosis c.
    pseudotumor c.
cerebritis
cerebro-oculo-facio-skeletal syndrome
cerebroprotection
cerebrospinal
    c. fluid (CSF)
    c. fluid analysis
    c. fluid shunt
cerebrovascular
    c. accident (CVA)
    c. disorder
cerium oxalate
certified
    board c.
cerumen
    c. impaction
    inspissated c.
cervical
    c. adenitis
    c. collar (C-collar)
    c. cord injury
    c. flexor muscle
    c. fracture
    c. iliocostal muscle
    c. immobilization device (CID)
    c. infection
    c. interspinal muscle
    c. laceration
    c. ligament
    c. motion tenderness
    c. rotator muscle
    c. sensory nerve
    c. spine
    c. spine immobilization
    c. spine injury
    c. spine protection
    c. spine stabilization
    c. splanchnic nerve
    c. strain
    c. subcutaneous emphysema
    c. suture
    c. sympathetic nerve

c. trochanteric displaced fracture
c. vascular organ injury
c. vein
c. vertebral bone
cervices (*pl. of* cervix)
cervicitis
chlamydial c.
gonococcal c.
cervicoocular reflex
cervicotrochanteric displaced fracture
cervix, pl. **cervices**
incompetent c.
strawberry c.
cesarean section
cestode
intestinal c.
Cetacaine spray
CFI
closed-fist injury
chaffeensis
Ehrlichia c.
Chagas disease
chain
lymphatic c.
c. of survival
c. suture
chair
combination stretcher c.
Sirocco evacuation c.
stair c.
chalazion
hordeolum and c.
chalk-stick fracture
chalk toxicity
chalky bone
challenge
fluid c.
chamber
bone growth c.
c. decompression
hyperbaric c.
Champion trauma score
Chance vertebral fracture
chancroid ulcer
chandelier sign
change
associated orthostatic c.
c. in bladder function
c. in bowel function
c. in bowel habit
c. in level of consciousness
c. in mental status

orthostatic blood pressure c.
ventilator circuit c.
visual c.
channel
amiloride-sensitive sodium c. (aEnaC)
chaotic atrial tachycardia
chaparral ingestion
Chaput fracture
characteristic
endpoint c.
historical c.
c. symptom
charcoal
Actidose activated c.
activated c.
c. hemoperfusion
InstaChar activated c.
LiquiChar activated c.
multiple-dose activated c. (MDAC)
SuperChar activated c.
Charcot fracture
chart
flow c.
Chassaignac muscle
chauffeur's fracture
check ligament
checkrein ligament
cheek
c. bone
c. muscle
cheesewiring of suture
cheesy
c. abscess
c. pus
cheilorrhaphy
chelating agent
chelation therapy
chemical
c. abuse
c. acne
c. antidote
c. asphyxiant
c. burn
c. cardioversion
c. decontamination
c. dependency unit (CDU)
c. detection equipment
c. formula
C. Transportation Emergency Center (CHEMTREC)
c. warfare agent

NOTES

chemical *(continued)*
    c. warfare mass casualty management
    c. weapon poisoning
chemistry
    clinical c.
    histological c.
chemoprophylaxis
chemotaxis
    negative c.
chemotherapy (CTx)
    c. toxicity
CHEMTREC
    Chemical Transportation Emergency Center
CHEPER
    Chest Pain Evaluation Registry
    CHEPER study
cherry
    c. kernel ingestion
    c. red lip
    c. red spot
chest
    barrel c.
    c. blast
    c. compression
    emphysematous c.
    c. excursion
    fissured c.
    flail c.
    c. heaviness
    hourglass c.
    c. pain
    C. Pain Evaluation Registry (CHEPER)
    c. pain observation unit (CPOU)
    c. physical therapy
    presence of flail c.
    c. PT
    rachitic c.
    c. radiograph
    c. radiography
    stove-in c.
    c. thrust
    c. tightness
    c. trauma
    c. tube insertion
    c. tube thoracostomy
    c. wall (CW)
    c. wall injury
    c. wall mechanics
    c. wound
    c. x-ray (CXR)
chevron
    c. bone
    c. fracture
    c. laceration
Cheyne-Stokes respiration

CHF
    congestive heart failure
CHI
    closed head injury
chickenpox
chief complaint (CC)
chilblain lupus erythematosus
child
    c. abuse
    C. cirrhosis classification
    c. maltreatment
    c. restraint seat
    c. sexual abuse
childbearing age
childhood fracture
children with special health care needs (CSHCN)
chill
    fevers and c.'s (F/C)
chin
    c. lift
    c. muscle
Chinese
    C. fingertrap suture
    C. herb nephropathy
    C. restaurant syndrome
    C. twisted silk suture
chin-lift maneuver
chip
    bone c.
    c. fracture
chiropractic
    c. treatment
    c. treatment of fracture
Chiropsalmus quadrumanus
chisel
    fracture c.
    c. fracture
Chlamydia
    C. pneumoniae
    C. trachomatis
    C. trachomatis infection
chlamydial
    c. cervicitis
    c. urethritis
chloracne grading system
chloral hydrate toxicity
chloramine catgut suture
chloramphenicol
chlordane
chlordiazepoxide
chlorhexidine
    c. gluconate
    c. toxicity
chloride
    Adrenalin C.
    calcium c.
    potassium c. (KOH)

pralidoxime c.
sodium c.
chloride-resistant alkalosis
chloride-wasting nephropathy
chlorine
c. gas
organ c.
chloroacetophenone (CN)
c., carbon tetrachloride, benzene (CNB)
c. in chloroform (CNC)
chlorocresol toxicity
chloroform
chloroacetophenone in c. (CNC)
chlorohydrate poisoning
chloroma
bone c.
chlorophenoxy herbicide poisoning
chlorophyll
chloropicrin
chloroquine
chlorothiazide
chlorpromazine
chlorpropamide
choanal atresia
choice
embarrassment of c.
study of c.
chokecherry kernel ingestion
cholangiopancreatography
endoscopic retrograde c. (ERCP)
cholangitis
ascending c.
bacterial c.
cholecalciferol
cholecystitis
acalculous c.
acute c.
chronic c.
emphysematous c.
evidence of c.
cholecystoduodenal ligament
cholecystography
choledocholithiasis
cholelithiasis
cholerae
Vibrio c.
cholesterol
c. elevation
c. embolism
cholesterolemia

cholinergic
c. agent
c. agonist
c. crisis
c. toxicity
cholinesterase chemical warfare agent
chondral fracture
chondritis
external ear c.
chondroid bone
chondropharyngeal muscle
chondroxiphoid ligament
Chopart
C. amputation
C. fracture
chorda tympani nerve
chorea
Huntington c.
choreic movement
choriomeningitis
lymphocytic c.
choroiditis
macular c.
choroid vein
Christmas tree pattern
chromated catgut suture
chromatography
high-performance liquid c.
liquid c.
chromic
c. blue dyed suture
c. catgut suture
c. collagen suture
c. gut suture
chromicized catgut suture
chromium picolinate abuse
chromogranin A
chronic
c. abscess
c. alcoholic
c. ambulatory peritoneal dialysis (CAPD)
c. anemia
c. bronchitis
c. caloric deficiency
c. cholecystitis
c. constipation
c. dacryocystitis
c. disease anemia
c. esophagitis
c. intoxication
c. lung disease (CLD)

NOTES

chronic *(continued)*
    c. lymphocytic leukemia
    c. malaria
    c. mastoiditis
    c. mountain sickness
    c. obstructive airways disease (COAD)
    c. obstructive pulmonary disease (COPD)
    c. pancreatitis
    c. pyelonephritis
    c. renal failure
    c. salicylate poisoning
    c. schizophrenia
    c. sinusitis
    c. ulcerative colitis
    c. urticaria
chronically elevated hypertension
chronicus
    lichen simplex c.
chronological age
chronotropic incompetence
chronotropy
    cardiac c.
Chrysaora quinquecirrha
Churg-Strauss syndrome
Chvostek sign
chylothorax
chylous
    c. ascites
    c. collection
chymotrypsin
CI
    cardiac index
cicatricial mass
cicatrix, pl. **cicatrices**
cicatrization stage
CICU
    cardiac intensive care unit
    cardiology intensive care unit
    coronary intensive care unit
Cicuta
    C. ingestion
    C. species
CID
    cervical immobilization device
cidofovir
cigarette toxicity
ciglitazone
ciguatera poisoning
ciguatoxin
cilastatin
ciliary
    c. ligament
    c. muscle
    c. nerve
    c. vein
cilioretinal vein
cimetidine

cinchonism
cinch suture
Cipro
ciprofloxacin
circinate balanitis
circular
    c. ciliary muscle
    c. dental ligament
    c. pharyngeal muscle
    c. suture
circulation
    airway, breathing, c. (ABC)
    fetal to neonatal c.
    c. management
    persistent fetal c. (PFC)
    return of spontaneous c. (ROSC)
circumcision
circumcisional suture
circumference
    abdominal c.
circumferential fracture
circumflex
    c. artery
    c. nerve
    c. vein
circumoral cyanosis
circumscribed infiltrate
circumstantiality
cirrhosis
    Laennec c.
    multilobular c.
    pipe stem c.
cirrhotic liver
CIS
    carcinoma in situ
cisapride
cisatracurium besylate
CISD
    critical incident stress debriefing
CISM
    critical incident stress management
    CISM program
cisplatin
citrate
    magnesium c.
    c. phosphate dextrose adenine
    c. toxicity
citric acid
Civinini ligament
CK-MB
    creatine kinase-myocardial band
Clado ligament
clammy skin
clamp
    antishock pelvic c.
    Kelly c.
    suture c.
clamping of umbilical cord
clamshell thoracotomy

clarithromycin
class
    C. IA, IB, IC antiarrhythmic agent
    C. II, IV, V antiarrhythmic agent
classic reflex sympathetic dystrophy (CRSD)
classification
    Ashhurst-Bromer ankle fracture c.
    Braunwald unstable angina c.
    Canadian Cardiovascular Society C. (CCSC)
    Child cirrhosis c.
    Danis-Weber malleolar fracture c.
    Denis Browne spinal fracture c.
    Denis spinal fracture c.
    Ellis tooth fracture c.
    Fielding-Magliato subtrochanteric fracture c.
    fracture c.
    Frykman hand fracture c.
    Gartland humeral supracondylar fracture c.
    Grantham femoral fracture c.
    Gustilo c.
    Hansen fracture c.
    Hawkins talar fracture c.
    Herbert scaphoid fracture c.
    Ingram-Bachynski hip fracture c.
    Jeffery radial fracture c.
    Jones diaphysial fracture c.
    Key-Conwell pelvic fracture c.
    Kilfoyle humeral medial condylar fracture c.
    Knight and North malar fracture c.
    LaGrange humeral supracondylar fracture c.
    Lauge-Hansen ankle fracture c.
    Mallampati sign and c.
    Mathews olecranon fracture c.
    Meyers-McKeever tibial fracture c.
    Milch humeral fracture c.
    Neer-Horowitz humeral fracture c.
    Newman radial neck and head fracture c.
    O'Brien radial fracture c.
    Ogden epiphysial fracture c.
    Ovadia-Beals tibial plafond fracture c.
    Palmer trapezial ridge fracture c.
    Papavasiliou olecranon fracture c.
    Pipkin femoral fracture c.
    Poland epiphysial fracture c.
    Quinby pelvic fracture c.
    Riseborough-Radin intercondylar fracture c.
    Rockwood c.
    Russe scaphoid fracture c.
    Sakellarides calcaneal fracture c.
    Salter-Harris epiphysial fracture c.
    Seinsheimer femoral fracture c.
    Sorbie calcaneal fracture c.
    Steele intraarticular fracture type I-III c.
    Thompson-Epstein femoral fracture c.
    Tronzo intertrochanteric fracture c.
    Vostal radial fracture c.
    Watson-Jones tibial tubercle avulsion fracture c.
    Wilkins radial fracture c.
    Winquist-Hansen femoral fracture c.
claudication
    intermittent c.
clavicle
    c. bone
    c. fracture
    c. shaft fracture
clavicular
    c. dislocation
    c. fracture
    c. venous cannulation
clavulanate
clavulanic acid
claw
    cat's c.
clay shoveler's fracture
CLD
    chronic lung disease
cleaner
    drain c.
cleanser
    wound c.
cleansing
    wound c.
clearance
    antigen c.
    creatine c.
cleavage fracture
Cleland ligament
clenbuterol abuse
click
    auditory c.
clindamycin

NOTES

clinical
- c. chemistry
- c. correlation
- c. course (CC)
- c. diagnosis
- c. neurology
- c. support tool (CST)
- c. toxicity

clinically sober

clinoid ligament

clip
- wound c.

cloacae
- *Enterobacter c.*

clonazepam

clonidine

clopidogrel

Cloquet ligament

clorgyline

closed
- c. ankle fracture
- c. break fracture
- c. chest compression
- c. fracture
- c. head injury (CHI)
- c. head trauma
- c. indirect fracture
- c. reduction
- c. reduction of fracture
- c. skull fracture
- c. wound

closed-fist injury (CFI)

close followup

clostridial myonecrosis

Clostridium
- *C. botulinum*
- *C. difficile*
- *C. perfringens*
- *C. tetani*

closure
- abdominal c.
- delayed c.
- layered c.
- premature c.
- primary c.
- secondary c.
- single-layer c.
- suture c.
- suture Strip Plus wound c.
- wound c.

clot
- passage of c.

clothesline injury

clothing drag technique

clotrimazole troche

clotting
- c. factor
- c. time

clouding of consciousness

cloud-to-ground lightning

clove-hitch suture

clozapine toxicity

clue
- c. cell
- historical c.

cluneal nerve

clupeotoxin fish poisoning

cluster headache

CMO
- comfort measures only

CMV
- conventional mechanical ventilation
- cytomegalovirus

CN
- chloroacetophenone
- cranial nerve
  - CN irritant

CNB
- chloroacetophenone, carbon tetrachloride, benzene
  - CNB irritant

CNC
- chloroacetophenone in chloroform
  - CNC irritant

CNS
- central nervous system

CO
- carbon monoxide
- cardiac output

CO$_2$
- carbon dioxide

COAD
- chronic obstructive airways disease

coagulant

coagulase-negative staphylococcus

coagulation
- c. cascade
- c. disorder
- disseminated intravascular c. (DIC)
- c. profile
- c. study
- zone of c.

coagulopathy
- consumption c.
- consumptive c.
- dilutional c.
- disseminated intravascular c. (DIC)

coal
- c. gas odor
- c. tar burn
- c. tar toxicity

coalesce

coalition of bone

coapt

coaptation
- nerve c.

coarctate

coarctation
  c. of aorta
  aortic c.
coarse
  c. crackle
  c. rhonchi
coated
  c. polyester suture
  c. Vicryl Rapide suture
cobblestone mucosa
cobra bite
cobweb pattern
cocaine
  c. poisoning
  tetracaine, adrenaline, c. (TAC)
  c. toxicity
cocaine-induced
  c.-i. myocardial infarction
  c.-i. seizure
cocci (*pl. of* coccus)
Coccidia
Coccidioides immitis
coccidioidomycosis
  bone c.
coccus, pl. **cocci**
  gram-positive cocci
  multiresistant gram-positive cocci
coccygeal
  c. bone
  c. fracture
  c. injury
  c. ligament
  c. muscle
  c. nerve
coccyx, pl. **coccyges**
  c. bone
  c. fracture
  c. spine injury
cochlear
  c. nerve
  c. vein
cochleovestibular nerve
Cockett communicating perforating vein
cocktail
  coma c.
  GI c.
cocoon thread suture
COD
  cause of death

codeine
  aspirin, phenacetin, caffeine with c. (APC-C)
  c. phosphate
coding
  diagnosis-related group c.
coefficient
  bone attenuation c.
coelenterate
  c. envenomation
  c. poisoning
Coe-Pak dressing
coexistent illness
coffee-bean sign
coffee enema
coffee-grounds
  c.-g. emesis
  c.-g. vomit
coffin bone
cognitive function
cognizant
coherent stream of thinking
cohosh plant ingestion
coin
  fracture en c.
  c. rubbing
Coiter muscle
Colchicum autumnale
cold
  c. agglutinin disease
  c. exposure
  c. pack
  c. zone
colectomy
coli
  Escherichia c.
colic
  biliary c.
  c. vein
colicky pain
colitis
  chronic ulcerative c.
  infectious c.
  ischemic c.
  mucous c.
  neutropenic c.
  parasitic c.
  radiation c.
  ulcerative c.
collagen
  c. absorbable suture

C

NOTES

65

collagen (continued)
    c. hemostatic material for wounds
    c. vascular disease
collapse
    bone graft c.
    cardiovascular c.
    hemodynamic c.
    lobar c.
    vasovagal c.
collar
    abrasion c.
    c. bone
    cervical c. (C-collar)
    hard cervical c.
    Philadelphia c.
    Philly Bloc-Head cervical c.
    Philly one-piece cervical c.
    soft cervical c.
    StediSpine c.
    tracheostomy c.
collarbone
collateral
    c. ligament
    c. vein
collecting
    c. duct
    c. vein
collection
    chylous c.
collector
    bone c.
    wound drainage c.
Colles
    C. fracture
    C. ligament
collicular fracture
collision
    traffic c. (TC)
colloid fluid therapy
cologne ingestion
colon
    ascending c.
    descending c.
    perforated c.
    pseudoobstruction of c.
    sigmoid c.
    transverse c.
    c. trauma
colonic
    c. bleeding
    c. circular muscle
    c. pseudoobstruction
colonization
    catheter c.
colonoscopy
    surveillance c.
colony-stimulating factor (CSF)
color
    urine c.

Coltart fracture
column
    spinal c.
3-column spinal stability theory
coma
    c. aberration
    c. cocktail
    diabetic c.
    hyperosmolar hyperglycemic
      nonketotic c.
    hypoglycemic c.
    Kussmaul c.
    myxedema c.
    nonketotic hyperosmolar c.
    pontine c.
    c. position
    Reed classification of c.
    c. scale
    subarachnoid c.
comatose patient
combative behavior
combativeness score
Combiguard II irrigation splash guard
combination
    c. headache
    c. stretcher chair
combined
    c. flexion-distraction injury and
      burst fracture
    c. fracture
    c. radial-ulnar-humeral fracture
Combitube
    C. airway device
    esophageal tracheal C. (ETC)
Combivent inhalation aerosol
combustion
    spontaneous c.
comfort
    c. measures only (CMO)
    c. zone
comfrey
coming
    death is c. (DIC)
comitant strabismus
commensurate
comminuted
    c. bursting fracture
    c. fracture
    c. intraarticular fracture
    c. orbital fracture
    c. skull fracture
    c. teardrop fracture
commission
    Consumer Product Safety C.
commitment
    psychiatric c.
common
    c. anterior facial vein
    c. anular tendon

c. basal vein
c. cardinal vein
c. digital nerve
c. extensor tendon
c. femoral vein
c. fibular nerve
c. iliac vein
c. modiolar vein
c. palmar digital nerve
c. peroneal nerve
c. plantar digital nerve

communicable disease
communicating vein
communis
Ricinus c.
c. tendon
community-acquired pneumonia (CAP)
community hospital
compact bone
companion vein
comparable worth
compartmental perfusion pressure
2-compartment model
compartment syndrome
compensatory
c. antiinflammatory response
syndrome
c. atrophy
c. renal metabolic alkalosis
competent elder patient
complaint
chief c. (CC)
current c. (CC)
plethora of c.'s
somatic c.
complete
c. abortion
c. airway obstruction
c. blood count (CBC)
c. disruption
c. fracture
c. hepatic failure
complex
c. access
AIDS dementia c.
anisoylated plasminogen
streptokinase activator c. (APSAC)
c. disaster
c. fracture
c. laceration
*Mycobacterium avium-
intracellulare* c. (MAC)

c. regional pain syndrome type 1
(CRPS-1)
c. simple fracture
compliance
left ventricular c.
pulmonary c.
complicated
c. fracture
c. labor
complication
cardiac transplantation c.
cardiac transportation c.
dialysis c.
Evaluation of 7E3 for the
Prevention of Ischemic C.'s
(EPIC)
feeding tube c.
infectious c.
mechanical c.
periesophageal c.
preeclampsia c.
transfusion c.
wound c.
composite fracture
compound
acyclic c.
ammonia c.
c. comminuted fracture
c. complex fracture
c. fracture
c. multiple fractures
c. skull fracture
c. suture
compressed fracture
compression
acute spinal cord c.
aortocaval c.
cauda equina c.
cerebral c.
chest c.
closed chest c.
c. dressing
external chest c.
c. fracture
intermittent pneumatic c. (IPC)
nerve c.
nerve root c.
c. stocking
c. suture
c. therapy
vein c.
compression-relaxation cycle

NOTES

compressor muscle
compromise
    airway c.
    cardiac c.
    maternal-fetal c.
    neurovascular c.
    neutropenia/immune c.
compromised host
computed
    c. axial tomography (CAT)
    c. tomographic scan
    c. tomography (CT)
computer
    sequential multiple analyzer plus c.
    (SMAC)
Computer-Aided Management of
  Emergency Operations (CAMEO)
computerized axial tomography (CAT)
conal papillary muscle
conation
concave temporalis muscle
concentrate
    factor VIII c.
concentration
    mean corpuscular hemoglobin c.
    (MCHC)
    minimum inhibitory c. (MIC)
    peak plasma c.
    plasma bicarbonate c.
    serum ethanol c.
    therapeutic plasma c.
concept
    golden hour c.
conception
    products of c. (POC)
concerned party
concomitant
    c. condition
    c. disease
    c. hemothorax
    c. medical problem
    c. symptom
concomitantly
concurrent
    c. alcohol withdrawal
    c. hepatic laceration
    c. osmolal gap
concussion
    brain c.
    cerebral c.
    myocardial c.
    spinal cord c.
condensation
    tube c.
condition
    abusive home c.
    concomitant c.
    grave c.

    life-threatening c.
    neglect home c.
conduction
    c. abnormality
    bone c.
    heat loss by c.
    nerve c.
conductive heat loss
condylar
    c. compression fracture
    c. emissary vein
    c. fracture
    c. process fracture
    c. split fracture
condyle bone
condyloma, pl. condylomata
    c. acuminata
    c. lata
cone shell poisoning
confidentiality
    patient c.
confined-space medicine
conflict
    armed c.
    c. of interest
confluence
    vein c.
Conform dressing
confusion
    mental c.
congenerous muscle
congenital
    c. adrenal hyperplasia
    c. disease
    c. fracture
    c. heart disease
    c. hypothyroidism
    c. myxedema
congestive heart failure (CHF)
congruence angle
congruent
    c. affect
    c. point
congruous hemianopia
conical cornea
coniotomy
Conium poisoning
conjoined tendon
conjugate
    c. gaze
    c. ligament
conjunctiva
    bulbar c.
conjunctival
    c. laceration
    c. vein
conjunctivitis
    allergic c.
    pinkeye c.

connective tissue disorder
Connell suture
conniventes
  valvulae c.
conoid ligament
Conrad-Bugg
  C.-B. trapping
  C.-B. trapping of soft tissue in
    ankle fracture
consanguinity
consciousness
  change in level of c.
  clouding of c.
  diminished c.
  level of c.
  loss of c. (LOC)
conscious sedation
consecutive symptom
consent
  age of c.
  expressed c.
  implied c.
  written c.
consequence
  dire c.
  hemodynamic c.
conservative
  c. medication
  c. surgery
  c. therapy
  c. treatment
consideration
  pediatric c.
consistency
  doughy c.
consolidation
  bone c.
  fracture line c.
constant abdominal wall pain
constellation of symptoms
constipated
constipation
  chronic c.
  c. prevention
constitutional symptom
constricted pupil
constricting band removal
constriction
  airway c.
constrictive pericarditis
constrictor pharyngeal muscle

consultant
  neurosurgical c.
  orthopaedic c.
consultation
  emergent surgical c.
  gynecologic c.
  neurosurgical c.
  orthopaedic c.
Consumer Product Safety Commission
consumption
  c. coagulopathy
  oxygen c.
consumptive coagulopathy
contact
  c. allergy
  c. dermatitis
  direct c.
  indirect c.
  c. rewarming
contagiosum
  molluscum c.
contagious
  c. disease
  not c.
contained hematoma
container failure shock
contamination from bowel contents
content
  aspiration of gastric c.'s
  bone mineral c.
  contamination from bowel c.'s
  gastric c.'s
contiguity
  appendicitis by c.
continuity of care
continuous
  c. arteriovenous hemodiafiltration
  c. arteriovenous hemodialysis
    (CAVHD)
  c. arteriovenous hemofiltration
    (CAVH)
  c. cardiac output
  c. hemodiafiltration
  c. over-and-over suture
  c. pain
  c. positive airway pressure (CPAP)
  c. renal replacement therapy
  c. running monofilament suture
  c. sling suture
  c. venovenous hemodiafiltration
    (CVVHD, CVVHDF)

NOTES

continuous (*continued*)
    c. venovenous hemodialysis
    c. venovenous hemofiltration
continuum
    critical care c.
contraception
    postcoital c.
contraceptive
    Depo-Provera injectable c.
    oral c.
contracted muscle
contractile reserve
contractility
    cardiac c.
    muscle c.
    c. of muscle
contraction
    atrial c.
    Braxton-Hicks c.
    eccentric c.
    junctional c.
    muscle c.
    premature atrial c. (PAC)
    premature junctional c. (PJC)
    premature ventricular c. (PVC)
    pressure generated by muscle c.
      (Pmus)
    wound c.
    wound matrix c.
contracture
    c. of interosseous muscle
    muscle c.
contractured muscle
contrafissura
contraindication
    relative c.
contrast
    c. effect
    c. esophagram
    intravenous c.
contrast-induced renal failure
contrecoup
    fracture by c.
    c. fracture
contributory cause of death
control
    bleeding c.
    c. bleeding
    direct medical c.
    flow c.
    lack of pain c.
    parasympathetic c.
    pressure c.
    tidal volume c.
controlled comminuted fracture
controlling behavior
controversial management
contused wound

contusion
    bone c.
    brain c.
    cardiac c.
    cerebral c.
    muscle c.
    myocardial c.
    pulmonary c.
    scalp c.
    temporal c.
contusion-laceration
conus
    c. ligament
    c. medullaris syndrome
convalescence
convalescent course
Convallaria majalis **ingestion**
convection
    heat loss by c.
convective heat loss
conventional
    c. mechanical ventilation (CMV)
    c. tomography
conversion
    c. disorder
    c. reaction
convexity
    cortical c.
convoluted bone
convulsion
    benign idiopathic neonatal c.
      (BINC)
Cook peel-away sheath
Cooley U suture
cooling
    c. measure
    nerve c.
cool skin
cooperation
    muscle c.
Cooper ligament
coordinated body movement
coordination
    hand-breath c.
co-oximetry
COPD
    chronic obstructive pulmonary disease
copper
coprine mushroom poisoning
coracoacromial ligament
coracobrachial
    c. bursa
    c. muscle
coracobrachialis muscle
coracoclavicular
    c. ligament
    c. ligament rupture
coracohumeral ligament

coracoid
    c. bursa
    c. fracture
coral
    c. poisoning
    c. snake
    c. snake envenomation
cord
    clamping of umbilical c.
    c. hemisection syndrome
    nuchal c.
    prolapsed umbilical c.
    umbilical c.
Cordarone
core
    c. body temperature
    bone c.
    c. region
    c. rewarming
    c. suture
    c. temperature after drop
cornea
    conical c.
corneal
    c. abrasion
    c. burn
    c. foreign body
    c. laceration
    c. nerve
    c. reflex
    c. rust stain
    c. ulceration
Cornelia de Lange syndrome
corneoscleral
    c. laceration
    c. suture
corner
    c. fracture
    c. suture
3-cornered bone
corniculopharyngeal ligament
corn lily ingestion
coronal
    c. split fracture
    c. suture
coronary
    c. angiography
    c. arteriosclerotic heart disease (CAHD)
    c. artery bypass graft (CABG)
    c. artery disease (CAD)
    c. artery vasospasm

    c. atherosclerotic heart disease (CAHD)
    c. bone
    café c.
    c. care unit (CCU)
    c. heart disease
    c. intensive care unit (CICU)
    c. ligament
    c. tendon
    c. vein
coroner
coronoid
    c. fracture
    c. process fracture
corpora (*pl. of* corpus)
corporeal
corporis
    tinea c.
corpse
cor pulmonale
corpus, pl. **corpora**
    c. callosum
corpuscle
    bone c.
    tendon c.
corpuscular volume
correct tube placement
correlation
    clinical c.
Corrigan sign
corrosive
    c. agent
    c. injury
    c. poison
corrugator muscle
cortex, pl. **cortices**
    bone c.
cortical
    c. blindness
    c. bone
    c. convexity
    c. fracture
    c. scarring
    c. vein
corticocancellous bone
corticospinal tract injury
corticosteroid injection
corticotropin deficiency
cortisol excretion
cortisol-releasing factor (CRF)
Corynebacterium jeikeium

C

NOTES

coryza
    allergic c.
costal
    c. bone
    c. margin
costoaxillary vein
costochondritis
costoclavicular ligament
costocolic ligament
costotransverse ligament
costovertebral
    c. angle (CVA)
    c. angle tenderness (CVAT)
    c. junction rupture
    c. ligament
costoxiphoid ligament
co-trimoxazole
cotton
    C. ankle fracture
    c. Deknatel suture
    c. fever
    c. nonabsorbable suture
    c. suture
cottonmouth
    c. bite
    c. water moccasin
cotton-tip applicator
cottony Dacron suture
Cotunnius
    nerve of C.
    C. nerve
cotyloid ligament
coudé catheter
cough fracture
coughing
    assisted c.
    pain exacerbated by movement
       and c.
Coumadin
coumarin necrosis
count
    absolute lymphocytic c. (ALC)
    bone marrow differential c.
    complete blood c. (CBC)
    platelet c.
    posttetanic c.
    red blood c. (RBC)
    white blood cell c.
    white cell c. (WCC)
counter
    Geiger-Müller c.
counterirritant
counterpulsation
    balloon c.
    intraaortic balloon pump c.
counterweight
coupling
    excitation-contraction c.

course
    clinical c. (CC)
    convalescent c.
    downhill c.
    hospital c.
    ICU c.
    treatment c.
coursing of gas
coved T wave
covering
    wound c.
cowl muscle
Cowper
    C. gland
    C. ligament
cowslip ingestion
COX-2
    cyclooxygenase-2
    COX-2 inhibitor
coxal bone
Coxiella burnetii
Coxsackie stomatitis
coxsackievirus
CPAP
    continuous positive airway pressure
    CPAP kit
CPB
    cardiopulmonary bypass
CPEM
    The Center for Pediatric Emergency
    Medicine
CPOU
    chest pain observation unit
CPP
    cerebral perfusion pressure
CPR
    cardiopulmonary resuscitation
    CPR Micromask
crack
    c. dancing
    c. fracture
    c. lung
crackle
    basilar c.
    coarse c.
cramp
    heat c.
    muscle c.
Crampton muscle
crampy pain
crania (*pl. of* cranium)
cranial
    c. bone
    caudad to c.
    c. fracture
    c. muscle
    c. nerve (CN)
    c. suture
    c. vault suture

craniofacial
    c. dysjunction fracture
    c. dysostosis
    c. fracture
craniotomy
    detached c.
    osteoplastic c.
cranium, pl. **crania**
crank amphetamine
crash cart
crater
    bone c.
crayon toxicity
CRC
    crisis resolution center
cream
    mafenide acetate c.
    Savlon antiseptic c.
    silver sulfadiazine c.
crease
    inguinal c.
    c. wound
creatine
    c. clearance
    c. kinase-myocardial band (CK-MB)
    c. monohydrate abuse
creeper
    Virginia c.
creeping
    c. eruption
    c. substitution of bone
cremasteric vein
cremaster muscle
creosote toxicity
crepitant
    c. rale
    c. wound
crepitation
    patellofemoral c.
crepitus
    bony c.
crescendo murmur
crescentic lesion
crescent sign
CREST
    calcinosis, Raynaud syndrome,
    esophageal dysmotility, scleroderma,
    and telangiectasia
    CREST syndrome
crest
    iliac c.
crestal cortical bone

Creutzfeld-Jakob disease
crew
    flight c.
CRF
    cardiac risk factor
    cortisol-releasing factor
crib
    bone c.
cribriform
    c. bone
    c. fascia
    c. fracture
    c. ligament
    c. plate
cricoarytenoid
    c. ligament
    c. muscle
cricoesophageal tendon
cricoid
    c. cartilage
    c. pressure
    c. ring
cricopharyngeal
    c. ligament
    c. muscle
cricosantorinian ligament
cricothyroid
    c. intubation
    c. ligament
    c. membrane
    c. muscle
    c. puncture
cricothyroidotomy
cricothyrotomy
cricotomy
cricotracheal ligament
criminal
    c. abortion
    c. sexual assault (CSA)
CR irritant
crisis, pl. **crises**
    abdominal c.
    adolescent c.
    adrenal c.
    bone c.
    cholinergic c.
    hypertensive c.
    renal c.
    c. resolution center (CRC)
criterion, pl. **criteria**
    admission criteria
    Brush ECG criteria

C

NOTES

criterion *(continued)*
    discharge criteria
    criteria for effective advance
        directive
    Gurd fat embolism syndrome
        criteria
    Ranson acute pancreatitis criteria
    Rochester febrile infant criteria
critical
    c. care
    c. care continuum
    c. care medicine
    c. care pharmacologist
    c. care specialist
    c. care team
    c. care unit (CCU)
    c. hemorrhage
    c. illness polyneuropathy
    c. incident stress debriefing (CISD)
    c. incident stress management
        (CISM)
Crohn disease
cromolyn sodium
crossed-finger technique
crossing
    nerve c.
cross ligament
crossmatch
    type and c.
crossmatched blood
crossmatching
    blood typing and c.
cross-section
    nerve c.-s.
crotalaria poisoning
crotalid envenomation
Crotalus
    C. antitoxin
    C. toxin
croup
    spasmodic c.
crowing inspiration
crown fracture
crowning of fetus
crown-root fracture
CRPS-1
    complex regional pain syndrome type 1
CRSD
    classic reflex sympathetic dystrophy
crucial angle of Gissane
cruciate
    c. ligament
    c. muscle
cruciform ligament
crunch
    Hamman c.
crural
    c. ligament
    c. vein

cruris
    tinea c.
crush
    c. fracture
    c. injury
    c. injury syndrome
    c. kidney
    c. line
    c. syndrome
crushed eggshell fracture
crushing chest pain
crush-type laceration
Cruveilhier ligament
crying
    intractable c.
cryoprecipitate
    c. therapy
    c. transfusion
cryopreserved vein
cryotherapy
cryptic tonsil tissue
cryptitis
    anal c.
cryptococcal
    c. meningoencephalitis
    c. pulmonary infection
cryptococcosis
Cryptococcus
    C. neoformans
    C. neoformans infection
cryptogenic
    c. infection
    c. sepsis
cryptorchidism
Cryptosporidium parvum
crystal-induced arthritis
crystalloid
    c. fluid
    c. infusion
    c. solution
crystalluria
CS
    orthochlorobenzylidene malononitrile
        CS irritant
C&S
    culture and sensitivity
CSA
    criminal sexual assault
CSD
    cat-scratch disease
CSF
    cerebrospinal fluid
    colony-stimulating factor
        CSF rhinorrhea
CSHCN
    children with special health care needs
CSP
    carotid sinus pressure
C-spine immobilization

CST
　　clinical support tool
CT
　　computed tomography
　　　abdominal CT
　　　bone quantitative CT
　　　intravenous contrast CT
　　　CT scan
　　　spiral CT
CT1 suture
CTx
　　chemotherapy
cubital
　　c. bone
　　c. nerve
　　c. vein
cuboid
　　c. bone
　　c. fracture
cuboideonavicular ligament
cuff
　　blood pressure c.
　　c. inflation
　　nerve c.
　　vein c.
culdocentesis
Cullen sign
cultural healing practice
culture
　　aerobic c.
　　anaerobic c.
　　blood c.
　　bone c.
　　bone marrow c.
　　pure c.
　　c. and sensitivity (C&S)
　　sputum c.
　　through-the-catheter c. (TTC)
　　wound c.
cumulative
　　c. action
　　c. effect
cuneiform
　　c. bone
　　c. fracture
　　c. ligament
cuneocuboid ligament
cuneometatarsal interosseous ligament
cuneonavicular ligament
curare toxicity
curdy pus

curettage
　　dilation and c.
currant jelly stool
current
　　c. ailment
　　c. complaint (CC)
　　direct c. (DC)
curve
　　forced velocity c.
　　muscle c.
　　oxyhemoglobin dissociation c.
　　pressure-volume c.
　　saddleback fever c.
curved blade
curvilinear laceration
Cushing
　　C. response
　　C. suture
　　C. syndrome
cushion
　　air c.
　　suture c.
cuspidata
　　Taxus c.
custodial care
Custodis suture
cutaneous
　　c. abscess
　　c. anthrax
　　c. bacterial infection
　　c. cellulitis
　　c. lesion
　　c. muscle
　　c. nerve
　　c. reaction pattern
　　c. tinea infection
　　c. vein
cutdown
　　venous c.
cutis marmorata
cutter
　　suture c.
cutting needle
CV
　　cardiovascular
CVA
　　cerebrovascular accident
　　costovertebral angle
CVAT
　　costovertebral angle tenderness
CVC
　　central venous catheter

NOTES

75

CVP
central venous pressure
CVR
cardiovascular-respiratory
CVS
cardiovascular surgery
cardiovascular system
CVVHD
continuous venovenous hemodiafiltration
CVVHDF
continuous venovenous hemodiafiltration
CW
chest wall
CXR
chest x-ray
cyanide
cyanogen chloride c.
hydrogen c.
c. poisoning
c. toxicity
cyanoacrylate
c. adhesive
c. glue
cyanocobalamin deficiency
cyanogen chloride cyanide
cyanosis
circumoral c.
cyanotic
c. congenital heart disease
c. extremity
c. heart disease
c. lip
cyclamate
calcium c.
cycle
compression-relaxation c.
pain-anxiety c.
cyclic
c. antidepressant
c. antidepressant intoxication
c. neutropenia
cyclobenzaprine
cyclooxygenase-2 (COX-2)
c.-2 inhibitor
cyclopeptide
cyclophosphamide
cycloplegic
cyclorotary muscle
cycloserine
cyclosporin A
cyclosporine
cyclovertical muscle
cylinder
muscle c.

oxygen (size D, E, M, G, and H) c.
Cyon nerve
cyproheptadine
cyst
Baker c.
Bartholin c.
bone c.
bone implantation c.
epidermoid inclusion c.
locular c.
nabothian c.
ovarian c.
pilonidal c.
sebaceous c.
subpleural air c.
cystectomy
radical c.
cystic
c. fibrosis
c. mastitis
c. vein
cysticercosis
cystitis
acute c.
cystoduodenal ligament
cystography
cystoid maculopathy
cystostomy
suprapubic c.
cytarabine
cytochrome P-450 biotransformation
cytogenetics
bone marrow c.
cytohistologic diagnosis
cytokine
antiinflammatory c.
proinflammatory c.
cytologic diagnosis
cytomegalovirus (CMV)
c. disease
c. infection
cytoprotection
cytoprotective
c. agent
c. antacid
cytotoxicity
antibody-dependent cellular c. (ADCC)
Cytovene
Czerny-Lembert suture
Czerny suture

daclizumab
Dacron
    D. bolstered suture
    D. synthetic ligament
    D. traction suture
dacryoadenitis
    infectious d.
dacryocystitis
    chronic d.
DAE
    dysbaric air embolism
daffodil ingestion
Dafilon suture
Dagrofil suture
DAI
    diffuse axonal injury
Dalmane
damage
    diffuse alveolar d.
    diffuse cortical anoxic d.
    hepatic d.
danazol
dancer's
    d. bone
    d. fracture
Dance sign
dancing
    crack d.
Dandy-Walker syndrome
Dane particle
danger space
Danis-Weber
    D.-W. fracture
    D.-W. malleolar fracture
      classification
dantrolene sodium
Daphne toxicity
dapsone
Darrach-Hughston-Milch fracture
dartos muscle
dashboard fracture
DAT
    diphtheria antitoxin
data (*pl. of* datum)
database
    APACHE III d.
    POISINDEX d.
date
    d. of birth (DB, DOB)
    d. rape drug
datum, pl. data
Datura
    D. *stramonium*
    D. *stramonium* ingestion
    D. toxicity

Davis-Geck suture
DAWN
    Drug Abuse Warning Network
day of the week
DB
    date of birth
DBP
    diastolic blood pressure
DC
    direct current
    discharge
DCAP-BTLS
    deformity, contusion, abrasion,
      puncture/penetrating wound, burn,
      tenderness, laceration, swelling
DD
    differential diagnosis
DDAVP
    1-desamino-8-didanosine-arginine
    vasopressin
ddI, ddi
    didanosine
D–dimer
    D–d. assay
    D–d. test
de
    de Lange syndrome
    De Musset sign
    de Quervain disease
    de Quervain fracture
    de Quervain stenosing tenosynovitis
DEA
    Drug Enforcement Agency
dead
    d. bone
    d. nerve
    d. on arrival (DOA)
    d. space
    d. time
dead-space
    d.-s. fraction
    d.-s. ventilation
deaf-mute
deaf-mutism
deafness
    bone conduction d.
    nerve d.
    traumatic d.
dearth
    d. of evidence
    d. of finding
    d. of symptoms
death
    associated cause of d.
    brain d.

D

death *(continued)*
    d. camas ingestion
    cause of d. (COD)
    cerebral d.
    contributory cause of d.
    dive-related d.
    intrauterine fetal d.
    d. is coming (DIC)
    nerve cell d.
    sudden d.
    sudden cardiac d.
    underlying cause of d.
debilitate
debilitation
debility
    profound d.
débride
débridement
    incision and d.
    d. of pseudomembrane
    wound d.
debriefing
    critical incident stress d. (CISD)
debris
    bone d.
    grumous d.
debrisoquine polymorphism
decay
    bone d.
deceleration
decerebrate posture
decompression
    bone graft d.
    chamber d.
    emergent d.
    d. of fracture
    fracture d.
    needle d.
    nerve d.
    nerve root d.
    NG d.
    d. sickness
    vein d.
decongestant
decontamination
    chemical d.
    gastric d.
    gastrointestinal d.
decorticate
    d. posture
    d. rigidity
decreased
    d. bowel sound
    d. exercise tolerance
    d. fetal heart tones
    d. gastrointestinal motility
    d. oxygen saturation
    d. salivation
decrement

decrepitate
decrepitation
decrudescence
decrustation
decubitus ulcer
decussation
    nerve d.
deep
    d. abscess
    d. cerebral vein
    d. cervical vein
    d. circumflex iliac vein
    d. dermal suture
    d. dorsal vein
    d. epigastric vein
    d. facial vein
    d. femoral vein
    d. flexor muscle
    d. flexor tendon
    d. hand injury
    d. inferior epigastric vein
    d. infrapatellar bursa
    d. lingual vein
    d. middle cerebral vein
    d. periorbital ecchymosis
    rapture of the d.
    d. respiration
    d. suspension suture
    d. temporal vein
    d. tendon reflex (DTR)
    d. tracheal suctioning
    d. vein thrombosis (DVT)
    d. venous thromboembolism
    d. venous thrombosis (DVT)
DEET
    diethyltoluamide
defasciculating dose
defecation
    obstructed d.
defect
    atrial septal d. (ASD)
    atrioventricular septal d.
    bone d.
    isolated atrial septal d.
    lateralization d.
defective acceleration
deferoxamine
    d. challenge test
    d. chelation therapy
defervescence
defervescent stage
defibrillation
    automated external d. (AED)
    automatic external d. (AED)
    ventricular d.
defibrillator
    AccessAED d.
    AccessALS d.
    automated external d. (AED)

cardiac d.
fully-automated d.
HeartStart d.
implantable d.
manual d.
semiautomated external d. (SAED)
shock-advisory d.
Zoll M Series Critical Care
transport d.
defibrillator/monitor
LIFEPAK 12 d./m.
deficiency
antithrombin III d.
bone d.
chronic caloric d.
corticotropin d.
cyanocobalamin d.
factor XI d.
folate d.
glucose-6-phosphate
dehydrogenase d.
immunologic d.
magnesium d.
mineralocorticoid d.
prolactin d.
vitamin B_{12} d.
deficit
base d.
focal d.
memory d.
motor d.
neurocognitive d.
neurologic d.
neurologic vascular d.
pulse d.
vascular d.
visual d.
definitive cause
definitively
deflection
fracture simple and depressed full-
scale d.
deformity
bird-beak d.
boutonnière d.
d., contusion, abrasion,
puncture/penetrating wound, burn,
tenderness, laceration, swelling
(DCAP-BTLS)
fracture d.
valgus d.
defuse

defusing
degenerative
d. arthritis
d. joint disease (DJD)
degloving
d. avulsion
d. injury
d. laceration
dehiscence
d. of fascia
suture line d.
wound d.
dehydration
d. fever
severe d.
Deklene
D. II cardiovascular suture
D. polypropylene suture
Deknatel silk suture
delay
intraventricular conduction d.
d. in seeking care
delayed
d. closure
d. closure of suture
d. organ system toxicity
d. presentation
d. suture
deleterious effect
delineate
delinquency
delinquent
juvenile d.
delirious mania
delirium
acute d.
alcohol withdrawal d.
d. tremens (DT)
delivery
aerosol d.
oxygen d.
spontaneous breech d.
uncomplicated d.
**delta-aminolevulinate dehydratase
activity**
deltoid
d. bursa
d. ligament
d. muscle
deltotrapezius fascial ligament
delusion of reference

D

NOTES

demand-valve
    d.-v. ventilation
    d.-v. ventilation device
demeclocycline
dementia
    dialysis d.
    paralytic d.
Demerol
demineralization
    bone d.
demise
demulcent
demyelinating
    d. disease
    d. polyneuropathy
demyelination
    brainstem d.
dendritic depolarization
denervated muscle
denervation
    muscle d.
dengue fever
denial and isolation
Denis
    D. Browne spinal fracture
      classification
    D. spinal fracture
    D. spinal fracture classification
denitrogenation
    absorption atelectasis d.
    d. absorption atelectasis
Denonvilliers ligament
dense bone
dens fracture
densitometer
    bone d.
densitometry
    bone d.
    bone mineral d.
    fracture site nonunion Norland
      bone d.
density
    bone d.
    bone mass d.
    bone mineral d.
dental
    d. avulsion
    d. care product ingestion
    d. caries
    d. disorder
    d. fracture
    d. infection
    d. nerve
    d. trauma
dentate
    d. fracture
    d. ligament
    d. line
    d. suture

denticulate
    d. ligament
    d. suture
dentinal intratubular nerve
dentoalveolar
    d. fracture
    d. ligament
    d. trauma
denudation
deodorant ingestion
deoxycholate
    amphotericin B d.
deoxygenated blood
deoxyspergualin
department
    emergency d. (ED)
    pediatric emergency d. (PED)
dependence
    financial d.
    physiologic determinants of
      ventilator d.
    ventilator d.
dependency
    alcohol d.
    caregiver d.
    victim d.
dependent
    alcohol d.
    d. lividity
    d. personality disorder
depilatory preparation ingestion
depletion
    sodium d.
    volume d.
depolarization
    dendritic d.
Depo-Provera injectable contraceptive
deposit
    atherosclerotic d.
deposition
    bone d.
    iron d.
deprenyl toxicity
depressant
    cardiac d.
depressed
    d. affect
    d. fontanelle
    d. fracture
    d. skull fracture
depression
    bone d.
    bone marrow d.
    endogenous d.
    d. fracture
    humeral d.
    myocardial d.
    neural d.
    stuporous d.

depression-type intraarticular fracture
depressive
    d. affect
    d. disorder
    d. stupor
    d. symptomatology
depressor
    d. nerve
    tongue d.
deprivation
    oxygen d.
depth
    adequate d.
    respiratory d.
derby hat fracture
derivative
    amphetamine d.
DERMABOND topical skin adhesive
Dermacentor **tick**
dermal
    d. bone
    d. muscle
    d. suture
Dermalene polyethylene suture
Dermalon cuticular suture
dermatitidis
    Blastomyces d.
dermatitis, pl. **dermatitides**
    allergic d.
    atopic d.
    carcinomatous d.
    contact d.
    eczema atopic d.
    exfoliative d.
    poison sumac d.
    rhus d.
    seborrheic d.
dermatome
dermatomyositis
dermatomyositis/polymyositis
dermis
1-desamino-8-didanosine-arginine
   vasopressin (DDAVP)
desaturation
    red d.
Desault fracture
descending
    d. aorta
    d. colon
    d. genicular vein
    d. nerve
    d. part of iliofemoral ligament

Descot fracture
desiccant
desiccate
designer
    d. drug
    d. fentanyl
desmopressin
desquamatic interstitial pneumonia
   (DIP)
destruction
    bone d.
Desyrel toxicity
detached craniotomy
detachment
    retinal d.
detailed physical examination
detection
    intimate partner violence d.
detector
    Easy Cap II CO_2 d.
detergent
    cationic d.
deterioration
    mental d.
determinant
    physiologic d.
determination
    bone age d.
    glucose d.
    d. of incompetence
    rapid hemoglobin d.
detox
    detoxification
detoxification (detox)
detritus bone
detrusor muscle
development
    bone d.
developmental
    d. age
    d. anomaly
deviation
    bilateral tonic d.
    fracture d.
    skew d.
    tracheal d.
    varus d.
device
    AutoPulse CPR d.
    bag-mask d.
    bag-valve d.
    bag-valve-mask d.

D

NOTES

device *(continued)*
    cardiac assist d.
    cervical immobilization d. (CID)
    Combitube airway d.
    demand-valve ventilation d.
    EGTA d.
    electric suction d.
    EOA d.
    esophageal detector d. (EDD)
    extrication d.
    flow restricted oxygen-powered
      ventilation d.
    fracture fixation d.
    hand-operated suction d.
    hand-powered suction d.
    implantable venous access d.
    Kendrick extrication d. (KED)
    left ventricular assist d. (LVAD)
    mechanical support d.
    portable suction d.
    Suture Lok d.
    traction d.
    ventricular assist d. (VAD)
    vest-type extrication d.
dexamethasone sodium phosphate
dexmedetomidine hydrochloride injection
Dexon
    D. absorbable synthetic polyglycolic
      acid suture
    D. Plus suture
    D. II suture
dextran
    low-molecular-weight d.
dextromethorphan
dextroposition
dextrose
    empirical d.
    d. therapy
    d. in water (D/W)
DF-2
    dysgonic fermenter-2
DG
    diagnosis
    DG Softgut suture
DHE
    dihydroergotamine
DI
    diabetes insipidus
diabetes
    borderline d.
    HHNK d.
    d. insipidus (DI)
    latent d.
    d. mellitus
    d. mellitus, juvenile
diabetic
    d. coma
    d. history
    d. ketoacidosis (DKA)

diacondylar fracture
diagnose
diagnosis (DG, Dx)
    admitting d. (AD)
    biological d.
    clinical d.
    cytohistologic d.
    cytologic d.
    differential d. (DD)
    pathologic d.
    Prospective Investigation of
      Pulmonary Embolism D.
      (PIOPED)
    provocative d.
    roentgen d.
    serum d.
diagnosis-related
    d.-r. group (DRG)
    d.-r. group coding
diagnostic
    d. laparotomy
    d. peritoneal lavage (DPL)
    d. results
    d. serology
    D. and Statistical Manual of
      Mental Disorders
    D. and Statistical Manual of
      Mental Disorders-IV (DSM-IV)
dial-a-flow IV line
dialysis
    acute intermittent peritoneal d.
      (AIPD)
    chronic ambulatory peritoneal d.
      (CAPD)
    d. complication
    d. dementia
    d. disequilibrium syndrome
    gastrointestinal d.
    intermittent peritoneal d.
    peritoneal d.
dialyzer
diameter
    aortic d.
    biparietal d. (BPD)
diametric pelvic fracture
diaper
    d. fluorescence
    d. rash
diaphoresis
diaphoretic
diaphragm
    d. laceration
    d. rupture
diaphragmatic
    d. hernia
    d. injury
    d. laceration
    d. ligament
    d. muscle

d. nerve
d. trauma
diaphysial fracture
diarrhea
adult d.
backpacker d.
mucous d.
nausea, vomiting, d. (NVD)
pediatric d.
diarthrodial
d. joint bursae
d. muscle
diastasis
fracture d.
suture d.
d. of suture
diastatic
d. lambdoid suture
d. skull fracture
diastolic
d. blood pressure (DBP)
d. pressure (DP)
diathermy
diathesis
diazepam
diazoxide therapy
dibenzofurans
toxic skin reaction to d.
DIC
death is coming
disseminated intravascular coagulation
disseminated intravascular coagulopathy
dicing abrasion
dicloxacillin
dicondylar fracture
didanosine (ddI, ddi)
d. therapy
Dieffenbachia toxicity
diencephalic vein
die punch fracture
diet
CAPS-free d.
high-protein d.
low-carbohydrate d.
reducing d.
warm water, analgesic, stool
softener, high-fiber d. (WASH)
dietary restriction
diet-controlled diabetes mellitus
dietetic

diethylamide
lysergic acid d. (LSD)
diethyltoluamide (DEET)
dieting
yo-yo d.
dietitian
differential
d. diagnosis (DD)
d. stethoscope
differentiate
difficile
Clostridium d.
difficult to wean patient
difficulty breathing
diffuse
d. abdominal pain
d. abscess
d. alveolar damage
d. axonal injury (DAI)
d. cortical anoxic damage
d. goiter
d. peritonitis
d. rhonchi
**diffusing capacity of lung for carbon
monoxide (DLCO)**
diffusion
d. hypoxia
d. impairment
Diflucan
digastric
d. muscle
d. nerve
DiGeorge syndrome
Digibind
digital
d. exploration
d. extensor tendon
d. flexor tendon
d. nerve
d. nerve block
d. retinacular ligament
d. subtraction angiography (DSA)
d. vein
digitalis
d. effect
d. glucoside
d. glycoside therapy
d. intoxication
d. toxicity
Digitalis purpurea
digitalization
digitize

D

NOTES

digoxin
    d. poisoning
    d. toxicity
digoxin-specific antibody fragment therapy
digoxin-toxic arrhythmia
dihydroergotamine (DHE)
Dilantin toxicity
dilated
    d. cardiomyopathy
    fixed and d. (F&D)
    d. pupil
    d. ureter
    d. vein
dilation, dilatation
    d. and curettage
    ductal d.
    vein d.
dilational anemia
dilator
    fascial d.
    d. muscle
    vein d.
dilemma
diltiazem hydrochloride
dilute hydrogen peroxide rinse
dilution
    dye d.
    d. therapy
dilutional
    d. acidosis
    d. coagulopathy
    d. hyponatremia
dimension
2-dimensional echocardiography
dimercaprol
dimercaptosuccinic acid (DMSA)
dimethyl
    d. iminodiacetic acid (HIDA)
    d. sulfoxide (DMSO)
diminished consciousness
diminution
dimpling
    skin d.
dinitrate
    topical isosorbide d.
dinitrophenol toxicity
dioxide
    carbon d. (CO_2)
    nitrous d.
    partial pressure of carbon d. (pCO_2)
dioxin toxicity
DIP
    desquamatic interstitial pneumonia
dipalmitoylphosphatidylcholine (DPPC)
diphenhydramine
diphenoxylate
diphenylhydantoin therapy

diphosgene
diphtheria
    d. antitoxin (DAT)
    d., pertussis, tetanus (DPT)
    d., tetanus, pertussis (DTP)
    d. toxin
diphtheric laryngitis
diploic vein
dipping
    ocular d.
Diprivan
dipstick test
dipyridamole thallium scintigraphy
dipyridyl herbicide poisoning
diquat poisoning
dire
    d. consequence
    d. strait
direct
    d. carry technique
    d. contact
    d. coronary artery bypass
    d. current (DC)
    d. force
    d. fracture
    d. ground lift technique
    d. lateral vein
    d. medical control
    d. medical direction
    d. orbital floor fracture
    d. pressure
direction
    caudal d.
    cephalad d.
    direct medical d.
    off-line medical d.
    on-line medical d.
directive
    advanced d. (AD)
    criteria for effective advance d.
director
    medical d.
disability
    permanent and total d.
disarticulation
    wrist d.
disaster
    complex d.
    d. medical assistance team (DMAT)
    d. medicine
    d. planning
    d. response
disc (*var. of* disk)
discharge (DC)
    d. after observation
    d. criteria
    nipple d.
    purulent d.

urethral d.
vaginal d.
wound d.
disciform process
disciplinary
discitis
iatrogenic d.
disclosing
disclosure
full d.
discoloration
skin d.
discomfort
threshold of d.
discontinuity
nerve d.
discord
marital d.
discordance
birth weight d.
discordant twin
discrepancy
d. in history
limb-length d.
discrete
d. disease
d. mass
d. nodule
d. organ enlargement
discrimination
2-point d.
disease
acute cardiovascular d.
acute respiratory d. (ARD)
acyanotic congenital heart d.
acyanotic heart d.
adrenal d.
adult polycystic kidney d.
advanced lung d.
airborne d.
aortic valve d.
arteriosclerotic cardiovascular d.
(ACVD)
Bartholin gland d.
Bassen-Kornzweig d.
Behçet d.
bilateral maxillary sinus d.
biliary tract d.
bloodborne d.
bone d.
Bornholm d.
Buerger d.

cat-scratch d. (CSD)
Chagas d.
chronic lung d. (CLD)
chronic obstructive airways d.
(COAD)
chronic obstructive pulmonary d.
(COPD)
cold agglutinin d.
collagen vascular d.
communicable d.
concomitant d.
congenital d.
congenital heart d.
contagious d.
coronary arteriosclerotic heart d.
(CAHD)
coronary artery d. (CAD)
coronary atherosclerotic heart d.
(CAHD)
coronary heart d.
Creutzfeld-Jakob d.
Crohn d.
cyanotic congenital heart d.
cyanotic heart d.
cytomegalovirus d.
degenerative joint d. (DJD)
demyelinating d.
de Quervain d.
discrete d.
diverticular d.
endemic d.
end-stage liver d.
end-stage renal d. (ESRD)
fibrocystic breast d.
fifth d.
findings reflect underlying d.
flight into d.
foodborne d.
fracture d.
Fragmin During Instability in
Coronary Artery D. (FRISC)
frontal sinus d.
gastroesophageal reflux d. (GERD)
gestational thromboblastic d.
Gilbert d.
gonococcal d.
graft versus host d. (GVHD)
Graves d.
hand-foot-and-mouth d.
Hirschsprung d.
iatrogenic drug-induced d.
inflammatory bowel d. (IBD)

D

NOTES

disease *(continued)*
    International Classification of D. (ICD)
    interstitial d.
    Kawasaki d.
    Köhler d.
    lactation d.
    Legg-Calvé-Perthes d.
    Legionnaires d.
    lipohyalinotic small vessel d.
    Lyme d.
    maxillary sinus d.
    Ménière d.
    metabolic d.
    metabolic bone d.
    Meyer-Betz d.
    moldy hay d.
    Mondor d.
    Monge d.
    multisystem d.
    muscle d.
    muscle d.
    muscle layer d.
    nosocomial d.
    obstructive airway d. (OAD)
    occupational d.
    Osgood-Schlatter d.
    Paget d.
    parathyroid d.
    Parkinson d.
    pelvic inflammatory d. (PID)
    peptic ulcer d.
    periodontal d.
    peripheral neuromuscular d.
    peripheral vascular d.
    polycystic kidney d.
    posttransplant lymphoproliferative d. (PTLD)
    primary cardiac d.
    psychosomatic d.
    reactive airway d.
    recalcitrant d.
    Reiter d.
    restrictive lung d.
    retinal manifestation of systemic d.
    sexually transmitted d. (STD)
    sickle cell d.
    silo filler's d.
    streptococcal d.
    suspected gestational thromboblastic d.
    systemic d.
    thoracic valvular d.
    thromboblastic d.
    thyroid d.
    transfusion-transmitted d. (TTD)
    underlying d.
    valvular heart d.
    venoocclusive d.
    vertebrobasilar atherothrombotic d.
    von Willebrand d.

disease-modifying antirheumatic drug (DMARD)
disentanglement
dishpan fracture
DISI
    dorsal intercalated segment instability
disinfect
disinfectant
disinfection
    high-level d.
    low-level d.
disinserted muscle
disintegration
disk, disc
    herniated d,
dislocated shoulder
dislocation
    ankle d.
    atlantooccipital d. (AOD)
    clavicular d.
    elbow d.
    d. fracture
    fracture d.
    hip d.
    knee d.
    late d.
    lens d.
    lunate d.
    perilunate d.
    shoulder d.
    spinal d.
    tendon d.
dismutase
    superoxide d.
disodium
    pamidronate d.
disopyramide
disorder
    acid-base d.
    adenohypophyseal d.
    adjustment d.
    altitude-related d.
    antisocial personality d.
    anxiety d.
    back d.
    biliary tract d.
    binge eating d.
    bipolar d.
    bipolar affective d.
    bleeding d.
    borderline personality d.
    cerebrovascular d.
    coagulation d.
    connective tissue d.
    conversion d.
    dental d.
    dependent personality d.

depressive d.
Diagnostic and Statistical Manual of Mental D.'s
Diagnostic and Statistical Manual of Mental D.'s-IV (DSM-IV)
eating d.
electrolyte d.
endocrine d.
inflammatory adnexal d.
lumbar disk d.
major depressive d.
manic-depressive d.
mixed acid-base d.
mood d.
movement d.
muscle inflammatory d.
muscle myotonic d.
muscle psychogenic d.
nutritional d.
obsessive-compulsive d. (OCD)
panic d.
personality d.
posttraumatic stress d. (PTSD)
primary glial d.
primary neuronal d.
tendon d.
thought d.
triple acid base d.
underlying d.
wound healing d.

disorganized
d. bone
d. language

disorientation
patient d.
spatial d.

disparate

dispatch

dispatcher
emergency medical d. (EMD)

displaced
d. fracture
d. intraarticular fracture
d. malar fracture
d. pilon fracture
d. tibia-fibula fracture
d. tooth
d. zygomatic fracture

displacement
anterior d.
fracture fragment d.
lens d.

posterior d.
tendon d.

disposition

disruption
aortic d.
biliary duct d.
complete d.
esophageal d.
d. of ligament
near complete d.
wound d.

dissecting thoracic aneurysm

dissection
adventitial d.
aortic d.
bone d.
carotid artery d.
International Registry of Acute Aortic D. (IRAD)
muscle d.
thoracic aortic d.
vertebral artery d.

dissector
nerve root laminectomy d.

disseminated
d. candidiasis
d. intravascular
d. intravascular coagulation (DIC)
d. intravascular coagulopathy (DIC)

dissipate

dissociation
electromechanical d.

dissociative anesthesia

dissolution

dissymmetry

distal
d. accessory nerve
d. femoral epiphysial fracture
d. humeral fracture
d. intestinal obstruction syndrome
d. intestinal obstruction syndrome of cystic fibrosis
d. muscle
d. pulse
d. radial fracture
d. shaft forearm fracture
d. ulnar collateral ligament

distance
muzzle-to-skin d.

distended
d. bursa
d. vein

D

NOTES

distention, distension
  abdominal d.
  gastric d.
  intestinal d.
  jugular venous d. (JVD)
  organ capsule d.
  visceral d.
  viscous d.
distraction
  d. of fracture
  fracture fragment d.
  muscle d.
  spine d.
  d. of spine
distraught
distress
  acute respiratory d. (ARD)
  fetal d.
  respiratory d.
distribution
  nerve d.
  skew d.
disturbance
  acid-base d.
  behavioral d.
  electrolyte d.
  fluid d.
  myocardial conduction d.
  myocardial contraction d.
  visual d.
disulfide
  carbon d.
disulfiram-alcohol syndrome
disulfiram-like toxin
disulfiram reaction
dithiocarbamate
dithionite urine test
diuresis, pl. diureses
  acid d.
  forced d.
  postobstructive d.
  postresuscitation d.
diuretic
  loop d.
  osmotic d.
  potassium-sparing d.
  thiazide d.
diurnal
dive-related
  d.-r. death
  d.-r. injury
  d.-r. stroke
divergent rectus muscle
diversion
  urinary d.
diverticula (*pl. of* diverticulum)
diverticular disease
diverticulitis

diverticulosis
  acute d.
diverticulum, pl. diverticula
  esophageal d.
  Meckel d.
diving emergency
divulsion
dizocilpine
dizziness
DJD
  degenerative joint disease
DKA
  diabetic ketoacidosis
DLCO
  diffusing capacity of lung for carbon
    monoxide
DLT
  double-lung transplantation
DMARD
  disease-modifying antirheumatic drug
DMAT
  disaster medical assistance team
DMSA
  dimercaptosuccinic acid
DMSO
  dimethyl sulfoxide
DNAR
  do not attempt resuscitation
DNR
  do not resuscitate
    DNR order
do
  do not attempt resuscitation
    (DNAR)
  do not resuscitate (DNR)
  do not resuscitate order
DOA
  dead on arrival
DOB
  date of birth
dobutamine
  d. stress echocardiography
  d. therapy
Docktor suture
doctrine
  emergency d.
docusate
  calcium d.
Dodd perforating vein
DOE
  dyspnea on exertion
dog bite
dog-leg fracture
dollop
  bone d.
doll's eye reflex
dome-binding suture
dome fracture
domestic violence

donation
　　organ d.
Donati suture
Done nomogram
donor
　　bone marrow d.
　　organ d.
Donovan body
door-to-balloon inflation time
door-to-drug time
dopamine
dopaminergic agonist
dope
dopexamine
Doppler
　　transcranial D. (TCD)
　　D. ultrasonography
d'orange
　　peau d'o.
dorsa (*pl. of* dorsum)
dorsal
　　d. antebrachial cutaneous nerve
　　d. aspect
　　d. calcaneocuboid ligament
　　d. calcaneonavicular ligament
　　d. callosal vein
　　d. carpal arcuate ligament
　　d. carpometacarpal ligament
　　d. cuboideonavicular ligament
　　d. cuneocuboid ligament
　　d. cuneonavicular ligament
　　d. intercalated segment instability (DISI)
　　d. intercarpal ligament
　　d. intercuneiform ligament
　　d. interosseous nerve
　　d. lateral cutaneous nerve
　　d. lingual vein
　　d. medial cutaneous nerve
　　d. metacarpal ligament
　　d. metacarpal vein
　　d. metatarsal ligament
　　d. metatarsal vein
　　d. muscle
　　d. nerve of penis
　　d. penile vein
　　d. radiocarpal ligament
　　d. rim distal radial fracture
　　d. sacroiliac ligament
　　d. scapular nerve
　　d. scapular vein
　　d. talonavicular bone

　　d. talonavicular ligament
　　d. tarsal ligament
　　d. tarsometatarsal ligament
　　d. wing fracture
　　d. wrist ligament
dorsalis
　　d. pedis artery
　　d. pedis pulse
　　d. pedis vein
dorsispinal vein
dorsomedial cutaneous nerve
dorsoradial ligament
dorsum, pl. **dorsa**
dose
　　bolus d.
　　bone marrow d.
　　defasciculating d.
　　incorrect d.
　　intravenous single d.
　　lethal d.
　　loading d.
　　toxic d.
dose-ranging study
dosimeter
dosimetry
　　x-ray d.
double
　　d. fracture
　　d. right-angle suture
　　d. sickening
　　d. strength (DS)
double-armed wire suture
double-blind
　　d.-b. edrophonium test
　　d.-b. study
double-lung transplantation (DLT)
double-rib fracture
double-running penetrating keratoplasty suture
douche
　　Betadine d.
doughy
　　d. abdomen
　　d. consistency
Douglas
　　D. ligament
　　pouch of D.
douloureux
　　tic d.
dowel
　　bone d.
downhill course

D

NOTES

downstroke
    inspiratory d.
Down syndrome
downward movement
doxacurium
doxycycline
DP
    diastolic pressure
DPL
    diagnostic peritoneal lavage
DPPC
    dipalmitoylphosphatidylcholine
DPT
    diphtheria, pertussis, tetanus
    DPT vaccine
drain
    d. cleaner
    wound d.
drainage
    incision and d. (I&D)
    lymphocele d.
    nasogastric d.
    percutaneous catheter d.
    postural d.
    splenic bed d.
    tube d.
    wound d.
draining vein
draw sheet
dream
    vivid d.
dressing
    adhesive-type d.
    bibulous d.
    Biobrane d.
    Bioclusive d.
    biological d.
    bulky d.
    Coe-Pak d.
    compression d.
    Conform d.
    DuoDerm d.
    hydrocolloid d.
    impregnated d.
    IntraSite d.
    Jones d.
    multitrauma d.
    occlusive d.
    OpSite d.
    Scarlet Red d.
    sterile d.
    sterile gauze d.
    Tegaderm d.
    Tegasorb d.
    universal d.
    wound d.
Dressler syndrome
DRG
    diagnosis-related group

drift
    antigenic d.
drill
    d. bit fracture
    suture hole d.
drip
    nitroglycerin d.
dromotropy
    negative d.
    positive d.
droop
    facial d.
drop
    benzocaine ear d.'s
    core temperature after d.
droperidol
droplet
    airborne d.
dropsy
drowning
    dry d.
    near d.
    wet d.
drug
    d. absorption
    d. abuse
    D. Abuse Warning Network
    (DAWN)
    d. allergy
    anorectic d.
    antiadrenergic d.
    antiarrhythmic d.
    anticholinergic d.
    antiepileptic d. (AED)
    antifibrinolytic d.
    antifungal d.
    antisense d.
    bactericidal d.
    date rape d.
    designer d.
    disease-modifying antirheumatic d.
    (DMARD)
    D. Enforcement Agency (DEA)
    enteral d.
    d. fever
    first-line d.
    d. half-life
    illicit d.
    LEAN d.
    d. listing
    nonsteroidal antiinflammatory d.
    (NSAID)
    d. paraphernalia
    street d.
    d. tolerance
    d. treatment
    vasotropic d.
    d. withdrawal
drug-drug interaction

drug-induced acute coronary syndrome
3-drug regimen
drumstick appearance
drunkenness
dry
- d. drowning
- d. mouth
- d. oxygen
- d. skin
- d. snow avalanche
- d. socket paste

dry-powder inhaler
DS
- double strength
- Bactrim DS

DSA
- digital subtraction angiography

DSM-IV
- Diagnostic and Statistical Manual of Mental Disorders-IV

DT
- delirium tremens

DTP
- diphtheria, tetanus, pertussis

DTR
- deep tendon reflex

Dubin-Johnson syndrome
Dubowitz score
duct
- alveolar d.
- bile d.
- collecting d.
- d. ectasia
- extrahepatic d.
- lacrimal d.

ductal dilation
ductus arteriosus
dulcamara
- Solanum d.

dullness
- bibasilar d.

dull pain
Dulox suture
dumbcane plant ingestion
dumb rabies
duodenal
- d. ligament
- d. trauma
- d. vein

duodenocolic ligament
duodenorenal ligament

duodenum
- perforated d.

DuoDerm dressing
duplex ultrasound
Dupuytren
- D. fracture
- D. suture

durable power of attorney for health care
Duraclon
dural
- d. ectasia
- d. ligament
- d. puncture headache
- d. tack-up suture

dura mater
duration of pain
Duroziez sign
dust
- angel d.
- d. exposure

duty
- breach of d.
- implied d.

Duverney
- D. fracture
- D. muscle

DVT
- deep vein thrombosis
- deep venous thrombosis

D/W
- dextrose in water

Dx
- diagnosis

dye
- d. dilution
- d. punch fracture

DynaCirc
dynamic
- d. hyperinflation
- d. ileus
- d. splinting

dysbaric air embolism (DAE)
dysbarism
dyschezia
- rectal d.

dysconjugate gaze
dyscrasia
- blood d.

dyscrasic fracture
dysenteriae
- Shigella d.

NOTES

dysequilibrium
dysesthesia
    palmar d.
dysfunction
    bone marrow d.
    end-organ d.
    primary graft d.
    reactive d.
    right ventricular d.
dysfunctional uterine bleeding
dysgonic fermenter-2 (DF-2)
dyshidrotic eczema
dyskinesia
    tardive d.
dyslipidosis
dysmenorrhea
dysmenorrheal
dysmotility
dysostosis
    craniofacial d.
dysoxia
dyspareunia
dyspepsia
dysphagia
dysplasia
    bone d.
    bronchopleural d. (BPD)
    bronchopulmonary d.
    fibromuscular d.
    fibrous bone d.
    nerve d.

dyspnea
    blunted perception of d.
    exertional d.
    nocturnal d.
    d. on exertion (DOE)
    paroxysmal nocturnal d. (PND)
dyspneic
dysreflexia
    autonomic d.
dysrhythmia
    life-threatening d.
    ventricular d.
dystocia
    shoulder d.
dystonia
    muscle d.
dystonic
    d. effect
    d. reaction
    d. tremor
dystrophy
    bone d.
    classic reflex sympathetic d.
      (CRSD)
    muscular d.
    oculopharyngeal d.
    reflex sympathetic d.
dysuria
    spastic d.

ε (*var. of* epsilon)
EACA
> epsilon aminocaproic acid

ear
> e. bone
> e. foreign body
> inner e.
> e., nose, throat (ENT)
> e. squeeze

earlobe
> bifid e.

early
> e. blood transfusion
> e. intubation

Early Retavase-Thrombolysis In Myocardial Infarction (ER-TIMI)
EAST
> Enlimomab Acute Stroke Trial

Easy Cap II CO$_2$ detector
EAT
> ectopic atrial tachycardia

eating disorder
Eaton-Lambert syndrome
EBBS
> equal bilateral breath sounds

Ebola virus infection
ebonation
Ebstein anomaly
ebullism
eburnated bone
eccentric contraction
ecchymosed
ecchymosis, pl. **ecchymoses**
> bilateral medial orbital e.
> deep periorbital e.
> old e.

ecchymotic mask
ECF
> extended care facility

ECG, EKG
> electrocardiogram
> electrocardiography

ECG-gated ventriculography
echinococcosis
> bone e.

Echinodermata envenomation
echinoderm envenomation
echocardiography
> 2-dimensional e.
> dobutamine stress e.
> stress e.
> transesophageal e. (TEE)

echoing
eclampsia

ECLS
> extracorporeal life support

ECMO
> extracorporeal membrane oxygenation

ecstasy
ectasia
> duct e.
> dural e.

ectethmoid bone
ectocuneiform bone
ectopic
> e. atrial tachycardia (EAT)
> e. beat
> e. bone
> e. pregnancy

ectopy
> ventricular e.

eczema
> e. atopic dermatitis
> dyshidrotic e.
> nummular e.

ED
> emergency department

EDD
> esophageal detector device

edema
> acute pulmonary e.
> airway e.
> ambulant e.
> angioneurotic e.
> bilateral leg e.
> bone marrow e.
> brawny e.
> cardiogenic pulmonary e.
> cerebral e.
> cerebral cytotoxic e.
> cerebral vasogenic e.
> flash pulmonary e.
> high-altitude cerebral e. (HACE)
> high-altitude pulmonary e.
> hypervolemic pulmonary e.
> interstitial e.
> ischemic e.
> laryngeal e.
> leg e.
> lower extremity e.
> negative-pressure pulmonary e.
> nerve root e.
> neurogenic pulmonary e.
> noncardiogenic pulmonary e.
> nonpitting e.
> pedal e.
> pulmonary e.

E

edema *(continued)*
    susceptibility to high-altitude
      pulmonary e. (HAPE-S)
    vasogenic e.
edematous bowel
edentulism
edentulous
    e. mandibular fracture
    e. patient
edge
    ligament reflecting e.
    ligament shelving e.
Edinburgh suture
EDOU
    emergency department observation unit
edrophonium
EDTA
    ethylenediamine tetraacetic acid
education
    level of e.
EEA Auto Suture
EENT
    eyes, ears, nose, throat
EF
    ejection fraction
effacement
    nerve root sheath e.
effect
    additive e.
    adverse e.
    anticonvulsant e.
    blast e.
    bone e.
    central anticholinergic e.
    contrast e.
    cumulative e.
    deleterious e.
    digitalis e.
    dystonic e.
    endocrine e.
    extrapyramidal e.
    flutter-valve e.
    Haldane e.
    local e.
    Mach e.
    muscle e.
    nephrotoxic e.
    Penumbra e.
    peripheral anticholinergic e.
    placebo e.
    positive end-expiratory pressure e.
    proarrhythmic e.
    second gas e.
    side e.
    systemic e.
    untoward e.
    vagal e.
effective breathing
effectiveness

effector cell function
efferent digital nerve
Effexor toxicity
efficacious
efficacy
    E. and Safety of Subcutaneous
      Enoxaparin in Non-Q-Wave
      Coronary Events (ESSENCE)
    therapeutic e.
efflux
effort
    e. of breathing
    respiratory e.
effusion
    malignant pleural e.
    pericardial e.
    pleural e.
    pulmonary e.
    septic e.
    tense joint e.
eggshell fracture
egophony
egress of blood
EGTA
    esophageal gastric tube airway
    esophagogastric tube airway
    EGTA device
EH
    essential hypertension
Ehlers-Danlos syndrome
Ehrlichia
    E. chaffeensis
    E. phagocytophilia
ehrlichiosis
Eikenella corrodens brain abscess
Eisenmenger syndrome
ejection
    e. fraction (EF)
    e. murmur (EM)
EKG *(var. of ECG)*
elaboration
elapid snake bite
elastance
elastic
    e. bandage
    e. suture
elasticity
    muscle e.
    ventricular e.
elastin
Elavil
elbow
    e. bone
    e. dislocation
    e. extensor tendon
    e. fracture
    e. injury
    nursemaid's e.
    pulled e.

elder abuse
elderly patient
elective
electric
    e. shock
    e. suction device
electrical
    e. air humidifier
    e. burn
    e. injury
electrocardiogram (ECG, EKG)
electrocardiographic
    e. manifestation
    e. wave (QRS)
electrocardiography (ECG, EKG)
    ambulatory e. (AECG)
electrocautery
    bipolar e.
electrocution
electrolyte
    e. abnormality
    e. altering medication
    e. disorder
    e. disturbance
    e. imbalance
    e. replacement
    serum e.
    urine e.
electrolytic
electromagnetic radiation injury
electromechanical dissociation
electronic
    e. patient care reporting system
    e. PCR system
    e. stethoscope
electrophysiologic action
electropyrexia
electrostimulation for nonunion of
    fracture
electrotherapy
element
    bone marrow e.
elementary fracture
elephant foot fracture
elevated acidosis
elevation
    cholesterol e.
elevator
    bone e.
    fracture reducing e.
elimination

ELISA
    enzyme-linked immunosorbent assay
elixir
Ellestad protocol
Ellis
    E. technique
    E. technique for Barton fracture
    E. tooth fracture classification
elongation
    ligament e.
    e. and tortuosity
elucidate
elude
EM
    ejection murmur
emaciated
embarrassment
    e. of choice
    nerve root e.
embed
embedding
    bone e.
embolectomy
    suction e.
emboli (pl. of embolus)
embolic
    e. stroke
    e. syndrome
embolism
    acute gas e.
    air e.
    amniotic fluid e. (AFE)
    arterial air e.
    arterial gas e. (AGE)
    bone marrow e.
    bullet e.
    cerebral arterial gas e. (CAGE)
    cholesterol e.
    dysbaric air e. (DAE)
    fat e.
    gas e.
    microbubble e.
    paradoxical e.
    pulmonary e. (PE)
    septic e.
    venous air e.
embolization
    angiographic e.
    bronchial artery e.
    splenic artery e.
    venous air e.
embolus, pl. emboli

E

NOTES

embolus *(continued)*
  bone marrow e.
  gas e.
embryo
embryonic
  e. bone
  e. sac
  e. umbilical vein
EMD
  emergency medical dispatcher
EMDR
  eye movement desensitization and
  reprocessing
emepronium bromide
emerge
emergency
  e. admission
  e. call service
  e. cardiac pacing
  e. care
  e. cesarean section
  e. department (ED)
  e. department observation unit
  (EDOU)
  diving e.
  e. doctrine
  hypertensive e.
  life-threatening e.
  e. medical dispatcher (EMD)
  e. medical radio service (EMRS)
  e. medical service (EMS)
  e. medical service system (EMSS)
  e. medical technician (EMT)
  e. medical technician–advanced
  (EMT-A)
  e. medical technician–basic (EMT-
  B)
  e. medical technician–intermediate
  (EMT-I)
  e. medical technician–paramedic
  (EMT-P)
  e. medicine
  non-life-threatening e.
  e. room (ER)
emergent
  e. angioplasty
  e. decompression
  e. laparotomy
  e. operative intervention
  e. surgical consultation
emesis
  e. basin
  coffee-grounds e.
  nausea and e.
  salivation, lacrimation, urination,
  diarrhea, gastric cramping, e.
  (SLUDGE)
emetic agent
emetocathartic

eminent
EMIP
  European Myocardial Infarction Project
emissary vein
EMIT
  enzyme multiplied immunoassay
  technique
EMLA
  eutectic mixture of local anesthetics
emollient
emotional
  e. abuse
  e. age
  e. catharsis
  e. immobilization
empathize
emphysema
  bullous e.
  centrilobar e.
  cervical subcutaneous e.
  panacinar e.
  panlobular e.
  pulmonary interstitial e. (PIE)
  pure e.
  subcutaneous e.
emphysematous
  e. chest
  e. cholecystitis
  e. pyelonephritis
empiric
  e. therapy
  e. treatment
  e. use of antibiotics
empirical dextrose
emptying
  gastric e.
empyema
  loculated e.
  thoracic e.
EMRS
  emergency medical radio service
EMS
  emergency medical service
    EMS Immobile-VAC pediatric
    universal mattress
EMSS
  emergency medical service system
EMT
  emergency medical technician
EMT-A
  emergency medical technician–advanced
EMT-B
  emergency medical technician–basic
EMT-I
  emergency medical
  technician–intermediate
EMT-P
  emergency medical technician–paramedic

emulsion
> wound dressing e.

en
> en bloc
> en bloc running locking suture

enalapril

enalaprilat

enamel fracture

encainide hydrochloride

encapsulated abscess

encased tumor

encephalic nerve

encephalitis
> herpes e.
> herpes simplex e.
> *Herpesvirus hominis* e.
> HVH e.
> varicella e.
> Venezuelan equine e.

encephalopathy
> hemorrhagic shock and e. (HSE)
> hepatic e.
> hypertensive e.
> hypoxic ischemic e.
> postshunt e.
> septic e.
> toxic-metabolic e.
> uremic e.
> Wernicke e.

encompass

encysted abscess

end
> bone e.
> e. point

endarterectomy
> carotid e.

end-diastolic pressure

endemic disease

Ender
> E. rod fixation
> E. rod fixation of fracture

end-expiratory
> e.-e. alveolar recruitment
> e.-e. pressure

ending
> nerve e.

end-inspiratory
> e.-i. pause
> e.-i. plateau

endocarditis
> acute infective e.
> bacterial e.

> candidal e.
> infectious e.
> infective e.
> e. prophylaxis
> prosthetic valve e. (PVE)
> staphylococcal prosthetic valve e.
> subacute bacterial e. (SBE)

endocardium

endocrine
> e. disorder
> e. effect
> e. effects of bedrest
> e. fracture

end-of-life issue

endogenous
> e. catecholamine release
> e. depression
> e. pyrogen
> e. transmission

EndoGrip endotracheal tube holder

Endoloop suture

endometrial lesion

endometriosis

endometritis

endomorph

endomorphic

endophthalmitis
> *Candida* e.

endoplasm

end-organ
> e.-o. dysfunction
> e.-o. infarction

endoscopic
> e. gastrostomy
> e. papillotomy
> e. retrograde
> cholangiopancreatography (ERCP)

endoscopy

endothelia permeability

endotoxin

endotracheal (ET)
> e. intubation (ETI)
> e. stylet
> e. tube (ETT)
> e. tube cuff stiffness
> e. tube management

Endotrol tracheal tube

endplate
> muscle e.

endpoint
> e. characteristic
> e. of motion

E

NOTES

end-stage
    e.-s. liver disease
    e.-s. renal disease (ESRD)
end-systolic pressure
end-to-end suture
end-to-side suture
enema
    analeptic e.
    barium e.
    coffee e.
energy
    kinetic e.
    muscle e.
engorge
engorged vein
engorgement
    breast e.
    macular venous e.
enhanced
    e. 911
    e. cardiac automaticity
enigmatci fever
enigmatic
enlargement
    aortic root e.
    discrete organ e.
    muscle e.
Enlimomab Acute Stroke Trial (EAST)
enoxaparin
ENT
    ear, nose, throat
entactogen
Entamoeba
    E. histolytica
    E. histolytica infection
enteral
    e. administration
    e. drug
    e. feeding
    e. nutrition
    e. perforation
enteric
    e. abscess
    e. fever
Enterobacter cloacae
Enterobacteriaceae infection
Enterobius
    E. vermicularis
    E. vermicularis infection
Enterococcus faecalis
enterocutaneous fistula
enteropathy
    necrotizing e.
    protein-losing e.
enterotoxin
    staphylococcal e. B
entocuneiform bone
entrainment
    jet e.

entrance
    wound e.
    e. wound
entrapment
    nerve plexus e.
    nerve root e.
    tendon e.
entrapped
    e. nerve
    e. plantar sesamoid bone
entropy
entry
    route of e.
entry-exit burn
entubulation
    nerve e.
enucleate
envenomation
    Annelida e.
    arthropod e.
    beaded lizard e.
    caterpillar e.
    catfish e.
    centipede e.
    coelenterate e.
    coral snake e.
    crotalid e.
    echinoderm e.
    Echinodermata e.
    Gila monster e.
    Hydrophiidae e.
    Hymenoptera e.
    jellyfish e.
    lion fish e.
    lizard e.
    mamba snake e.
    marine e.
    millipede e.
    octopus e.
    pit viper e.
    scorpion e.
    snake e.
    stingray e.
environment
    patient e.
    physical e.
environmental
    e. illness
    E. Protection Agency (EPA)
    e. stressor
enzymatic therapy
enzyme
    angiotensin-converting e. (ACE)
    cardiac e.
    e. multiplied immunoassay
       technique (EMIT)
    muscle e.
enzyme-linked immunosorbent assay
    (ELISA)

EOA
esophageal obturator airway
EOA device
eosinophil
eosinophilic granuloma of bone
EPA
Environmental Protection Agency
eparsalgia
ephedrine
aminophylline, phenobarbital, e.
(APE)
ephemeral fever
EPIC
Evaluation of 7E3 for the Prevention of
Ischemic Complications
epicondylar avulsion fracture
epicranial muscle
epidemic vertigo
epidemiologic
epidermic cell
epidermis
epidermoid inclusion cyst
epididymitis and orchitis
epidural
e. abscess
e. brain abscess
e. hematoma
e. infection
e. local anesthesia block
e. meningitis
e. puncture
epigastric
e. calcification
e. chest pain
e. inferior vein
e. vein
epigastrium
epiglottiditis
epiglottis
epiglottitis
adult e.
pediatric e.
epihyal ligament
epihyoid bone
epilepsy
adult-onset e.
epileptic seizure
epilepticus
status e.
epinephrine
e. auto-injector

bupivacaine with e.
lidocaine with e.
e. therapy
epineurial suture
EpiPen Jr
epiperineurial suture
epiphysial
e. growth plate fracture
e. injury
e. plate
e. slip fracture
e. tibial fracture
epiphysis
e. bone
bone lesion e.
slipped capital femoral e.
epipteric bone
episcleral vein
episcleritis
episiotomy
episode
syncopal e.
transient cerebral ischemic e.
(TCIE)
transient ischemic e. (TIE)
Epistat
E. balloon
E. nasal catheter
E. II nasal catheter
epistatic
epistaxis
anterior e.
posterior e.
episternal bone
episternum
epitendinous suture
epitenon suture
epithelialization
epithelium, pl. **epithelia**
muscle e.
epitrochleoanconeus muscle
eponym
epoprostenol
epoxy resin
epsilon, ε
e. aminocaproic acid (EACA)
Epstein-Barr infection
EPTFE
expanded polytetrafluoroethylene
EPTFE vascular suture
eptifibatide

E

NOTES

equal
> e. bilateral breath sounds (EBBS)
> bilateral, symmetrical, and e. (BSE)

equality
> respiratory e.

equipment
> chemical detection e.
> personal protective e. (PPE)

Equisetene suture

equivalent
> metabolic e.'s (METS)

equivocal
> e. finding
> e. symptom

ER
> emergency room

ERCP
> endoscopic retrograde
> cholangiopancreatography

erector spinae muscle

ergonovine therapy

ergot
> e. alkaloid
> e. fungus toxicity

ergotamine
> e. tartrate toxicity
> e. therapy

erosio interdigitalis

erosion
> bone e.
> esophageal e.

erosive

error
> inborn e.'s

ER-TIMI
> Early Retavase-Thrombolysis In
> Myocardial Infarction

eructation

eruption
> creeping e.
> papulosquamous e.
> seabather's e.

eruptive fever

ERV
> expiratory reserve volume

erysipelas
> surgical e.

erythema
> e. infectiosum
> e. multiforme
> e. nodosum
> pharyngeal e.
> varying degrees of e.

erythematosus
> chilblain lupus e.
> systemic lupus e. (SLE)

erythematous mucous membrane

erythrityl tetranitrate

erythroderma

erythrohepatic porphyria

erythromelalgia
> primary e.

erythromycin ophthalmic preparation

erythropoietin abuse

escape loop

eschar

escharotomy

Escherichia coli

esmolol

esodic nerve

esophageal
> e. candidiasis
> e. capnometry
> e. detector device (EDD)
> e. disruption
> e. diverticulum
> e. erosion
> e. fistula
> e. foreign body
> e. gastric tube airway (EGTA)
> e. injury
> e. luminal pCO_2
> e. obturator
> e. obturator airway (EOA)
> e. obturator intubation technique
> e. perforation
> e. rupture
> e. stenting
> e. tracheal Combitube (ETC)
> e. trauma
> e. variceal bleeding
> e. vein

esophagi (*pl. of* esophagus)

esophagitis
> chronic e.
> reflux e.

esophagocardiac junction

esophagogastric tube airway (EGTA)

esophagoscopy
> flexible e.

esophagram
> contrast e.

esophagus, pl. **esophagi**
> Barrett e.
> nutcracker e.

ESRD
> end-stage renal disease

ESSENCE
> Efficacy and Safety of Subcutaneous
> Enoxaparin in Non-Q-Wave Coronary
> Events
> ESSENCE trial

essential
> e. hypertension (EH)
> e. thrombocytopenia

Essex-Lopresti joint depression fracture

ester anesthetic

estimated time of arrival (ETA)

estradiol
  ethinyl e.
estrogen
ET
  endotracheal
ETA
  estimated time of arrival
ETC
  esophageal tracheal Combitube
ethambutol
ethanol
  e. abuse
  e. intoxication
ethanolamine
ethchlorvynol toxicity
ether
  bischloromethyl e.
Ethibond
  E. extra polyester suture
  E. polybutylate-coated polyester
  suture
Ethicon
  E. micropoint suture
  E. Sabreloc suture
  E. silk suture
Ethicon-Atraloc suture
Ethiflex retention suture
Ethilon nylon suture
ethinyl estradiol
ethmoid
  e. bone
  perpendicular plate of e.
  e. sinus
ethmoidal
  e. nerve
  e. vein
ethmoidolacrimal suture
ethmoidomaxillary suture
ethosuximide
ethyl
  e. acrylate
  e. alcohol (EtOH, ETOH)
  e. chloride spray
ethylene
  e. glycol
  e. glycol intoxication
  e. glycol poisoning
  e. thiourea
ethylenediamine tetraacetic acid (EDTA)
ethylnebis
ETI
  endotracheal intubation

etiologic
etiology, pl. **etiologies**
  infectious e.
  nonemergent e.
ETKM
  every test known to man
EtOH, ETOH
  ethyl alcohol
etomidate
ETT
  endotracheal tube
euphoria
euphoriant
euphoric affect
eupnea
eupneic
European Myocardial Infarction Project (EMIP)
eustachian muscle
eutectic mixture of local anesthetics (EMLA)
euthanasia
euthyroid
Eutonyl
evacuation
evaluation
  Acute Physiology and Chronic
  Health E. (APACHE)
  E. of 7E3 for the Prevention of
  Ischemic Complications (EPIC)
  Glycoprotein Receptor Antagonist
  Patency E. (GRAPE)
  need for aggressive e.
  normal laboratory e.
  objective e.
  patient e. (PE)
  radiographic e.
  suicide risk e.
  trauma room e.
evaporation
  heat loss by e.
evaporative heat loss
event
  apparent life-threatening e. (ALTE)
  Efficacy and Safety of
  Subcutaneous Enoxaparin in Non-
  Q-Wave Coronary E.'s
  (ESSENCE)
  potassium-associated acute
  transfusion e.
eversion
  wound e.

E

NOTES

evert
everting mattress suture
every test known to man (ETKM)
evidence
    e. of cholecystitis
    dearth of e.
    powerful e.
evident bruising
eviscerated bowel
evisceration
    abdominal e.
evulsion
    nerve e.
Ewald tube
Ewing sarcoma
exacerbate
exacerbation
    abrupt e.
    explained e.
    sudden e.
exam
    examination
examination (exam)
    bimanual e.
    bone marrow e.
    cardiovascular e.
    detailed physical e.
    focused history and physical e.
    frequent abdominal e.
    mental status e. (MSE)
    muscle e.
    negative e.
    papillary e.
    physical e. (PE)
    slit-lamp e.
    sputum e.
exanthema, exanthem
    pediatric e.
    e. subitum
    viral e.
excess
    acetylcholine e.
    base e.
    mineralocorticoid e.
excess/deficit
    base e./d.
excessive
    e. extension
    e. flexion
exchange
    alveolar-capillary gas e.
    capillary-cellular gas e.
    gas e.
    guidewire e.
    plasma e.
    therapeutic plasma e.
exchanger
    intravascular blood gas e.

excision
    bone cyst e.
    wound e.
excitability
    cardiac e.
excitation-contraction coupling
excitatory amino acid neurotransmitter
excitoreflex nerve
excitor nerve
excitotoxicity
excrement
excrescence
excretion
    cortisol e.
    fractional e.
excursion
    chest e.
    tendon e.
exenteration
exercise
    e. bone
    isotonic e.
    e. tolerance
exertion
    dyspnea on e. (DOE)
exertional
    e. dyspnea
    e. headache
    e. heart stroke
exfoliative dermatitis
exhaustion
    heat e.
    salt depletion heat e.
    water depletion heat e.
exhilarated
exit wound
exoccipital bone
exodic nerve
exogenous obesity
exophytic
exotoxin
    staphylococcal e.
expanded
    e. polytetrafluoroethylene (EPTFE)
    e. polytetrafluoroethylene suture
expander
    blood volume e.
    plasma e.
expansion
    bone e.
    symmetrical chest e.
expectancy
expectant treatment
expected course and prognosis
expectorant
expediency
expiration
expiratory
    inspiratory to e. (I:E)

e. muscle
e. reserve volume (ERV)
e. rhonchi
e. upstroke
e. wheeze

explained exacerbation
explanation
vague e.

exploration
digital e.
local e.
local wound e.

exploratory
e. laparotomy
e. surgery

explosion fracture
exposure
airway, breathing, circulation,
disability, and e. (ABCDE)
asbestos e.
body fluid e.
bone e.
cadmium e.
cold e.
dust e.
hazardous material e.
heat e.
ingestion e.
inhalation e.
irritant gas e.
radiation e.
soap e.
time of e.
toxin e.

expressed
e. consent
e. skull fracture

expressive aphasia
expulsion
high-altitude flatus e. (HAFE)

exsanguination
extended
e. care
e. care facility (ECF)

extensibility
muscle e.

extension
excessive e.
e. teardrop fracture

extensive
e. gingival involvement
e. hepatic metabolism

extensor
e. back muscle
e. carpi radialis brevis muscle
e. carpi radialis longus muscle
e. carpi ulnaris muscle
e. communis muscle
e. digiti minimi muscle
e. digiti quinti muscle
e. digitorum brevis muscle
e. digitorum communis muscle
e. digitorum longus muscle
e. hallucis brevis muscle
e. hallucis longus muscle
e. indicis proprius muscle
e. pollicis brevis muscle
e. pollicis longus muscle
e. tendon
e. tendon central slip
e. wad of 3 muscles

externa
malignant otitis e.
otitis e.

external
e. abdominal muscle
e. anal sphincter muscle
e. auditory canal
e. auditory canal irrigation
e. auditory meatus
e. bleeding
e. calcaneoastragaloid ligament
e. carotid nerve
e. carotid vein
e. chest compression
e. cruciate ligament
e. ear abscess
e. ear cellulitis
e. ear chondritis
e. ear chondritis abscess
e. fixation
e. flash over
e. iliac vein
e. intercostal muscle
e. jugular vein
e. lateral ligament
e. mammary vein
e. naris
e. nasal nerve
e. nasal vein
e. oblique muscle
e. obturator muscle
e. orbital fracture
e. pacemaker

E

NOTES

external (*continued*)
 e. palatine vein
 e. popliteal nerve
 e. pterygoid muscle
 e. pterygoid nerve
 e. pterygoid vein
 e. pudendal vein
 e. pudic vein
 e. radial vein
 e. rectus muscle
 e. rotator muscle
 e. saphenous nerve
 e. spermatic nerve
 e. spermatic vein
 e. sphincter ani profundus muscle
 e. sphincter muscle
 e. temporary pacing
 e. transcutaneous cardiac pacing
extraabdominal radiation
extraalveolar gas
extraarticular
 e. fracture
 e. knee ligament
extracapsular
 e. fracture
 e. ligament
extracardiac obstructive shock
extracerebral
extrachromic suture
extracorporeal
 e. CO_2 removal
 e. life support (ECLS)
 e. membrane oxygenation (ECMO)
 e. method
 e. renal replacement therapy
extracostal muscle
extract
 allergenic e.
extraction
 partial breech e.
 total breech e.
extractor
 bone e.
 Sawyer e.
extradural
 e. hematoma
 e. hemorrhage
extrahepatic
 e. duct
 e. portal vein

extralaryngeal muscle
extraoctave fracture
extraocular
 e. movement
 e. muscle
extrapolate
extrapyramidal effect
extrarenal
 e. fluid removal
 e. loss
extravasation
extravascular lung water
extreme apathy
extremity
 both upper e.'s (BUE)
 cyanotic e.
 e. fracture
 left lower e. (LLE)
 left upper e. (LUE)
 e. lift technique
 right lower e. (RLE)
 right upper e. (RUE)
 e. trauma
extrication device
extrinsic
 e. coagulation pathway
 e. foot muscle
 e. ligament
 e. nerve
extrusion
 bone graft e.
extubate
extubation protocol
exuberance
exuberant tumor
exudate
 seropurulent e.
exudative bronchiolitis
eye
 e.'s, ears, nose, throat (EENT)
 e. movement desensitization and
  reprocessing (EMDR)
 raccoon e.'s
 red e.
 tender e.
eyebrow laceration
eyelid
 e. crease suture
 e. laceration
 e. muscle

fabellofibular ligament
facet
    vitreous hemorrhage f.
facial
    f. abrasion
    f. asymmetry
    f. bone
    f. droop
    f. fracture
    f. mimetic muscle
    f. muscle
    f. nerve
    f. nerve injury
    f. paralysis
    f. soft tissue avulsion
    f. soft tissue injury
    f. symmetry
    f. trauma
    f. vein
facilitated percutaneous coronary intervention
facility
    acute care f. (ACF)
    adult congregate living f.
    extended care f. (ECF)
    hyperbaric f.
    skilled nursing f. (SNF)
factitious wound
factor
    cardiac risk f. (CRF)
    clotting f.
    colony-stimulating f. (CSF)
    cortisol-releasing f. (CRF)
    Hageman f.
    hemorrhagic stress-induced serum f.
    institutional f.
    f. IX replacement therapy
    nerve f.
    nerve growth f.
    palliative f.
    predisposing f.
    provocative f.
    Rh f.
    tumor necrosis f.
    f. VIII:C level
    f. VIII concentrate
    f. VIII replacement therapy
    f. V Leiden (FVL)
    von Willebrand f.
    wind-chill f.
    f. XI deficiency
Faden suture
faecalis
    Enterococcus f.
failed airway

failure
    acute alveolar hyperventilation on chronic ventilatory f.
    acute renal f. (ARF)
    acute respiratory f. (ARF)
    bone marrow f.
    cardiac f.
    chronic renal f.
    complete hepatic f.
    congestive heart f. (CHF)
    contrast-induced renal f.
    fluid f.
    fulminant hepatic f. (FHF)
    heart f. (HF)
    hemodialysis for renal f.
    hepatic f.
    left heart f.
    left-sided heart f.
    left ventricular f.
    liver f.
    multiple organ f. (MOF)
    multiple organ system f.
    myoglobinuric renal f.
    organ f.
    f. to progress
    pulmonary f.
    renal f.
    respiratory f.
    suture f.
    f. to thrive
    treatment f.
    ventilatory f.
    wound f.
faint rhonchi
faith healing
falciform ligament
falciparum
    Plasmodium f.
fall
    f. onto outstretched hand (FOOSH)
    symmetric chest wall rise and f.
fallen
    f. lung
    f. lung sign
fallopian
    f. ligament
    f. tube
Fallot
    tetralogy of F.
    F. tetralogy
false
    f. aneurysm
    f. ligament
    f. lumen
    f. rib

F

false *(continued)*
    f. suture
    f. tendon
falx laceration
famciclovir
familial
    f. hypoparathyroidism
    f. varicose vein
family
    f. history (FH)
    f. practice (FP)
famotidine
Fansidar
FAS
    fetal alcohol syndrome
fascia, pl. **fasciae**
    cribriform f.
    dehiscence of f.
    muscle f.
    muscular f.
fascial
    f. dilator
    f. interconnection
    f. involvement
    f. sheath
    f. suture
fascicle
    muscle f.
    nerve f.
fascicular block
fasciculation
    muscle f.
fasciculus
fasciitis
    necrotizing f.
    plantar f.
    proliferative f.
fasciotomy
FAST
    focused abdominal sonography for
      trauma
fast
    f. muscle
    protein-sparing modified f. (PSMF)
fasting ketoacidosis
fast-track care
fast-twitch muscle
fat
    f. embolism
    f. embolism syndrome (FES)
    f. fracture
    f. necrosis
fatigability
fatigue
    f. fracture
    muscle f.
    suture f.
fatty liver

FB
    foreign body
F/C
    fevers and chills
F&D
    fixed and dilated
FDA
    Food and Drug Administration
FDP
    fibrin degradation product
Fe
    iron
febrile
    f. illness
    f. nonhemolytic transfusion reaction
    f. reaction
    f. seizure
fecal impaction
feces
federal
    F. Emergency Management Agency
      (FEMA)
    F. Hazardous Substance Act
      (FHSA)
feeblemindedness
feeble pulse
feeder vein
feeding
    f. button
    enteral f.
    tube f.
    f. tube
    f. tube complication
felon
    bone f.
felonious assault
FEMA
    Federal Emergency Management Agency
female
    African-American f.
    Asian f. (AF)
    black f.
    Caucasian f.
    Hispanic f.
    middle-aged f.
    Oriental f.
    sexually active f.
    white middle-aged f.
femoral
    f. artery
    f. bone
    f. cutaneous nerve
    f. diaphysial fracture
    f. fracture
    f. head
    f. intertrochanteric fracture
    f. ligament
    f. muscle
    f. neck fracture

f. nerve
f. pulse
f. shaft fracture
f. supracondylar fracture
f. vein
femorofemoral bypass
femoropopliteal vein
femur fracture
FENa
  fractional excretion of sodium
fencer's bone
fender fracture
fenestrated
  f. oculomotor nerve
  f. sheath
fenestration
fenofibrate
fenoldopam mesylate
fentanyl
  designer f.
fermenter-2
  dysgonic f.-2 (DF-2)
Fermi vaccine
Ferrein ligament
ferric chloride test
fervescence
FES
  fat embolism syndrome
fetal
  f. alcohol syndrome (FAS)
  f. beat-to-beat variability
  f. bone fracture
  f. distress
  f. fracture
  f. heart tones
  f. intrahepatic vein
  f. lie
  f. malnutrition
  f. monitoring
  f. to neonatal circulation
  f. Y suture
fetid
fetomaternal
  f. hemorrhage
  f. transfusion
fetoplacental anasarca
fetus
  crowning of f.
  nonviable f.
  viability of f.
FEV$_1$
  forced expiratory volume in 1 second

fever
  adult f.
  f. adult
  artificial f.
  aseptic f.
  biphasic f.
  carbuncular f.
  cat-scratch f.
  f.'s and chills (F/C)
  cotton f.
  dehydration f.
  dengue f.
  drug f.
  enigmatci f.
  enteric f.
  ephemeral f.
  eruptive f.
  fracture f.
  glandular f.
  hay f.
  hemorrhagic f.
  hyperpyrexial f.
  intermittent f.
  low grade f.
  pediatric f.
  f. phobia
  polyfume f.
  pyogenic f.
  Q f.
  recrudescence of f.
  rheumatic f.
  Rocky Mountain spotted f.
  scarlet f.
  tactile f.
  transitory f.
  typhoid f.
  f. of undetermined origin (FUO)
  undulating f.
  f. of unknown origin (FUO)
  viral hemorrhagic f.
  wound f.
  yellow f.
feverfew
FEVT
  forced expired volume timed
FFP
  fresh frozen plasma
FH
  family history
FHF
  fulminant hepatic failure

F

NOTES

FHSA
Federal Hazardous Substance Act
fiber
muscle f.
nerve f.
fiberglass splint
fiberoptic
f. bronchoscope intubation
f. bronchoscopy
f. intubation
f. laryngoscope
f. laryngoscope intubation
f. laryngoscopy
fibril
nerve f.
fibrillation
atrial f.
recurrent atrial f.
synchronized atrial f.
ventricular f. (VF)
fibrin
f. degradation product (FDP)
f. formulation
f. gel
f. glue
fibrinogen
f. degradation product
f. level
fibrinogen-fibrin conversion syndrome
fibrinolysis
fibroblast
bone marrow f.
wound f.
fibrocystic breast disease
fibroid tumor
fibrolipomatous hamartoma nerve
fibroma
fibromuscular dysplasia
fibromyalgia
fibrosarcoma
bone f.
fibrosed muscle
fibrosing alveolitis
fibrosis
bone marrow f.
cystic f.
distal intestinal obstruction
syndrome of cystic f.
idiopathic pulmonary f. (IPF)
interstitial f.
interstitial pulmonary f. (IPF)
muscle f.
pulmonary f.
fibrositis
fibrous bone dysplasia
fibula
fibular
f. collateral ligament
f. diaphysial fracture

f. muscle
f. nerve
f. sesamoidal ligament
f. sesamoid bone
f. shaft fracture
f. vein
fibularis
f. brevis muscle
f. longus muscle
f. tertius muscle
fibulocalcaneal ligament
fibulotalar ligament
fibulotalocalcaneal ligament
Fick
F. method
F. principle
F. technique
field
f. block
high-power f. (HPF)
nerve f.
f. triage
Fielding-Magliato subtrochanteric
fracture classification
fifth
f. disease
f. metatarsal base fracture
fifth-day fit
fighter's fracture
figure-of-8 suture
filament suture
filariasis
file
bone f.
filling
muscle f.
film
long bone f.
plain f.
filter
IVC f.
muscle f.
vena caval f.
filtration
HEPA f.
plasma f.
fimbriated fold
fimbriation
financial
f. abuse
f. dependence
f. dependence upon patient
finding
dearth of f.
equivocal f.
incongruous f.
physical exam f.
f.'s reflect underlying disease
salient f.

fine
    f. chromic suture
    f. silk suture
fine-needle aspiration (FNA)
finger
    baseball f.
    f. flexor muscle
    f. fracture
    mallet f.
    f. oximeter
    f. oximetry
    f. splint
    f. sweep
    f. sweep technique
    f. trap
fingerbreadth
fingernail cosmetic ingestion
fingertip injury
fingertrap suture
FIO_2
    fractional concentration of inspired
    oxygen
fire
    f. ant bite
    f. ant sting
fire-induced cyanide toxicity
fireworks injury
first
    f. aid
    f. aid kit
    f. carpometacarpal joint fracture
    f. cuneiform bone
    f. dorsal interosseous muscle
    f. intention
    f. intermetacarpal ligament
    f. palmar interosseous muscle
    f. responder
    f. trimester
first-degree
    f.-d. atrioventricular block
    f.-d. AV block
    f.-d. burn
    f.-d. hyperthermia
    f.-d. injury
    f.-d. laceration
first-line drug
first-order kinetics
fish botulism
fishhook removal
fishmouth
    f. end-to-end suture

    f. fracture
    f. wound
fissure
    anal f.
    f. in ano
    f. fracture
    genital f.
fissured chest
fistula, pl. **fistulae, fistulas**
    anal f.
    anorectal f.
    aortoenteric f. (AEF)
    biliary f.
    bronchopleural f. (BPF)
    cavernous sinus f.
    enterocutaneous f.
    esophageal f.
    perilymph f.
    postoperative ileal f.
    postoperative jejunal f.
    f. test
    tracheoinnominate f.
    transesophageal f.
    urinary tract f.
fit
    fifth-day f.
Fitz-Hugh-Curtis syndrome
fixation
    bone suture f.
    Ender rod f.
    external f.
    fracture f.
    internal f.
    open reduction and internal f.
    (ORIF)
    suture f.
    f. suture
fixator muscle
fixed
    f. and dilated (F&D)
    f. suction unit
fixed-dose oral contraceptive tablet
flaccid
flagellate protozoa
Flagg blade
Flagyl
flail
    f. chest
    f. chest sign
    f. segment
flake hamate fracture

F

NOTES

flank
   f. bone
   f. gunshot wound
   f. hematoma
   f. pain
flap
   bone f.
   muscle f.
   V f.
   vein f.
   V-Y advancement f.
flare
   asthma f.
flaring
   grunting and f.
   nasal f.
flash
   f. burn
   light f.
   peripheral light f.
   f. pulmonary edema
flat
   f. affect
   f. frontal bone
   f. muscle
   f. neck vein
   f. suture
flatulence
Flaxedil suture
flecainide acetate
fleck
   f. fracture
   f. sign
Fleischmann bursa
flesh
   proud f.
flexibility
flexible
   f. esophagoscopy
   f. plastic catheter
   f. plastic suction catheter
   f. stretcher
flexion
   excessive f.
   f. teardrop fracture
flexion-burst fracture
flexion-compression fracture
flexion-distraction fracture
Flexitone suture
flexor
   f. accessorius muscle
   f. bursa
   f. carpi radialis muscle
   f. carpi ulnaris muscle
   f. digiti quinti brevis muscle
   f. digitorum brevis muscle
   f. digitorum longus muscle
   f. digitorum profundus muscle
   f. digitorum sublimis muscle

   f. digitorum superficialis muscle
   f. hallucis brevis muscle
   f. hallucis longus muscle
   f. muscle
   f. pollicis brevis
   f. pollicis brevis muscle
   f. pollicis longus muscle
   f. tendon
   f. tendon injury
   f. tendon laceration
   f. tenosynovitis
flight
   f. crew
   f. into disease
   F. for Life
   f. team
Flight-for-Life transfer
floater
floating
   f. arch fracture
   f. black speck
   f. ligament
   f. shoulder
flocculus, pl. flocculi
Flood ligament
floor fracture
floribunda
   Pieris f.
florid infection
flow
   antegrade f.
   blood f.
   cerebral blood f. (CBF)
   f. chart
   f. control
   inspiratory f.
   laminar f.
   peak blood f.
   f. rate
   f. rate value
   f. restricted oxygen-powered
      ventilation device
   skin blood f. (SkBF)
   turbulent f.
flow-cycled ventilator
flower bone
flowmeter
**flow-restricted oxygen powered
   ventilation**
fluconazole
fluctuant
flucytosine
fludrocortisone
fluid
   amniotic f.
   bone f.
   bronchoalveolar lavage f. (BALF)
   cerebrospinal f. (CSF)
   f. challenge

crystalloid f.
f. disturbance
f. failure
free f.
hypertonic f.
inability to tolerate oral f.
intraperitoneal f.
oral f.
f. overload
pericholecystic f.
f. replacement
f. resuscitation
serosanguineous f.
f. therapy
turbid f.
wound f.
fluke infection
Flumadine
flumazenil
fluoresce
fluorescein
fluorescence
diaper f.
fluorescens
Pseudomonas f.
fluoride
fluoroquinolone antibiotic
fluoroscope
fluoxetine
fluphenazine
flurazepam
flushed skin
fluticasone propionate
flutter
atrial f.
synchronized atrial f.
ventricular f.
flutter-valve effect
FNA
fine-needle aspiration
foam
Allevyn f.
LYOfoam f.
Synthaderm f.
focal
f. deficit
f. lesion
f. region
focus, pl. **foci**
Ghon f.
focused
f. abdominal sonography

f. abdominal sonography for
trauma (FAST)
f. history and physical examination
f. medical assessment
f. trauma assessment
Fogarty vascular catheter
fogging
tube f.
folate deficiency
fold
alar f.
fimbriated f.
intragluteal f.
mucobuccal f.
folding fracture
Foley catheter
folic acid
Folius muscle
follicle
folliculitis
followup (FU)
f. care
close f.
fomepizole
fontanelle
anterior f.
bulging f.
depressed f.
posterior f.
retracted f.
sunken f.
food
f. additive
f. allergen
caffeine, alcohol, pepper, spicy f.
(CAPS)
F. and Drug Administration (FDA)
f. particle
f. poisoning
foodborne
f. disease
f. toxin
food-drug interaction
FOOSH
fall onto outstretched hand
foot
f. bone
f. fracture
f. phalangeal injury
f. puncture wound
trench f.

F

NOTES

footprint
    tibial f.
force
    direct f.
    indirect f.
    nerve f.
    twisting f.
forced
    f. diuresis
    f. duction test
    f. expiratory volume
    f. expiratory volume in 1 second
      (FEV_1)
    f. expired volume timed (FEVT)
    f. respiration
    f. velocity curve
    f. vital capacity (FVC)
forced-air technique
forceps
    Adson f.
    alligator f.
    apposition f.
    Asch f.
    bayonet f.
    bone f.
    f. fracture
    Magill f.
    McGill f.
    mosquito f.
    nontoothed f.
    suture clip f.
    suture grasper f.
    suture tag f.
    toothed f.
    wound f.
forearm fracture
foreign
    f. body (FB)
    f. body aspiration
    f. body ingestion
    f. body obstruction
    f. body removal
    f. object
forensic psychiatry
formaldehyde
    f. catgut suture
    f. inhalation injury
    f. odor
formalin toxicity
formation
    bone f.
    bone matrix f.
    callous f.
    slab avalanche f.
    vesicle f.
formic acid
formula, pl. **formulae, formulas**
    chemical f.

Galveston fluid needs f.
Parkland fluid resuscitation f.
formulary
formulation
    fibrin f.
Fortaz
foscarnet
Foscavir
Foster suture
Fothergill suture
foul breath
Fournier gangrene
fourth
    f. carpometacarpal joint fracture
    f. turbinated bone
fourth-degree
    f.-d. burn
    f.-d. hyperthermia
    f.-d. laceration
fourth-layer spinal muscle
fovea centralis bone
foveal ligament
foveola, pl. **foveolae**
Fowler
    F. dead space
    F. position
foxglove toxicity
FP
    family practice
FRACAS
    fracture computer-aided surgery
fraction
    dead-space f.
    ejection f. (EF)
    plasma protein f.
    right ventricular ejection f.
    ventricular ejection f.
fractional
    f. concentration of inspired oxygen
      (FIO_2)
    f. excretion
    f. excretion of sodium (FENa)
fracture
    abduction f.
    abduction-external rotation f.
    accessory navicular f.
    accessory ossicle f.
    acetabular posterior wall f.
    acetabular rim f.
    acute f.
    acute avulsion f.
    acute on chronic f.
    adduction f.
    adult-type III TIE f.
    agenetic f.
    AIIS avulsion f.
    Aitken classification of
      epiphysial f.

Allen open reduction of
  calcaneal f.
alveolar f.
alveolar bone f.
alveolar process f.
alveolar socket wall f.
anatomic f.
anatomic neck f.
Anderson-Hutchins unstable tibial
  shaft f.
angle f.
angulated f.
angulation f.
ankle f.
ankle mortise f.
anterior f.
anterior calcaneal process f.
anterior column f.
anterior rib f.
anteroinferior corner f.
anterolateral compression f.
anular f.
AO classification of ankle f.
apex f.
apophysial f.
arch f.
articular mass separation f.
articular pillar f.
artificial f.
Atkin epiphysial f.
atlantal f.
atlas-axis combination f.
atlas burst f.
f. at rhinion
atrophic f.
avulsion f.
avulsion chip f.
avulsion stress f.
axial compression f.
axial loading f.
axial load teardrop f.
axial load three-part, two-plane f.
axis f.
axis-atlas combination f.
backfire f.
banana f.
f. band
Bankart f.
f. bar
Barton f.
Barton-Smith f.
basal neck f.

basal skull f. (BSF)
baseball finger f.
basicervical f.
basilar femoral neck f.
basilar skull f.
bayonet position of f.
beak f.
f. bed
bedroom f.
bend f.
bending f.
Bennett basic hand f.
Bennett comminuted f.
Berndt-Hardy classification of
  transchondral f.
bicolumn f.
bicondylar T-shaped f.
bicondylar Y-shaped f.
bicycle spoke f.
bilateral condylar f.
bimalleolar f.
bimalleolar ankle f.
bipartite f.
birth f.
f. blister
blow-in f.
blowout f.
bone shaft f.
f. boot
boot-top f.
Bosworth f.
both-bone f.
both-column f.
bowing f.
f. box
boxer's punch f.
Boyd type II f.
f. bracing
Broberg-Morrey f.
bronchial f.
bucket-handle f.
buckle f.
bumper f.
bunk bed f.
Burkhalter-Reyes method
  phalangeal f.
burst f.
bursting f.
butterfly f.
buttonhole f.
calcaneal avulsion f.
calcaneal displaced f.

NOTES

fracture *(continued)*
  calcaneal stress f.
  calcaneal type I–III f.
  calcaneus tongue f.
  f. callus
  f. callus loading
  calvarial f.
  Canale-Kelly talar neck f.
  capillary f.
  capitate f.
  capitellar f.
  capitulum f.
  carpal bone f.
  carpal bone stress f.
  carpal navicular f.
  carpal scaphoid bone f.
  carpometacarpal joint f.
  cartwheel f.
  Cedell f.
  cementum f.
  central f.
  cephalomedullary nail f.
  cerebral palsy pathological f.
  cervical f.
  cervical trochanteric displaced f.
  cervicotrochanteric displaced f.
  chalk-stick f.
  Chance vertebral f.
  Chaput f.
  Charcot f.
  chauffeur's f.
  chevron f.
  childhood f.
  chip f.
  chiropractic treatment of f.
  chisel f.
  f. chisel
  chondral f.
  Chopart f.
  circumferential f.
  f. classification
  clavicle f.
  clavicle shaft f.
  clavicular f.
  clay shoveler's f.
  cleavage f.
  f. in close apposition
  closed f.
  closed ankle f.
  closed break f.
  closed indirect f.
  closed reduction of f.
  closed skull f.
  coccygeal f.
  coccyx f.
  Colles f.
  collicular f.
  Coltart f.
  combined f.

  combined flexion-distraction injury
    and burst f.
  combined radial-ulnar-humeral f.
  comminuted f.
  comminuted bursting f.
  comminuted intraarticular f.
  comminuted orbital f.
  comminuted skull f.
  comminuted teardrop f.
  complete f.
  complex f.
  complex simple f.
  complicated f.
  composite f.
  compound f.
  compound comminuted f.
  compound complex f.
  compound multiple f.'s
  compound skull f.
  compressed f.
  compression f.
  f. computer-aided surgery
    (FRACAS)
  f. computer-aided surgery system
  condylar f.
  condylar compression f.
  condylar process f.
  condylar split f.
  congenital f.
  Conrad-Bugg trapping of soft
    tissue in ankle f.
  f. by contrecoup
  contrecoup f.
  controlled comminuted f.
  coracoid f.
  corner f.
  coronal split f.
  coronoid f.
  coronoid process f.
  cortical f.
  Cotton ankle f.
  cough f.
  crack f.
  cranial f.
  craniofacial f.
  craniofacial dysjunction f.
  cribriform f.
  crown f.
  crown-root f.
  crush f.
  crushed eggshell f.
  cuboid f.
  cuneiform f.
  dancer's f.
  Danis-Weber f.
  Darrach-Hughston-Milch f.
  dashboard f.
  f. decompression
  decompression of f.

f. deformity
Denis spinal f.
dens f.
dental f.
dentate f.
dentoalveolar f.
depressed f.
depressed skull f.
depression f.
depression-type intraarticular f.
de Quervain f.
derby hat f.
Desault f.
Descot f.
f. deviation
diacondylar f.
diametric pelvic f.
diaphysial f.
f. diastasis
diastatic skull f.
dicondylar f.
die punch f.
direct f.
direct orbital floor f.
f. disease
dishpan f.
dislocation f.
f. dislocation
displaced f.
displaced intraarticular f.
displaced malar f.
displaced pilon f.
displaced tibia-fibula f.
displaced zygomatic f.
distal femoral epiphysial f.
distal humeral f.
distal radial f.
distal shaft forearm f.
distraction of f.
dog-leg f.
dome f.
dorsal rim distal radial f.
dorsal wing f.
double f.
double-rib f.
drill bit f.
Dupuytren f.
Duverney f.
dye punch f.
dyscrasic f.
edentulous mandibular f.
eggshell f.

elbow f.
electrostimulation for nonunion
 of f.
elementary f.
elephant foot f.
Ellis technique for Barton f.
enamel f.
f. en coin
Ender rod fixation of f.
endocrine f.
f. en rave
epicondylar avulsion f.
epiphysial growth plate f.
epiphysial slip f.
epiphysial tibial f.
Essex-Lopresti joint depression f.
explosion f.
expressed skull f.
extension teardrop f.
external orbital f.
extraarticular f.
extracapsular f.
extraoctave f.
extremity f.
facial f.
fat f.
fatigue f.
femoral f.
femoral diaphysial f.
femoral intertrochanteric f.
femoral neck f.
femoral shaft f.
femoral supracondylar f.
femur f.
fender f.
fetal f.
fetal bone f.
f. fever
fibular diaphysial f.
fibular shaft f.
fifth metatarsal base f.
fighter's f.
finger f.
first carpometacarpal joint f.
fishmouth f.
fissure f.
f. fixation
f. fixation device
flake hamate f.
fleck f.
flexion-burst f.
flexion-compression f.

NOTES

fracture *(continued)*
flexion-distraction f.
flexion teardrop f.
floating arch f.
floor f.
folding f.
foot f.
forceps f.
forearm f.
fourth carpometacarpal joint f.
fragility f.
f. fragment
f. fragment displacement
f. fragment distraction
f. fragment nonunion
f. fragment separation
f. frame
framework f.
Freiberg f.
frontal orbital nasoethmoidal f.
frontal sinus f.
Frykman hand f.
fulcrum f.
Gaenslen f.
Galeazzi radical f.
f. gap
Garden femoral neck f.
glabellar f.
glenoid rim f.
Gosselin f.
graft f.
greater trochanteric femoral f.
greater tuberosity f.
greenstick f.
greenstick Le Fort f.
grenade thrower's f.
gross f.
growing skull f.
growth plate f.
Guérin f.
gunshot f.
Gustilo-Anderson open clavicular f.
Gustilo tibial f.
gutter f.
Hahn-Steinthal f.
hairline f.
hamate body f.
hamate hook f.
hamate tail f.
hand f.
hangman's f.
Hawkins talus f.
head f.
head-splitting humeral f.
healed f.
f. healing
healing f.
heat f.
hemicondylar f.
hemitransverse f.
Henderson f.
Herbert scaphoid bone f.
Hermodsson f.
hickory-stick f.
high-energy f.
Hill-Sachs posterolateral
  compression f.
hindfoot f.
hip avulsion f.
hockey-stick f.
Hoffa f.
Holstein-Lewis f.
hook of the hamate f.
hoop stress f.
horizontal maxillary f.
horizontal oblique f.
humeral condylar f.
humeral head f.
humeral head-splitting f.
humeral physeal f.
humeral shaft f.
humeral supracondylar f.
humerus f.
Hunt-Hess hand f.
Hutchinson f.
hyoid bone f.
hyperextension teardrop f.
hyperflexion teardrop f.
ice skater's f.
idiopathic f.
impacted articular f.
impacted subcapital f.
impacted valgus f.
impaction f.
implant f.
impression f.
impure blowout f.
incomplete compound f.
incomplete vertical root f.
indented f.
indirect orbital floor f.
inflammatory f.
infraction f.
infraorbital f.
insufficiency f.
interarticular f.
intercondylar femoral f.
intercondylar humeral f.
intercondylar tibial f.
internal fixation f.
internally fixed f.
interperiosteal f.
intertrochanteric f.
intertrochanteric femoral f.
intertrochanteric hip f.
intertrochanteric 4-part f.
F. Intervention Trial
intraarticular calcaneal f.

intraarticular proximal tibial f.
intracapsular femoral neck f.
intraoperative f.
intraorbital f.
intraperiosteal f.
intrauterine f.
inverted-Y f.
ipsilateral acetabular f.
ipsilateral femoral neck f.
ipsilateral femoral shaft f.
ipsilateral pelvic f.
ipsilateral tibial f.
irreducible f.
ischioacetabular f.
isolated hook f.
Jefferson cervical burst f.
Jefferson radial f.
joint depression f.
Jones stress f.
J retention wire f.
Judet epiphysial f.
junctional f.
juvenile Tillaux f.
juxtaarticular f.
juxtacortical f.
Kapandji radical f.
Kocher f.
Kocher-Lorenz f.
Köhler f.
labral and anterior inferior glenoid
  rim f.
laminar f.
lap seat belt f.
laryngeal f.
laryngeal cartilage f.
larynx f.
lateral column calcaneal f.
lateral condylar f.
lateral condylar humeral f.
lateral humeral condyle f.
laterally displaced f.
lateral malleolus f.
lateral mass f.
lateral talar process f.
lateral tibial plateau f.
lateral wedge f.
Lauge-Hansen stage II supination-
  eversion f.
Laugier f.
lead pipe f.
Le Fort I-III f.
Le Fort mandibular f.

Le Fort-Wagstaffe f.
lesser trochanter f.
f. line
linear skull f.
f. line consolidation
Lisfranc f.
Lloyd-Roberts f.
local compression f.
local decompression f.
long bone f.
longitudinal f.
longitudinal tibial fatigue f.
long oblique f.
loose f.
Looser zone in insufficiency f.
lorry driver's f.
low-energy f.
lower extremity f.
lower frontal bone f.
low lumbar spine f.
low T humerus f.
lumbar spine f.
lumbar spine burst f.
lumbosacral junction f.
lunate f.
Maisonneuve fibular f.
malar complex f.
Malgaigne pelvic f.
malleolar chip f.
mallet f.
f. malreduction
malunited calcaneus f.
malunited forearm f.
malunited radial f.
mandibular f.
mandibular body f.
mandibular condyle f.
mandibular ramus f.
mandibular symphysis f.
march f.
marginal ridge f.
Marmor-Lynn f.
Mason f.
mastoid bone f.
maternal f.
maxillary f.
maxillofacial f.
medial column calcaneal f.
medial epicondyle humeral f.
f. medialization
medial malleolar f.
medial orbital wall f.

F

NOTES

117

fracture *(continued)*

mesiodistal f.
metacarpal head f.
metacarpal neck f.
metacarpal shaft f.
metaphysial avulsion f.
metaphysial tibial f.
metatarsal base f.
metatarsal neck f.
metatarsal stress f.
micronized purified flavonoid f.
middle tibial shaft f.
midface f.
midfacial f.
midfoot f.
midnight f.
midshaft f.
midwaist scaphoid f.
milkman's f.
minimally displaced f.
mini-pilon f.
missed f.
Moberg-Gedda f.
molar tooth f.
monomalleolar ankle f.
Monteggia forearm f.
Montercaux f.
Moore f.
Mouchet f.
multangular ridge f.
multilevel f.
multipartite f.
multiple f.'s
multiray f.
nasal f.
nasal-septal f.
nasoethmoidal f.
nasomaxillary f.
nasoorbital f.
navicular f.
navicular body f.
navicular dorsal lip f.
navicular hand f.
navicular tuberosity f.
naviculocapitate f.
neck f.
Neer type I-III shoulder f.
neoplastic f.
neural arch f.
neurogenic f.
neuropathic f.
neurotrophic f.
nightstick f.
night-walker f.
NOE f.
nonaccidental spiral tibial f.
nonarticular distal radial f.
nonarticular radial head f.
noncomminuted f.

noncontiguous f.
nondepressed skull f.
nondisplaced f.
nonpathologic f.
nonphyseal f.
nonrotational burst f.
nonunion of f.
f. nonunion
nonunion horse-hoof f.
nonunion torsion wedge f.
nonunited f.
nutcracker f.
oblique f.
oblique spiral f.
obliquity shoulder f.
obturator avulsion f.
occipital condyle f.
occult f.
occult osseous f.
occult scaphoid f.
odontoid condyle f.
odontoid neck f.
old f.
olecranon tip f.
open f.
open book f.
open break f.
open clavicular f.
open reduction of f.
open skull f.
orbital f.
orbital blow-in f.
orbital blowout f.
orbital floor f.
orbital nasoethmoidal f.
orbital rim f.
orbital roof f.
orbital wall f.
ossification-associated f.
osteochondral slice f.
osteoporotic compression f.
os trigonum f.
outlet strut f.
overlapping f.
pacemaker lead f.
Pais f.
palatal alveolar f.
palate f.
Palmer primary f.
pancraniomaxillofacial f.
panfacial f.
parasymphysis f.
paratrooper's f.
parry f.
pars interarticularis f.
1-part f.
2-part f.
3-part f.
4-part f.

patellar sleeve f.
pathological f.
f. pattern
Pauwels femoral neck f.
pediatric f.
pedicle f.
pelvic f.
pelvic avulsion f.
pelvic insufficiency f.
pelvic rim f.
pelvic ring f.
pelvic straddle f.
pelvis f.
penetrating f.
penile shaft f.
penis f.
perforating f.
periarticular f.
perinatal clavicle f.
perinatal humerus f.
peripheral f.
periprosthetic f.
peritrochanteric f.
PER-IV f.
pertrochanteric f.
petrous pyramid f.
phalangeal diaphysial f.
physeal f.
physeal plate f.
physis f.
Piedmont f.
pillar f.
pillow f.
pilon f.
pilon ankle f.
ping-pong f.
pisiform f.
plafond f.
plaque f.
plastic bowing f.
plastic deformation f.
plate f.
plateau f.
plateau tibia f.
pond f.
porcelain f.
Posada f.
posterior f.
posterior arch f.
posterior column f.
posterior element f.
posterior process f.

posterior rib f.
posterior ring f.
posterior talar process f.
posterior wall f.
postirradiation f.
postmortem f.
postoperative f.
Pott ankle f.
Pouteau f.
pressure f.
Prevent Recurrence of
    Osteoporotic F.'s (PROOF)
profundus artery f.
pronation-abduction f.
pronation-eversion f.
pronation-eversion/external
    rotation f.
prosthetic f.
proximal end tibia f.
proximal femoral f.
proximal humeral f.
proximal humeral stress f.
proximal shaft f.
proximal tibial metaphysial f.
pseudo-Jefferson f.
pseudo-Jones f.
pubic ramus stress f.
pubic symphysis f.
puncture f.
pure blowout f.
pyramidal f.
Quervain f.
radial head f.
radial neck f.
radial styloid f.
radical f.
radiographically occult f.
ramus f.
f. reducing elevator
reduction of f.
f. reduction
f. remodeling
f. repair
resecting f.
retrodisplaced f.
reverse Barton f.
reverse Bennett f.
reverse Colles f.
reverse Monteggia f.
reverse obliquity f.
reverse Segond f.
rib f.

NOTES

119

fracture *(continued)*
ring f.
ring-disrupting f.
Rockwood classification of
  clavicular f.
Rolando f.
Rolando-type f.
roof f.
root f.
rotation f.
rotational burst f.
Ruedi f.
Ruedi-Allgower tibial plafond f.
f. running length of bone
sacral f.
sacral insufficiency f.
sacroiliac f.
sacrum f.
sagittal slice f.
sagittal splitting f.
Salter-Harris epiphysial f.
Salter-Harris type I–VI f.
sandbagging long bone f.
Sanders f.
Sangeorzan navicular f.
scaphoid f.
scaphoid hand f.
scapular f.
scotty dog f.
seat belt f.
secondary f.
segmental f.
Segond tibial avulsion f.
senile subcapital f.
sentinel spinous process f.
septal f.
SER-IV f.
sesamoid f.
shaft forearm f.
shear f.
shearing f.
Shepherd f.
short oblique f.
sideswipe elbow f.
silver fork f.
simple f.
f. simple and depressed full-scale
  deflection
simple skull f.
single f.
single-column f.
f. site
f. site nonunion Norland bone
  densitometry
skier's f.
Skillern f.
skull f.
sleeve f.
slice f.

slot f.
small f.
Smith ankle f.
Sneppen talar f.
snowboarder's f.
sphenoid bone f.
spinal f.
spinal compression f.
spine f.
spinous process f.
spiral f.
spiral oblique f.
spiral tibial f.
f. splint
splintered f.
split compression f.
split-heel f.
splitting f.
spontaneous f.
sprain f.
Springer f.
sprinter's f.
stability of f.
f. stabilization
stable burst f.
stairstep f.
stellate f.
stellate skull f.
stellate undepressed f.
stepoff of f.
sternal f.
sternum f.
Stieda f.
straddle f.
strain f.
stress f.
strut f.
styloid f.
subcapital f.
subcapital hip f.
subchondral f.
subcondylar f.
subcutaneous f.
subperiosteal f.
subtrochanteric f.
subtrochanteric femoral f.
supination-adduction f.
supination-eversion f.
supination-external rotation f.
supracondylar f.
supracondylar femoral f.
supracondylar humeral f.
supracondylar Y-shaped f.
supraorbital f.
suprasyndesmotic f.
surgical neck f.
sustentaculum tali f.
symphysial f.
synchondritic f.

T f.
f. table
talar avulsion f.
talar dome f.
talar neck f.
talar osteochondral f.
talus body f.
tarsal bone f.
T condylar f.
teacup f.
teardrop burst f.
teardrop-shaped flexion-
  compression f.
telescoping septal f.
temporal bone f.
tennis f.
tension f.
testis f.
thalamic f.
thoracic spine f.
thoracolumbar burst f.
thoracolumbar junction f.
thoracolumbar spine f.
threatened pathologic f.
f. threshold
through-and-through f.
thrower's f.
thumb f.
Thurston Holland f.
tibia-fibula f.
tibial bending f.
tibial condyle f.
tibial diaphysial f.
tibial-fibular shaft f.
tibial open f.
tibial pilon f.
tibial plafond f.
tibial plateau f.
tibial shaft f.
tibial stress f.
tibial triplane f.
tibial tuberosity f.
tibiofibular f.
Tillaux f.
f. of Tillaux
Tillaux-Chaput f.
Tillaux-Kleiger f.
toddler's f.
tongue f.
tongue-type intraarticular f.
tooth f.
Torg f.

torsion f.
torsional f.
torus f.
total condylar depression f.
total talus f.
trabecular bone f.
tracheal f.
traction f.
trampoline f.
transcaphoid f.
transcapitate f.
transcervical femoral f.
transchondral talar f.
transcondylar f.
transepiphysial f.
transhamate f.
transiliac f.
translational f.
transsacral f.
transscaphoid dislocation f.
transtriquetral f.
transverse f.
transverse f.
transverse comminuted f.
transverse facial f.
transversely oriented endplate
  compression f.
transverse maxillary f.
transverse process f.
trapezial ridge f.
trapezium f.
traumatic f.
traversing the f.
trimalar f.
trimalleolar ankle f.
triplane f.
triplane tibial f.
tripod f.
triquetral f.
trophic f.
T-shaped f.
tuberosity f.
tuberosity avulsion f.
tuft f.
ulnar styloid f.
unciform f.
uncinate process f.
uncommon f.
undepressed skull f.
underlying rib f.
undisplaced f.
unexplained f.

F

NOTES

fracture *(continued)*
    unicondylar f.
    unilateral condylar f.
    unimalleolar f.
    unstable f.
    unstable tibial shaft f.
    unstable zygomatic complex f.
    ununited f.
    upper thoracic spine f.
    valgus f.
    vertebral body f.
    vertebral compression f.
    vertebral stable burst f.
    vertebral wedge compression f.
    vertebra plana f.
    vertical oblique pattern f.
    vertical shear f.
    vertical tooth f.
    volar rim distal radial f.
    volar shear f.
    Volkmann f.
    V-shaped f.
    wagon wheel f.
    Wagstaffe f.
    Wagstaffe-Le Fort f.
    waist f.
    Walther f.
    Watson-Jones navicular f.
    Weber (B, C) f.
    wedge compression f.
    wedge flexion-compression f.
    wedge-shaped uncomminuted tibial
     plateau f.
    western boot in open f.
    willow f.
    Wilson f.
    f. with malunion
    f. with nonunion
    f. with scoliosis
    Y f.
    Y-shaped f.
    Y-T f.
    Zickel f.
    Zingg type A1 zygomatic arch f.
    ZMC f.
    f. zone
    zygoma f.
    zygomatic f.
    zygomatic arch f.
    zygomatic body f.
    zygomatic complex f.
    zygomatic maxillary complex f.
    zygomaticomalar complex f.
    zygomaticomaxillary complex f.
fracture-dislocation
    ankle f.-d.
    f.-d. with anterior ligament
fractured tooth
fragile bone

fragilis
    Bacteroides f.
fragility
    bone f.
    f. fracture
fragment
    bone f.
    fracture f.
    f. wound
fragmentation
Fragmin During Instability in Coronary Artery Disease (FRISC)
frame
    fracture f.
framework fracture
Framingham Heart Study
FRC
    functional residual capacity
free
    f. fluid
    f. intraperitoneal air
    seizure f.
free-wall rupture
Freiberg fracture
fremitus
    tactile f.
French
    F. catheter
    F. nasogastric tube
Frenzel maneuver
frequent abdominal examination
fresh
    f. frozen plasma (FFP)
    f. wound
friction
    f. burn
    f. rub
FRISC
    Fragmin During Instability in Coronary
    Artery Disease
    FRISC trial
frog toxin
frontal
    f. bone
    f. diploic vein
    f. nerve
    f. orbital nasoethmoidal fracture
    f. plane
    f. sinus
    f. sinus disease
    f. sinus fracture
    f. sinusitis
    f. suture
    f. vein
    f. view
frontoethmoidal suture
frontolacrimal suture
frontomalar suture
frontomaxillary suture

frontonasal suture
frontoparietal suture
frontosphenoid suture
frontotemporal muscle
frontozygomatic suture
frostbite
Frost suture
frothy sputum
fruity breath odor
Frykman
    F. hand fracture
    F. hand fracture classification
FU
    followup
Fudaka stepping test
fulcrum fracture
fulgurate
fulguration
full
    f. body spinal immobilization
    f. cardiopulmonary arrest
    f. disclosure
    f. pulse
    f. spinal immobilization
full-jacketed bullet wound
fullness
    pelvic f.
full-term gestation
full-thickness
    f.-t. burn
    f.-t. corneal laceration
fully-automated defibrillator
fulminant
    f. glomerulonephritis
    f. hepatic failure (FHF)
fulminating appendicitis
function
    bladder f.
    bone marrow f.
    bowel f.
    brainstem f.
    cardiac f.
    change in bladder f.
    change in bowel f.
    cognitive f.
    effector cell f.

    gross motor f.
    liver f.
    motor f.
    muscle f.
    organ f.
    sensory f.
functional
    f. age
    f. funduscopy
    f. residual capacity (FRC)
fundiform ligament
fundoplication
    Nissen f.
funduscopy
    functional f.
fungal infection
fungating wound
fungemia
fungicide poisoning
fungus, pl. **fungi**
funnel web spider
FUO
    fever of undetermined origin
    fever of unknown origin
furazolidone
furcal nerve
Furnas suture
furosemide
furrier suture
further workup
furuncle
furunculosis
Fusarium oxysporum
fused papillary muscle
fusible
fusidic acid
fusiform
    f. muscle
    f. periosteal new bone
fusimotor nerve
fusion
    bone block f.
FVC
    forced vital capacity
FVL
    factor V Leiden

F

NOTES

γ (*var. of* gamma)
GABA
  gamma-aminobutyric acid
GABA-mediated inhibition
GABHS
  group A beta-hemolytic streptococcus
Gaenslen fracture
gag reflex
Gaillard-Arlt suture
gait
  g. ataxia
  g. and station
galactorrhea
galea aponeurotica muscle
Galeazzi radical fracture
Galen
  G. nerve
  G. vein
gallbladder (GB)
  g. obstruction
gallium
  g. nitrate
  g. scan
gallium-67 scanning
gallstone ileus
gallstone-solubilizing agent
Galveston fluid needs formula
Gambee suture
Gambierdiscus toxicus
gamekeeper's thumb
gamma, γ
  g. hydroxybutyrate
  g. radiation
gamma-aminobutyric acid (GABA)
gamma-hydroxybutyrate
Gamow bag
ganciclovir
gangliated nerve
ganglion
  nerve g.
ganglionic motor neuron
gangrene
  abdominal g.
  Fournier g.
  gas g.
  postoperative synergistic
    abdominal g.
  scrotal g.
  synergistic g.
gangrenous
  g. appendicitis
  g. limb
  g. stomatitis
Gantzer muscle

gap
  anion g.
  concurrent osmolal g.
  fracture g.
  increased anion g.
  nerve g.
  osmolar g.
  urine anion g.
  urine osmolal g.
gape
  wound g.
gaping wound
Garden femoral neck fracture
garlic
  g. capsule
  g. odor
garment
  pneumatic antishock g. (PASG)
garrulous personality
Gartland humeral supracondylar
  fracture classification
gas
  g. abscess
  arterial blood g. (ABG)
  arterial venous blood g.
  blood g.
  carbamate poisoning extraalveolar g.
  chlorine g.
  coursing of g.
  g. embolism
  g. embolus
  g. exchange
  extraalveolar g.
  g. gangrene
  g. inhalation
  mixed venous blood g.
  mustard g.
  nerve g.
  g. peritonitis
  tear g.
  g. ventilation
gaseous pulse
Gaskell nerve
gasp reflex
gastric
  g. acid inhibitor
  g. atony
  g. bleeding
  g. contents
  g. contents aspiration
  g. decontamination
  g. decontamination poisoning
  g. distention
  g. emptying
  g. emptying study

G

gastric *(continued)*
    g. lavage
    g. nerve
    g. outlet obstruction (GOO)
    g. tonometry
    g. tube (GT)
    g. vein
gastrinoma
gastritis
    acute g.
gastrocnemius
    g. bursa
    g. muscle
gastrocnemius-semimembranosus bursa
gastrocnemius-soleus muscle
gastrocolic ligament
gastrodiaphragmatic ligament
gastroenteritis
gastroepiploic vein
gastroesophageal
    g. reflux
    g. reflux disease (GERD)
    g. variceal bleeding
gastrogavage
Gastrografin swallow
gastrohepatic ligament
gastrointestinal (GI)
    g. anthrax
    g. bleed
    g. bleeding
    g. decontamination
    g. dialysis
    g. hemorrhage
    g. malignancy
    g. motility
    g. obstruction
    g. smooth muscle
    g. surgical gut suture
    g. surgical linen suture
    g. surgical silk suture
    g. system (GIS)
gastrolienal ligament
gastropancreatic ligament
gastroparesis
gastrophrenic ligament
gastroschisis
gastrosplenic ligament
gastrostomy
    endoscopic g.
    percutaneous g.
    percutaneous endoscopic g. (PEG)
    surgical g.
    g. tube (G-tube)
Gatch bed
gated radionuclide angiography
gatifloxacin
gauge

gauze
    g. pad
    g. roll
Gavard muscle
gaze
    conjugate g.
    dysconjugate g.
    sustained conjugate upward g.
    upward g.
GB
    gallbladder
GCS
    Glasgow coma scale
    graduated compression stocking
gear
    turnout g.
Geiger-Müller counter
gel
    adsorbent g.
    amethocaine g.
    fibrin g.
    wound g.
Gelsemium
    G. sempervirens
    G. sempervirens ingestion
gemellus
    g. inferior muscle
    g. superior muscle
gemfibrozil
geminate
GEMS CAREpoint EMS workstation
general
    g. closure suture
    g. medical problem
    g. medicine (GM)
    g. stimulant
    g. surgery (GS)
    g. symptom
generalized
    g. anxiety disorder and phobia
    g. gingival inflammation
    g. mouth pain
generator
    small-particle aerosol g.
genicular vein
genioglossal muscle
geniohyoid muscle
genital
    g. area
    g. fissure
    herpes g.
    g. ligament
    g. mutilation
    g. wart
genitalia
genitalis
    herpes g.
genitocrural nerve
genitofemoral nerve

genitoinguinal ligament
genitourinary (GU)
  g. system (GUS)
  g. trauma
gentamicin therapy
gentian violet
GERD
  gastroesophageal reflux disease
GERD-associated asthma
Gerlach anular tendon
germander ingestion
German measles
gestation
  full-term g.
gestational
  g. hypertension
  g. thromboblastic disease
gesture
  suicidal g.
GFR
  glomerular filtration rate
GHB-hydroxybutyrate poisoning
Ghon focus
GI
  gastrointestinal
  GI bleed
  GI cocktail
  GI popoff silk suture
  GI symptom
Giampapa suture
giant
  g. aneurysm
  g. cell interstitial pneumonia (GIP)
Giardia
  G. lamblia
  G. lamblia infection
giardiasis
Gila monster envenomation
Gilbert disease
Gillette suspensory ligament
Gilliam round ligament
Gillies horizontal dermal suture
Gimbernat reflex ligament
gingival
  g. ligament
  g. nerve
  g. pseudomembrane
  g. tissue loss
gingivitis
  acute g.
  acute necrotizing ulcerative g.
  (ANUG)

gingivodental ligament
gingivostomatitis
  herpetic g.
ginkgo biloba
ginseng
GIP
  giant cell interstitial pneumonia
girdle
  shoulder g.
GIS
  gastrointestinal system
Gissane
  crucial angle of G.
glabellar
  g. fracture
  g. muscle
glabrata
  Candida g.
  Torulopsis g.
glancing wound
gland
  accessory g.
  bulbourethral g.
  Cowper g.
  hematopoietic g.
  lacrimal g.
  mammary g.
  parathyroid g.
  salivary g.
  thyroid g.
glandular
  g. abscess
  g. fever
Glasgow
  G. coma scale (GCS)
  G. coma score
  G. Outcome Score
  G. Pediatric Coma Score
glauca
  Nicotiana g.
glaucoma
  acute angle closure g.
  narrow-angle g.
  open-angle g.
glenohumeral ligament
glenoid
  g. ligament
  g. rim fracture
gliomatosis cerebri
globe rupture
globulin
  antilymphocyte g.

G

NOTES

127

globulin *(continued)*
    antithymocyte g. (ATG)
    hyperimmune anti-D g.
    tetanus immune g.
glomerular filtration rate (GFR)
glomerulonephritis
    fulminant g.
glossoepiglottic ligament
glossopalatine muscle
glossopharyngeal
    g. muscle
    g. nerve
glottis
glove
    N-DEX non-latex g.
    puncture-proof g.
    Supreno EC one tough nitrile g.
glovelike burn
glucagon
    g. stimulation test
    g. therapy
glucocorticoid replacement
gluconate
    calcium g.
    chlorhexidine g.
glucose
    blood g.
    g. determination
    g. insulin potassium infusion
    g. metabolism
    oral g.
    serum g.
    g. tolerance test (GTT)
glucose-6-phosphate dehydrogenase deficiency
glucoside
    digitalis g.
glucosuria
glucuronidation
glue
    cyanoacrylate g.
    fibrin g.
    Krazy G.
    skin g.
    tissue g.
    g. toxicity
glue-in suture
glue-sniffing
glutamate
glutamine
gluteal
    g. muscle
    g. nerve
    g. vein
gluteofemoral bursa
gluteus
    g. maximus muscle
    g. medius bursa
    g. medius muscle

    g. minimus bursa
    g. minimus muscle
Glutose
glycerin laxative abuse
glycerol metabolism
glyceryl trinitrate (GTN)
glycine vasopressin
glycol
    ethylene g.
glycopeptide antibiotic
glycoprotein
    alpha-1 acid g.
    G. Receptor Antagonist Patency Evaluation (GRAPE)
glycopyrrolate
glycoside
    cardiac g.
Glypressin
GM
    general medicine
GnRH
    gonadotrophin releasing hormone
Goethe
    suture of G.
goiter
    diffuse g.
    multinodular g.
golden
    g. hour
    g. hour concept
Goldenhar syndrome
Goldfrank-Hoffman cocaine toxicity model
Goldman method
Goldmann
    G. applanation tonometry
    G. tonometer
Golgi tendon
gonadal
    g. ligament
    g. vein
gonadotrophin releasing hormone (GnRH)
gonadotropin
    beta-human chorionic g. (beta-hCG, beta-HCG)
    human chorionic g. (hCG, HCG)
gondii
    Toxoplasma g.
gonococcal
    g. cervicitis
    g. disease
    g. urethritis
gonorrhea
GOO
    gastric outlet obstruction
Goodpasture syndrome
goose bumps

Gore-Tex
>G.-T. anterior cruciate ligament
>G.-T. nonabsorbable suture

gossamer silk suture
Gosselin fracture
gouge
>bone g.

Gould inverted mattress suture
gout
>hyperuricemic g.
>saturnine g.

grabber
>tendon g.

gracile bone
gracilis
>g. muscle
>g. tendon

gradient
>pressure g.

grading
>wound 1-6 g.

graduated compression stocking (GCS)
graft
>bone g.
>bone autogenous g.
>bone block g.
>bone chip g.
>bone graft substitute g.
>bone peg g.
>coronary artery bypass g. (CABG)
>g. fracture
>g. function assessment and optimization
>ligament g.
>muscle pedicle bone g.
>nerve g.
>g. stenosis
>tendon g.
>g. thrombosis
>g. tunnel
>vein g.
>g. versus host disease (GVHD)

grafting
>bone g.
>tendon g.
>g. vein

grain alcohol
gram-negative bacillus
gram-positive cocci
Gram stain
grand mal seizure
granny battering

Grantham femoral fracture classification
granulate
granulation tissue
granulocytopenia
granuloma
>annulare g.
>pyogenic g.
>suture g.

granulomatis
>*Calymmatobacterium g.*

granulose
GRAPE
>Glycoprotein Receptor Antagonist Patency Evaluation
>GRAPE pilot study

grasping suture
Grassi
>nerve of G.
>G. nerve

grave
>g. condition
>g. illness

Graves disease
gravida
gravidarum
>hyperemesis g.

gravis
>myasthenia g.

gravity
>line of g.

Grayson ligament
gray-white gingival pseudomembrane
grease gun injury
great
>g. adductor muscle
>g. auricular nerve
>g. sciatic nerve
>g. toe sesamoid bone

greater
>g. occipital nerve
>g. palatine nerve
>g. pectoral muscle
>g. petrosal nerve
>g. psoas muscle
>g. rhomboid muscle
>g. saphenous vein
>g. splanchnic nerve
>g. superficial petrosal nerve
>g. trochanter
>g. trochanteric bursa
>g. trochanteric femoral fracture
>g. trochanter muscle

G

NOTES

greater (continued)
  g. tuberosity fracture
  g. zygomatic muscle
greatest gluteal muscle
green
  g. braided suture
  g. Mersilene suture
  g. monofilament polyglyconate
  suture
  g. pus
  g. sputum
greenstick
  g. fracture
  g. Le Fort fracture
Gregg phenomenon
grenade thrower's fracture
Grey Turner sign
grip
  power g.
groove suture
gross
  g. fracture
  g. motor function
group
  g. A beta-hemolytic streptococcus
  (GABHS)
  diagnosis-related g. (DRG)
  HACEK g.
  muscle g.
  Rh blood g.
growing skull fracture
growth
  bone g.
  carbunculoid g.
  g. plate fracture
Gruber
  G. ligament
  G. suture
grumous debris
grunting
  g. breath sound
  g. and flaring
  g. respiration
GS
  general surgery
G-suit
GSW
  gunshot wound
GT
  gastric tube
GTN
  glyceryl trinitrate
  GTN ointment
GTT
  glucose tolerance test
G-tube
  gastrostomy tube
GU
  genitourinary

guaiac
  rectal g.
guanfacine overdose
guanidine hydrochloride
guard
  Combiguard II irrigation splash g.
guardian ad litem
guarding
  involuntary g.
  muscle g.
gubernacular vein
Guedel airway
Guérin fracture
guide
  bone wire g.
  SAM OnScene patient
  assessment g.
  suture g.
  wound measuring g.
guideline
  bone marrow exposure g.
guidewire exchange
Guillain-Barré syndrome
guilliermondii
  Candida g.
guillotine amputation
gum
  blue line on g.'s
  spontaneously bleeding g.'s
gunshot
  g. fracture
  g. wound (GSW)
gun wound
Gurd fat embolism syndrome criteria
gurgling
  g. bowel sound
  g. breath sound
gurney
  SafetySure transfer g.
GUS
  genitourinary system
Gussenbauer suture
Gustilo
  G. classification
  G. classification of puncture wound
  G. open fracture scoring
  G. tibial fracture
**Gustilo-Anderson open clavicular
  fracture**
gut
  g. motor hypothesis
  g. starter hypothesis
  g. suture
Guthrie muscle
gut-liver axis
gutter
  g. fracture
  paracolic g.

g. splint
g. wound
Guyton-Friedenwald suture
GVHD
graft versus host disease
gynecologic
g. consultation
g. history

Gyne-Lotrimin
Gyromitra toxin
gyromitrin

NOTES

G

habit
> bowel h.
> change in bowel h.

habitual

HACE
> high-altitude cerebral edema

HACEK
> *Haemophilus aphrophilus, Actinobacillus actinomycetemcomitans, Cardiobacterium hominis, Eikenella corrodens, Kingella kingae*
> HACEK group

Haemonetics Cell Saver

Haemophilus
> *H. aphrophilus, Actinobacillus actinomycetemcomitans, Cardiobacterium hominis, Eikenella corrodens, Kingella kingae* (HACEK)
> *H. influenzae*
> *H. influenzae* infection
> *H. influenzae* type B (Hib)

HAFE
> high-altitude flatus expulsion

Hageman factor

HAH
> high-altitude headache

Hahn-Steinthal fracture

Haines-McDougall medial sesamoid ligament

hair
> h. dye toxicity
> h. product ingestion

hairline fracture

Haldane effect

Haldol

half backboard

half-buried mattress suture

half-life
> drug h.-l.

halitosis

Hall-Pike maneuver

hallucination
> auditory h.
> visual h.

hallucinogenic

hallucinogen poisoning

hallucinosis
> alcoholic h.

hallucis longus laceration

hallux sesamoid bone

halogenated hydrocarbon ingestion

haloperidol therapy

halothane

halo traction

Halsted
> H. epitendinous suture
> H. interrupted mattress suture
> H. interrupted quilt suture

hamate
> h. body fracture
> h. bone
> h. hook fracture
> h. ligament
> h. tail fracture

hamatometacarpal ligament

Hamman crunch

hammock ligament

Hampton hump

hamstring
> h. muscle
> h. tendon

hand
> fall onto outstretched h. (FOOSH)
> h. fracture
> h. infection
> ipsilateral h.
> h. phalangeal injury

hand-breath coordination

hand-foot-and-mouth disease

hand-held aerosol inhaler

hand-operated suction device

hand-powered suction device

hanging
> h. drop sign
> h. injury
> neck injury by h.

hangman's fracture

Hansen fracture classification

Hantaan virus

Hantavirus **cardiopulmonary syndrome**

HAPE-S
> susceptibility to high-altitude pulmonary edema

hard
> h. cervical collar
> h. palate

hardening
> bone h.

harelip suture

harmonic suture

harsh
> h. breath sound
> h. rhonchi

harvest
> stem cell h.

harvested vein

harvesting
> bone h.

Hatch suture

H

haunch bone
HAV
    hepatitis A virus
haversian bone
Hawkins
    H. talar fracture classification
    H. talus fracture
hay fever
hazardous
    h. material (HazMat)
    h. material exposure
HazMat
    hazardous material
    HazMat team
HBC
    hepatitis C virus
HBO
    hyperbaric oxygen
    HBO therapy
HBV
    hepatitis B virus
hCG, HCG
    human chorionic gonadotropin
    serum hCG
HCl
    hydrochloride
HCTZ
    hydrochlorothiazide
HDV
    hepatitis D virus
head
    aftercoming fetal h.
    h., eyes, ears, nose, throat
      (HEENT)
    femoral h.
    h. fracture
    h. injury
    subluxed radial h.
    h. trauma
headache
    cluster h.
    combination h.
    dural puncture h.
    exertional h.
    high-altitude h. (HAH)
    meningeal h.
    migraine h.
    muscle contraction h.
    muscle tension h.
    postconcussional h.
    tension h.
    thunderclap h.
    traumatic h.
    vascular h.
head-down position
2-headed muscle
3-headed muscle
4-headed muscle
headlamp

head-lift maneuver
head-splitting humeral fracture
head-tilt-chin lift
head-tilt maneuver
Heaf tuberculosis test
healed fracture
healing
    faith h.
    h. by first intention
    fracture h.
    h. fracture
    h. by primary intention
    h. by secondary intention
    h. by second intention
    h. by third intention
    tissue h.
    wound h.
health
    h. maintenance organization (HMO)
    National Institute of Occupational
      Safety and H. (NIOSH)
    h. risk appraisal
healthy individual
Heaney suture
heart
    h. attack
    h. auscultation
    h. block
    h. failure (HF)
    h. murmur
    h. muscle
    h. pill
    h. rate (HR)
    h. rate variability
    h. sound
    total artificial h. (TAH)
    h. transplant
    h. transplant recipient
    h. valve
    h. valve injury
heart-lung
    h.-l. transplant
    h.-l. transplantation (HLT)
HeartStart defibrillator
heat
    h. cramp
    h. exhaustion
    h. exposure
    h. fracture
    h. illness
    h. loss by conduction
    h. loss by convection
    h. loss by evaporation
    h. loss by radiation
    h. loss by respiration
    h. stroke (*var. of* heatstroke)
heatstroke, heat stroke, heat stroke
heaviness
    chest h.

heavy
    h. bleeding
    h. metal
    h. metal poisoning
    h. monofilament suture
    h. retention suture
    h. silk retention suture
    h. silk suture
    h. wire suture
heavy-gauge suture
Hector tendon
heel
    h. bone
    h. tendon
HEENT
    head, eyes, ears, nose, throat
Heimlich
    H. catheter
    H. maneuver
helical suture
helicis
    h. major muscle
    h. minor muscle
Helicobacter pylori
heliox
helium-oxygen therapy
hellebore
    American h.
HELLP
    hemolysis, elevated liver enzymes, low
    platelets
        HELLP syndrome
helmet
    traction h.
Helmholtz axis ligament
helminthic
    h. appendicitis
    h. worm
Helvetius ligament
hemangioma
    bone h.
    bone capillary h.
hemarthrosis
hematemesis
hematinics
hematochezia
hematocrit
hematogenous abscess
hematoma
    auricular h.
    brain h.
    central retroperitoneal h.

    cerebral h.
    contained h.
    epidural h.
    extradural h.
    flank h.
    intracerebral h.
    intraparenchymal h.
    pulsatile h.
    retroperitoneal h.
    subdural h.
    subperichondrial h.
    subungual h.
    wound h.
hematopoietic gland
hematuria
    microscopic h.
    profound h.
    h. and proteinuria
heme
hemianopia, hemianopsia
    congruous h.
    homonymous h.
    unilateral h.
hemiazygos vein
hemicondylar fracture
hemiparesis
hemipelvis
hemiplegia
hemisphere
    intact cerebral h.
hemispheric vein
hemitransverse fracture
hemlock
    ingestion of h.
    h. poisoning
hemobilia
hemochromatosis
hemodiafiltration
    arteriovenous h.
    continuous h.
    continuous arteriovenous h.
    continuous venovenous h.
        (CVVHD, CVVHDF)
hemodialysis
    continuous arteriovenous h.
        (CAVHD)
    continuous venovenous h.
    h. for renal failure
    h. vascular access
    venovenous h.
hemoductal surgical treatment

NOTES

H

135

hemodynamic
- h. collapse
- h. consequence
- h. instability
- h. monitoring

hemodynamically stable

hemodynamics

hemofiltration
- continuous arteriovenous h. (CAVH)
- continuous venovenous h.

hemoglobin
- mean corpuscular h. (MCH)
- muscle h.
- h. toxin

hemolysis
- h., elevated liver enzymes, low platelets (HELLP)
- immune h.

hemolytic
- h. anemia
- h. splenomegaly
- h. transfusion reaction
- h. uremic syndrome (HUS)

hemoperfusion
- charcoal h.

hemopericardium

hemoperitoneum
- traumatic h.

hemophagocytic syndrome

hemophilia
- h. A, B
- type A, B h.

hemopneumothorax,
  pl. **hemopneumothoraces**

hemoptysis

hemopump
- Nimbus h.

hemorrhage
- accidental h.
- acute intracerebral h.
- cerebellar h.
- cerebral h.
- critical h.
- extradural h.
- fetomaternal h.
- gastrointestinal h.
- intracerebral h.
- intracranial h. (ICH)
- intraventricular h. (IVH)
- major external h.
- neonatal h.
- nerve fiber layer h.
- pontine h.
- posterior fossa h.
- postpartum h.
- punctate h.
- putamen h.
- recalcitrant h.

- severe h.
- subarachnoid h.
- thalamic h.
- variceal h.
- vitreous h.

hemorrhagic
- h. abscess
- h. arthritis
- h. fever
- h. fever with renal syndrome (HFRS)
- h. hypotension
- h. shock
- h. shock and encephalopathy (HSE)
- h. stress-induced serum factor
- h. stroke

hemorrhoid
- anorectal h.
- thrombosed h.

hemorrhoidal
- h. bleeding
- h. nerve
- h. vein

hemostasis
- local h.

hemostat

hemostatic suture

hemosuccus

hemothorax
- concomitant h.
- massive h.
- recurrent h.

hemotympanum

Henderson fracture

Henle ligament

Hennebert pressure test

Henoch-Schönlein purpura

Hensing ligament

HEPA
- high-efficiency particulate air
  - HEPA filtration
  - HEPA respirator

heparin
- adjusted-dose unfractionated h.
- low molecular weight h. (LMWH)
- h. therapy

heparinization

hepatectomy

hepatic
- h. abscess
- h. artery
- h. artery aneurysm
- h. damage
- h. encephalopathy
- h. failure
- h. gunshot wound
- h. injury
- h. ligament
- h. portal vein

h. resection
h. transplantation
h. vein
hepatitis
h. A, B, C, D, E
h. A virus (HAV)
h. B virus (HBV)
h. C virus (HBC)
h. D virus (HDV)
hepatocolic ligament
hepatocystocolic ligament
hepatoduodenal ligament
hepatoesophageal ligament
hepatogastric ligament
hepatogastroduodenal ligament
hepatomegaly
hepatophrenic ligament
hepatorenal
h. ligament
h. syndrome
hepatosplenomegaly
hepatotoxicity
acute onset h.
hepatotoxic level
hepatotoxin
indirect h.
intrinsic h.
hepatoumbilical ligament
Hep-B-Gammagee
herald patch
herb
herbal toxicity
Herbert
H. scaphoid bone fracture
H. scaphoid fracture classification
Herculon suture
hereditary angioedema
Hering sinus nerve
Hermodsson fracture
hernia
diaphragmatic h.
incarcerated h.
inguinal h.
irreducible h.
muscle h.
reducible h.
wound h.
herniated
h. disk
h. stomach
herniation
brain h.

cardiac h.
central cerebral h.
cerebellar h.
cerebellotonsillar h.
muscle h.
h. syndrome
tonsillar h.
transtentorial h.
uncal h.
heroin
h. usage
h. vapor inhalation
herpangina
herpes
h. encephalitis
h. genital
h. genitalis
h. simplex
h. simplex encephalitis
h. simplex virus (HSV)
h. zoster
h. zoster ophthalmicus
h. zoster oticus
Herpesvirus
H. hominis (HVH)
H. hominis encephalitis
herpetic
h. gingivostomatitis
h. keratoconjunctivitis
h. whitlow
herring
red h.
Hesselbach ligament
heterologous bone
heterotopic
h. bone
h. ossification
h. transplant
h. transplantation
hexachlorobenzene
Hey ligament
HF
heart failure
HFFI
high-frequency flow interrupted
HFJV
high-frequency jet ventilation
HFOV
high-frequency oscillatory ventilation
HFRS
hemorrhagic fever with renal syndrome

NOTES

H

HFV
    high-frequency ventilation
H1, H2 antagonist
HHNK
    hyperosmolar hyperglycemia nonketotic
    HHNK diabetes
Hib
    Haemophilus influenzae type B
hibernating myocardium
Hibiclens antiseptic solution
hiccup, hiccough
hickory-stick fracture
HIDA
    dimethyl iminodiacetic acid
    HIDA scan
hidradenitis suppurativa
high
    h. blood sugar
    h. frontal bone
    h. incidence
    h. incidence of relapse
    h. index of suspicion
    h. output
    h. T$_4$ syndrome
high-altitude
    h.-a. cerebral edema (HACE)
    h.-a. flatus expulsion (HAFE)
    h.-a. headache (HAH)
    h.-a. illness
    h.-a. pulmonary edema
    h.-a. sickness
high-efficiency particulate air (HEPA)
high-energy
    h.-e. fracture
    h.-e. gunshot wound
higher trauma unit
highest
    h. intercostal vein
    h. turbinated bone
high-flow
    h.-f. oxygen
    h.-f. priapism
high-frequency
    h.-f. flow interrupted (HFFI)
    h.-f. jet ventilation (HFJV)
    h.-f. oscillatory ventilation (HFOV)
    h.-f. ventilation (HFV)
high-level disinfection
highly
    h. agitated
    h. protein-bound medication
high-performance liquid chromatography
high-pitched
    h.-p. breath sound
    h.-p. rhonchi
high-power field (HPF)
high-pressure
    h.-p. hand injury
    h.-p. injection injury

high-protein diet
high-riding
    h.-r. prostate
    h.-r. testis
high-tension burn
high-velocity gunshot wound
Hill-Sachs posterolateral compression fracture
Hilton muscle
hindfoot fracture
hinge joint
hip
    h. adductor muscle
    h. avulsion fracture
    h. bone
    h. dislocation
    h. injury
    h. joint
hippocampus infarct
Hirschsprung disease
hirudin
Hispanic
    H. female
    H. male
histamine
    h. antagonist
    h. cephalgia
histamine-2 receptor antagonist
histological chemistry
histology
    bone h.
histolytica
    Entamoeba h.
histomorphometry
    bone h.
Histoplasma capsulatum
histoplasmosis
historical
    h. characteristic
    h. clue
history (Hx, hx)
    birth h.
    case h.
    diabetic h.
    discrepancy in h.
    family h. (FH)
    gynecologic h.
    incongruous h.
    ingestion exposure with
        suspicious h.
    medial h.
    occupational h.
    h. of past injury
    past medical h. (PMH)
    past surgical h. (PSH)
    h. of present illness (HPI)
    psychiatric h.
    social h.
    substance abuse h.

surgical h.
suspicious h.
toxin exposure with suspicious h.
h. of trauma
violence h.

hitch
ankle h.

HIV
human immunodeficiency virus
HIV infection

hives

HLT
heart-lung transplantation

HMO
health maintenance organization

hoarseness
hobble restraint
hockey-stick fracture
Hoffa fracture
hold
postinflation h.

holder
bone h.
EndoGrip endotracheal tube h.
nerve h.
suture h.
Thomas endotracheal tube h.

holding room treatment
hole
tattoo h.

holistic
Holl ligament
hollow
h. organ
h. viscus injury

holly toxicity
Holstein-Lewis fracture
Holter monitor
home health care
homeostasis
protein h.
water h.

homicidal ideation
homicide
hominis
Herpesvirus h. (HVH)
Trichomonas h.

homogeneous, homogenous
homogeneously
homonymous
h. hemianopia
h. muscle

hook
bone h.
h. of the hamate fracture
muscle h.
nerve h.
nerve pull h.
suture pickup h.

hookworm
hoop stress fracture
hordeolum and chalazion
horizontal
h. dermal suture
h. length
h. length of mandible
h. mattress stitch
h. mattress suture
h. maxillary fracture
h. oblique fracture
h. plane

hormone
adrenocorticotropic h. (ACTH)
antidiuretic h. (ADH)
gonadotrophin releasing h. (GnRH)
parathyroid h.
syndrome of inappropriate
antidiuretic h. (SIADH)
thyroid h.

horn
bone graft shoe h.

Horner
H. muscle
H. syndrome

Horsley suture
hospital
community h.
h. course
h. security
h. stay
h. triage

hospital-acquired
h.-a. infection
h.-a. pneumonia

hospitalist
host
compromised h.

hot
h. abscess
h. appendix
h. joint
H. Tap portable hot shower

hotline
24-hour emergency h.

NOTES

H

139

hour
    golden h.
24-hour emergency hotline
hourglass chest
household
    h. industrial poison
    h. injury
Houston muscle
HPF
    high-power field
HPI
    history of present illness
HPV
    human papillomavirus
    hypoxic pulmonary vasoconstriction
HR
    heart rate
HSE
    hemorrhagic shock and encephalopathy
    HSE syndrome
H substance
HSV
    herpes simplex virus
5-HT antagonist
HTS
    hypertonic saline
Hueck ligament
Hu-Friedy PermaSharp suture
human
    h. bite
    h. chorionic gonadotropin (hCG, HCG)
    h. immunodeficiency virus (HIV)
    h. papillomavirus (HPV)
    h. umbilical vein
humboldtriana
    Karwinski h.
humeral
    h. bone
    h. condylar fracture
    h. depression
    h. head fracture
    h. head-splitting fracture
    h. physeal fracture
    h. shaft fracture
    h. supracondylar fracture
humerus fracture
humidification
humidified oxygen
humidifier
    electrical air h.
humor
    aqueous h.
    vitreous h.
hump
    Hampton h.
Humphry ligament
hunger
    bone h.

hungry bone
Hunter ligament
Hunt-Hess
    H.-H. hand fracture
    H.-H. scale
Huntington chorea
Hurler syndrome
Hurricaine spray
HUS
    hemolytic uremic syndrome
Huschke ligament
Hutchinson fracture
HVH
    Herpesvirus hominis
    HVH encephalitis
HVR
    hypoxic ventilatory response
HVS
    hyperviscosity syndrome
Hx, hx
    history
hyalinization
hyalocapsular ligament
hyaloideocapsular ligament
hyaluronidase
hydantoin
hydatidiform mole
hydralazine
hydration
    able to maintain h.
    maintain h.
hydrocarbon
    aliphatic halogenated h.
    h. insecticide
    h. poisoning
hydrocele repair
hydrocephalus
hydrochloride (HCl)
    amiodarone h.
    diltiazem h.
    encainide h.
    guanidine h.
    methadone h.
    mexiletine h.
    moricizine h.
    naloxone h.
    nicardipine h.
    tocainide h.
hydrochlorothiazide (HCTZ)
hydrocolloid dressing
hydrofluoric
    h. acid
    h. acid burn
    h. acid ingestion
hydrogen
    h. cyanide
    h. fluoride poisoning
    h. fluoride toxicity
    h. peroxide

h. sulfide
h. sulfide gas poisoning
h. sulfide inhalation injury
h. sulfide poisoning
h. sulfide toxicity
hydromorphone
hydronephrosis
Hydrophiidae envenomation
hydrophila
    Aeromonas h.
hydrophilic medication
hydroxide
aluminum h.
hydroxyapatite bone
hydroxybutyrate
gamma h.
hydroxyephedrine
carbon-11 h.
Hydrozoa poisoning
hygiene
oral h.
poor oral h.
hygienist
industrial h.
Hymenoptera
H. bite
H. envenomation
H. sting
hyoepiglottic ligament
hyoglossal muscle
hyoid
h. bone
h. bone fracture
h. bursa
h. muscle
hypaxial muscle
hyperactive
h. muscle
h. reflex
hyperacusis
hyperacute rejection
hyperammonemia
hyperbaric
h. chamber
h. facility
h. medicine
h. oxygen (HBO)
h. oxygen therapy
h. saline ventilation
hypercalcemia
idiopathic h.

hypercapnia
permissive h.
hypercarbia
hyperoxic h.
hypercoagulable state
hypercyanotic
hyperdynamic sepsis
hyperemesis gravidarum
hyperemia
zone of h.
hyperestrogenism
hyperextension teardrop fracture
hyperfibrinogenemia
reactive h.
hyperflexion teardrop fracture
hyperglycemia
rebound h.
hyperimmune anti-D globulin
hyperinflation
dynamic h.
hyperintense muscle
hyperintensity
muscle h.
hyperkalemia
shift-related h.
hyperketonemia
hyperketonuria
hyperkinesia
hyperkinesis
hyperkinetic syndrome
hypermagnesemia
hypermetabolic phase
hypermetabolism
hypermobile joint
hypernatremia
hyperosmolar
    h. hyperglycemia nonketotic (HHNK)
    h. hyperglycemic nonketotic coma
    h. state
    h. syndrome
hyperoxic hypercarbia
hyperparathyroidism
hyperparathyroid syndrome
hyperphosphatemia
hyperpigmentation
hyperplasia
adrenal h.
benign prostatic h. (BPH)
congenital adrenal h.

NOTES

H

hyperplastic
  h. bone
  h. inflammation
hyperpnea
  central reflex h.
hyperpyretic
hyperpyrexia
  malignant h.
hyperpyrexial fever
hyperreflexia
  autonomic h.
hypersensitivity reaction
hypersplenism
hypertension
  abdominal h.
  accelerated h.
  acute intracranial h.
  benign intracranial h.
  chronically elevated h.
  essential h. (EH)
  gestational h.
  idiopathic h.
  intraabdominal h.
  intracranial h.
  labile h.
  malignant h.
  maternal h.
  portal h.
  pregnancy-induced h. (PIH)
  pulmonary h.
  systolic h.
hypertensive
  h. crisis
  h. emergency
  h. encephalopathy
hyperthermia
  first-degree h.
  fourth-degree h.
  malignant h. (MH)
  second-degree h.
  third-degree h.
hyperthyroidism
  apathetic h.
  primary h.
hypertonia
  internal fissure h.
hypertonic
  h. fluid
  h. muscle
  h. saline (HTS)
  h. saline solution
hypertonicity
  muscle h.
hypertrophic
  h. cardiomyopathy
  h. ligament
  h. pyloric stenosis
hypertrophied corneal nerve

hypertrophy
  asymmetric septal h. (ASH)
  benign prostatic h. (BPH)
  bone h.
  muscle h.
hyperuricemia
hyperuricemic gout
hyperventilation
  central neurogenic h.
  h. maneuver
  h. syndrome
hyperviscosity syndrome (HVS)
hypervitaminosis
hypervolemia
hypervolemic
  h. hyponatremia
  h. pulmonary edema
  h. shock
hypha, pl. **hyphae**
hyphema
hypnotic state
hypoadrenalism
hypocalcemia
hypocapnia
hypocapnia-induced vasoconstriction
hypochlorite
  sodium h.
hypochondriac
hypochromic
  h. anemia
  h. microcytic anemia
hypodermic needle
hypofibrinogenemia
hypofunction
hypogammaglobulinemia
hypogastric
  h. nerve
  h. region
  h. vein
hypoglossal nerve
hypoglycemia
  ketotic h.
hypoglycemic
  h. agent poisoning
  biguanide h.
  h. coma
  h. drug overdose
  h. shock
hypohydration
hypokalemia
hypomagnesemia
hyponatremia
  dilutional h.
  hypervolemic h.
  hypovolemic h.
  isovolemic h.
hypoparathyroidism
  familial h.
hypoperfusion

hypopexia
hypophosphatemia
hypophyseoportal vein
hypopituitarism
hypoplasia
hypoproteinemia
hypotension
    hemorrhagic h.
    iatrogenic h.
    orthostatic h.
    postural h.
hypothalamus
hypothenar muscle
hypothermia
    accidental h.
    profound h.
hypothermic blanket
hypothesis, pl. **hypotheses**
    gut motor h.
    gut starter h.
    Monro-Kelly h.
hypothyroidism
    congenital h.
    secondary h.
hypotonia
    muscle h.

hypotonic muscle
hypotoxicity
hypotrophy
hypoventilation
hypovolemia
    severe h.
hypovolemic
    h. hyponatremia
    h. patient
    h. shock
hypoxemia test
hypoxia
    cerebral h.
    diffusion h.
    ischemic h.
    tissue h.
    wound h.
hypoxic
    h. ischemic encephalopathy
    h. pulmonary vasoconstriction (HPV)
    h. ventilatory response (HVR)
hypsiloid ligament
hysteric

NOTES

H

IABP
  intraaortic balloon pump
IAC-CPR
  interposed abdominal compression-
    cardiopulmonary resuscitation
IAP
  intraabdominal pressure
iatrogenesis
iatrogenic
    i. cause
    i. discitis
    i. drug-induced disease
    i. hypotension
    i. morbidity
    i. pneumothorax
IBD
  inflammatory bowel disease
ibotenic acid mushroom poisoning
IBS
  irritable bowel syndrome
ibuprofen
ibutilide
IC
  intensive care
ICC
  intensive coronary care
ICCU
  intensive coronary care unit
ICD
  implantable cardioverter-defibrillator
  internal cardioverter-defibrillator
  International Classification of Disease
ice
    i. pack
    i. skater's fracture
    i. water caloric test
ICH
  intracranial hemorrhage
ichthyism
ichthyismus
ichthyoacanthotoxism
ichthyohemotoxism
ichthyoid
ichthyosarcotoxin
ichthyotoxism
ICI
  intracranial injury
ICM
  intercostal margin
ICP
  intracranial pressure
ictal
icteric
icterus

ICU
  intensive care unit
    ICU course
    ICU psychosis
    ICU stay
    ICU treatment
I&D
  incision and drainage
IDDM
  insulin-dependent diabetes mellitus
ideation
    homicidal i.
    suicidal i.
identification
    snake i.
    toxin i.
identifier
    bracelet i.
    necklace i.
    wallet card i.
idiogenic osmole
idiopathic
    i. abscess
    i. fracture
    i. hypercalcemia
    i. hypertension
    i. hypertrophic subaortic obstruction
    i. hypertrophic subaortic stenosis
    i. pulmonary fibrosis (IPF)
    i. thrombocytopenic purpura (ITP)
idiopathy
idiosyncrasy
idiosyncratic reaction
idioventricular rhythm
IDS
  intubation difficulty scale
I:E
  inspiratory to expiratory
    I:E ratio
ifosfamide
IgE-mediated allergic reaction
IKI catgut suture
ileac
ileal
    i. artery
    i. loop
    i. loop obstruction
    i. loop urostomy
    i. vein
ileocecal syndrome
ileocolic vein
ileofemoral vein
ileum
ileus
    adynamic i.

ileus *(continued)*
> dynamic i.
> gallstone i.
> paralytic i.

iliac
> i. artery
> i. bone
> i. bursa
> i. cancellous bone
> i. crest
> i. muscle
> i. vein

iliacus minor muscle
iliococcygeal muscle
iliocostal muscle
iliofemoral
> i. ligament
> i. vein

iliohypogastric
> i. muscle
> i. nerve

ilioinguinal
> i. nerve
> i. vein

iliolumbar
> i. ligament
> i. vein

iliopatellar ligament
iliopectineal
> i. bursa
> i. ligament

iliopsoas
> i. bursa
> i. muscle
> i. tendon

iliopubic
> i. ligament
> i. nerve

iliotibial ligament
iliotrochanteric ligament
ilium bone
illicit drug
illness
> acute on chronic i.
> altitude i.
> coexistent i.
> environmental i.
> febrile i.
> grave i.
> heat i.
> high-altitude i.
> history of present i. (HPI)
> present i.
> refractory i.
> sign/symptom, allergy, medications, pertinent past medical history, last oral intake, event leading up to the injury or i. (SAMPLE)

illusion of reperfusion

ILM
> intubating laryngeal mask

ILV
> independent lung ventilation

IM
> intramuscular

image
> bone phase i.

imaging
> abdominal trauma i.
> bone i.
> bone age i.
> bone density i.
> bone length i.
> bone mineral content i.
> bone phase i.
> bone scintiscan i.
> magnetic resonance i. (MRI)
> i. modality
> i. study

imbalance
> electrolyte i.
> muscle i.

imbed
imbricated stitch
^{131}**I-MIBG**
> iodine-131 metaiodobenzylguanidine
> ^{131}I-MIBG scintigraphy

imine
> *N*-acetyl-*p*-benzoquinone i.

imipenem
Imitrex
immature
> i. bone
> i. cataract

immediate reduction
immersion
> i. burn
> i. scald

immitis
> *Coccidioides* i.

immobility
immobilization
> adequate i.
> bone mineral i.
> cervical spine i.
> C-spine i.
> emotional i.
> full body spinal i.
> full spinal i.
> in-line i.
> manual i.
> sling i.
> spinal i.

immobilize
immobilizer
> STA-BLOCK head i.

immune hemolysis

immunity
    cell-mediated i.
immunization
    Rh i.
immunoassay test
immunocompromised
    i. patient
    i. pneumonia
immunodeficiency
immunoglobulin
immunologic deficiency
immunomodulation
immunosuppressant
immunosuppression
immunotherapy
IMPACT-AMI
    Integrilin to Minimize Platelet
    Aggregation and Coronary Thrombosis-
    Acute Myocardial
    IMPACT-AMI trial
impacted
    i. articular fracture
    i. subcapital fracture
    i. valgus fracture
IMPACT-II
    Integrilin to Minimize Platelet
    Aggregation and Coronary Thrombosis-
    II
    IMPACT-II study
impaction
    cerumen i.
    fecal i.
    i. fracture
    mucus i.
impact seizure
impaired
    i. affect
    i. mental performance
impairment
    acute neurologic i.
    diffusion i.
impaled foreign object
impalement injury
impedance
    aortic i.
    i. monitor
    i. plethysmography (IPG)
imperfecta
    osteogenesis i.
imperforate anus
impetigo

impingement
    nerve i.
    nerve root i.
    i. syndrome
implant
    bone i.
    i. fracture
    tendon i.
implantable
    i. cardioverter-defibrillator (ICD)
    i. defibrillator
    i. venous access device
implantation
    autogenous cartilage i.
    muscle i.
    nerve i.
implied
    i. consent
    i. duty
impotency
impregnated dressing
impression fracture
impulse
    nerve i.
    point of maximal i. (PMI)
impure blowout fracture
IMS
    incident management system
Imuran
IMV
    intermittent mandatory ventilation
in
    in toto
    in vivo
inability
    i. to accommodate
    i. to handle secretions
    i. to tolerate oral fluid
inadequate air movement
inadvertent laceration
inappropriate
    i. affect
    i. antidiuretic hormone secretion
    i. behavior
inborn
    i. errors
    i. errors of metabolism
incarcerated hernia
incarial bone
incentive spirometry
incessant atrial tachycardia

NOTES

inch
   pounds per square i. (psi)
incidence
   high i.
   low i.
incident
   i. command system
   i. management system (IMS)
   mass casualty i. (MCI)
   multiple casualty i. (MCI)
incised wound
incision
   i. and débridement
   i. and drainage (I&D)
   paramedian i.
   thoracoabdominal i.
incisive
   i. bone
   i. muscle
   i. nerve
   i. suture
incompatibility
   ABO i.
   Rh i.
incompetence
   chronotropic i.
   determination of i.
incompetent cervix
incomplete
   i. abortion
   i. compound fracture
   i. vertical root fracture
incongruent nystagmus
incongruous
   i. finding
   i. history
incontinence
   urinary i.
incontinent
incorporation
   bone graft i.
incorrect dose
increase in bleeding
increased
   i. anion gap
   i. maternal age
   i. parity
   i. plasma volume
   i. risk of toxicity
   i. work of breathing
incudal ligament
incus bone
indemnity benefit
indented fracture
independence
   ventricular i.
independent lung ventilation (ILV)
Inderal
index, pl. **indices**

   cardiac i. (CI)
   i. extensor muscle
   oxygen i. (OI)
   oxygenation i. (OI)
   pulmonary vascular resistance i.
      (PVRI)
   risk i.
   stroke i. (SI)
   systemic vascular resistance i.
      (SVRI)
India rubber suture
indications for immediate reduction
indicator muscle
indices (*pl. of* index)
indinavir
indirect
   i. contact
   i. force
   i. hepatotoxin
   i. orbital floor fracture
individual
   healthy i.
indoleacetic acid
indolent ulcer
Indole poisoning
indomethacin
indrawing
   intercostal i.
   suprasternal i.
induced
   i. abortion
   i. symptom
induction
   paralysis i.
   rapid sequence i.
industrial hygienist
inebriation
inevitable abortion
infant
   irritable i.
   poorly explained death of i.
   unexplained death of i.
infantile
   i. myxedema
   i. spasm
infantum
   roseola i.
infarct
   amygdaloid i.
   bone i.
   brainstem i.
   cerebellar i.
   hippocampus i.
   lacunar i.
   muscle i.
infarcted heart muscle
infarction
   acute myocardial i. (AMI)
   acute Q-wave myocardial i.

anteroinferior myocardial i.
anterolateral myocardial i.
bone i.
brain i.
brainstem i.
cocaine-induced myocardial i.
Early Retavase-Thrombolysis In Myocardial I. (ER-TIMI)
end-organ i.
myocardial i. (MI)
non-Q-wave myocardial i.
Q-wave myocardial i.
right ventricular i.
rule out myocardial i.
ST-elevation myocardial i. (STEMI)
watershed i.
infarctive purpura
infected bone
infection
    Acinetobacter i.
    adnexal i.
    adult urinary tract i.
    anaerobic i.
    anorectal herpes simplex i.
    anthrax i.
    arbovirus i.
    Bacillus i.
    bacterial i.
    Bacteroides i.
    Blastomyces dermatitidis i.
    bone i.
    Borrelia burgdorferi i.
    botulism bacterial i.
    Candida i.
    catheter-associated urinary tract i. (CAUTI)
    cervical i.
    Chlamydia trachomatis i.
    i. control procedure
    cryptococcal pulmonary i.
    Cryptococcus neoformans i.
    cryptogenic i.
    cutaneous bacterial i.
    cutaneous tinea i.
    cytomegalovirus i.
    dental i.
    Ebola virus i.
    Entamoeba histolytica i.
    Enterobacteriaceae i.
    Enterobius vermicularis i.
    epidural i.
    Epstein-Barr i.

florid i.
fluke i.
fungal i.
Giardia lamblia i.
Haemophilus influenzae i.
hand i.
HIV i.
hospital-acquired i.
intraperitoneal i.
Legionella i.
MAC i.
mycobacterial i.
Mycobacterium avium complex i.
Mycobacterium tuberculosis i.
myocarditis bacterial i.
necrotizing soft tissue i.
Nocardia i.
nosocomial urinary tract i.
opportunistic i.
pediatric urinary tract i.
pericarditis bacterial i.
periorbital i.
port i.
postengraftment i.
postpartum adnexal i.
pretransplant to engraftment i.
Pseudomonas i.
reservoir i.
respiratory bacterial i.
rickettsial i.
Salmonella i.
sexually transmitted i. (STI)
Shigella i.
shunt i.
small bowel bacterial i.
soft tissue i.
spinal cord i.
spirochetal bacterial i.
subdural i.
tendon sheath space i.
tinea cutaneous i.
Treponema pallidum i.
upper respiratory i. (URI)
upper respiratory tract i. (URTI)
Ureaplasma urealyticum i.
urinary tract i. (UTI)
vaginal bacterial i.
vascular access i.
viral i.
wound i.
infectiosum
    erythema i.

NOTES

infectious
    i. arthritis
    i. cause of adnexal mass
    i. colitis
    i. complication
    i. dacryoadenitis
    i. endocarditis
    i. etiology
    i. low back pain
infective endocarditis
inferior
    i. adrenal vein
    i. alveolar nerve
    i. alveolar vein
    i. anal nerve
    i. anastomotic vein
    i. basal vein
    i. calcaneal nerve
    i. calcaneonavicular ligament
    i. cardiac vein
    i. cerebellar vein
    i. cerebral vein
    i. choroid vein
    i. cluneal nerve
    i. constrictor pharyngeal muscle
    i. dental nerve
    i. dorsal radioulnar ligament
    i. epigastric vein
    i. gemellus muscle
    i. glenohumeral ligament
    i. gluteal nerve
    i. gluteal vein
    i. hemiazygos vein
    i. hemorrhoidal nerve
    i. hemorrhoidal vein
    i. ilioischial ligament
    i. labial vein
    i. laryngeal nerve
    i. laryngeal vein
    i. lateral brachial cutaneous nerve
    i. lingual muscle
    i. maxillary bone
    i. maxillary nerve
    i. mesenteric vein
    i. nasal nerve
    i. nasal vein
    i. oblique extraocular muscle
    i. oblique muscle
    i. ophthalmic vein
    i. palpebral nerve
    i. palpebral vein
    i. phrenic vein
    i. posterior serratus muscle
    i. pubic ligament
    i. pulmonary ligament
    i. pulmonary vein
    i. radicular vein
    i. recess of omental bursa
    i. rectal nerve

    i. rectal vein
    i. rectus extraocular muscle
    i. tarsal muscle
    i. temporal vein
    i. thalamostriate vein
    i. thyroid vein
    i. transverse scapular ligament
    i. turbinate bone
    i. vena cava (IVC)
    i. ventricular vein
    i. vesical nerve
inferolateral margin
infestation
    tapeworm i.
infiltrate
    circumscribed i.
infiltration
    i. anesthesia
    i. suture
inflammation
    generalized gingival i.
    hyperplastic i.
    tendon i.
    vein i.
inflammatory
    i. abdominal aortic aneurysm
    i. adnexal disorder
    i. bowel disease (IBD)
    i. fracture
    i. response
inflation
    cuff i.
in-flight assessment
influenzae
    Haemophilus i.
    Haemophilus i. type B (Hib)
influenza-related pneumonia
influenza virus
information
    anatomic i.
infracardiac bursa
infraclavicular
    i. cannulation
    i. retraction
infraction fracture
infradiaphragmatic vein
infraepitrochlear nerve
infrahyoid
    i. bursa
    i. strap muscle
infrainguinal reconstruction
infraoccipital nerve
infraorbital
    i. fracture
    i. nerve
    i. suture
    i. vein
infrapatellar
    i. bursa

i. ligament
i. tendon
infrasegmental vein
infraspinatus
i. bursa
i. muscle
i. tendon
infraspinous muscle
infratrochlear nerve
infundibuloovarian ligament
infundibulopelvic ligament
infuser
rapid i.
infusion
crystalloid i.
glucose insulin potassium i.
intraosseous i.
nerve block i.
stem cell i.
ingestion
acid i.
alkali i.
American yew i.
ammonia i.
anticonvulsant drug i.
Arisaema triphyllum i.
autumn crocus i.
azalea i.
baneberry i.
battery i.
black locust tree i.
bleach i.
bloodroot plant i.
Boston ivy i.
Brugmansia i.
buckthorn i.
bufalin i.
Caladium i.
Callipesis laureola i.
Caltha palustris i.
cardiac glycoside i.
Carolina jessamine plant i.
castor bean i.
caustic i.
cement i.
chaparral i.
cherry kernel i.
chokecherry kernel i.
Cicuta i.
cohosh plant i.
cologne i.
Convallaria majalis i.

corn lily i.
cowslip i.
daffodil i.
Datura stramonium i.
death camas i.
dental care product i.
deodorant i.
depilatory preparation i.
dumbcane plant i.
i. exposure
i. exposure with suspicious history
fingernail cosmetic i.
foreign body i.
Gelsemium sempervirens i.
germander i.
i. of golden chain tree
hair product i.
halogenated hydrocarbon i.
i. of hemlock
hydrofluoric acid i.
inorganic arsenic i.
Jack-in-the-pulpit i.
Japanese yew i.
jequirity bean i.
Jin Bu Huan i.
Lanatana camera shrub i.
larkspur i.
locoweed i.
marigold i.
Nerium oleander i.
Nicotiana glauca i.
Nicotiana tabacum i.
pesticide i.
Phytolacca americana i.
pine oil i.
pokeweed i.
Rhododendron i.
rhubarb leaf blade i.
skin lightener i.
talc i.
toxic i.
turpentine i.
Ingram-Bachynski hip fracture
classification
ingrown toenail
ingrowth
bone i.
inguinal
i. crease
i. hernia
i. ligament

NOTES

inguinal (*continued*)
    i. nerve
    i. region
inhalant abuse
inhalation
    ammonia gas i.
    arsine gas i.
    i. exposure
    gas i.
    heroin vapor i.
    i. injury
    smoke i.
    toxic gas i.
    vapor i.
inhalational
    i. anesthesia
    i. anthrax
inhaled nitric oxide (iNO)
inhaler
    Atrovent i.
    dry-powder i.
    hand-held aerosol i.
    metered-dose i. (MDI)
    Proventil i.
inherited anemia
inhibited muscle
inhibition
    GABA-mediated i.
    mediated i.
    platelet i.
inhibitor
    ACE i.
    acetylcholinesterase i.
    adenosine triphosphatase i.
    5-alpha reductase i.
    angiotensin-converting enzyme i.
    aromatase i.
    carbonic anhydrase i.
    COX-2 i.
    cyclooxygenase-2 i.
    gastric acid i.
    monoamine oxidase i. (MAOI)
    phosphodiesterase i.
    platelet i.
    protease i.
inhibitory nerve
initial
    i. airway support
    i. assessment
    i. injury
    i. location
    i. location of pain
    i. stabilization
    i. therapy
injection
    corticosteroid i.
    dexmedetomidine hydrochloride i.
    intrathecal i.
    nerve root sleeve i.

    Nimbex i.
    Precedex i.
    Protopam I.
    i. sclerotherapy
    i. site
    i. therapy
injured brain
injury
    Achilles tendon i.
    acrolein inhalation i.
    acromioclavicular i.
    acromioclavicular joint i.
    acute intracranial i.
    acute lung i. (ALI)
    adult cerebrospinal i.
    aerodigestive tract i.
    air bag i.
    airway i.
    alkaline caustic i.
    anoxic brain i.
    anterior cruciate ligament i.
    assaultive i.
    axonal i.
    ballistic i.
    bicycle i.
    bladder i.
    blast i.
    blunt cardiac i. (BCI)
    bony i.
    brachial plexus i.
    brain i.
    caustic i.
    celiac axis i.
    cerebral i.
    cervical cord i.
    cervical spine i.
    cervical vascular organ i.
    chest wall i.
    closed-fist i. (CFI)
    closed head i. (CHI)
    clothesline i.
    coccygeal i.
    coccyx spine i.
    corrosive i.
    corticospinal tract i.
    crush i.
    deep hand i.
    degloving i.
    diaphragmatic i.
    diffuse axonal i. (DAI)
    dive-related i.
    elbow i.
    electrical i.
    electromagnetic radiation i.
    epiphysial i.
    esophageal i.
    facial nerve i.
    facial soft tissue i.
    fingertip i.

fireworks i.
first-degree i.
flexor tendon i.
foot phalangeal i.
formaldehyde inhalation i.
grease gun i.
hand phalangeal i.
hanging i.
head i.
heart valve i.
hepatic i.
high-pressure hand i.
high-pressure injection i.
hip i.
history of past i.
hollow viscus i.
household i.
hydrogen sulfide inhalation i.
impalement i.
inhalation i.
initial i.
intracranial i. (ICI)
isocyanate inhalation i.
isolated i.
joint i.
knee i.
lap seat belt i.
light-induced i.
lightning i.
lumbar spine i.
mechanism of i. (MOI)
medial meniscus i.
metacarpal i.
metatarsal i.
minor i.
multiple associated i.'s
muscle crushing i.
nailbed i.
near-drowning i.
nerve crush i.
neutrophil-dependent lung i.
occult i.
open i.
ozone inhalation i.
parenchymal i.
past i.
patella i.
patellar i.
pediatric cerebrospinal i.
penetrating i.
pericardial i.
periorbital soft tissue i.

peripheral vascular i.
peroneal tendon i.
phalangeal i.
pressure gun i.
radiation i.
renal i.
reperfusion i.
roller-type i.
rotation i.
rotator cuff i.
seat belt i.
severe head i.
severity of i.
I. Severity Score
shearing i.
small bowel i.
soft tissue hand i.
solid organ i.
solid viscus i.
specific organ i.
spinal cord i.
spinothalamic tract i.
splenic i.
sternoclavicular joint i.
straddle i.
submersion i.
tarsal i.
temporomandibular joint i.
tendon i.
thoracic great vessel i.
thoracic spine i.
tibial plateau i.
tracheobronchial tree i.
traumatic axonal shear i.
traumatic brain i. (TBI)
unexplained i.
unstable i.
urogenital i.
vascular i.
ventilator-induced lung i.
wringer-type i.
zipper i.

in-line immobilization
inner ear
innermost intercostal muscle
innervated muscle
innervation
autonomic i.
muscle i.
innominate
i. artery

NOTES

innominate *(continued)*
    i. bone
    i. cardiac vein
Innsbruck Coma Scale
iNO
    inhaled nitric oxide
Inocor
inorganic arsenic ingestion
inotrope
inotropic
    i. agent
    i. therapy
inpatient unit (IPU)
input nerve
input/output (I/O)
insect
    i. bite
    i. sting
insecticide
    hydrocarbon i.
insertion
    bony i.
    chest tube i.
    tendon i.
    i. trauma
insipidus
    diabetes i. (DI)
inspiration
    crowing i.
inspiratory
    i. downstroke
    i. to expiratory (I:E)
    i. flow
    i. muscle
    i. rhonchi
    i. time (Ti)
Inspiron nebulizer
inspissated cerumen
instability
    dorsal intercalated segment i.
      (DISI)
    hemodynamic i.
    joint i.
    ligamentous i.
InstaChar activated charcoal
Insta-Glucose
instillation
institutional factor
institutionalize
    threat to i.
instrument
    acute cardiac ischemia-time
      insensitive predictive i. (ACI-TIPI)
    bone abduction i.
    Suture Assistant i.
insufficiency
    acute adrenal i.
    adrenal i.
    adrenocortical i.

    aortic valve i.
    arterial i.
    cardiac i.
    i. fracture
    limb-threatening arterial i.
    mitral i.
    muscle i.
    pulmonary i.
    tricuspid i.
    venous i.
insufflation
    jet i.
    nasal i.
    percutaneous transtracheal i.
insular
    i. artery
    i. vein
insulin
    i. abuse
    i. lipoatrophy
    i. shock
insulin-dependent diabetes mellitus
   (IDDM)
insulinoma
intact cerebral hemisphere
integration
Integrilin
    I. to Minimize Platelet Aggregation
      and Coronary Thrombosis-Acute
      Myocardial (IMPACT-AMI)
    I. to Minimize Platelet Aggregation
      and Coronary Thrombosis-II
      (IMPACT-II)
    I. therapy
integument
integumentary system
intelligence quotient (IQ)
intensity
    point of maximal i. (PMI)
intensive
    i. care (IC)
    i. care unit (ICU)
    i. care unit monitoring
    i. care unit stay
    i. coronary care (ICC)
    i. coronary care unit (ICCU)
intensivist
intention
    first i.
    healing by first i.
    healing by primary i.
    healing by second i.
    healing by secondary i.
    healing by third i.
    primary i.
    second i.
    secondary i.
    third i.

interaction
    acetaminophen-alcohol i.
    drug-drug i.
    food-drug i.
    interpersonal i.
interarticular fracture
interarytenoid muscle
interatrial septum
intercapital
    i. ligament
    i. vein
intercapitular vein
intercarotid nerve
intercarpal ligament
interchondral ligament
interclavicular ligament
interclinoid ligament
intercom
    ultrasound i.
intercondylar
    i. femoral fracture
    i. humeral fracture
    i. tibial fracture
interconnection
    fascial i.
    ligamentous i.
intercornual ligament
intercostal
    i. indrawing
    i. ligament
    i. margin (ICM)
    i. muscle
    i. nerve
    i. nerve block
    i. retraction
    i. space
    i. vein
intercostobrachial nerve
intercostohumeral nerve
intercourse
    anal i.
    sexual i.
intercrural-septal suture
intercuneiform ligament
interdental ligament
interdependence
    ventricular i.
interdigital
    i. ligament
    i. nerve
interdigitalis
    erosio i.

interdomal suture
interendognathic suture
interest
    conflict of i.
interfascicular guide suture
interference
    nerve i.
interferon alpha
interfoveolar
    i. ligament
    i. muscle
interim
interleukin-6
interleukin-10
interligamentous bursa
interlobar vein
intermaxillary
    i. bone
    i. suture
intermediary nerve
intermediate
    i. antebrachial vein
    i. basilic vein
    i. bursa
    i. cephalic vein
    i. cubital vein
    i. cuneiform bone
    i. dorsal cutaneous nerve
    i. great muscle
    i. hepatic vein
    i. supraclavicular nerve
    i. tendon
    i. vastus muscle
intermedius nerve
intermetacarpal ligament
intermetatarsal
    i. bursa
    i. ligament
    i. nerve
    i. vein
intermetatarsophalangeal bursa
intermittent
    i. claudication
    i. fever
    i. mandatory ventilation (IMV)
    i. peritoneal dialysis
    i. pneumatic compression (IPC)
    i. positive-pressure breathing (IPPB)
    i. ventilation
intermuscular gluteal bursa
internal
    i. abdominal muscle

NOTES

internal *(continued)*
  i. auditory vein
  i. bleeding
  i. calcaneoastragaloid ligament
  i. cardiac massage
  i. cardioverter-defibrillator (ICD)
  i. carotid nerve
  i. cerebral vein
  i. collateral ligament
  i. fissure hypertonia
  i. fixation
  i. fixation fracture
  i. iliac vein
  i. intercostal muscle
  i. jugular vein
  i. jugular vein cannulation
  i. lateral ligament
  i. lesion
  i. maxillary vein
  i. oblique muscle
  i. obturator muscle
  i. popliteal nerve
  i. pterygoid muscle
  i. pudendal vein
  i. rectal nerve
  i. rotator muscle
  i. saphenous nerve
  i. sphincter
  i. suture
  i. thoracic vein
internally fixed fracture
internasal suture
international
  I. Classification of Disease (ICD)
  I. Knee Ligament
  I. Registry of Acute Aortic Dissection (IRAD)
  i. relief assistance
interosseous
  i. cubital bursa
  i. cuneocuboid ligament
  i. cuneometatarsal ligament
  i. intercuneiform ligament
  i. metacarpal ligament
  i. metatarsal ligament
  i. muscle
  i. nerve
  i. sacroiliac ligament
  i. talocalcaneal ligament
  i. tendon
  i. tibiofibular ligament
  i. vein
interpalatine suture
interpalpebral suture
interparietal
  i. bone
  i. suture
interperiosteal fracture
interpersonal interaction

interphalangeal collateral ligament
interposed abdominal compression-cardiopulmonary resuscitation (IAC-CPR)
interproximal bone
interrogans
  Leptospira i.
interrupted
  high-frequency flow i. (HFFI)
  i. loop mattress suture
  i. manual mucomucosal absorbable suture
  i. nylon suture
  i. pledgeted suture
  i. quilt suture
  i. seromuscular suture
  i. stitch
interruption
  caval i.
intersesamoid ligament
intersphincteric
  i. abscess
  i. space
interspinal
  i. ligament
  i. muscle
interspinous ligament
interstice
  bone i.
interstitial
  i. disease
  i. edema
  i. fibrosis
  i. nephritis
  i. pneumonia (IP)
  i. pulmonary fibrosis (IPF)
intertransverse
  i. ligament
  i. muscle
intertrigo
intertrochanteric
  i. femoral fracture
  i. fracture
  i. hip fracture
  i. 4-part fracture
interval
  lucid i.
intervening muscle
intervention
  emergent operative i.
  facilitated percutaneous coronary i.
  need for operative i.
  operative i.
  surgical i.
  therapeutic i.
  triage i.
interventional radiologist
interventricular vein

intervertebral
 i. ligament
 i. vein
interview
 patient-centered i.
 triad model i.
intervolar plate ligament
intestinal
 i. atresia
 i. cestode
 i. distention
 i. muscularis fiber spasm
 i. obstruction syndrome
 i. pseudoobstruction
 i. sepsis
 i. transport
 i. vein
intima
intimal
 i. proliferation
 i. tear
intimate
 i. partner abuse (IPA)
 i. partner violence (IPV)
 i. partner violence detection
intolerance
 lactose i.
intoxication
 acute i.
 alcohol i.
 antipsychotic i.
 aspirin i.
 barbiturate i.
 central nervous system i.
 chronic i.
 cyclic antidepressant i.
 digitalis i.
 ethanol i.
 ethylene glycol i.
 isopropyl alcohol i.
 lithium i.
 poisonous plant i.
 substance i.
 sympathomimetic i.
 theophylline i.
 tricyclic antidepressant i.
 valproic acid i.
intraabdominal
 i. abscess
 i. hypertension
 i. mass
 i. pathology

 i. pressure (IAP)
 i. sepsis
intraaortic
 i. balloon pump (IABP)
 i. balloon pump counterpulsation
 i. counterpulsation balloon
intraarticular
 i. calcaneal fracture
 i. cartilage
 i. ligament
 i. proximal tibial fracture
intraatrial reentrant tachycardia
intraauricular muscle
intrabuccal wound
intracameral suture
intracapsular
 i. femoral neck fracture
 i. ligament
intracardiac shunt
intracartilaginous bone
intracellular water
intracerebral
 i. aneurysm
 i. hematoma
 i. hemorrhage
 i. pressure
intracoronary
 i. laser therapy
 i. stent
intracranial
 i. abscess
 i. hemorrhage (ICH)
 i. hypertension
 i. injury (ICI)
 i. pressure (ICP)
intractable
 i. crying
 i. pain
intracuticular running suture
intradermal continuous suture
intradural draining vein
intrafascicular suture
intraforaminal vein
intragluteal fold
intrahepatic
 i. shunt
 i. umbilical vein
intraligamentous bursa
intraluminal
 i. balloon
 i. suture
intramedullary rodding

NOTES

intramembranous bone
intramuscular (IM)
    i. conscious sedation
intranasal palpation test
intraocular muscle
intraoperative fracture
intraoral
    i. anesthetic
    i. muscle
intraorbital fracture
intraosseous
    i. infusion
    i. line
    i. tibiofibular ligament
    i. venous access
intrapancreatic nerve
intraparenchymal hematoma
intrapatellar bursa
intraperiosteal fracture
intraperitoneal
    i. fluid
    i. infection
intrapleural pressure
intraportal vein
intrapulmonary shunt
intrarenal vein
intrascapular ligament
IntraSite dressing
intraspinous muscle
intratendinous olecranon bursa
intrathecal injection
intrathoracic abdomen
intrauterine
    i. fetal death
    i. fracture
    i. resuscitation
intravascular
    i. blood gas exchanger
    disseminated i.
    i. oxygenator (IVOX)
    i. volume
intravenous (I.V.)
    i. access
    i. antibiotic
    i. conscious sedation
    i. contrast
    i. contrast CT
    i. drug abuser (IVDA)
    i. drug use (IVDU)
    i. line
    i. pyelogram (IVP)
    i. pyelography
    i. single dose
    i. tissue plasminogen activator
    i. urography
intraventricular
    i. conduction delay
    i. hemorrhage (IVH)

intrinsic
    i. hepatotoxin
    i. ligament
    i. muscle
Introcan Safety IV catheter
introducer
    percutaneous sheath i.
intubate
intubating laryngeal mask (ILM)
intubation
    blind nasotracheal i. (BNTI)
    cricothyroid i.
    i. difficulty scale (IDS)
    early i.
    endotracheal i. (ETI)
    fiberoptic i.
    fiberoptic bronchoscope i.
    fiberoptic laryngoscope i.
    main stem bronchus i.
    nasoduodenal i.
    nasogastric i.
    nasojejunal i.
    nasotracheal i.
    oral awake i.
    orotracheal i.
    rapid sequence i. (RSI)
    retrograde i. (RI)
    retrograde tracheal i.
    tracheal i.
    transillumination i.
    i. tube
intussusception
    vein i.
invaginate
invasive
    i. core rewarming
    i. pressure monitoring
inverse
    i. ratio (IR)
    i. ratio ventilation (IRV)
inversion stress
inverted
    i. mattress suture
    i. subcuticular suture
inverted-Y fracture
inverting suture
Investa suture
involuntary
    i. guarding
    i. movement
    i. muscle
involutional melancholia
involvement
    extensive gingival i.
    fascial i.
    perirectal i.
    spontaneous i.
    systemic i.

I/O
> input/output

iodide
>> potassium i. (KI)
>> saturated solution of potassium i. (SSKI)

iodine
>> i. catgut suture
>> povidone i.
>> i. toxicity

iodine-131 metaiodobenzylguanidine (^{131}I-MIBG)
iodized surgical gut suture
iodochromic catgut suture
iodothymol toxicity
ion
>> I. Tester KST-900
>> i. trapping

ionizing radiation
IP
> interstitial pneumonia

IPA
> intimate partner abuse

IPC
> intermittent pneumatic compression
>> IPC boot

ipecac
>> syrup of i.
>> i. syrup

IPF
> idiopathic pulmonary fibrosis
> interstitial pulmonary fibrosis

IPG
> impedance plethysmography

IPPB
> intermittent positive-pressure breathing

ipratropium bromide
ipsilateral
>> i. acetabular fracture
>> i. femoral neck fracture
>> i. femoral shaft fracture
>> i. hand
>> i. lateral rectus muscle
>> i. pelvic fracture
>> i. tibial fracture

IPU
> inpatient unit

IPV
> intimate partner violence

IQ
> intelligence quotient

IR
> inverse ratio

IRAD
> International Registry of Acute Aortic Dissection

iridial muscle
iridodialysis
iris
>> i. scissors
>> i. sphincter muscle
>> i. suture

iritis
iron (Fe)
>> i. deficiency anemia
>> i. deposition
>> i. poisoning
>> i. toxicity

irradiated bone
irradiation
irreducible
>> i. fracture
>> i. hernia

irregular
>> i. bone
>> i. pulse

irregularity
>> luminal i.
>> tendon i.

irreversible shock
irrigation
>> external auditory canal i.
>> tendon sheath i.
>> whole bowel i. (WBI)
>> wound i.

irritability
>> muscle i.
>> nerve root i.

irritable
>> i. bowel
>> i. bowel syndrome (IBS)
>> i. infant
>> i. somnolence

irritant
>> CA i.
>> CN i.
>> CNB i.
>> CNC i.
>> CR i.
>> CS i.
>> i. gas exposure
>> i. laxative

NOTES

irritant *(continued)*
    peritoneal i.
    PS i.
irritation
    nerve root i.
    peritoneal i.
    vulvar i.
IRV
    inverse ratio ventilation
ischemia
    abdominal i.
    acute limb i.
    acute mesenteric i.
    asymptomatic cardiac i. (ACI)
    bowel i.
    cerebral i.
    limb i.
    mesenteric i.
    muscle i.
    myocardial i.
    prolonged warm i.
    suspicion of bowel i.
    tissue i.
    tourniquet i.
    traumatic i.
    visceral i.
    wound i.
ischemic
    i. bowel
    i. brain lesion
    i. colitis
    i. edema
    i. hypoxia
    i. optic neuropathy
    i. stroke
ischiadic nerve
ischial
    i. bone
    i. bursa
    i. strap
    i. tuberosity
ischioacetabular fracture
ischiocapsular ligament
ischiocavernous muscle
ischiococcygeus muscle
ischiofemoral ligament
ischiogluteal bursa
ischiorectal
    i. abscess
    i. space
ischium
isethionate
    pentamidine i.
ISIS-3
    Third International Study of Infarct
    Survival
    ISIS-3 trial
island
    bone i.

islet of Langerhans
isoantigen
    Rh i.
isocarboxazid
isocyanate inhalation injury
isoetharine
isograft
    bone i.
isolated
    i. atrial septal defect
    i. hook fracture
    i. injury
    i. lung transplant
isolation
    body substance i. (BSI)
    denial and i.
isoniazid poisoning
isonitrile
    technetium 99m i.
isopropanol poisoning
isopropyl
    i. alcohol intoxication
    i. alcohol toxicity
    i. alcohol treatment
isoproterenol therapy
isoquinoline
isotonia
isotonic exercise
isotope
    bone mineralization i.
isovolemic
    i. blood loss
    i. hyponatremia
isradipine
issue
    end-of-life i.
ITP
    idiopathic thrombocytopenic purpura
itraconazole
I.V.
    intravenous
    Protonix I.V.
    I.V. t-PA
Ivalon suture
IVC
    inferior vena cava
    IVC filter
IVDA
    intravenous drug abuser
IVDU
    intravenous drug use
IVH
    intraventricular hemorrhage
ivory bone
IVOX
    intravascular oxygenator
IVP
    intravenous pyelogram

ivy
  Boston i.
  poison i.

Ixodes scapularis

NOTES

jacket
    Weathertech EMS 3-in-1 systems j.
Jack-in-the-pulpit ingestion
Jacobson nerve
Jamaican vomiting sickness
Japanese yew ingestion
japonica
    Pieris j.
Jarjavay ligament
JAS
    juvenile ankylosing spondylitis
jaundice
    neonatal j.
jaundiced skin
jaw
    j. bone
    j. thrust
jaw-thrust
    j.-t. maneuver
    j.-t. method
Jefferson
    J. cervical burst fracture
    J. radial fracture
Jeffery radial fracture classification
Jehovah's Witness
jeikeium
    Corynebacterium j.
jejunostomy
    percutaneous j.
    surgical j.
jelly
    K-Y j.
jellyfish envenomation
jequirity bean ingestion
jerk
    tendon j.
jerking
    myoclonic j.
jerky nystagmus
jet
    j. entrainment
    j. insufflation
    j. nebulizer
    j. ventilator
jimson
    j. weed
    j. weed poisoning
Jin Bu Huan ingestion
Jobert de Lamballe suture
joint
    j. abnormality
    acromioclavicular j.
    ball-and-socket j.
    j. depression fracture
    hinge j.

    hip j.
    hot j.
    hypermobile j.
    j. injury
    j. instability
    locking of j.
    metacarpophalangeal j.
    metatarsal j.
    metatarsophalangeal j. (MPJ, MTPJ)
    j. space
    j. space air
    splinting of j.
    suture pusher talofibular j.
    j. synovium
    temporomandibular j. (TMJ)
    j. wound
Jones
    J. diaphysial fracture classification
    J. dressing
    J. stress fracture
joule
Jr
    EpiPen Jr
J retention wire fracture
Judet epiphysial fracture
judgment
    poor j.
jugal
    j. bone
    j. ligament
jug-handle view
jugular
    j. foramen muscle
    j. nerve
    j. vein (JV)
    j. vein cannulation
    j. venous distention (JVD)
    j. venous pressure (JVP)
    j. venous pulse (JVP)
    j. venous saturation
jugulocephalic vein
junction
    esophagocardiac j.
    neuromuscular j.
junctional
    j. arrhythmia
    j. contraction
    j. fracture
    j. rhythm
juncturae tendinum
Jung muscle
juvenile
    j. ankylosing spondylitis (JAS)
    j. delinquent
    diabetes mellitus, j.

J

juvenile *(continued)*
- j. idiopathic arthritis
- j. insulin-dependent type 1 diabetes mellitus
- j. rheumatoid arthritis
- j. Tillaux fracture

juxtaarticular fracture
juxtacortical fracture
juxtahepatic vein

juxtalimbal suture
juxtaposition
JV
- jugular vein

JVD
- jugular venous distention

JVP
- jugular venous pressure
- jugular venous pulse

K
  potassium
Kal-Dermic suture
Kalmia latifolia
kangaroo tendon suture
Kapandji radical fracture
Kaposi sarcoma
Karwinski humboldtriana
kava kava
Kawasaki
  K. disease
  K. syndrome
Kayexalate therapy
KED
  Kendrick extrication device
Kehr sign
Kelly clamp
keloid
Kendrick extrication device (KED)
keratitis
  ulcerative k.
  ultraviolet k.
keratoacanthoma
keratoconjunctivitis
  herpetic k.
keraunoparalysis
Kernig sign
Kessler
  K. grasping suture
  K. stitch
Kessler-Kleinert suture
Kessler-Tajima suture
Ketalar
ketamine
ketoacidosis
  alcoholic k. (AKA)
  diabetic k. (DKA)
  fasting k.
  metabolic k.
ketoconazole
ketone
ketorolac
ketotic hypoglycemia
Kety-Schmidt blood flow measurement method
Key-Conwell pelvic fracture classification
key vein
KI
  potassium iodide
kidney
  k. basin
  crush k.
  multicystic k.
  multilobar k.

parenchymal injury of k.
  k. rejection
  k. transplantation
  k. trauma
  k.'s, ureters, bladder (KUB)
Kiesselbach
  K. area
  K. plexus
Kilfoyle humeral medial condylar fracture classification
kinase
  acetate k.
kinematics
kinetic energy
kinetics
  first-order k.
  Michaelis-Menten k.
  zero-order k.
kingae
  Haemophilus aphrophilus, Actinobacillus actinomycetemcomitans, Cardiobacterium hominis, Eikenella corrodens, Kingella k. (HACEK)
Kirschner suture
kissing burn
kit
  CPAP k.
  first aid k.
  nitrite-thiosulfate k.
  peel-away sheath cystostomy k.
  rape k.
  Xpouch emergency k.
Klebsiella pneumoniae
Kleihauer-Betke test
Klein muscle
Klippel-Feil syndrome
knee
  k. arthrocentesis
  k. bone
  k. dislocation
  k. injury
  k. ligament
  k. splint
kneecap stabilizer
knee-to-chest position
knife wound
Knight and North malar fracture classification
knot
  buried k.
  muscle k.
known trigger
knuckle bone

K

Kocher fracture
Kocher-Lorenz fracture
KOH
  potassium chloride
  KOH smear
Köhler
  K. disease
  K. fracture
Kohlrausch
  K. muscle
  K. vein
Korotkoff sound
Korsakoff
  K. psychosis
  K. syndrome
Koyter muscle
Krackow suture
Krause
  K. ligament

  K. muscle
  suture of K.
Krazy Glue
Krukenberg vein
krusei
  Candida k.
KST-900
  Ion Tester KST-900
KUB
  kidneys, ureters, bladder
  KUB and upright
Kuhnt postcentral vein
Kussmaul
  K. coma
  K. respiration
  K. sign
Küstner suture
K-Y jelly

L-25 absorbable surgical suture
Labeling of Art Materials Act
labetalol
labia (*pl. of* labium)
labial
    l. nerve
    l. vein
labile
    l. affect
    l. hypertension
labioglossopharyngeal nerve
labiomandibular ligament
labium, pl. labia
    labia majora
    l. majus
    l. majus muscle
    labia minora
    l. minus
    l. minus muscle
labor
    complicated l.
    preterm l.
labored
    l. breathing
    l. respiration
labral and anterior inferior glenoid rim fracture
lab results
Laburnum anagyroides
labyrinthine vein
labyrinthitis
    acute vestibular l.
lacerate
lacerated
    l. tendon
    l. wound
lacerating wound
laceration
    anal sphincter l.
    aortic l.
    avulsed l.
    birth canal l.
    bladder l.
    boot-top l.
    brain l.
    burst-type l.
    canalicular l.
    central stellate l.
    cerebral l.
    cervical l.
    chevron l.
    complex l.
    concurrent hepatic l.
    conjunctival l.
    corneal l.

    corneoscleral l.
    crush-type l.
    curvilinear l.
    degloving l.
    diaphragm l.
    diaphragmatic l.
    eyebrow l.
    eyelid l.
    falx l.
    first-degree l.
    flexor tendon l.
    fourth-degree l.
    full-thickness corneal l.
    hallucis longus l.
    inadvertent l.
    lid margin l.
    linear l.
    liver l.
    longitudinal l.
    lower pole l.
    lung l.
    Mallory-Weiss l.
    l. management
    nail bed l.
    otologic l.
    parenchymal l.
    partial-thickness corneal l.
    penile l.
    perineal l.
    peripheral l.
    pharyngeal l.
    posterior pharyngeal l.
    rectal l.
    scalp l.
    second-degree l.
    shallow l.
    spinal cord l.
    spleen l.
    splenic l.
    stellate nail bed l.
    suture penile l.
    tarsal l.
    tendon l.
    tentorial l.
    third-degree l.
    through-and-through l.
    trap-door l.
    vaginal l.
    vascular l.
    zigzag l.
lacidem suture
lacinate ligament
laciniate ligament
lack of pain control

L

lacrimal
  l. bone
  l. duct
  l. gland
  l. nerve
  l. vein
lacrimation
lacrimoconchal suture
lacrimoethmoidal suture
lacrimomaxillary suture
lacrimoturbinal suture
lactated
  l. Ringer (LR)
  l. Ringer solution (LRS)
Lactate Pro LT-1710 portable lactate analyzer
lactation disease
lactic acidosis
lactose intolerance
lactulose abuse
lacuna, pl. **lacunae**
  bone l.
lacunar
  l. infarct
  l. ligament
  l. stroke
Laennec cirrhosis
LaGrange humeral supracondylar fracture classification
lambdoidal cranial suture
lambdoid suture
Lambert-Eaton myasthenic syndrome
lamblia
  Giardia l.
laminar
  l. bone
  l. flow
  l. fracture
lamivudine
lamp
  slit l.
Lanatana camera shrub ingestion
lancet
  suture l.
  l. suture
lancinating pain
Lancisi
  L. muscle
  L. nerve
Landry-Guillain-Barré syndrome
Landsmeer ligament
Langerhans
  islet of L.
Langer muscle
Langley nerve
Lang suture
language
  disorganized l.
  rambling l.

Lannelongue ligament
Lanoxin
lap
  l. seat belt fracture
  l. seat belt injury
laparoscopic trocar wound
laparoscopy
  pelvic l.
laparotomy
  blind l.
  diagnostic l.
  emergent l.
  exploratory l.
Lapra-Ty suture
large
  l. bowel obstruction
  l. intestine obstruction
  l. saphenous vein
large-bore
  l.-b. intravenous line
  l.-b. suction catheter
large-caliber nonabsorbable suture
larkspur ingestion
laryngeal
  l. bursa
  l. cartilage fracture
  l. edema
  l. fracture
  l. mask
  l. mask airway (LMA)
  l. muscle
  l. nerve
  l. nerve paralysis
  l. spasm
  l. vein
laryngectomy
larynges (*pl. of* larynx)
laryngitis
  diphtheric l.
laryngopharynx
laryngoscope
  l. blade
  fiberoptic l.
  rigid l.
laryngoscopy
  fiberoptic l.
  reflex sympathetic response to l. (RSRL)
laryngospasm
  reflex glottic closure and l.
laryngotracheal
  l. separation
  l. trauma
laryngotracheobronchitis
larynx, pl. **larynges**
  l. fracture
lashing suture
Lasix

lassitude
last menstrual period (LMP)
lata (*pl. of* latum)
Latarjet
    L. nerve
    L. vein
late dislocation
latency
latent diabetes
lateral
    l. abdominal region
    l. accessory ligament
    l. approach
    l. arcuate ligament
    l. atlantooccipital ligament
    l. atrial vein
    l. bending
    l. canthal tendon
    l. canthus
    l. circumflex femoral vein
    l. collateral ligament
    l. column calcaneal fracture
    l. condylar fracture
    l. condylar humeral fracture
    l. condyle bone
    l. costotransverse ligament
    l. cricoarytenoid muscle
    l. cuneiform bone
    l. direct vein
    l. dorsal cutaneous nerve
    l. epicondylar bursa
    l. femoral cutaneous nerve
    l. great muscle
    l. humeral condyle fracture
    l. interosseous ligament
    l. lumbar intertransverse muscle
    l. lumbosacral ligament
    l. malleolar subcutaneous bursa
    l. malleolus
    l. malleolus bursa
    l. malleolus fracture
    l. malleolus muscle
    l. mammary vein
    l. mass fracture
    l. mastoid bone
    l. maxillary ligament
    l. palpebral ligament
    l. pectoral nerve
    l. plantar nerve
    l. plantar vein
    l. popliteal nerve
    l. pressure syndrome

    l. pterygoid muscle
    l. pterygoid nerve
    l. puboprostatic ligament
    l. rectal ligament
    l. rectus extraocular muscle
    l. rectus tendon
    l. recumbent position
    l. sacral vein
    l. sacrococcygeal ligament
    l. sesamoid bone
    l. spring ligament
    l. superior genicular nerve
    l. supraclavicular nerve
    l. sural cutaneous nerve
    l. talar process fracture
    l. talocalcaneal ligament
    l. temporomandibular ligament
    l. thoracic vein
    l. thyrohyoid ligament
    l. thyroid ligament
    l. tibial plateau fracture
    l. trap suture
    l. two lumbricals, opponens
      pollicis, abductor pollicis brevis,
      flexor pollicis brevis (LOAF)
    l. ulnar collateral ligament
    l. umbilical ligament
    l. vastus muscle
    l. wedge fracture
    l. wound
lateralization defect
laterally displaced fracture
latex allergy
latifolia
    Kalmia l.
latissimus dorsi muscle
latum, pl. lata
    condyloma lata
laudable pus
Lauge-Hansen
    L.-H. ankle fracture classification
    L.-H. stage II supination-eversion
      fracture
    L.-H. system
Laugier fracture
Lauth ligament
lavage
    bone l.
    bronchoalveolar l. (BAL)
    bronchopulmonary l.
    diagnostic peritoneal l. (DPL)
    gastric l.

L

NOTES

lavage *(continued)*
 orogastric l.
 peritoneal l.
 pulmonary l.
laxative
 l. abuse
 bulk-producing l.
 irritant l.
 saline l.
 stimulant l.
 surfactant l.
lax ligament
layer
 arachnoid l.
 membranous l.
 multiform l.
 nerve fiber bundle l.
 subcuticular l.
layered closure
LCM
 left costal margin
Le
 Le Dentu suture
 Le Fort I-III fracture
 Le Fort mandibular fracture
 Le Fort suture
 Le Fort-Wagstaffe fracture
lead
 l. pipe fracture
 l. poisoning
 precordial l.
 l. suture
 tooth l.
leader
 medical unit l. (MUL)
 tendon l.
lead-shot tie suture
leaf of broad ligament
leaking
 l. ascites
 l. vein
LEAN
 lidocaine, epinephrine, atropine, naloxone
 LEAN drug
least
 l. gluteal muscle
 l. splanchnic nerve
Lee-Jones
 L.-J. test
 L.-J. test for cyanide toxicity
left
 l. brachiocephalic vein
 l. colic vein
 l. coronary vein
 l. costal margin (LCM)
 l. gastric vein
 l. gastroepiploic vein
 l. gastroomental vein
 l. gonadal vein

 l. heart failure
 l. hepatic vein
 l. hypogastric nerve
 l. inferior pulmonary vein
 l. inferior rectus muscle
 l. internal jugular vein
 l. lateral recumbent position
 l. lower extremity (LLE)
 l. lower quadrant (LLQ)
 l. mainstem bronchus
 l. marginal vein
 l. median vein
 l. ovarian vein
 l. pericardiacophrenic vein
 l. phrenic vein
 l. pulmonary vein
 l. recurrent laryngeal nerve
 l. respiratory nerve
 l. retroaortic renal vein
 l. rhomboid muscle
 l. sternal border (LSB)
 l. subclavian vein
 l. superior gluteal vein
 l. superior intercostal vein
 l. superior pulmonary vein
 l. superior rectus muscle
 l. suprarenal vein
 l. testicular vein
 l. triangular ligament
 l. umbilical vein
 l. upper extremity (LUE)
 l. upper quadrant (LUQ)
 l. ventricular assist device (LVAD)
 l. ventricular compliance
 l. ventricular end-diastolic pressure (LVEDP)
 l. ventricular failure
 l. ventricular muscle
 l. ventricular preload
 l. vertical vein
left-sided heart failure
left-to-right intracardiac shunt
legal causation
leg edema
Legg-Calvé-Perthes disease
Legionella
 L. infection
 L. pneumophila
Legionnaires disease
Leiden
 factor V L. (FVL)
leiomyoma
leiomyosarcoma
leishmaniasis
Lembert
 L. inverting seromuscular suture
 L. running suture
length
 horizontal l.

muscle moment arm l.
vertical l.
lengthening
muscle l.
tendon l.
lens
l. dislocation
l. displacement
suture of l.
l. suture
lenticular bone
lentiform bone
Lepidoptera **poisoning**
Leptospira interrogans
leptospirosis
lesion
acneiform l.
bone surface l.
brain l.
brainstem l.
bullous skin l.
caustic l.
cerebral vascular l.
crescentic l.
cutaneous l.
endometrial l.
focal l.
internal l.
ischemic brain l.
midbrain l.
nerve root l.
l. repair
space-occupying l.
subtentorial l.
supratentorial l.
lesser
l. internal cutaneous nerve
l. occipital nerve
l. ovarian vein
l. palatine nerve
l. rhomboid muscle
l. saphenous vein
l. splanchnic nerve
l. superficial petrosal nerve
l. trochanter fracture
l. trochanter pubic bone
l. zygomatic muscle
LET
lidocaine, epinephrine, tetracaine
LET anesthesia
LET solution
let-go threshold

lethal dose
lethargic
lethargy
leukemia
adult T-cell l.
chronic lymphocytic l.
lymphoblastic l.
leukocyte-depleted blood product
leukocytosis
mild l.
leukodepleted blood
leukoencephalopathy
progressive multifocal l.
leukopenia
leukotriene receptor
levalbuterol
Levaquin
levarterenol
levator
l. ani muscle
l. check ligament
level
air-fluid l. (AFL)
albumin l.
bone conduction l.
catecholamine l.
l. of consciousness
l. of education
factor VIII:C l.
fibrinogen l.
hepatotoxic l.
l. I trauma center
muscle l.
muscle enzyme serum l.
salicylate l.
levoatriocardinal vein
levodopa
levofloxacin
lewisite
LFPPV
low-frequency positive pressure
ventilation
Lhermitte sign
lice
lichen
l. planus
l. simplex chronicus
lid margin laceration
lidocaine
l. anesthesia
l., epinephrine, atropine, naloxone
(LEAN)

L

NOTES

171

lidocaine *(continued)*
l., epinephrine, tetracaine (LET)
l. toxicity
viscous l.
l. with epinephrine

lie
fetal l.
transverse l.

lienal vein
lienophrenic ligament
lienorenal ligament
life
Flight for L.
L. SoftPac AED companion oxygen unit
l. support

LIFEPAK 12 defibrillator/monitor
life-saving skill
life-threatening
l.-t. condition
l.-t. dysrhythmia
l.-t. emergency

lift
chin l.
head-tilt-chin l.
precordial l.

lifting
no heavy l.

ligament
abdominal triangular l.
accessory l.
accessory atlantoaxial l.
accessory lateral collateral l.
accessory plantar l.
accessory volar l.
acromioclavicular l.
acromiocoracoid l.
adipose l.
alar l.
alveolodental l.
ankle inferior transverse l.
anococcygeal l.
anterior anular l.
anterior collateral l.
anterior commissure l.
anterior costotransverse l.
anterior cruciate l. (ACL)
anterior fibular l.
anterior inferior tibiofibular l.
anterior longitudinal l.
anterior mallear l.
anterior medial ankle l.
anterior meniscofemoral l.
anterior oblique l.
anterior sacrococcygeal l.
anterior sacroiliac l.
anterior sacrosciatic l.
anterior spinal l.
anterior sternoclavicular l.

anterior suspensory l.
anterior talocalcaneal l.
anterior talofibular l.
anterior talotibial l.
anterior tibiofibular l.
anular l.
apical dental l.
Arantius l.
arcuate popliteal l.
arcuate pubic l.
arterial l.
artificial l.
atlantal l.
atlantoaxial l.
atlantoepistrophic l.
atlantooccipital l.
attenuated l.
auricular l.
avulsed l.
l. avulsion
axis l.
Bardinet l.
Barkow l.
l. barrier
beak l.
Bellini l.
Berry l.
Bertin l.
Bichat l.
bifurcate l.
bifurcated l.
Bigelow l.
Botallo l.
Bourgery l.
brachioradial l.
broad l.
broad uterine l.
Brodie l.
Broyle l.
Burns l.
l. button
calcaneoastragaloid l.
calcaneoclavicular l.
calcaneocuboid l.
calcaneofibular l.
calcaneonavicular l.
calcaneotibial l.
Caldani l.
Campbell l.
Camper l.
canthal l.
capital l.
capitolunate l.
capsular l.
Carcassonne l.
cardinal l.
caroticoclinoid l.
carpal l.
carpometacarpal l.

Casser l.
casserian l.
caudal l.
cemental l.
ceratocricoid l.
cervical l.
check l.
checkrein l.
cholecystoduodenal l.
chondroxiphoid l.
ciliary l.
circular dental l.
Civinini l.
Clado l.
Cleland l.
clinoid l.
Cloquet l.
coccygeal l.
collateral l.
Colles l.
conjugate l.
conoid l.
conus l.
Cooper l.
coracoacromial l.
coracoclavicular l.
coracohumeral l.
corniculopharyngeal l.
coronary l.
costoclavicular l.
costocolic l.
costotransverse l.
costovertebral l.
costoxiphoid l.
cotyloid l.
Cowper l.
cribriform l.
cricoarytenoid l.
cricopharyngeal l.
cricosantorinian l.
cricothyroid l.
cricotracheal l.
cross l.
cruciate l.
cruciform l.
crural l.
Cruveilhier l.
cuboideonavicular l.
cuneiform l.
cuneocuboid l.
cuneometatarsal interosseous l.
cuneonavicular l.

cystoduodenal l.
Dacron synthetic l.
deltoid l.
deltotrapezius fascial l.
Denonvilliers l.
dentate l.
denticulate l.
dentoalveolar l.
descending part of iliofemoral l.
diaphragmatic l.
digital retinacular l.
disruption of l.
distal ulnar collateral l.
dorsal calcaneocuboid l.
dorsal calcaneonavicular l.
dorsal carpal arcuate l.
dorsal carpometacarpal l.
dorsal cuboideonavicular l.
dorsal cuneocuboid l.
dorsal cuneonavicular l.
dorsal intercarpal l.
dorsal intercuneiform l.
dorsal metacarpal l.
dorsal metatarsal l.
dorsal radiocarpal l.
dorsal sacroiliac l.
dorsal talonavicular l.
dorsal tarsal l.
dorsal tarsometatarsal l.
dorsal wrist l.
dorsoradial l.
Douglas l.
duodenal l.
duodenocolic l.
duodenorenal l.
dural l.
l. elongation
epihyal l.
external calcaneoastragaloid l.
external cruciate l.
external lateral l.
extraarticular knee l.
extracapsular l.
extrinsic l.
fabellofibular l.
falciform l.
fallopian l.
false l.
femoral l.
Ferrein l.
fibular collateral l.
fibular sesamoidal l.

NOTES

L

ligament *(continued)*
    fibulocalcaneal l.
    fibulotalar l.
    fibulotalocalcaneal l.
    first intermetacarpal l.
    floating l.
    Flood l.
    foveal l.
    fracture-dislocation with anterior l.
    fundiform l.
    gastrocolic l.
    gastrodiaphragmatic l.
    gastrohepatic l.
    gastrolienal l.
    gastropancreatic l.
    gastrophrenic l.
    gastrosplenic l.
    genital l.
    genitoinguinal l.
    Gillette suspensory l.
    Gilliam round l.
    Gimbernat reflex l.
    gingival l.
    gingivodental l.
    glenohumeral l.
    glenoid l.
    glossoepiglottic l.
    gonadal l.
    Gore-Tex anterior cruciate l.
    l. graft
    Grayson l.
    Gruber l.
    Haines-McDougall medial
      sesamoid l.
    hamate l.
    hamatometacarpal l.
    hammock l.
    Helmholtz axis l.
    Helvetius l.
    Henle l.
    Hensing l.
    hepatic l.
    hepatocolic l.
    hepatocystocolic l.
    hepatoduodenal l.
    hepatoesophageal l.
    hepatogastric l.
    hepatogastroduodenal l.
    hepatophrenic l.
    hepatorenal l.
    hepatoumbilical l.
    Hesselbach l.
    Hey l.
    Holl l.
    Hueck l.
    Humphry l.
    Hunter l.
    Huschke l.
    hyalocapsular l.

hyaloideocapsular l.
hyoepiglottic l.
hypertrophic l.
hypsiloid l.
iliofemoral l.
iliolumbar l.
iliopatellar l.
iliopectineal l.
iliopubic l.
iliotibial l.
iliotrochanteric l.
incudal l.
inferior calcaneonavicular l.
inferior dorsal radioulnar l.
inferior glenohumeral l.
inferior ilioischial l.
inferior pubic l.
inferior pulmonary l.
inferior transverse scapular l.
infrapatellar l.
infundibuloovarian l.
infundibulopelvic l.
inguinal l.
intercapital l.
intercarpal l.
interchondral l.
interclavicular l.
interclinoid l.
intercornual l.
intercostal l.
intercuneiform l.
interdental l.
interdigital l.
interfoveolar l.
intermetacarpal l.
intermetatarsal l.
internal calcaneoastragaloid l.
internal collateral l.
internal lateral l.
International Knee L.
interosseous cuneocuboid l.
interosseous cuneometatarsal l.
interosseous intercuneiform l.
interosseous metacarpal l.
interosseous metatarsal l.
interosseous sacroiliac l.
interosseous talocalcaneal l.
interosseous tibiofibular l.
interphalangeal collateral l.
intersesamoid l.
interspinal l.
interspinous l.
intertransverse l.
intervertebral l.
intervolar plate l.
intraarticular l.
intracapsular l.
intraosseous tibiofibular l.
intrascapular l.

intrinsic l.
ischiocapsular l.
ischiofemoral l.
Jarjavay l.
jugal l.
knee l.
Krause l.
labiomandibular l.
lacinate l.
laciniate l.
lacunar l.
Landsmeer l.
Lannelongue l.
lateral accessory l.
lateral arcuate l.
lateral atlantooccipital l.
lateral collateral l.
lateral costotransverse l.
lateral interosseous l.
lateral lumbosacral l.
lateral maxillary l.
lateral palpebral l.
lateral puboprostatic l.
lateral rectal l.
lateral sacrococcygeal l.
lateral spring l.
lateral talocalcaneal l.
lateral temporomandibular l.
lateral thyrohyoid l.
lateral thyroid l.
lateral ulnar collateral l.
lateral umbilical l.
Lauth l.
lax l.
leaf of broad l.
left triangular l.
levator check l.
lienophrenic l.
lienorenal l.
Lisfranc l.
Lockwood l.
longitudinal l.
lumbocostal l.
lumbodorsal l.
lunotriquetral l.
Luschka l.
Mackenrodt l.
macroscopic hemorrhage l.
Maissiat l.
mamilloaccessory l.
mandibular osteocutaneous l.
Marshall l.

masseteric cutaneous l.
Mauchart l.
maxillary l.
Meckel l.
medial arcuate l.
medial canthal l.
medial capsular l.
medial collateral l.
medial palpebral l.
medial patellofemoral l.
medial puboprostatic l.
medial rectus check l.
medial talocalcaneal l.
medial thyroid l.
medial ulnar collateral l.
medial umbilical l.
median arcuate l.
median cricothyroid l.
median cruciate l.
median thyrohyoid l.
median thyroid l.
median umbilical l.
meniscofemoral l.
meniscotibial l.
metacarpal l.
metacarpoglenoidal l.
metacarpophalangeal l.
metatarsal interosseous l.
metatarsosesamoid l.
middle costotransverse l.
middle glenohumeral l.
middle umbilical l.
midline l.
mucosal suspensory l.
nasolabial l.
nasomandibular l.
natatory l.
navicular cuneiform l.
naviculocuneiform l.
nephrocolic l.
nuchal l.
oblique popliteal l.
oblique retinacular l.
occipitoaxial l.
odontoid l.
olecranon l.
orbicular l.
orbitomalar l.
Osborne l.
osseocutaneous l.
ovarian suspensory l.
palmar beak l.

L

NOTES

ligament *(continued)*

palmar carpal l.
palmar carpometacarpal l.
palmar intercarpal deltoid l.
palmar metacarpal l.
palmar midcarpal l.
palmar radiocarpal l.
palmar radioulnar l.
palmar ulnocarpal l.
l. palpation
palpebral l.
pancreaticosplenic l.
patellar l.
patellofemoral l.
patellomeniscal l.
patellotibial l.
pectinate l.
pectineal l.
pelvic l.
pericardiosternal l.
peridental l.
periimplant l.
periodontal l.
peritoneal l.
periurethral l.
Petit l.
petroclinoid l.
petrosphenoid l.
petrosphenoidal l.
phalangeal glenoidal l.
phrenicocolic l.
phrenicoesophageal l.
phrenicolienal l.
phrenicosplenic l.
phrenoesophageal l.
phrenogastric l.
phrenosplenic l.
pisiform metacarpal l.
pisohamate l.
pisometacarpal l.
pisounciform l.
pisouncinate l.
plantar calcaneocuboid l.
plantar calcaneonavicular l.
plantar cuboideonavicular l.
plantar cuneocuboid l.
plantar cuneonavicular l.
plantar intercuneiform l.
plantar metatarsal l.
plantar spring l.
plantar tarsal l.
plantar tarsometatarsal l.
Poirier l.
popliteal l.
posterior anular l.
posterior costotransverse l.
posterior cricoarytenoid l.
posterior cruciate l.
posterior false l.

posterior incudal l.
posterior inferior tibiofibular l.
posterior leaf of broad l.
posterior longitudinal l.
posterior meniscofemoral l.
posterior oblique l.
posterior occipitoaxial l.
posterior sacroiliac l.
posterior sacrosciatic l.
posterior sternoclavicular l.
posterior suspensory l.
posterior talocalcaneal l.
posterior talofibular l.
posterior talotibial l.
posterior tibiotalar part of
    deltoid l.
posterior uterosacral l.
Poupart l.
pterygomandibular l.
pterygospinal l.
pterygospinous l.
pubic arcuate l.
pubocapsular l.
pubocervical l.
pubofemoral l.
puboprostatic l.
pubourethral l.
pubovesical l.
pulmonary l.
quadrate l.
radial carpal collateral l.
radial metacarpal l.
radiate carpal l.
radiate sternocostal l.
radiocapitate l.
radiocarpal l.
radiolunate l.
radiolunotriquetral l.
radioscaphocapitate l.
radioscaphoid l.
radioscapholunate l.
radiotriquetral l.
radioulnar l.
rearfoot l.
l. reconstruction
rectosacral l.
rectouterine l.
reflected inguinal l.
l. reflecting edge
reflex l.
l. reinsertion
l. replacement
retinacular l.
Retzius l.
rhomboid l.
right prostatic l.
right triangular l.
ring l.
Robert l.

round uterine l.
Rouviere l.
l. rupture
l. rupture sprain
sacrococcygeal l.
sacrodural l.
sacrogenital l.
sacroiliac l.
sacrospinal l.
sacrospinous l.
sacrotuberal l.
sacrotuberous l.
sacrouterine l.
Santorini l.
Sappey l.
scapholunate interosseous l.
scaphotrapezoid interosseous l.
scaphotriquetral l.
scapular l.
scapulohumeral l.
Scarpa l.
Schlemm l.
serous l.
sesamoid l.
sesamophalangeal l.
sheath l.
l. shelving edge
short calcaneocuboid l.
short plantar l.
short radiolunate l.
Simonart l.
skin l.
Soemmerring l.
sphenomandibular l.
spinal posterior l.
spinal transverse l.
spinoglenoid l.
spinous tarsus l.
spiral oblique retinacular l.
splenocolic l.
splenopancreatic l.
splenorenal l.
spring l.
stabilizing l.
Stanley cervical l.
stellate l.
sternoclavicular l.
sternocostal l.
sternopericardial l.
l. stress testing
stretched out l.
Struthers l.

stylohyoid l.
stylomandibular l.
stylomaxillary l.
subtalar interosseous l.
superficial dorsal sacrococcygeal l.
superficial medial l.
superficial posterior
  sacrococcygeal l.
superficial tibiotalar l.
superficial transverse metacarpal l.
superficial transverse metatarsal l.
superior astragalonavicular l.
superior costotransverse l.
superior incudal l.
superior mallear l.
superior pubic l.
superior transverse scapular l.
superomedial calcaneonavicular l.
suprascapular l.
supraspinal l.
supraspinous l.
suspensory l.
sutural l.
syndesmotic l.
synovial l.
talocalcaneal interosseous l.
talocalcaneonavicular l.
talofibular l.
talonavicular l.
tarsal interosseous l.
tarsometatarsal l.
l. tear
tectoral l.
temporomandibular l.
tendinotrochanteric l.
Teutleben l.
Thompson l.
thyroepiglottic l.
thyrohyoid l.
tibial collateral l.
tibial lateral l.
tibial sesamoid l.
tibiocalcaneal l.
tibiofibular l.
tibionavicular l.
Toldt l.
torn meniscotibial l.
transcarpal l.
transseptal l.
transverse acetabular l.
transverse atlantal l.
transverse atlas l.

L

NOTES

177

ligament *(continued)*

transverse carpal l.
transverse cervical l.
transverse crural l.
transverse genicular l.
transverse humeral l.
transverse intertarsal l.
transverse metacarpal l.
transverse metatarsal l.
transverse part of iliofemoral l.
transverse perineal l.
transverse retinacular l.
transverse scapular l.
transverse spinal l.
transverse tibiofibular l.
trapezoid l.
traumatized l.
Treitz l.
triangular deltoid l.
triquetrohamate l.
triquetroscaphoid l.
true collateral l.
Tuffier inferior l.
ulnar carpal collateral l.
ulnocarpal l.
ulnolunate l.
ulnotriquetral l.
umbilical l.
urachal l.
urethropelvic l.
uterine l.
uteroovarian l.
uteropelvic l.
uterosacral l.
uterovesical l.
vaginal hand l.
Valsalva l.
venous l.
ventral sacrococcygeal l.
ventral sacroiliac l.
ventricular l.
vertebropelvic l.
vesical l.
vesicosacral l.
vesicoumbilical l.
vesicouterine l.
vestibular l.
vocal l.
volar beak l.
volar carpal l.
volar radiocarpal l.
volar radiotriquetral l.
Waldeyer preurethral l.
Walther oblique l.
web l.
Weigert l.
Weitbrecht l.
Whitnall l.
Wieger l.

Winslow l.
Wrisberg l.
xiphicostal l.
xiphoid l.
yellow l.
Y-shaped l.
Zaglas l.
Zenotech biomaterial-synthetic l.
Zenotech synthetic l.
Zinn l.
zygomatic osteocutaneous l.
zygomatic retaining l.

ligamentous

l. instability
l. interconnection
l. pain
l. weakness

ligamentum arteriosum
Ligapak suture
ligated

suture l.

ligation

suture l.

ligator

McGivney l.

ligature

suture l.

light

l. flash
pupils equal and react to l.
(PERL)
l. touch
l. wand
Wood l.

lighted stylet
lightheadedness
light-induced injury
lightning

cloud-to-ground l.
l. injury
l. splash
l. stroke

limb

acyanotic l.
anacrotic l.
gangrenous l.
l. ischemia
l. presentation
l. replantation

limbal suture
limb-length discrepancy
limbous suture
limb-threatening arterial insufficiency
limbus of sphenoid bone
LIMIT-2

Second Leicester Intravenous Magnesium
Intervention Trial

limited study

limp
> psychogenic l.

Linatrix suture
lincosamide antibiotic
lindane poisoning
Lindner corneoscleral suture
line
> arterial l.
> central l.
> crush l.
> dentate l.
> dial-a-flow IV l.
> fracture l.
> l. of gravity
> intraosseous l.
> intravenous l.
> large-bore intravenous l.
> midaxillary l.
> midclavicular l. (MCL)
> midsternal l. (MSL)
> pectinate l.
> peripherally inserted central
>   catheter l.
> PICC l.
> l. sepsis
> Shenton l.
> skin tension l.
> suture l.

linear
> l. laceration
> l. skull fracture

linen thread suture
linezolid
lingual
> l. alveolar bone
> l. muscle
> l. nerve
> l. vein

lingular vein
linguofacial vein
liniment
Linvatec meniscal BioStinger anchor suture
lion fish envenomation
LIP
> lymphocytic interstitial pneumonia

lip
> cherry red l.
> cyanotic l.

lipase
> serum l.

lipid solubility

lipoatrophy
> insulin l.

lipohyalinotic small vessel disease
lipoma
> bone l.

Liponyssus bursa
lipopolysaccharide
liquefaction
> bone l.
> l. necrosis

LiquiChar activated charcoal
liquid
> l. chromatography
> oxygenated perfluorochemical l.
> l. substance aspiration
> l. ventilation

LiquiVent
Lisfranc
> L. fracture
> L. ligament

lisinopril
lisofylline
Listeria monocytogenes
listing
> drug l.

litem
> guardian ad l.

liters per minute (LPM)
lithium
> l. intoxication
> l. poisoning

liver
> acute fatty l.
> cirrhotic l.
> l. failure
> fatty l.
> l. function
> l. laceration
> l. transplant
> l. transplantation
> l. trauma
> triangular ligament of l.
> venoocclusive disease of l.

lividity
> dependent l.

living
> activities of daily l. (ADL)
> l. will

lizard
> l. bite
> l. envenomation

NOTES

LLE
   left lower extremity
Lloyd-Roberts fracture
LLQ
   left lower quadrant
LMA
   laryngeal mask airway
LMN
   lower motor neuron
LMP
   last menstrual period
LMWH
   low molecular weight heparin
loading
   axial l.
   l. dose
   fracture callus l.
LOAF
   lateral two lumbricals, opponens pollicis,
      abductor pollicis brevis, flexor pollicis
      brevis
   LOAF muscles
lobar collapse
lobe
   caudate l.
   occipital l.
lobular carcinoma
lobulization
LOC
   loss of consciousness
local
   l. anesthesia
   l. anesthetic
   l. compression fracture
   l. decompression fracture
   l. effect
   l. exploration
   l. hemostasis
   l. police
   l. symptom
   l. tetanus
   l. wound exploration
localized
   l. pain
   l. peritonitis
localizing symptom
location
   bruise in suspicious l.
   initial l.
   supraumbilical l.
   suspicious l.
locator
   automatic vehicle l. (AVL)
loci (*pl. of* locus)
locked-in syndrome
locking
   l. horizontal mattress suture
   l. of joint

lockout suture
lock-stitch suture
Lockwood
   L. ligament
   L. tendon
locoweed ingestion
locular cyst
loculated empyema
loculation
locus, pl. **loci**
   l. of brain abscess
log roll technique
lomustine
long
   l. abductor muscle
   l. abductor tendon
   l. ACTH stimulation test
   l. adductor muscle
   l. backboard
   l. bone
   l. bone film
   l. bone fracture
   l. buccal nerve
   l. ciliary nerve
   l. extensor muscle
   l. fibular muscle
   l. flexor muscle
   l. head biceps tendon
   l. levatores costarum muscle
   l. oblique fracture
   l. palmar muscle
   l. peroneal muscle
   l. radial extensor muscle
   l. rotator muscle
   l. saphenous nerve
   l. saphenous vein
   l. subscapular nerve
   l. thoracic nerve
   l. thoracic vein
longissimus
   l. capitis muscle
   l. cervicis muscle
   l. colli muscle
   l. thoracis muscle
longitudinal
   l. ciliary muscle
   l. fracture
   l. laceration
   l. ligament
   l. nerve
   l. pharyngeal muscle
   l. scan
   l. split biceps tendon
   l. suture
   l. tibial fatigue fracture
longitudinalis
   l. inferior muscle
   l. superior muscle

longus
- l. capitis muscle
- l. cervicis muscle

Look suture

loop
- l. diuretic
- escape l.
- ileal l.
- l. mattress suture
- l. stoma

looped polypropylene suture

loose
- l. body
- l. fracture

Looser
- L. zone
- L. zone in insufficiency fracture

Lopid

LOQ
- lower outer quadrant

lorazepam

lorry driver's fracture

Losartan

loss
- blood l.
- bone l.
- conductive heat l.
- l. of consciousness (LOC)
- convective heat l.
- evaporative heat l.
- extrarenal l.
- gingival tissue l.
- isovolemic blood l.
- memory l.
- nerve l.
- ongoing blood l.
- sensory l.
- soft tissue l.
- visual l.

Louis angle

loupe
- ocular l.

Lovenox

low
- l. air loss bed
- l. blood sugar
- l. flow state
- l. grade fever
- l. incidence
- l. lumbar spine fracture
- l. molecular weight heparin (LMWH)
- l. output
- l. T humerus fracture

low-carbohydrate diet

low-energy fracture

lower
- l. airway
- l. airway obstruction
- l. back pain
- l. esophageal sphincter circular muscle
- l. extremity aneurysm
- l. extremity edema
- l. extremity fracture
- l. frontal bone fracture
- l. gastrointestinal bleeding
- l. genitourinary trauma
- l. motor neuron (LMN)
- l. outer quadrant (LOQ)
- l. pole laceration
- l. respiratory tract

lowest splanchnic nerve

low-flow priapism

low-frequency positive pressure ventilation (LFPPV)

low-level disinfection

low-molecular-weight dextran

low-oxygen area

loxoscelism
- viscerocutaneous l.

LP
- lumbar puncture

LPM
- liters per minute

LR
- lactated Ringer

LRS
- lactated Ringer solution

LSB
- left sternal border

LSD
- lysergic acid diethylamide

lucid interval

lucidity

Ludiomil

Ludloff sign

Ludwig
- L. angina
- L. nerve

LUE
- left upper extremity

Luer-type syringe

Lukens catgut suture

L

NOTES

lumbar
l. disk disorder
l. erector spinae muscle
l. extensor muscle
l. iliocostal muscle
l. interspinal muscle
l. puncture (LP)
l. quadrate muscle
l. rotator muscle
l. spine burst fracture
l. spine fracture
l. spine injury
l. splanchnic nerve
l. suture
l. vein
l. vertebra
lumbocostal ligament
lumbodorsal ligament
lumboinguinal nerve
lumbosacral junction fracture
lumbrical
l. muscle
l. tendon
lumbricoides
Ascaris l.
lumen
false l.
vein l.
luminal irregularity
lunate
l. bone
l. dislocation
l. fracture
lung
l. blast
burst l.
crack l.
fallen l.
l. laceration
l. squeeze
l. transplant
lunocapitate bone
lunotriquetral ligament

lupuslike syndrome
LUQ
left upper quadrant
Luschka
L. bursa
L. ligament
L. muscle
L. nerve
lusitaniae
Candida l.
luxated bone
LVAD
left ventricular assist device
LVEDP
left ventricular end-diastolic pressure
Lyme disease
lymphadenectomy
retroperitoneal l.
lymphadenitis
regional l.
lymphadenopathy
painful regional l.
regional l.
lymphangiogram
lymphangitis
lymphatic chain
lymphoblastic leukemia
lymphocele drainage
lymphocyte
lymphocytic
l. choriomeningitis
l. interstitial pneumonia (LIP)
lymphogranuloma venereum
lymphoma
bone l.
malignant l.
nodular l.
LYOfoam foam
lysergic acid diethylamide (LSD)
lysis
l. of adhesion
muscle l.

3M
>3M Healthcare particulate respirator
>3M Healthcare surgical mask

MAC
>*Mycobacterium avium-intracellulare* complex
>MAC infection

mace
maceration
Mach effect
machine
>suction m.

MacIntosh blade
Mackenrodt ligament
mackerel poisoning
macrocytic anemia
macrodactyly
>nerve territory oriented m.

macroglossia
macrolide antibiotic
macroscopic hemorrhage ligament
macular
>m. choroiditis
>m. venous engorgement

maculopathy
>cystoid m.

mafenide
>m. acetate
>m. acetate cream

magic mouthwash
Magill forceps
magnesium
>m. citrate
>m. deficiency
>m. salt
>m. sulfate
>m. therapy
>m. and thermite incendiary agent

magnetic
>m. resonance angiography (MRA)
>m. resonance imaging (MRI)

mahogany stool
main
>m. renal vein
>m. stem bronchus intubation

maintain hydration
maintenance
>bone mass m.

Maisonneuve fibular fracture
Maissiat ligament
majalis
major
>m. bronchi rupture
>m. depressive disorder
>m. external hemorrhage

>m. muscle
>m. surgery
>m. trauma
>m. vessel

majus, pl. **majora**
>labia majora
>labium m.

malabsorption
malacia
malady
malaise
malar
>m. bone
>m. complex fracture
>m. periosteum-SMAS flap fixation suture

malaria
>cerebral m.
>chronic m.

maldistribution of blood
male
>African-American m.
>black m.
>Caucasian m.
>Hispanic m.
>middle-aged m.
>Oriental m.
>m. pattern baldness
>sexually active m.
>white middle-aged m.

malfeasance
malformation
>arteriovenous m. (AVM)
>bone occipital m.

Malgaigne pelvic fracture
malignancy
>gastrointestinal m.

malignant
>m. hyperpyrexia
>m. hypertension
>m. hyperthermia (MH)
>m. lymphoma
>m. otitis externa
>m. pleural effusion

malingering
Mallampati
>M. difficult intubation scale
>M. sign and classification

malleable
malleolar chip fracture
malleolus
>lateral m.
>medial m.
>m. muscle

M

mallet
    bone m.
    m. finger
    m. fracture
Mallory-Weiss
    M.-W. laceration
    M.-W. syndrome
    M.-W. tear
malnourished patient
malnutrition
    fetal m.
malomaxillary suture
malononitrile
    orthochlorobenzylidene m. (CS)
malreduction
    fracture m.
malrotation of bowel
maltreatment
    child m.
malunion
    fracture with m.
malunited
    m. calcaneus fracture
    m. forearm fracture
    m. radial fracture
MalvP
    mean alveolar pressure
6-MAM
    6-monoacetylmorphine
mamba snake envenomation
mamillary suture
mamilloaccessory ligament
mammal bite
mammary
    m. gland
    m. vein
man
    every test known to m. (ETKM)
management
    airway m.
    biological warfare mass casualty m.
    breathing m.
    chemical warfare mass casualty m.
    circulation m.
    controversial m.
    critical incident stress m. (CISM)
    endotracheal tube m.
    laceration m.
    mass casualty m.
    pain m.
    topical pain m.
    m. of violence
mandated reporter
mandatory minute ventilation (MMV)
mandible
    horizontal length of m.
mandibular
    m. body fracture

    m. bone
    m. condyle fracture
    m. fracture
    m. nerve
    m. osteocutaneous ligament
    m. ramus fracture
    m. symphysis fracture
maneuver
    BURP m.
    chin-lift m.
    Frenzel m.
    Hall-Pike m.
    head-lift m.
    head-tilt m.
    Heimlich m.
    hyperventilation m.
    jaw-thrust m.
    Mauriceau m.
    McRoberts m.
    neck-lift m.
    neck-thrust m.
    Pringle m.
    Sellick m.
    vagal antiarrhythmic m.
    Valsalva m.
    Woods corkscrew m.
    Zavanelli m.
manganese
mangled extremity severity scoring (MESS)
mania
    delirious m.
manic-depressive disorder
manifestation
    electrocardiographic m.
    retinal m.
    systemic inflammatory m.
    vasomotor m.
manner
    aggressive m.
Mannis suture
mannitol
man-of-war poisoning
MANTRELS
    migration of pain, anorexia, nausea,
    tenderness in right lower quadrant,
    rebound, elevated temperature,
    leukocytosis, shift
    MANTRELS acute appendicitis
    score
manual
    m. defibrillator
    m. immobilization
    m. jet ventilator
    m. resuscitator
manubrium
MAOI
    monoamine oxidase inhibitor

MAP
  mean airway pressure
  mean arterial pressure
Mapleson D breathing system
maple sugar odor
mapping
  nerve m.
maprotiline toxicity
marasmus syndrome
marble bone
Marcacci muscle
marcescens
  Serratia m.
march fracture
Marfan syndrome
margin
  bone m.
  costal m.
  inferolateral m.
  intercostal m. (ICM)
  left costal m. (LCM)
  right costal m. (RCM)
  m. of safety
  wound m.
marginal
  m. abrasion
  m. abscess
  m. branch
  m. mandibular nerve
  m. ridge fracture
  m. vein
marigold ingestion
marijuana
  m. addiction
  m. toxicity
marine
  m. envenomation
  m. organism bite
  m. organism sting
marital discord
marked rhonchi
marker
  bone formation m.
  bone resorption m.
Marlex suture
marmorata
  cutis m.
Marmor-Lynn fracture
Marplan
marrow
  bone m.

Marshall
  M. ligament
  M. U-stitch suture
  M. vein
  M. V-suture
marsupialization
mask
  aerosol m.
  air entrainment face m.
  air entrapment m.
  bag and m.
  bag-valve m.
  BLB m.
  Boothby m.
  ecchymotic m.
  intubating laryngeal m. (ILM)
  laryngeal m.
  3M Healthcare surgical m.
  nonbreather m.
  nonrebreather m.
  nonrebreathing face m.
  m. oxygenation
  partial rebreathing face m.
  pocket m.
  Venti m.
  m. ventilation
  Venturi m.
Mason-Allen suture
Mason fracture
mass
  adnexal m.
  bone mineral m.
  breast m.
  m. casualty incident (MCI)
  m. casualty management
  cicatricial m.
  discrete m.
  infectious cause of adnexal m.
  intraabdominal m.
  muscle m.
  m. poisoning accident
  pulsatile m.
  m. spectroscopy
massage
  cardiac m.
  internal cardiac m.
  uterine m.
masseter
  m. muscle
  m. tendon
masseteric
  m. cutaneous ligament

M

NOTES

masseteric *(continued)*
    m. nerve
    m. vein
massive
    m. blood transfusion
    m. facial trauma
    m. hemothorax
    m. overdose
    m. transfusion syndrome
MAST
    military antishock trousers
masticator nerve
masticatory
    m. bone
    m. muscle
mastitis
    cystic m.
mastocytosis
    bone m.
    systemic m.
mastoid
    m. bone
    m. bone fracture
    m. emissary vein
    m. suture
mastoid-conchal suture
mastoiditis
    chronic m.
MAT
    multifocal atrial tachycardia
mater
    arachnoid m.
    dura m.
    pia m.
material
    bone grafting m.
    bone implant m.
    hazardous m. (HazMat)
    Omnipaque contrast m.
    suture m.
maternal
    m. cortical vein
    m. fracture
    m. hypertension
    m. morbidity
    m. stabilization
maternal-fetal compromise
Mathews olecranon fracture classification
matrix
    bone tumor m.
matted
    m. bowel
    m. omentum
mattress
    EMS Immobile-VAC pediatric universal m.
    m. suture

maturation
    bone m.
maturity
    bone m.
Mauchart ligament
Mauriceau maneuver
Maxam suture
maxillary
    m. bone
    m. fracture
    m. ligament
    m. nerve
    m. sinus
    m. sinus disease
    m. vein
maxillofacial fracture
maxillofrontal suture
maxillojugal suture
maxillonasal suture
maximal voluntary ventilation (MVV)
maximum
    m. hospital benefit
    m. medical benefit
    m. temperature
Maxipime
Maxon
    M. absorbable suture
    M. delayed-absorbable suture
Mayo
    M. linen suture
    M. vein
MCA
    multiple casualty accident
McBurney sign
McCannel suture
McGill forceps
McGivney ligator
MCH
    mean corpuscular hemoglobin
MCHC
    mean corpuscular hemoglobin concentration
MCI
    mass casualty incident
    multiple casualty incident
MCL
    midclavicular line
McLaughlin modification of Bunnell pull-out suture
McLean suture
McMurray test
MCP
    metacarpophalangeal
McRoberts maneuver
MCS
    multiple casualty situation
MDAC
    multiple-dose activated charcoal

MDI
metered-dose inhaler
MDMA
methylenedioxy-n-methylamphetamine
meal
bone m.
mean
m. airway pressure (MAP)
m. alveolar pressure (MalvP)
m. arterial pressure (MAP)
m. corpuscular hemoglobin (MCH)
m. corpuscular hemoglobin
concentration (MCHC)
m. systemic pressure (MSP)
measles
German m.
measure
ancillary m.
cooling m.
radical m.
supportive m.
temporizing m.
toxin-specific m.
measured serum osmolality
measurement
anthropometric m.
bone density m.
bone mass m.
bone mineral m.
bone strength m.
midflow m.
muscle m.
Measuroll suture
meatus
external auditory m.
mechanic
body m.'s
chest wall m.'s
mechanical
m. complication
m. low back pain
m. obstruction
m. purpura
m. reserve
m. support
m. support device
m. ventilation
m. ventilator actuator
mechanism
m. of action
m. of injury (MOI)

Meckel
M. diverticulum
M. ligament
meclofenamate
meconium aspiration
media
barotitis m.
bilateral otitis m. (BOM)
otitis m. (OM)
medial
m. antebrachial cutaneous nerve
m. anterior thoracic nerve
m. approach
m. arcuate ligament
m. articular nerve
m. atrial vein
m. border
m. brachial cutaneous nerve
m. calcaneal branch of tibial nerve
m. canthal ligament
m. canthal tendon
m. canthus
m. capsular ligament
m. circumflex femoral vein
m. cluneal nerve
m. collateral ligament
m. collateral ligament strain
m. column calcaneal fracture
m. crural cutaneous branch of
saphenous nerve
m. crural suture
m. cuneiform bone
m. dorsal cutaneous nerve
m. epicondylar bursa
m. epicondyle humeral fracture
m. genicular vein
m. great muscle
m. history
m. lumbar intertransverse muscle
m. malleolar fracture
m. malleolar subcutaneous bursa
m. malleolus
m. meniscus
m. meniscus injury
m. metacarpal bone
m. orbital wall fracture
m. palpebral ligament
m. palpebral muscle
m. papillary muscle
m. patellofemoral ligament
m. pectoral nerve
m. plantar nerve

M

NOTES

medial *(continued)*
    m. plantar vein
    m. popliteal nerve
    m. pterygoid muscle
    m. pterygoid nerve
    m. puboprostatic ligament
    m. rectus check ligament
    m. rectus extraocular muscle
    m. sesamoid bone
    m. supraclavicular nerve
    m. sural cutaneous nerve
    m. talocalcaneal ligament
    m. thyroid ligament
    m. turbinate bone
    m. ulnar collateral ligament
    m. umbilical ligament
    m. vastus muscle
medialization
    fracture m.
median
    m. antebrachial vein
    m. arcuate ligament
    m. artery
    m. basilic vein
    m. cephalic vein
    m. cricothyroid ligament
    m. cruciate ligament
    m. cubital vein
    m. fascicular block
    m. nerve
    m. nerve block
    m. palatine suture
    m. sacral vein
    m. sternotomy
    m. thyrohyoid ligament
    m. thyroid ligament
    m. umbilical ligament
mediastinal
    m. pleurisy
    m. shift
    m. vein
    m. widening
mediastinitis
    postoperative m.
mediastinum
    widened m.
mediated inhibition
medical
    m. bridge
    m. director
    m. intensive care unit (MICU)
    m. psychosis
    m. unit leader (MUL)
medication *(See also* medicine)
    aerosolized m.
    antianxiety m.
    conservative m.
    electrolyte altering m.
    highly protein-bound m.

    hydrophilic m.
    m. noncompliance
    over-the-counter m.
    primary pain m.
    psychotropic m.
    sublingual m.
    vasoactive m.
medication-induced dystonic reaction
medicine *(See also* medication)
    acute care m.
    adolescent m.
    American Academy of
      Emergency M.
    confined-space m.
    critical care m.
    disaster m.
    emergency m.
    general m. (GM)
    hyperbaric m.
    Society of Critical Care M.
      (SCCM)
    Standard Nomenclature of M.
      (SNOMED)
    The Center for Pediatric
      Emergency M. (CPEM)
mediolateral
Medi-Pac rescue seat
medium vein
medius muscle
Medrafil wire suture
medroxyprogesterone
Med Spec prosplint
medullary
    m. bone
    m. vein
mefenamic acid
megacolon
    aganglionic m.
    toxic m.
megaloblastic anemia
Meigs suture
meiopragic bone
melancholia
    involutional m.
melancholy
melanoma
melanotic pigment
melatonin
melena
melenic stool
melioidosis
Melker cuffed emergency
  cricothyrotomy catheter
Mellaril
mellitus
    diabetes m.
    diet-controlled diabetes m.
    insulin-dependent diabetes m.
      (IDDM)

juvenile insulin-dependent type 1 diabetes m.
non-insulin-dependent diabetes m. (NIDDM)
melphalan
membranaceous tendon
membrane
boggy mucous m.
cricothyroid m.
erythematous mucous m.
mucous m.
m. oxygenator
premature rupture of m.'s
purple mucous m.
membranous layer
memory
m. deficit
m. loss
Ménière disease
meningeal
m. headache
m. nerve
m. vein
meninges (*pl. of* meninx)
meningitidis
Neisseria m.
meningitis, pl. *meningitides*
anthrax m.
aseptic m.
bacterial m.
carcinoid m.
epidural m.
Mollaret m.
viral m.
meningococcal arthritis
meningococcemia
meningoencephalitis
cryptococcal m.
viral m.
meningorachidian vein
meninx, pl. **meninges**
meniscal bone
meniscofemoral ligament
meniscotibial ligament
meniscus
medial m.
menorrhagia
primary m.
menstruation
anovular m.
mental
m. age

m. confusion
m. deterioration
m. muscle
m. nerve
m. status
m. status examination (MSE)
mentalis muscle
mentally unstable patient
mentation
altered m.
meperidine
mepivacaine
meprobamate poisoning
meralgia paresthetica
mercury
millimeters of m. (mmHg)
m. poisoning
m. toxicity
Merkel muscle
Merocel self-expanding packing
meropenem
Merrem
Mersilene braided nonabsorbable suture
Mersilk black silk suture
mescaline
mesencephalic vein
mesenteric
m. adenitis
m. ischemia
m. superior vein
m. vasculitis
mesh suture
mesiodistal fracture
mesocuneiform bone
mesothenar muscle
MESS
mangled extremity severity scoring
MESS system
mesylate
fenoldopam m.
metabolic
m. abnormality
m. abnormality resolution
m. acidosis
m. alkalemia
m. alkalosis
m. bone disease
m. cause
m. disease
m. equivalents (METS)
m. ketoacidosis
m. need

M

NOTES

metabolism
  bone mineral m.
  cerebral m.
  extensive hepatic m.
  glucose m.
  glycerol m.
  inborn errors of m.
  oxidative m.
  oxygen m.
metacarpal
  m. amputation
  m. bone
  m. head fracture
  m. injury
  m. ligament
  m. neck fracture
  m. shaft fracture
  m. vein
metacarpoglenoidal ligament
metacarpophalangeal (MCP)
  m. joint
  m. ligament
metaiodobenzylguanidine
  iodine-131 m, (^{131}I-MIBG)
metal
  m. band suture
  m. casting toxicity
  heavy m.
  m. oxide fume syndrome
  m. splint
metallic
  m. foreign body
  m. suture
Metamucil abuse
metaphysial
  m. avulsion fracture
  m. tibial fracture
metarteriole
metastasis, pl. metastases
  bone m.
metastasize
metastatic mumps
metatarsal
  m. base fracture
  m. injury
  m. interosseous ligament
  m. joint
  m. neck fracture
  m. stress fracture
metatarsophalangeal joint (MPJ, MTPJ)
metatarsosesamoid ligament
metered-dose inhaler (MDI)
methadone hydrochloride
methamphetamine
methanol poisoning
methaqualone toxicity
methemoglobinemia
methemoglobin reductase

methicillin-resistant *Staphylococcus aureus* (MRSA)
method
  Burkhalter-Reyes m.
  extracorporeal m.
  Fick m.
  Goldman m.
  jaw-thrust m.
  Kety-Schmidt blood flow measurement m.
methohexital
methotrexate
methylamine
  carboprost m.
methyldopa
methylene blue
methylenedioxy-n-methylamphetamine (MDMA)
methylprednisolone
methylxanthine
metoclopramide
metocurine
metopic suture
metronidazole
METS
  metabolic equivalents
mexiletine hydrochloride
Meyer-Betz disease
Meyers-McKeever tibial fracture classification
Mezlin
mezlocillin
MH
  malignant hyperthermia
MI
  myocardial infarction
MIC
  minimum inhibitory concentration
Michaelis-Menten kinetics
miconazole
Micrins microsurgical suture
microaerosol
microangiopathy
  thrombotic m.
microaspiration
microbubble embolism
microcirculation
  nerve root m.
microcytic anemia
microdose
microemboli
Micro-Glide corneal suture
micrognathia
microhyphema
microinjection
Micromask
  CPR M.
MicroMite anchor suture
micronized purified flavonoid fracture

micronutrient
microphone
> Bluetooth remote wireless technology m.

micropoint suture
microscopic hematuria
Microsporidia
Microstream capnography
microsurgical reimplantation
microtrauma
MICU
> medical intensive care unit

midaxillary line
midazolam
midbrain lesion
midclavicular line (MCL)
middle
> m. cardiac cervical nerve
> m. cardiac vein
> m. cervical cardiac nerve
> m. cluneal nerve
> m. colic vein
> m. constrictor pharyngeal muscle
> m. costotransverse ligament
> m. cuneiform bone
> m. ear squeeze
> m. genicular vein
> m. glenohumeral ligament
> m. gluteal muscle
> m. hemorrhoidal vein
> m. hepatic vein
> m. lobe vein
> m. meningeal vein
> m. palatine suture
> m. rectal vein
> m. sacral vein
> m. scalene muscle
> m. supraclavicular nerve
> m. temporal vein
> m. thyroid vein
> m. tibial shaft fracture
> m. turbinate bone
> m. umbilical ligament

middle-aged
> m.-a. female
> m.-a. male

midface fracture
midfacial fracture
midflow measurement
midfoot
> m. amputation
> m. fracture

midline
> m. ligament
> m. scar
> m. shift

midnight fracture
midpatellar tendon
midsagittal plane
midshaft fracture
midsternal line (MSL)
midwaist scaphoid fracture
migraine
> atypical m.
> basilar m.
> m. headache
> m. variant

migrating abscess
migration
> m. of pain, anorexia, nausea, tenderness in right lower quadrant, rebound, elevated temperature, leukocytosis, shift (MANTRELS)

migratory pneumonia
Milch humeral fracture classification
mild
> m. chromic suture
> m. lactic acidosis
> m. leukocytosis

miliary abscess
milieu therapy
military antishock trousers (MAST)
milk
> m. abscess
> breast m.

milk-alkali syndrome
milkman's fracture
Miller blade
millimeters of mercury (mmHg)
millipede envenomation
Millipore suture
millisecond (msec)
milrinone
mimetic muscle
mineral
> bone m.

mineralization
> bone m.

mineralocorticoid
> m. deficiency
> m. excess

M

NOTES

191

mini
    m. stroke
    m. tracheostomy
MiniCorr digital oximeter
minimally
    m. displaced fracture
    m. invasive direct coronary artery
      bypass
minimum
    m. inhibitory concentration (MIC)
    m. temperature
minimus muscle
mini-pilon fracture
minocycline
minor
    m. injury
    m. muscle
minora
    labia m.
minoxidil
minus, pl. **minora**
    labium m.
minute
    liters per m. (LPM)
    m. volume
miosis
miotic
mirabilis
    Proteus m.
MiraLax
Miralene suture
miscarriage
    spontaneous m.
misdiagnosis
mismatch
    ventilation/perfusion m.
    V/Q m.
misoprostol
missed
    m. abortion
    m. fracture
missile-caused wound
missile wound
misuse
    substance m.
mitral
    m. insufficiency
    m. regurgitation
    m. regurgitation murmur
    m. stenosis
    m. valve
    m. valve prolapse
mittelschmerz
Mivacron
mivacurium
Mivazerol
mixed
    m. acid-base disorder
    m. drug abuse

    m. nerve
    m. pressor agent
    m. venous blood gas
    m. venous saturation
M&M
    morbidity and mortality
mmHg
    millimeters of mercury
MMV
    mandatory minute ventilation
Moberg-Gedda fracture
mobile response unit
mobility
    muscle tissue m.
Mobitz
    M. atrioventricular block
    M. I, II AV block
    M. I, II second-degree AV block
moccasin
    cottonmouth water m.
modality
    imaging m.
model
    2-compartment m.
    Goldfrank-Hoffman cocaine
      toxicity m.
modified
    m. Frost suture
    m. jaw thrust
    m. Kessler suture
    m. Kessler-Tajima suture
MODS
    multiple organ dysfunction score
    multiple organ dysfunction syndrome
MOF
    multiple organ failure
Mohs wound
MOI
    mechanism of injury
Mojave rattlesnake
molar
    m. pregnancy
    m. region
    m. tooth fracture
moldy hay disease
mole
    hydatidiform m.
Mollaret meningitis
molluscum contagiosum
mollusk poisoning
molybdenum
monarticular arthritis
Mondor disease
Monge disease
monitor
    cardiac m.
    Holter m.
    impedance m.

monitoring
    brain m.
    fetal m.
    hemodynamic m.
    intensive care unit m.
    invasive pressure m.
    neurosurgical m.
    respiratory m.
    rewarming hemodynamic m.
    train-of-4 m.
    uterine tocographic m.
    venous saturation m.
6-monoacetylmorphine (6-MAM)
monoamine
    m. oxidase inhibitor (MAOI)
    m. oxidase inhibitor poisoning
    m. oxidase inhibitor toxicity
monobactam
monocortical bone
Monocryl poliglecaprone suture
monocytogenes
    Listeria m.
monofascicular nerve
monofilament
    m. absorbable suture
    m. clear suture
    m. green suture
    m. nonabsorbable suture
    m. nylon suture
    m. polypropylene suture
    m. skin suture
    m. steel suture
    m. wire suture
monomalleolar ankle fracture
mononucleosis
Monosof suture
Monospot test
monoxide
    carbon m. (CO)
    diffusing capacity of lung for
        carbon m. (DLCO)
Monro bursa
Monro-Kelly hypothesis
mons pubis
Monteggia forearm fracture
Montercaux fracture
mood disorder
Moore fracture
Moraxella catarrhalis
morbidity
    iatrogenic m.
    maternal m.

    m. and mortality (M&M)
    m. rate
morbid obesity
morcellation
morcellized bone
moribund
moricizine hydrochloride
Morison pouch
morning-after
    m.-a. pill
    m.-a. seizure
morning sniff position
morphine sulfate (MS)
morphology
mortality
    morbidity and m. (M&M)
    perinatal m.
mortis
    rigor m.
mortise
    bone m.
Morton neuroma
mosquito forceps
moth
    m. repellent
    venomous m.
mothball odor
motility
    decreased gastrointestinal m.
    gastrointestinal m.
motion
    endpoint of m.
    paradoxical m.
    range of m. (ROM)
    reduced range of m.
motivation
    patient m.
motor
    m. deficit
    m. function
    m. nerve
    m. unit muscle
    m. vehicle accident (MVA)
mottled
Mouchet fracture
mountain sickness
mouth
    dry m.
    m. pain
mouth-to-mask
    m.-t.-m. breathing
    m.-t.-m. ventilation

M

NOTES

mouth-to-mouth
 m.-t.-m. breathing
 m.-t.-m. respiration
 m.-t.-m. resuscitation
mouth-to-nose resuscitation
mouth-to-stoma resuscitation
mouthwash
 magic m.
movement
 adversive m.
 athetoid m.
 bowel m.
 choreic m.
 coordinated body m.
 m. disorder
 downward m.
 extraocular m.
 inadequate air m.
 involuntary m.
 observation of chest wall m.
 paradoxical m.
 vermicular m.
MPJ, MTPJ
 metatarsophalangeal joint
MRA
 magnetic resonance angiography
MRI
 magnetic resonance imaging
MRSA
 methicillin-resistant *Staphylococcus aureus*
MS
 morphine sulfate
MSBP
 Münchausen syndrome by proxy
MSE
 mental status examination
msec
 millisecond
MSL
 midsternal line
MSP
 mean systemic pressure
MTPJ (*var. of* MPJ)
mucin clot test
mucobuccal fold
mucociliary transport
mucocutaneous muscle
mucolytic
mucormycosis
 bone m.
mucosa
 buccal m.
 cobblestone m.
 oral m.
mucosal
 m. barrier
 m. suspensory ligament
mucosanguineous

mucositis
 oral m.
mucous
 m. colitis
 m. diarrhea
 m. membrane
mucoviscidosis
mucus impaction
MUL
 medical unit leader
multangular
 m. bone
 m. ridge fracture
multicystic kidney
multidisciplinary
multidrug resistance
multifactorial
multifidus muscle
multifilament steel suture
multifocal atrial tachycardia (MAT)
multiforme
 erythema m.
multiform layer
multilevel fracture
multilobar kidney
multilobular cirrhosis
multinodular goiter
multiorgan
 m. dysfunction syndrome
 m. toxicity
multipartite fracture
multipennate muscle
multiple
 m. associated injuries
 m. bruises
 m. casualty accident (MCA)
 m. casualty incident (MCI)
 m. casualty situation (MCS)
 m. drug resistance
 m. fractures
 m. fragment wound
 m. myeloma
 m. organ dysfunction score (MODS)
 m. organ dysfunction syndrome (MODS)
 m. organ failure (MOF)
 m. organ system failure
 m. sclerosis
 m. stab wounds
 m. therapy
multiple-dose activated charcoal (MDAC)
multiple-vehicle response
multiray fracture
multiresistant gram-positive cocci
multistrand suture
multisystem disease
multitrauma dressing

multivisceral transplantation
multocida
    Pasteurella m.
mumps
    metastatic m.
Münchausen
    M. syndrome
    M. syndrome by proxy (MSBP)
mupirocin
mural
    m. abscess
    m. thrombus
muriatic acid
murmur
    crescendo m.
    ejection m. (EM)
    heart m.
    mitral regurgitation m.
Murphy sign
muscarine
muscimol
muscle
    abdominal m.
    abdominis m.
    abduction m.
    abductor digiti minimi m.
    abductor digiti quinti m.
    abductor hallucis brevis m.
    abductor magnus m.
    abductor pollicis brevis m.
    abductor pollicis longus m.
    m. absence
    absence of rectal m.'s
    accessory m.
    accessory flexor m.
    accessory inspiratory m.
    accessory soleus m.
    m. actin
    m. action potential
    m. activity
    adductor brevis m.
    adductor hallucis m.
    adductor magnus m.
    adductor minimus m.
    adductor pollicis longus m.
    agonist m.
    agonistic m.
    airway smooth m.
    alar m.
    Albinus m.
    m. analysis
    anconeus m.

anomalous m.
anorectoperineal m.
antagonist m.
anterior auricular m.
anterior papillary m.
anterior rectus m.
anterior scalene m.
anterior serratus m.
anterior splenis m.
anterior superficialis m.
anterior tibial m.
antigravity m.
antitragicus m.
antitragus m.
appendicular skeletal m.
articular m.
m. artifact
aryepiglottic m.
arytenoid m.
m. asthenia
asynchrony of respiratory m.
m. atonia
m. atrophy
auricular m.
axial m.
axillary arch m.
banding of m.
Bell m.
2-bellied m.
m. belly
bicipital m.
m. biomechanics
m. biopsy
bipennate m.
bladder neck detrusor m.
bladder smooth m.
Bochdalek m.
Bovero m.
Bowman ciliary m.
brachial m.
brachioradial m.
branchiomeric m.
Braune m.
m. breakdown
brevis m.
m. bridge
bronchial smooth m.
bronchoesophageal m.
buccal m.
buccinator m.
bulbocavernous m.
m. bulk

M

NOTES

muscle *(continued)*

m. bundle
m. cachexia
capillary m.
cardiac m.
Casser m.
casserian m.
m. catabolism
ceratocricoid m.
ceratopharyngeal m.
cervical flexor m.
cervical iliocostal m.
cervical interspinal m.
cervical rotator m.
Chassaignac m.
cheek m.
chin m.
chondropharyngeal m.
ciliary m.
circular ciliary m.
circular pharyngeal m.
coccygeal m.
Coiter m.
colonic circular m.
compressor m.
conal papillary m.
concave temporalis m.
congenerous m.
constrictor pharyngeal m.
contracted m.
m. contractile protein
contractility of m.
m. contractility
m. contraction
m. contraction headache
m. contracture
contractured m.
contracture of interosseous m.
m. contusion
m. cooperation
coracobrachial m.
coracobrachialis m.
corrugator m.
cowl m.
m. cramp
Crampton m.
cranial m.
cremaster m.
cricoarytenoid m.
cricopharyngeal m.
cricothyroid m.
cruciate m.
m. crushing injury
m. curve
cutaneous m.
cyclorotary m.
cyclovertical m.
m. cylinder
dartos m.

deep flexor m.
deltoid m.
denervated m.
m. denervation
dermal m.
detrusor m.
diaphragmatic m.
diarthrodial m.
digastric m.
dilator m.
m. disease
m. disease
disinserted m.
m. dissection
distal m.
m. distraction
divergent rectus m.
dorsal m.
Duverney m.
m. dystonia
m. effect
m. elasticity
m. endplate
m. energy
m. enlargement
m. enzyme
m. enzyme serum level
m. enzyme test
epicranial m.
m. epithelium
epitrochleoanconeus m.
erector spinae m.
m. ergo receptor
eustachian m.
m. examination
expiratory m.
m. extensibility
extensor back m.
extensor carpi radialis brevis m.
extensor carpi radialis longus m.
extensor carpi ulnaris m.
extensor communis m.
extensor digiti minimi m.
extensor digiti quinti m.
extensor digitorum brevis m.
extensor digitorum communis m.
extensor digitorum longus m.
extensor hallucis brevis m.
extensor hallucis longus m.
extensor indicis proprius m.
extensor pollicis brevis m.
extensor pollicis longus m.
extensor wad of 3 m.'s
external abdominal m.
external anal sphincter m.
external intercostal m.
external oblique m.
external obturator m.
external pterygoid m.

external rectus m.
external rotator m.
external sphincter m.
external sphincter ani profundus m.
extracostal m.
extralaryngeal m.
extraocular m.
extrinsic foot m.
eyelid m.
facial m.
facial mimetic m.
m. fascia
m. fascicle
m. fasciculation
fast m.
fast-twitch m.
m. fatigue
femoral m.
m. fiber
m. fiber action potential
m. fiber conduction velocity
m. fiber type
m. fiber wasting
fibrosed m.
m. fibrosis
fibular m.
fibularis brevis m.
fibularis longus m.
fibularis tertius m.
m. filling
m. filter
finger flexor m.
m. firing pattern
first dorsal interosseous m.
first palmar interosseous m.
fixator m.
m. flap
flat m.
flexor m.
flexor accessorius m.
flexor carpi radialis m.
flexor carpi ulnaris m.
flexor digiti quinti brevis m.
flexor digitorum brevis m.
flexor digitorum longus m.
flexor digitorum profundus m.
flexor digitorum sublimis m.
flexor digitorum superficialis m.
flexor hallucis brevis m.
flexor hallucis longus m.
flexor pollicis brevis m.
flexor pollicis longus m.

Folius m.
fourth-layer spinal m.
frontotemporal m.
m. function
fused papillary m.
fusiform m.
galea aponeurotica m.
Gantzer m.
gastrocnemius m.
gastrocnemius-soleus m.
gastrointestinal smooth m.
Gavard m.
gemellus inferior m.
gemellus superior m.
genioglossal m.
geniohyoid m.
glabellar m.
glossopalatine m.
glossopharyngeal m.
gluteal m.
gluteus maximus m.
gluteus medius m.
gluteus minimus m.
gracilis m.
great adductor m.
greater pectoral m.
greater psoas m.
greater rhomboid m.
greater trochanter m.
greater zygomatic m.
greatest gluteal m.
m. group
m. guarding
Guthrie m.
hamstring m.
2-headed m.
3-headed m.
4-headed m.
heart m.
helicis major m.
helicis minor m.
m. hemoglobin
m. hernia
m. herniation
Hilton m.
hip adductor m.
homonymous m.
m. hook
Horner m.
Houston m.
hyoglossal m.
hyoid m.

NOTES

M

muscle *(continued)*
    hypaxial m.
    hyperactive m.
    hyperintense m.
    m. hyperintensity
    hypertonic m.
    m. hypertonicity
    m. hypertrophy
    hypothenar m.
    m. hypotonia
    hypotonic m.
    iliac m.
    iliacus minor m.
    iliococcygeal m.
    iliocostal m.
    iliohypogastric m.
    iliopsoas m.
    m. imbalance
    m. implantation
    incisive m.
    index extensor m.
    indicator m.
    m. infarct
    infarcted heart m.
    inferior constrictor pharyngeal m.
    inferior gemellus m.
    inferior lingual m.
    inferior oblique m.
    inferior oblique extraocular m.
    inferior posterior serratus m.
    inferior rectus extraocular m.
    inferior tarsal m.
    m. inflammatory disorder
    infrahyoid strap m.
    infraspinatus m.
    infraspinous m.
    inhibited m.
    innermost intercostal m.
    innervated m.
    m. innervation
    inspiratory m.
    m. insufficiency
    interarytenoid m.
    intercostal m.
    interfoveolar m.
    intermediate great m.
    intermediate vastus m.
    internal abdominal m.
    internal intercostal m.
    internal oblique m.
    internal obturator m.
    internal pterygoid m.
    internal rotator m.
    interosseous m.
    interspinal m.
    intertransverse m.
    intervening m.
    intraauricular m.
    intraocular m.

intraoral m.
intraspinous m.
intrinsic m.
involuntary m.
ipsilateral lateral rectus m.
iridial m.
iris sphincter m.
m. irritability
m. ischemia
ischiocavernous m.
ischiococcygeus m.
jugular foramen m.
Jung m.
Klein m.
m. knot
Kohlrausch m.
Koyter m.
Krause m.
labium majus m.
labium minus m.
Lancisi m.
Langer m.
laryngeal m.
lateral cricoarytenoid m.
lateral great m.
lateral lumbar intertransverse m.
lateral malleolus m.
lateral pterygoid m.
lateral rectus extraocular m.
lateral vastus m.
latissimus dorsi m.
m. layer disease
least gluteal m.
left inferior rectus m.
left rhomboid m.
left superior rectus m.
left ventricular m.
m. lengthening
lesser rhomboid m.
lesser zygomatic m.
levator ani m.
m. level
lingual m.
LOAF m.'s
long abductor m.
long adductor m.
long extensor m.
long fibular m.
long flexor m.
longissimus capitis m.
longissimus cervicis m.
longissimus colli m.
longissimus thoracis m.
longitudinal ciliary m.
longitudinalis inferior m.
longitudinalis superior m.
longitudinal pharyngeal m.
long levatores costarum m.
long palmar m.

long peroneal m.
long radial extensor m.
long rotator m.
longus capitis m.
longus cervicis m.
lower esophageal sphincter
  circular m.
lumbar erector spinae m.
lumbar extensor m.
lumbar iliocostal m.
lumbar interspinal m.
lumbar quadrate m.
lumbar rotator m.
lumbrical m.
Luschka m.
m. lysis
major m.
malleolus m.
Marcacci m.
m. mass
masseter m.
masticatory m.
m. measurement
medial great m.
medial lumbar intertransverse m.
medial palpebral m.
medial papillary m.
medial pterygoid m.
medial rectus extraocular m.
medial vastus m.
medius m.
mental m.
mentalis m.
Merkel m.
mesothenar m.
middle constrictor pharyngeal m.
middle gluteal m.
middle scalene m.
mimetic m.
minimus m.
minor m.
m. mobilizing technique
m. moment arm length
motor unit m.
mucocutaneous m.
multifidus m.
multipennate m.
mylohyoid m.
mylopharyngeal m.
myocardial m.
myometrial smooth m.
m. myotonic disorder

nasal m.
nasolabial m.
m. necrosis
nonstriated m.
nuchal m.
oblique abdominal m.
oblique arytenoid m.
oblique auricular m.
oblique capitis m.
obturator internus m.
occipitofrontal m.
Ochsner m.
ocular m.
oculorotatory m.
Oddi m.
Oehl m.
omohyoid m.
opponens digiti minimi m.
opponens digiti quinti m.
opponens pollicis m.
opposing m.
orbicularis oculi m.
orbicularis oris m.
orbicular oculi m.
orbital m.
orbitalis m.
organic m.
palatal m.
palatoglossal m.
palatopharyngeal m.
m. palpation
palpebral m.
papillary m.
paralaryngeal m.
paraspinal m.
paraspinous m.
paravertebral m.
Passavant m.
m. pathology
m. patterning sequence
pectinate m.
pectoral m.
pectoralis major m.
pectoralis minor m.
pectorodorsal m.
pectorodorsalis m.
m. pedicle bone graft
pelvic floor m.
pelvis m.
pennate m.
penniform m.
perineal m.

M

NOTES

muscle *(continued)*

m. periodic paralysis
perioral m.
periurethral striated m.
peroneal m.
peroneus brevis m.
peroneus longus m.
peroneus quartus m.
peroneus tertius m.
pharyngeal constrictor m.
pharyngopalatine m.
phasic m.
Phillips m.
m. phosphorylase
physical elasticity of m.
physiologic elasticity of m.
piriform m.
piriformis m.
plantar interossei interosseous m.
plantar interosseous m.
plantaris m.
plantar quadrate m.
plantar tendon sheath of fibularis
  longus m.
plantar tendon sheath of peroneus
  longus m.
m. plate
platysma m.
m. play
m. pleasure
pleuroesophageal m.
pleuroesophageus m.
pollicis longus m.
popliteal m.
popliteus m.
postaxial m.
posterior auricular m.
posterior cervical intertransverse m.
posterior cricoarytenoid m.
posterior deltoid m.
posterior digastric m.
posterior papillary m.
posterior scalene m.
posterior serratus m.
posterior tibial m.
postural m.
Pozzi m.
preaxial m.
procerus m.
profundus m.
pronator quadratus m.
pronator teres m.
m. proprioceptor
m. protein synthesis
m. proteolysis
m. pseudohypertrophy
psoas major m.
psoas minor m.
m. psychogenic disorder

pterygoid m.
puboanalis m.
pubococcygeal m.
puboprostatic m.
puborectal m.
puborectalis m.
pubovaginal m.
pubovesical m.
pupillary constrictor m.
pupillary sphincter m.
pyloric m.
pyramidal auricular m.
pyramidalis m.
quadrate pronator m.
quadratus m.
quadriceps m.
radial dilator m.
radial extensor m.
radial flexor m.
m. recruitment pattern
rectococcygeal m.
rectourethral m.
rectouterine m.
rectovesical m.
rectus abdominis m.
rectus capitis lateralis m.
rectus capitis posterior major m.
rectus capitis posterior minor m.
rectus femoris m.
red m.
Reisseisen m.
m. relaxant
m. relaxation
m. relaxing agent
m. repositioning
m. resection
m. reserve
respiratory m.
m. retraining
retronuchal m.
rhabdosphincter m.
rhomboideus major m.
rhomboid major m.
rhomboid minor m.
ribbon m.
rider's m.
m. rigidity
Riolan m.
risorius m.
rotator cuff m.
Rouget m.
round m.
Ruysch m.
sacrococcygeal m.
sacrospinal m.
salpingopharyngeal m.
Santorini m.
m. sarcoma
sartorius m.

scalene m.
scalenus anterior m.
scalenus medius m.
scalenus minimus m.
scalenus posterior m.
scalloped m.
scalp m.
scapular m.
scapulohumeral m.
scapulothoracic m.
Sebileau m.
second tibial m.
semimembranosus m.
semipennate m.
semispinal m.
semitendinous m.
m. sense
m. sensory receptor
septal papillary m.
serratus anterior m.
serratus posterior m.
m. serum
shawl m.
m. sheath
short abductor m.
short adductor m.
short anconeus m.
shortened psoas m.
short extensor m.
short fibular m.
short flexor m.
short levator m.
short palmar m.
short peroneal m.
short radial extensor m.
short rotator m.
shoulder m.
shunt m.
Sibson m.
skeletal m.
m. slide
m. sliding operation
m. sling
slow m.
slow-twitch m.
smaller pectoral m.
smaller psoas m.
smallest scalene m.
smooth m.
Soemmerring m.
soleus m.
somatic m.

m. sound
m. spasm
m. spasm pain
spastic m.
sphincter m.
spinal m.
m. spindle
m. spindle reflex
spindle-shaped m.
m. splitting
spurt m.
square m.
stapedius m.
static m.
sternal m.
sternochondroscapular m.
sternoclavicular m.
sternocleidomastoid m.
sternohyoid m.
sternomastoid m.
sternothyroid m.
m. stiffness
m. strain
strap m.
m. strength
m. strength testing
m. stretch reflex
striated m.
striped m.
styloauricular m.
styloglossus m.
stylohyoid m.
stylopharyngeal m.
subaortic m.
subclavian m.
subcostal m.
subcrural m.
submucosal vaginal m.
suboccipital m.
subquadricipital m.
subscapular m.
subtendinous bursae of
  gastrocnemius m.
subvertebral m.
sucking m.
superciliary m.
superficial m.
supinator m.
supraclavicular m.
suprahyoid m.
supramediastinal m.
supraspinatus m.

M

NOTES

muscle *(continued)*
    supraspinous m.
    m. surgery
    suspensory m.
    m. sympathetic nerve activity
    synergic m.
    synergistic m.
    tailor's m.
    tarsal m.
    temporal m.
    temporalis m.
    temporoparietal m.
    m. tension
    m. tension headache
    teres major m.
    teres minor m.
    Theile m.
    thenar m.
    m. therapy
    thigh m.
    third fibular m.
    third peroneal m.
    thoracic interspinal m.
    thoracic intertransverse m.
    thoracic longissimus m.
    thoracic rotator m.
    thoracoappendicular m.
    thyroarytenoid m.
    thyroepiglottic m.
    thyrohyoid m.
    thyroid m.
    thyropharyngeal m.
    tibial m.
    tibialis anterior m.
    tibialis posterior m.
    m. tissue
    m. tissue mobility
    Todd m.
    m. toe
    toe extensor m.
    toe flexor m.
    m. tone
    m. tone inhibitor system
    tonic m.
    m. tonicity
    m. tonus
    total elasticity of m.
    Toynbee m.
    m. trabeculation
    tracheal m.
    trachealis m.
    tracheloclavicular m.
    trachelomastoid m.
    tragicus m.
    tragus m.
    m. transfer
    transpalpebral corrugator m.
    m. transposition

    transverse abdominal m.
    transverse arytenoid m.
    transverse auricular m.
    transverse perineal m.
    transverse rectus abdominis m.
    transversospinal m.
    transversus abdominis m.
    trapezius m.
    Treitz m.
    triangular m.
    triceps brachii m.
    triceps coxae m.
    triceps surae m.
    tricipital m.
    trigonal m.
    trigone m.
    m. trimming
    trochlear m.
    true m.
    trunk m.
    m. twitch
    twitch m.
    tympanic m.
    ulnar flexor m.
    underlying chest m.
    unilateral hypoplastic pectoral m.
    unipennate m.
    unstriated m.
    unstriped m.
    upper trapezius m.
    m. uptake
    uptight m.
    urogenital sphincter m.
    uterine m.
    uvular m.
    vaginal m.
    Valsalva m.
    vascular smooth m.
    vastus intermedius m.
    vastus lateralis m.
    vastus medialis m.
    venous smooth m.
    ventral sacrococcygeal m.
    vertebral column m.
    vertical m.
    visceral m.
    vocal m.
    voluntary m.
    m. wasting
    m. weakness
    white m.
    Wilson m.
    wrinkler m.
    yoked m.
    zygomatic m.
    zygomaticus major m.
    zygomaticus minor m.
muscle-to-bone suture

muscular
    m. dystrophy
    m. fascia
muscularity
musculocutaneous nerve
musculospiral nerve
mushroom
    Amanita muscaria m.
    Amanita phalloides m.
    m. poisoning
    m. toxicity
musical rhonchi
Mustardé suture
mustard gas
mutilating wound
mutilation
    genital m.
mutism
    akinetic m.
muzzle-to-skin distance
muzzle velocity
MVA
    motor vehicle accident
MVV
    maximal voluntary ventilation
myalgia
myasthenia gravis
Mycelex-G
mycobacterial infection
Mycobacterium
    M. avium
    M. avium complex infection
    M. avium-intracellulare complex
      (MAC)
    M. tuberculosis
    M. tuberculosis infection
Mycoplasma
    M. pneumonia
    M. pneumoniae
mycotic aneurysm
mycotoxin
    T-2 m.
mydriasis
    unreactive m.
mydriatic
myelinated nerve
myelination
    nerve fiber m.
myelinolysis
    central pontine m.
myelitis
    transverse m.

myeloma
    multiple m.
myiasis
    wound m.
mylohyoid
    m. muscle
    m. nerve
mylopharyngeal muscle
myocardial
    m. cell action potential
    m. concussion
    m. conduction disturbance
    m. contraction disturbance
    m. contusion
    m. depression
    m. infarction (MI)
    m. infarction/heart attack
    Integrilin to Minimize Platelet
      Aggregation and Coronary
      Thrombosis-Acute M. (IMPACT-
      AMI)
    m. ischemia
    m. membrane stabilizing
    m. muscle
    m. stunning
myocarditis bacterial infection
myocardium
    hibernating m.
    reversibly injured m.
myoclonic
    m. jerking
    m. status
myoglobinuria
myoglobinuric renal failure
myometrial smooth muscle
myonecrosis
    clostridial m.
    nonclostridial m.
myopathy
    steroid m.
myositis ossificans
myringitis
    bullous m.
myringotomy
myxedema
    m. coma
    congenital m.
    infantile m.
myxoglobulosis appendicitis
myxoma
    atrial m.
    nerve sheath m.

M

NOTES

nabothian cyst
NAEPP
    National Asthma Education and
    Prevention Program
    NAEPP algorithm
nafcillin
nail
    n. bed laceration
    n. plate
    n. suture
nailbed injury
nalmefene
naloxone
    n. hydrochloride
    lidocaine, epinephrine, atropine, n.
    (LEAN)
napalm
naphthalene toxicity
Naproxen
Narcan
narcosis
    carbon dioxide n.
    nitrogen n.
narcostimulant
narcotic
    n. agonist
    n. agonist-antagonist
    n. analgesic
    neuroaxial n.
    n. poison
narcotize
Nardil
naris, pl. **nares**
    external n.
narrow-angle glaucoma
nasal
    n. balloon tamponade
    n. bone
    n. cannula
    n. flaring
    n. foreign body
    n. fracture
    n. insufflation
    n. muscle
    n. nerve
    n. septum
    n. suture
    n. trumpet
    n. turbinate
    n. vein
nasal-septal fracture
NASCIS
    National Acute Spinal Cord Injury Study
nasociliary nerve
nasoduodenal intubation

nasoethmoidal fracture
nasofrontal
    n. suture
    n. vein
nasogastric (NG)
    n. drainage
    n. intubation
    n. suction
    n. tube (NGT)
nasojejunal intubation
nasolabial
    n. ligament
    n. muscle
nasomandibular ligament
nasomaxillary
    n. fracture
    n. suture
nasoorbital fracture
nasopalatine nerve
nasopharyngeal
    n. airway (NPA)
    n. bursa
nasopharynx
nasoscope
nasotracheal
    n. intubation
    n. tube
natatory ligament
national
    N. Acute Spinal Cord Injury Study
    (NASCIS)
    N. Asthma Education and
    Prevention Program (NAEPP)
    N. Emergency Airway Registry
    (NEAR)
    N. Emergency X-Radiography
    Utilization Study (NEXUS)
    N. Highway Traffic Safety
    Administration (NHTSA)
    N. Institute of Occupational Safety
    and Health (NIOSH)
    N. Institute on Drug Abuse
    (NIDA)
    N. Registry of Emergency Medical
    Technicians (NREMT)
native portal vein
natriuretic peptide
natural
    n. resistance
    n. suture
nature of onset of pain
nausea
    n. and emesis
    n. and vomiting
    n., vomiting, diarrhea (NVD)

N

nauseous
Navane
navicular
- n. body fracture
- n. bone
- n. cuneiform ligament
- n. dorsal lip fracture
- n. fracture
- n. hand fracture
- n. tuberosity fracture

naviculocapitate fracture
naviculocuneiform ligament
NC
- noncontributory

N-DEX non-latex glove
NEAR
- National Emergency Airway Registry

near
- n. complete disruption
- n. drowning
- n. infrared spectroscopy

near-drowning
- n.-d. asphyxiation
- n.-d. injury

near-miss SIDS
nebulization treatment
nebulizer
- Inspiron n.
- jet n.
- small-volume n.
- ultrasonic n.

neck
- bone n.
- n. fracture
- n. injury by hanging
- n. injury by strangulation
- n. trauma
- n. vein

necklace identifier
neck-lift maneuver
neck-thrust maneuver
necrolysis
- toxic epidermal n. (TEN)

necrosis
- acute tubular n. (ATN)
- ammonia liquefaction n.
- aseptic n.
- avascular n. (AVN)
- bone aseptic n.
- bone avascular n.
- breast fat n.
- caseous n.
- coumarin n.
- fat n.
- liquefaction n.
- muscle n.
- nonoliguric acute tubular n.
- oliguric acute tubular n.
- tendon n.

- tubular n.
- warfarin skin n.
- wound n.

necrotic bone
necrotizing
- n. enteropathy
- n. fasciitis
- n. soft tissue infection
- n. vasculitis

need
- n. for aggressive evaluation
- children with special health care n.'s (CSHCN)
- metabolic n.
- n. for operative intervention
- n. for transfusion

needed to treat
needle
- cutting n.
- n. decompression
- hypodermic n.
- Potts-Cournand n.
- seeker n.
- n. stick
- tendon n.
- n. thoracentesis
- n. thoracostomy

needle-catheter cricothyroid ventilation
needleless injection site (NIS)
Needle-Less Suture
Neer-Horowitz humeral fracture classification
Neer type I-III shoulder fracture
nefazodone
negative
- n. chemotaxis
- n. dromotropy
- n. examination
- pertinent n.
- Rh n.

negative-pressure pulmonary edema
neglectful burn
neglect home condition
negligence
Neisseria meningitidis
neoadjuvant therapy
neoformans
- *Cryptococcus n.*

neonatal
- n. hemorrhage
- n. intensive care unit (NICU)
- n. jaundice
- n. resuscitation
- n. sepsis
- n. withdrawal

neonate
neonatorum
- ophthalmia n.

neoplasia

neoplasm
    bone n.
neoplastic
    n. fracture
    n. pericardial tamponade
Neo-Synephrine
neovascularization
nephrectomy
    radical n.
nephritic syndrome
nephritis
    acute interstitial n.
    acute tubular interstitial n. (ATIN)
    analgesic n.
    interstitial n.
nephrocolic ligament
nephronic syndrome
nephropathy
    Chinese herb n.
    chloride-wasting n.
    nephrotoxic vasomotor n.
    vasomotor n.
nephrostomy
    percutaneous n.
nephrotic syndrome
nephrotoxic
    n. effect
    n. vasomotor nephropathy
nephrotoxicity
    aminoglycoside n.
nephrotoxin
Nerium
    N. oleander
    N. oleander ingestion
nerve
    abducent n.
    accessory phrenic n.
    acoustic n.
    acousticofacial n.
    n. action potential
    afferent digital n.
    afferent renal n.
    n. allografting
    alveolar n.
    anal n.
    n. anastomosis
    Andersch n.
    anococcygeal n.
    anterior alveolar n.
    anterior antebrachial n.
    anterior ethmoidal n.
    anterior femoral cutaneous n.

anterior interosseous n.
anterior labial n.
anterior palatine n.
anterior scrotal n.
anterior supraclavicular n.
anterior thoracic n.
anterior tibial n.
anterolateral intercostal n.
anteromedial intercostal n.
aortic n.
n. approximator
Arnold n.
articular n.
articular recurrent n.
auditory tube n.
augmentor n.
auricular n.
auriculotemporal n.
autonomic n.
axillary n.
baroreceptor n.
basal epithelial n.
Bell respiratory n.
n. biopsy
block n.
n. block anesthesia
n. block infusion
Bock n.
brachial cutaneous n.
brachial plexus n.
n. branch
branchial n.
buccal n.
buccinator n.
buffer n.
calcaneal n.
n. cap
cardiac sensory n.
cardiopulmonary splanchnic n.
caroticotympanic n.
carotid sinus n.
cavernosal n.
cavernous n.
celiac n.
n. cell
n. cell body
n. cell death
n. cell survival
n. cell tumor
n. center
centrifugal n.
centripetal n.

N

NOTES

nerve *(continued)*
    cerebral n.
    cervical sensory n.
    cervical splanchnic n.
    cervical sympathetic n.
    chorda tympani n.
    ciliary n.
    circumflex n.
    cluneal n.
    n. coaptation
    coccygeal n.
    cochlear n.
    cochleovestibular n.
    common digital n.
    common fibular n.
    common palmar digital n.
    common peroneal n.
    common plantar digital n.
    n. compression
    n. compression-degeneration
      syndrome
    n. compression syndrome
    n. compression test
    n. conduction
    n. conduction velocity
    n. conduction velocity study
    n. conduction velocity test
    n. cooling
    corneal n.
    Cotunnius n.
    n. of Cotunnius
    cranial n. (CN)
    n. crossing
    n. cross-section
    n. crush injury
    cubital n.
    n. cuff
    cutaneous n.
    Cyon n.
    dead n.
    n. deafness
    n. decompression
    n. decussation
    dental n.
    dentinal intratubular n.
    depressor n.
    descending n.
    diaphragmatic n.
    digastric n.
    digital n.
    n. discontinuity
    distal accessory n.
    n. distribution
    dorsal antebrachial cutaneous n.
    dorsal interosseous n.
    dorsal lateral cutaneous n.
    dorsal medial cutaneous n.
    dorsal scapular n.
    dorsomedial cutaneous n.

    n. dysplasia
    efferent digital n.
    encephalic n.
    n. ending
    n. entrapment neuralgia
    n. entrapment site
    n. entrapment syndrome
    entrapped n.
    n. entubulation
    esodic n.
    ethmoidal n.
    n. evulsion
    n. excitability test
    excitor n.
    excitoreflex n.
    exodic n.
    external carotid n.
    external nasal n.
    external popliteal n.
    external pterygoid n.
    external saphenous n.
    external spermatic n.
    extrinsic n.
    facial n.
    n. factor
    n. fascicle
    femoral n.
    femoral cutaneous n.
    fenestrated oculomotor n.
    n. fiber
    n. fiber action potential
    n. fiber analyzer
    n. fiber bundle
    n. fiber bundle layer
    n. fiber layer hemorrhage
    n. fiber myelination
    n. fibril
    fibrolipomatous hamartoma n.
    fibular n.
    n. field
    n. force
    frontal n.
    furcal n.
    fusimotor n.
    Galen n.
    gangliated n.
    n. ganglion
    n. gap
    n. gas
    Gaskell n.
    gastric n.
    genitocrural n.
    genitofemoral n.
    gingival n.
    glossopharyngeal n.
    gluteal n.
    n. graft
    Grassi n.
    n. of Grassi

great auricular n.
greater occipital n.
greater palatine n.
greater petrosal n.
greater splanchnic n.
greater superficial petrosal n.
great sciatic n.
n. growth factor
n. growth factor antiserum
n. growth factor receptor
hemorrhoidal n.
Hering sinus n.
n. holder
n. hook
hypertrophied corneal n.
hypogastric n.
hypoglossal n.
iliohypogastric n.
ilioinguinal n.
iliopubic n.
n. impingement
n. implantation
n. impulse
incisive n.
inferior alveolar n.
inferior anal n.
inferior calcaneal n.
inferior cluneal n.
inferior dental n.
inferior gluteal n.
inferior hemorrhoidal n.
inferior laryngeal n.
inferior lateral brachial
  cutaneous n.
inferior maxillary n.
inferior nasal n.
inferior palpebral n.
inferior rectal n.
inferior vesical n.
infraepitrochlear n.
infraoccipital n.
infraorbital n.
infratrochlear n.
inguinal n.
inhibitory n.
input n.
intercarotid n.
intercostal n.
intercostobrachial n.
intercostohumeral n.
interdigital n.
n. interference

intermediary n.
intermediate dorsal cutaneous n.
intermediate supraclavicular n.
intermedius n.
intermetatarsal n.
internal carotid n.
internal popliteal n.
internal rectal n.
internal saphenous n.
interosseous n.
intrapancreatic n.
n. involvement testing
ischiadic n.
Jacobson n.
jugular n.
labial n.
labioglossopharyngeal n.
lacrimal n.
Lancisi n.
Langley n.
laryngeal n.
Latarjet n.
lateral dorsal cutaneous n.
lateral femoral cutaneous n.
lateral pectoral n.
lateral plantar n.
lateral popliteal n.
lateral pterygoid n.
lateral superior genicular n.
lateral supraclavicular n.
lateral sural cutaneous n.
least splanchnic n.
left hypogastric n.
left recurrent laryngeal n.
left respiratory n.
lesser internal cutaneous n.
lesser occipital n.
lesser palatine n.
lesser splanchnic n.
lesser superficial petrosal n.
lingual n.
long buccal n.
long ciliary n.
longitudinal n.
long saphenous n.
long subscapular n.
long thoracic n.
n. loss
lowest splanchnic n.
Ludwig n.
lumbar splanchnic n.
lumboinguinal n.

NOTES

N

nerve *(continued)*
Luschka n.
mandibular n.
n. mapping
marginal mandibular n.
masseteric n.
masticator n.
maxillary n.
medial antebrachial cutaneous n.
medial anterior thoracic n.
medial articular n.
medial brachial cutaneous n.
medial calcaneal branch of
 tibial n.
medial cluneal n.
medial crural cutaneous branch of
 saphenous n.
medial dorsal cutaneous n.
medial pectoral n.
medial plantar n.
medial popliteal n.
medial pterygoid n.
medial supraclavicular n.
medial sural cutaneous n.
median n.
meningeal n.
mental n.
middle cardiac cervical n.
middle cervical cardiac n.
middle cluneal n.
middle supraclavicular n.
mixed n.
monofascicular n.
motor n.
musculocutaneous n.
musculospiral n.
myelinated n.
mylohyoid n.
nasal n.
nasociliary n.
nasopalatine n.
nociceptive sensory n.
noncholinergic n.
nonmyelinated n.
nonrecurrent laryngeal n.
obturator n.
occipital n.
ocular n.
oculomotor n.
olfactory cranial n.
olivocochlear n.
Oort n.
ophthalmic recurrent n.
optic n.
orbital optic n.
output n.
n. pain
palatine n.
palmar cutaneous n.

palmar digital n.
n. palsy
n. papilla
n. paralysis
parasympathetic n.
parotid n.
pathetic n.
pectineus n.
pectoral n.
pelvic autonomic n.
pelvic floor n.
pelvic splanchnic n.
perforating cutaneous n.
pericardiophrenic n.
perineal n.
peripapillary retinal n.
peripheral motor n.
peripheral oculomotor n.
periradicular n.
peritonsillar n.
perivascular n.
peroneal communicating n.
petrosal n.
phrenic n.
phrenicoabdominal n.
pilomotor n.
pinched n.
piriform n.
plantar digital n.
n. plexus
n. plexus entrapment
pneumogastric n.
polyfascicular n.
popliteal communicating n.
postauricular n.
posterior ampullar n.
posterior ampullary n.
posterior antebrachial cutaneous n.
posterior auricular n.
posterior brachial cutaneous n.
posterior communicating n.
posterior cutaneous femoral n.
posterior ethmoidal n.
posterior femoral cutaneous n.
posterior inferior nasal n.
posterior labial n.
posterior palatine n.
posterior scapular n.
posterior scrotal n.
posterior superior alveolar n.
posterior superior nasal n.
posterior supraclavicular n.
posterior thoracic n.
posterior tibial n.
posterosuperior alveolar n.
postganglionic cholinergic n.
postganglionic short ciliary n.
postganglionic sympathetic n.
preauricular n.

prechiasmal optic n.
predentinal n.
prelaminar optic n.
presacral n.
pressor n.
pressoreceptor n.
proprioception n.
pterygoid n.
pterygopalatine n.
pudendal n.
pudic n.
n. pull hook
radial digital n.
radial sensory n.
rectal n.
recurrent laryngeal n.
recurrent meningeal n.
n. regeneration
n. regrowth
renal afferent n.
renal sympathetic n.
right common iliac n.
right hypogastric n.
right recurrent laryngeal n.
n. root
n. root avulsion
n. root axillary pouch
n. root block
n. root compression
n. root decompression
n. root edema
n. root embarrassment
n. root entrapment
n. root impingement
n. root irritability
n. root irritation
n. root laminectomy dissector
n. root lesion
n. rootlet
n. rootlet ablation
n. root microcirculation
n. root retractor
n. root sheath
n. root sheath effacement
n. root sleeve
n. root sleeve injection
n. root stimulation
n. root syndrome
n. root tumor
rostral cervical n.
saccular n.
sacral splanchnic n.

saphenous n.
sartorius n.
scapular n.
Scarpa n.
sciatic n.
scrotal n.
secretomotor n.
secretory n.
sensorimotor n.
sensory n.
n. separator
n. separator spatula
n. sharing
n. sheath malignant tumor
n. sheath myxoma
short ciliary n.
short saphenous n.
n. signal
sinocarotid n.
sinovertebral n.
sinus n.
sinuvertebral n.
somatic n.
spermatic n.
sphenopalatine n.
spinal accessory n.
splanchnic n.
splayed facial n.
n. sprouting
statoacoustic n.
n. stimulator
n. stimulator anesthetic technique
n. stretching
n. stroma
n. stump
stylohyoid n.
stylopharyngeal n.
subclavian n.
subcostal n.
subcutaneous temporal n.
sublingual n.
submandibular n.
submaxillary n.
suboccipital n.
subscapular n.
sudomotor n.
supraclavicular n.
supraorbital n.
suprascapular n.
supraspinatus n.
supratrochlear n.
supreme cardiac n.

NOTES

nerve *(continued)*
    sural n.
    n. suture
    n. suture technique
    sympathetic n.
    taste n.
    temporal n.
    temporomalar n.
    temporomandibular n.
    tentorial n.
    terminal n.
    n. territory oriented macrodactyly
    n. thickening
    thoracic cardiac branch of vagus n.
    thoracic spinal n.
    thoracic splanchnic n.
    thoracoabdominal n.
    thoracodorsal n.
    thoracolumbar sympathetic n.
    tibial communicating n.
    Tiedemann n.
    n. tissue
    n. tracing
    n. tract
    transcutaneous n.
    n. transfer
    n. transmission
    n. transsection
    transverse cervical n.
    transverse colli n.
    trifacial n.
    trigeminal n.
    trochlear n.
    n. trunk
    n. trunk action potential
    n. twig
    tympanic n.
    ulnar n.
    unmyelinated n.
    upper cervical n.
    upper subscapular n.
    upper thoracic splanchnic n.
    utricular n.
    utriculoampullar n.
    vaginal n.
    vagus n.
    Valentin n.
    variant n.
    vascular n.
    vasoconstrictor n.
    vasodilator n.
    vasomotor n.
    vasosensory n.
    vertebral n.
    vestibular n.
    vestibulocochlear n.
    vidian n.
    visceral n.
    volar interosseous n.
    vomeronasal n.
    Willis n.
    n. wrapping
    Wrisberg n.
    zygomatic n.
    zygomaticofacial n.
    zygomaticotemporal n.

nervosa
    anorexia n.
    bulimia n.

Nesacaine

netilmicin sulfate

network
    Drug Abuse Warning N. (DAWN)

neural
    n. arch fracture
    n. depression
    n. tube

neuralgia
    nerve entrapment n.
    trigeminal n.

neurapraxia

neurasthenia

neuritis
    optic n.

neuroaxial narcotic

neuroblastoma

neurocardiogenic syncope

neurocentral suture

neurocognitive deficit

neurofibromatosis
    abortive n.

neurogenic
    n. bladder
    n. fracture
    n. pulmonary edema
    n. shock

neurohormonal
    n. activation
    n. response

neuroleptic
    n. agent
    n. malignant syndrome (NMS)
    n. poisoning

neurologic
    n. deficit
    n. status
    n. vascular deficit

neurological intensive care unit (NICU)

neurology
    clinical n.

neuroma
    acoustic n.
    Morton n.

neuromimetic

neuromuscular (NM)
    n. blocking agent (NMBA)
    n. junction

neuromyopathy
    carcinomatous n.
neuron
    ganglionic motor n.
    lower motor n. (LMN)
    vagal preganglionic cardiomotor n.
neuronitis
    vestibular n.
neuropathic fracture
neuropathy
    acute compressive optic n.
    ischemic optic n.
    peripheral n.
    strangulation n.
    traumatic optic n. (TON)
neuroprotectant
neuropsychiatric sign
neurosurgical
    n. consultant
    n. consultation
    n. monitoring
    n. suture
neurotmesis
neurotoxic shellfish poisoning
neurotransmitter
    AA n.
    excitatory amino acid n.
neurotrauma
neurotrophic fracture
neurovascular compromise
neutralizer
    bromate hair n.
neutralizing agent
neutropenia
    cyclic n.
neutropenia/immune compromise
neutropenic colitis
neutrophil-dependent lung injury
new
    N. Injury Severity Score (NISS)
    n. onset angina
newborn resuscitation
newly woven bone
Newman radial neck and head fracture classification
newt toxin
NEXUS
    National Emergency X-Radiography Utilization Study
NG
    nasogastric

NG decompression
NG tube
NGT
    nasogastric tube
NHTSA
    National Highway Traffic Safety Administration
nicardipine hydrochloride
nicking
    vein n.
Nicoladoni suture
Nicotiana
    N. glauca
    N. glauca ingestion
    N. tabacum
    N. tabacum ingestion
nicotinate
    aluminum n.
NICU
    neonatal intensive care unit
    neurological intensive care unit
NIDA
    National Institute on Drug Abuse
NIDDM
    non-insulin-dependent diabetes mellitus
nidus, pl. nidi
nifedipine
nightmare
nightstick fracture
night-walker fracture
Nikolsky sign
Nimbex injection
Nimbus hemopump
nimodipine
NIOSH
    National Institute of Occupational Safety and Health
NIP
    nonspecific interstitial pneumonia
nipple discharge
NIS
    needleless injection site
NISS
    New Injury Severity Score
Nissen
    N. fundoplication
    N. suture
nitrate
    amyl n.
    gallium n.
    silver n.
    n. toxicity

NOTES

nitric
    n. acid
    n. oxide (NO)
nitrite-thiosulfate kit
nitrite toxicity
nitrofurantoin
nitrofurazone
nitrogen
    blood urea n. (BUN)
    n. narcosis
    n. oxide
nitroglycerin
    n. drip
    n. ointment
    n. paste
    sublingual n.
nitroprusside
    sodium n.
    n. therapy
nitrosourea
nitrous
    n. dioxide
    n. oxide
nitro vasodilator
Nizoral
NKA
    no known allergy
NM
    neuromuscular
NMBA
    neuromuscular blocking agent
NMS
    neuroleptic malignant syndrome
NO
    nitric oxide
no
    no heavy lifting
    no known allergy (NKA)
    no obtainable blood pressure
    no prolonged standing
Nocardia
    N. asteroides
    N. infection
nociceptive sensory nerve
nocturia
nocturnal
    n. dyspnea
    n. ventilation
nodal tachycardia
node
    atrioventricular n.
    sinoatrial n.
nodosum
    erythema n.
nodularity
    tendon n.
    vein n.
    n. vein
nodular lymphoma

nodule
    discrete n.
    singer's n.
    tendon n.
NOE fracture
noisy breathing
nomogram
    Done n.
    Rumack-Matthew acetaminophen
      poisoning n.
nonabsorbable
    n. mattress suture
    n. surgical suture
nonaccidental spiral tibial fracture
nonarticular
    n. distal radial fracture
    n. radial head fracture
nonbreather mask
noncardiogenic pulmonary edema
noncholinergic nerve
nonclostridial myonecrosis
noncomminuted fracture
noncompliance
    medication n.
    patient n.
    serious n.
noncontiguous fracture
noncontrast CT scan
noncontributory (NC)
nondepolarizing neuromuscular blocking
    agent
nondepressed skull fracture
nondisplaced fracture
nonemergent etiology
nonfeasance
nonfunctioning stent
nonfusion of cranial suture
nonhealing wound
non-insulin-dependent diabetes mellitus
    (NIDDM)
noninvasive
    n. nocturnal ventilation
    n. positive pressure ventilation
      (NPPV)
nonionizing radiation
nonketotic
    n. hyperosmolar coma
    hyperosmolar hyperglycemia n.
      (HHNK)
nonlamellar bone
nonlamellated bone
non-life-threatening emergency
nonmyelinated nerve
nonnecrotic tissue
nonobstructive appendicitis
nonoliguric acute tubular necrosis
nonoperative approach
nonparoxysmal atrioventricular
    junctional tachycardia

nonpathologic fracture
nonpenetrating wound
nonphyseal fracture
nonpitting edema
non-Q wave
non-Q-wave myocardial infarction
nonrebreather mask
nonrebreathing face mask
nonrecurrent laryngeal nerve
nonresorbable suture
nonrotational burst fracture
nonshivering thermogenesis
nonspecific
    n. interstitial pneumonia (NIP)
    n. tenderness
    n. vaginitis
nonsteroidal
    n. antiinflammatory agent
    n. antiinflammatory drug (NSAID)
    n. antiinflammatory drug overdose
    n. antiinflammatory drug poisoning
    n. antiinflammatory toxicity
nonstriated muscle
nonsustained ventricular tachycardia
nonthermal burn
nontoothed forceps
nonunion
    fracture n.
    n. of fracture
    fracture fragment n.
    fracture with n.
    n. horse-hoof fracture
    n. torsion wedge fracture
nonunited fracture
nonviable fetus
nonweightbearing (NWB)
Noonan syndrome
Norcuron
no-reflow phenomenon
norepinephrine
normal
    n. laboratory evaluation
    upper limits of n. (ULN)
    n. vital signs
normochromic normocytic anemia
nosocomial
    n. disease
    n. pneumonia
    n. urinary tract infection
    n. ventriculitis

notch
    suprasternal n.
not contagious
Novafil suture
Novocain
NPA
    nasopharyngeal airway
NPPV
    noninvasive positive pressure ventilation
NREMT
    National Registry of Emergency Medical
    Technicians
NSAID
    nonsteroidal antiinflammatory drug
nuchal
    n. cord
    n. ligament
    n. muscle
    n. rigidity
nuclear magnetic resonance spectroscopy
nummular eczema
Nurolon suture
Nuromax
nursemaid's elbow
nurse's aide
nutcracker
    n. esophagus
    n. fracture
nutrition
    adequate n.
    enteral n.
    parenteral n.
    n. status
    total parenteral n. (TPN)
    total peripheral parenteral n.
    (TPPN)
nutritional disorder
NVD
    nausea, vomiting, diarrhea
NWB
    nonweightbearing
nylon
    n. monofilament suture
    n. retention suture
    n. strap
    n. 66 suture
nystagmus
    incongruent n.
    jerky n.
Nystatin

N

NOTES

O2
    oxygen
OAD
    obstructive airway disease
oak
    poison o.
obesity
    exogenous o.
    morbid o.
object
    foreign o.
    impaled foreign o.
objective
    o. evaluation
    o. sign
    o. symptom
oblique
    o. abdominal muscle
    o. arytenoid muscle
    o. auricular muscle
    o. capitis muscle
    o. fracture
    o. popliteal ligament
    o. retinacular ligament
    o. spiral fracture
    o. tendon
    o. vein
    o. view
obliquity shoulder fracture
obliterans
    appendicitis o.
    bronchiolitis o. (BO)
obliterated vein
obliteration
O'Brien radial fracture classification
observation
    admission for o.
    o. of chest wall movement
    discharge after o.
obsessive-compulsive disorder (OCD)
obsolescence
obstetric level of care
obstipation
obstructed defecation
obstruction
    acute airway o.
    airway o.
    bowel o.
    complete airway o.
    foreign body o.
    gallbladder o.
    gastric outlet o. (GOO)
    gastrointestinal o.
    idiopathic hypertrophic subaortic o.
    ileal loop o.

    large bowel o.
    large intestine o.
    lower airway o.
    mechanical o.
    ostial o.
    partial airway o.
    small bowel o.
    small intestine o.
    total upper airway o.
    upper airway o.
    ureteral o.
    urinary tract o.
    vein o.
    visceral ischemic o.
obstructive
    o. airway disease (OAD)
    o. shock
obtund
obtundation
obtunded patient
obturator
    o. avulsion fracture
    esophageal o.
    o. internus muscle
    o. nerve
    o. sign
    o. vein
obtuse
occasional rhonchi
occipital
    o. bone
    o. cerebral vein
    o. condyle fracture
    o. diploic vein
    o. emissary vein
    o. lobe
    o. nerve
    o. region
    o. suture
    o. view
occipitoaxial ligament
occipitofrontal muscle
occipitomastoid suture
occipitoparietal suture
occipitosphenoidal suture
occipitosphenoid suture
occiput bone
occlusion
    arterial o.
    optic artery o.
    pulmonary artery o.
    retinal artery o.
    retinal vein o.
    vascular o.
    vein graft o.

O

occlusive
  o. bandage
  o. dressing
occult
  o. bleeding
  o. blood
  o. fracture
  o. injury
  o. osseous fracture
  o. scaphoid fracture
occupational
  o. asthma
  o. cancer
  o. disease
  o. history
  O. Safety and Health
    Administration (OSHA)
occupationally induced asthma
OCD
  obsessive-compulsive disorder
Ochsner muscle
octopus envenomation
octreotide
ocular
  o. abnormality
  o. bobbing
  o. burn
  o. dipping
  o. loupe
  o. muscle
  o. nerve
  o. tendon
oculomotor
  o. nerve
  o. nerve palsy
oculopharyngeal dystrophy
oculorotatory muscle
OD
  overdose
Oddi muscle
O-desmethylvenlafaxine (ODV)
odontoid
  o. bone
  o. condyle fracture
  o. ligament
  o. neck fracture
  open-mouth o. (OMO)
odor
  almond o.
  ammonia o.
  bitter almond o.
  burned rope o.
  carrot o.
  coal gas o.
  formaldehyde o.
  fruity breath o.
  garlic o.
  maple sugar o.
  mothball o.

  paste o.
  peanut o.
  pear o.
  pine oil o.
  rotten egg o.
  shoe polish o.
  urine o.
  vinegar o.
  vinyl shower curtain o.
  violet o.
  wintergreen o.
ODT
  oral disintegrating tablet
  Zofran ODT
ODV
  O-desmethylvenlafaxine
Oehl muscle
off-line medical direction
off-pump coronary artery bypass
ofloxacin
Ogden epiphysial fracture classification
Ogilvie syndrome
OI
  oxygenation index
  oxygen index
oiled silk suture
ointment
  GTN o.
  nitroglycerin o.
OKT3
  ornithine-ketoacid transaminase
  orthoclone
OLB
  open lung biopsy
old
  o. ecchymosis
  o. fracture
oleander
  Nerium o.
oleate-condensate
  triethanolamine polypeptide o.-c.
olecranon
  o. bursa
  o. ligament
  o. tip fracture
olfactory cranial nerve
oligemic shock
oligodipsia
oliguria
oliguric acute tubular necrosis
olivocochlear nerve
OLTx
  orthotopic liver transplantation
OM
  otitis media
omental
  o. bursa
  o. vein

omentum
matted o.
omeprazole
Omnipaque contrast material
omnivorous
OMO
open-mouth odontoid
OMO view
omohyoid muscle
omovertebral bone
OMPA
otitis media, purulent, acute
omphalomesenteric vein
oncotic pressure
ondansetron
ongoing
o. assessment
o. blood loss
on-line medical direction
only
comfort measures o. (CMO)
onset
acuteness of o.
o. of pain
o., provocation, quality,
region/radiation, severity, time
(OPQRST)
rapidity of o.
Ontario Prehospital Advanced Life Support (OPALS)
onychomycosis
Oort nerve
O&P
ova and parasite
OPA
oropharyngeal airway
OPALS
Ontario Prehospital Advanced Life Support
OPALS study
opaque wire suture
open
o. book fracture
o. break fracture
o. clavicular fracture
o. fracture
o. injury
o. lung biopsy (OLB)
o. pneumothorax
o. reduction
o. reduction of fracture

o. reduction and internal fixation (ORIF)
o. skull fracture
o. wound
open-angle glaucoma
open-mouth odontoid (OMO)
open-sky cataract wound
operating room
operation
Computer-Aided Management of Emergency O.'s (CAMEO)
muscle sliding o.
operative
o. intervention
o. repair
o. team
o. therapy
o. treatment
ophthalmia
o. neonatorum
sympathetic o.
ophthalmic
Polysporin O.
o. recurrent nerve
o. vein
ophthalmicus
herpes zoster o.
ophthalmomeningeal vein
ophthalmoplegia
Ophthalon suture
opiate
o. overdose
o. poisoning
o. withdrawal
opioid
o. addiction
o. overdose
opponens
o. digiti minimi muscle
o. digiti quinti muscle
o. pollicis muscle
opportunistic infection
opposing muscle
OPQRST
onset, provocation, quality, region/radiation, severity, time
OpSite dressing
optic
o. artery occlusion
o. nerve
o. nerve aplasia
o. neuritis

O

NOTES

opticociliary shunt vein
optimal positive end-expiratory pressure
optimization
    graft function assessment and o.
optimum ventilation
oral
    o. antibiotic
    o. anticoagulant toxicity
    o. awake intubation
    o. candidiasis
    o. conscious sedation
    o. contraceptive
    o. disintegrating tablet (ODT)
    o. fluid
    o. glucose
    o. hygiene
    o. mucosa
    o. mucositis
    o. suspension
    o. temperature
orange
    Agent O.
orbicular
    o. bone
    o. ligament
    o. oculi muscle
orbicularis
    o. oculi muscle
    o. oris muscle
orbit
orbital
    o. blow-in fracture
    o. blowout fracture
    o. bone
    o. cellulitis
    o. floor fracture
    o. fracture
    o. muscle
    o. nasoethmoidal fracture
    o. optic nerve
    o. rim fracture
    o. roof fracture
    o. stepoff
    o. varix ophthalmic vein
    o. wall fracture
orbitalis muscle
orbitomalar ligament
orbitosphenoidal bone
orchitis
    epididymitis and o.
order
    DNR o.
    do not resuscitate o.
orellanine
organ
    accessory o.
    o. capsule distention
    o. chlorine
    o. donation

    o. donor
    o. failure
    o. function
    hollow o.
    O. Injury Scale
    o. perfusion
    solid o.
organic
    o. bound iodide toxicity
    o. muscle
organism
    pathogenic o.
organization
    health maintenance o. (HMO)
organochlorine
organomegaly
organophosphate poisoning
Oriental
    O. female
    O. male
oriented
    awake, alert, and o. ×3 (AAO3)
ORIF
    open reduction and internal fixation
orifice
    vein o.
origin
    bleeding of undetermined o. (BUO)
    fever of undetermined o. (FUO)
    fever of unknown o. (FUO)
Orlowski score
ornithine-ketoacid transaminase
    orthoclone (OKT3)
Ornithonyssus bursa
orogastric
    o. feeding tube
    o. lavage
oropharyngeal
    o. airway (OPA)
    o. candidiasis
    o. flora aspiration
    o. swelling
orotracheal
    o. intubation
    o. suctioning
    o. tube
orphenadrine
orthochlorobenzylidene malononitrile
    (CS)
orthoclone
    ornithine-ketoacid transaminase o.
    (OKT3)
orthodeoxia
orthodromic tachycardia
orthopaedic
    o. consultant
    o. consultation
    o. referral
    o. specialist

o. stretcher
o. surgery
orthopnea
2-pillow o.
3-pillow o.
orthostatic
o. blood pressure
o. blood pressure change
o. hypotension
orthotopic
o. heart transplant
o. heart transplantation
o. liver transplantation (OLTx)
os
os calcis bone
os trigonum fracture
Osborne ligament
oscillate
oscillating vein
oscillometry
oseltamivir
Osgood-Schlatter disease
OSHA
Occupational Safety and Health
Administration
Osler-Weber-Rendu syndrome
osmolality
measured serum o.
serum o.
osmolar gap
osmolarity
osmole
idiogenic o.
osmotherapy
osmotic diuretic
osseocutaneous ligament
ossificans
myositis o.
ossification
heterotopic o.
ossification-associated fracture
ossiform
osteal resonance
osteitis
bone flap o.
osteoarthritis
osteochondral slice fracture
osteoclastic bone
osteogenesis imperfecta
osteolysis
osteomalacia
osteomyelitis

osteonal lamellar bone
osteonic bone
osteopenic bone
osteopetrosis-stricken facial bone
osteoplastic craniotomy
osteoporosis
osteoporotic
o. bone
o. compression fracture
ostial obstruction
ostium, pl. **ostia**
OTC
over-the-counter
oticus
herpes zoster o.
otitis
o. externa
o. media (OM)
o. media, purulent, acute (OMPA)
otologic
o. avulsion
o. laceration
o. trauma
Ottawa ankle rules
OURQ
outer upper right quadrant
outcome
weaning o.
outer upper right quadrant (OURQ)
outlet strut fracture
outpatient
o. therapy
o. treatment
output
bioimpedance-determined cardiac o.
cardiac o. (CO)
continuous cardiac o.
high o.
low o.
o. nerve
reduced cardiac o.
right-sided cardiac o.
thermodilution cardiac o.
Ovadia-Beals tibial plafond fracture classification
ovale
patent foramen o.
ova and parasite (O&P)
ovarian
o. bursa
o. cyst
o. suspensory ligament

O

NOTES

ovarian *(continued)*
    o. torsion
    o. vein
over
    external flash o.
over-and-over suture
overdevelopment
    bone o.
overdose (OD)
    ACE inhibitor o.
    calcium channel blocker o.
    guanfacine o.
    hypoglycemic drug o.
    massive o.
    nonsteroidal antiinflammatory
      drug o.
    opiate o.
    opioid o.
    paregoric o.
    phencyclidine o.
    salicylate o.
    sedative-hypnotic o.
    toxic o.
overflow
overlapping
    o. fracture
    o. suture
overload
    fluid o.
overpressure
overriding of suture
over-the-counter (OTC)
    o.-t.-c. medication
oviduct
ovulation
    spontaneous o.
oxacillin
oxalate
    cerium o.
oxalosis
    bone o.
oxazepam
oxazolidinediones
oxazolidinones
oxidase
    tyramine o.
oxidative
    o. metabolism
    o. phosphorylation
oxide
    inhaled nitric o. (iNO)
    nitric o. (NO)
    nitrogen o.
    nitrous o.
oxidize

oxime
    phosgene o.
oximeter
    Capnocheck II CO_2/pulse o.
    finger o.
    MiniCorr digital o.
    PalmSAT digital handheld pulse o.
    pulse o.
oximetry
    finger o.
    pulse o.
    transcutaneous o.
    venous o.
oxygen (O2)
    blow-by o.
    o. consumption
    o. delivery
    o. deprivation
    dry o.
    fractional concentration of
      inspired o. (FIO_2)
    high-flow o.
    humidified o.
    hyperbaric o. (HBO)
    o. index (OI)
    o. metabolism
    o. pressure tension
    o. (size D, E, M, G, and H)
      cylinder
    o. source
    supplemental o.
    O. Tank Lift Systems
    o. toxicity
    o. utilization
oxygenated
    o. blood
    o. perfluorochemical liquid
oxygenation
    extracorporeal membrane o.
    (ECMO)
    o. index (OI)
    mask o.
    venovenous extracorporeal
      membrane o.
oxygenator
    intravascular o. (IVOX)
    membrane o.
oxyhemoglobin dissociation curve
Oxylator positive pressure resuscitation
    and inhalation system
oxysporum
    Fusarium o.
oxytocin
Oyloidin suture
ozone inhalation injury

PA
    pulmonary artery
        PA catheter
P & A
    percussion and auscultation
PAC
    premature atrial contraction
Pac
    Smart Triage P.
pacemaker
    atrial p.
    cardiac p.
    external p.
    p. lead fracture
    runaway p.
    temporary p.
    wandering atrial p.
    Zoll M Series defibrillator
      monitor p.
pacemaker-mediated tachycardia
pacer spike
pacing
    cardiac p.
    emergency cardiac p.
    external temporary p.
    external transcutaneous cardiac p.
    permanent cardiac p.
    transcutaneous cardiac p. (TCP)
    transvenous temporary p.
pack
    cold p.
    ice p.
    subfascial gauze p.
packed red blood cell (PRBC)
packer
    body p.
packing
    abdominal p.
    Merocel self-expanding p.
    wound p.
paclitaxel
PACU
    postanesthesia care unit
PACWP
    pulmonary artery catheter wedge pressure
pad
    gauze p.
padding
    cast p.
Pagenstecher linen thread suture
Paget disease
pagetic bone
pagetoid bone
pain
    abdominal wall p.

aching abdominal wall p.
aching chest p.
anginal p.
back p.
bearing-down p.
bone p.
burning chest p.
chest p.
colicky p.
constant abdominal wall p.
continuous p.
crampy p.
crushing chest p.
diffuse abdominal p.
dull p.
duration of p.
epigastric chest p.
p. exacerbated by movement and
    coughing
flank p.
generalized mouth p.
infectious low back p.
initial location of p.
intractable p.
lancinating p.
ligamentous p.
localized p.
lower back p.
p. management
mechanical low back p.
mouth p.
muscle spasm p.
nature of onset of p.
nerve p.
onset of p.
parietal p.
pleuritic chest p.
presentation of p.
pressing chest p.
quality of p.
rebound p.
recrudescent p.
referred p.
sharp p.
smothering chest p.
somatic nerve transmitted p.
squeezing chest p.
substernal chest p.
testicular p.
p. threshold
time of onset of p.
visceral p.
viselike chest p.
well-localized p.
writhing with p.

P

pain-anxiety cycle
painful
    p. regional lymphadenopathy
    p. weightbearing
painless ulcer
paired skull bone
Pais fracture
palatability
palatal
    p. alveolar fracture
    p. muscle
    p. vein
palate
    p. fracture
    hard p.
    soft p.
palatine
    p. bone
    p. nerve
    perpendicular plate of p.
    p. suture
    p. vein
palatoethmoidal suture
palatoglossal muscle
palatomaxillary suture
palatopharyngeal muscle
Palfyn suture
palisade-type vein
palliate
palliative
    p. factor
    p. surgery
    p. therapy
    p. treatment
pallidum
    Treponema p.
pallor
palmar
    p. beak ligament
    p. carpal ligament
    p. carpometacarpal ligament
    p. cutaneous nerve
    p. cutaneous vein
    p. digital nerve
    p. digital vein
    p. dysesthesia
    p. intercarpal deltoid ligament
    p. metacarpal ligament
    p. metacarpal vein
    p. midcarpal ligament
    p. radiocarpal ligament
    p. radioulnar ligament
    p. ulnocarpal ligament
palmaris
    p. brevis tendon
    p. longus tendon
Palmer
    P. primary fracture

    P. trapezial ridge fracture
      classification
PalmSAT digital handheld pulse
  oximeter
palpable tenderness
palpate
palpation
    ligament p.
    muscle p.
    suture p.
    tendon p.
    vein p.
palpebral
    p. ligament
    p. muscle
    p. vein
palpitation
    paroxysmal p.
PALS
    pediatric advanced life support
palsy
    Bell p.
    nerve p.
    oculomotor nerve p.
    seventh nerve p.
palustris
    Caltha p.
pamidronate disodium
pampiniform vein
panacinar emphysema
Panacryl suture
Panalok absorbable suture
Pancoast suture
pancraniomaxillofacial fracture
pancreatic
    p. abscess
    p. arteriole
    p. pseudocyst
    p. trauma
    p. vein
pancreaticoduodenal vein
pancreaticosplenic ligament
pancreatitis
    acute hemorrhagic p.
    chronic p.
pancuronium
pancytopenia
panel
    basic metabolic p. (BMP)
    urine drug p.
panfacial fracture
panhidrosis (*var. of* panidrosis)
panhyperemia
panic
    p. attack
    p. disorder
paniculatis
    Zygadenus p.
panidrosis, panhidrosis

panlobular emphysema
pantoprazole
PAP
    positive airway pressure
papain
**Papavasiliou olecranon fracture
  classification**
papilla, pl. **papillae**
    anal p.
    nerve p.
papillary
    p. examination
    p. muscle
    p. muscle rupture (PMR)
papillomavirus
    human p. (HPV)
papillotomy
    endoscopic p.
papulosquamous eruption
paraben toxicity
paracentesis
    abdominal p.
paracolic gutter
paradichlorobenzene
paradoxical
    p. acidosis
    p. embolism
    p. motion
    p. movement
    p. movement of chest wall
paradoxic pulse
paradoxus
    pulsus p.
paraesophageal collateral vein
paralaryngeal muscle
paraldehyde toxicity
paralysis, pl. **paralyses**
    alternobaric facial p.
    arsenical p.
    Bell cruciate p.
    facial p.
    p. induction
    laryngeal nerve p.
    muscle periodic p.
    nerve p.
    therapeutic p.
    tick p.
    Todd p.
paralytic
    p. agent
    p. dementia
    p. ileus

paramedian
    p. approach
    p. incision
paramedic base
parameter
    setup p.
paranoia
paraphernalia
    drug p.
paraphimosis
paraplegia
paraproteinemia
parasite
    ova and p. (O&P)
parasitic colitis
paraspinal muscle
paraspinous muscle
parasternal short axis view
parasympathetic
    p. control
    p. nerve
parasympathomimetic
parasymphysis fracture
parathyroid
    p. disease
    p. gland
    p. hormone
    p. vein
paratonsillar vein
paratrooper's fracture
paraumbilical vein
paraventricular vein
paravertebral
    p. blockade
    p. muscle
paregoric
    p. overdose
    p. poisoning
parenchyma
parenchymal
    p. bleed
    p. injury
    p. injury of kidney
    p. laceration
parenteral
    p. administration
    p. alimentation
    p. nutrition
parent vein
paresis
    alcoholic p.
paresthesia

NOTES

P

paresthetica
  meralgia p.
Paré suture
pargyline
parietal
  p. emissary vein
  p. pain
  p. peritoneum
  p. pleura
  p. skull bone
  p. suture
parietomastoid suture
parietooccipital suture
parietosquamous suture
parietotemporal suture
Parinaud syndrome
Paris
  plaster of P.
parity
  increased p.
Parker-Kerr basting suture
Parkinson disease
Parkland
  P. fluid resuscitation formula
  P. formula for fluid replacement
Parnate
paronychia
parotid
  p. nerve
  p. vein
parotitis
  acute suppurative p.
paroxysm
paroxysmal
  p. atrial tachycardia (PAT)
  p. nocturnal dyspnea (PND)
  p. palpitation
  p. reentrant supraventricular
    tachycardia
  p. supraventricular tachycardia
    (PSVT)
parry fracture
pars interarticularis fracture
part
  aftercoming fetal p.
  amputated p.
1-part fracture
2-part fracture
3-part fracture
4-part fracture
partial
  p. airway obstruction
  p. anomalous pulmonary veins
  p. breech extraction
  p. liquid ventilation
  p. pressure of carbon dioxide
    (pCO$_2$)
  p. rebreathing face mask
  p. thromboplastin time (PTT)

partial-thickness
  p.-t. burn
  p.-t. corneal laceration
particle
  bone p.
  Dane p.
  food p.
party
  concerned p.
  rave p.
parvum
  Cryptosporidium parvum
PASG
  pneumatic antishock garment
passage of clot
Passavant muscle
passer
  suture p.
  tendon p.
passing suture
passive
  p. rewarming
  p. vasodilation
past
  p. injury
  p. medical history (PMH)
  p. surgical history (PSH)
paste
  bone p.
  calcium hydroxide p.
  dry socket p.
  nitroglycerin p.
  p. odor
Pasteurella multocida
Pastia sign
PAT
  paroxysmal atrial tachycardia
patch
  herald p.
  shagreen p.
  vein p.
patella, pl. patellae
  p. bone
  p. injury
patellar
  p. bursa
  p. injury
  p. ligament
  p. sleeve fracture
  p. tendon
patellofemoral
  p. crepitation
  p. ligament
patellomeniscal ligament
patellotibial ligament
patency
  assessment of p.
  vein graft p.

patent
- p. ductus arteriosus
- p. foramen ovale
- p. portal vein
- p. suture

pathetic nerve

pathogen
- airborne p.
- bloodborne p.

pathogenesis

pathogenic organism

pathognomonic symptom

pathologic
- p. cause
- p. diagnosis

pathological fracture

pathology
- bone p.
- intraabdominal p.
- muscle p.

pathophysiology

pathway
- accessory p.
- extrinsic coagulation p.

patient
- p. advocate
- p. agitation
- aphasic p.
- atraumatic p.
- p. care reporting (PCR)
- comatose p.
- competent elder p.
- p. confidentiality
- difficult to wean p.
- p. disorientation
- edentulous p.
- elderly p.
- p. environment
- p. evaluation (PE)
- financial dependence upon p.
- hypovolemic p.
- immunocompromised p.
- malnourished p.
- mentally unstable p.
- p. motivation
- p. noncompliance
- obtunded p.
- recalcitrant p.
- stable p.
- unstable p.

patient-centered interview

patient-controlled analgesia (PCA)

patient-provider relation

patient-triggered anesthesia

pattern
- Christmas tree p.
- cobweb p.
- cutaneous reaction p.
- fracture p.
- muscle firing p.
- muscle recruitment p.
- rugal p.

patterned bruise

patulous abdomen

pause
- end-inspiratory p.

Pauwels femoral neck fracture

PAV
- proportional assist ventilation

Pavulon

PAW
- pulmonary artery wedge

PAWP
- pulmonary artery wedge pressure

PBS
- protected brush specimen

PCA
- patient-controlled analgesia

PCC
- poison control center

PCIR
- pressure-controlled inverse ratio
  - PCIR ventilation

pCO$_2$
- partial pressure of carbon dioxide
  - esophageal luminal pCO$_2$

PCP
- phencyclidine

PCR
- patient care reporting
- prehospital care report

PCU
- progressive care unit

PDS
- polydioxanone suture
  - PDS II Endoloop suture
  - PDS Vicryl suture

PDT
- percutaneous dilational tracheostomy

PE
- patient evaluation
- physical examination
- pulmonary embolism

NOTES

P

PEA
    pulseless electrical activity
peak
    p. blood flow
    p. expiratory flow rate (PEFR)
    p. inspiratory pressure (PIP)
    p. plasma concentration
    p. pressure
peaked T wave
peanut odor
pear odor
Pearsall
    P. Chinese twisted suture
    P. silk suture
peau d'orange
pectinate
    p. ligament
    p. line
    p. muscle
pectineal ligament
pectineus nerve
pectoral
    p. muscle
    p. nerve
    p. vein
pectoralis
    p. major muscle
    p. minor muscle
    p. minor tendon
pectoris
    angina p.
pectorodorsalis muscle
pectorodorsal muscle
PED
    pediatric emergency department
pedal
    p. bone
    p. edema
pediatric
    p. abuse
    p. advanced life support (PALS)
    p. asthma
    p. casualty
    p. cerebrospinal injury
    p. consideration
    p. diarrhea
    p. emergency department (PED)
    p. epiglottitis
    p. exanthema
    p. feeding problem
    p. fever
    p. fracture
    p. intensive care unit (PICU)
    p. pneumonia
    p. poisoning
    p. rash
    p. resuscitation
    p. seizure
    p. trauma

    p. trauma center
    p. urinary tract infection
    p. vomiting
pedicle fracture
pediculosis pubis
pedis
    tinea p.
peduncular vein
pedunculated polyp
peel-away sheath cystostomy kit
PEEP
    positive end-expiratory pressure
PEFR
    peak expiratory flow rate
PEG
    percutaneous endoscopic gastrostomy
    PEG tube
peg
    bone p.
pegging
    bone p.
pellucidum
    posterior vein of septum p.
peltatum
    Podophyllum p.
pelvic
    p. autonomic nerve
    p. avulsion fracture
    p. bone
    p. cellulitis
    p. floor muscle
    p. floor nerve
    p. fracture
    p. fullness
    p. inflammatory disease (PID)
    p. insufficiency fracture
    p. laparoscopy
    p. ligament
    p. region
    p. rest
    p. rim fracture
    p. ring fracture
    p. splanchnic nerve
    p. straddle fracture
    p. trauma
    p. ultrasound
pelvis
    p. fracture
    p. muscle
    plain film of p.
    p. radiograph
pemphigus
pendulous breast
penetrating
    p. abdominal trauma
    p. anterior neck trauma
    p. cardiac trauma
    p. chest trauma
    p. extremity trauma

p. fracture
p. head trauma
p. injury
p. injury of brain
p. neck wound
penetration syndrome
penicillin G
penile
p. laceration
p. shaft fracture
p. vein
p. venous cannulation
penis
dorsal nerve of p.
p. fracture
pennate muscle
penniform muscle
pentamidine isethionate
Pentastarch
pentazocine
pentoxifylline
Penumbra effect
PEP
postexposure prophylaxis
peptic
p. ulcer
p. ulcer disease
p. ulcer perforation
peptide
atrial natriuretic p. (ANP)
natriuretic p.
per
p. nasogastric tube (PNGT)
p. rectum
perception
blunted p.
percussion
p. and auscultation (P & A)
auscultatory p.
percutaneous
p. catheter drainage
p. coronary angioplasty
p. dilational tracheostomy (PDT)
p. endoscopic gastrostomy (PEG)
p. femoral vein
p. gastrostomy
p. internal jugular vein
catheterization
p. jejunostomy
p. nephrostomy
p. sheath introducer

p. transluminal coronary angioplasty
(PTCA)
p. transtracheal insufflation
p. transtracheal ventilation (PTV)
perflubron
perfluorocarbon
perfluorochemical
perforated
p. colon
p. duodenum
p. stomach
p. ulcer
p. viscus
perforating
p. appendicitis
p. cutaneous nerve
p. fracture
p. vein
p. wound
perforation
bowel p.
enteral p.
esophageal p.
peptic ulcer p.
p. of pulmonary artery
tympanic membrane p.
perforative appendicitis
performance
impaired mental p.
perfringens
Clostridium p.
perfusion
organ p.
p. pressure
systemic p.
perianal
p. abscess
p. condyloma acuminata
p. suture
periapical abscess
periareolar pursestring suture
periarticular fracture
pericallosal vein
pericardiacophrenic vein
pericardiac vein
pericardial
p. effusion
p. injury
p. rub
p. tamponade
p. vein
p. window

NOTES

P

229

pericardiocentesis
pericardiophrenic nerve
pericardiosternal ligament
pericarditis
    p. bacterial infection
    constrictive p.
    serofibrinous p.
    suppurative p.
pericardium
pericardotomy
pericholecystic fluid
perichondral bone
pericoronitis
pericostal suture
peridental ligament
periesophageal
    p. collateral vein
    p. complication
periimplant ligament
perilunate dislocation
perilymph fistula
perimortem cesarean section
perinatal
    p. clavicle fracture
    p. humerus fracture
    p. mortality
perineal
    p. laceration
    p. muscle
    p. nerve
    p. pouch
perinephric abscess
perineum
perineurial suture
period
    last menstrual p. (LMP)
    quiescent p.
    refractory p.
    relative refractory p.
periodontal
    p. abscess
    p. disease
    p. ligament
perioral muscle
periorbital
    p. cellulitis
    p. infection
    p. soft tissue injury
periosteal bone
periotic bone
peripancreatic vein
peripapillary retinal nerve
peripartum cardiomyopathy
peripheral
    p. acinar vein
    p. anticholinergic effect
    p. arterial aneurysm
    p. fracture
    p. laceration

    p. light flash
    p. motor nerve
    p. nerve block
    p. nervous system (PNS)
    p. neuromuscular disease
    p. neuropathy
    p. oculomotor nerve
    p. pulse
    p. vascular disease
    p. vascular injury
    p. vasodilator
    p. vertigo
peripherally
    p. inserted central catheter (PICC)
    p. inserted central catheter line
    p. inserted central venous catheter
periprosthetic fracture
periradicular nerve
perirectal
    p. abscess
    p. involvement
peristalsis
perithyroid vein
peritoneal
    p. abscess
    p. dialysis
    p. irritant
    p. irritation
    p. lavage
    p. ligament
    p. sign
    p. vein
peritoneovenous shunt
peritoneum
    parietal p.
peritonitis
    diffuse p.
    gas p.
    localized p.
    spontaneous bacterial p. (SBP)
peritonsillar
    p. abscess
    p. nerve
peritrochanteric fracture
peritumoral vein
periurethral
    p. ligament
    p. striated muscle
    p. vein
perivascular nerve
PER-IV fracture
PERL
    pupils equal and react to light
PERLA
    pupils equal and react to light and
    accommodation
Perlon suture
Perma-Hand braided silk suture

permanent
    p. cardiac pacing
    p. mattress suture
    p. and total disability
PermaSharp PGA suture
permeability
    endothelia p.
permissive hypercapnia
pernicious anemia
peroneal
    p. bone
    p. communicating nerve
    p. muscle
    p. tendon injury
    p. vein
peroneus
    p. brevis muscle
    p. longus muscle
    p. quartus muscle
    p. tertius muscle
peroxide
    carbamide p.
    hydrogen p.
perpendicular
    p. plate of ethmoid
    p. plate of palatine
perphenazine
PERRLA
    pupils equal, round, and reactive to light
    and accommodation
persistent
    p. fetal circulation (PFC)
    p. frontal suture
    p. metopic suture
    p. right umbilical vein
personal
    p. protective equipment (PPE)
    p. stressor
personality
    addictive p.
    p. disorder
    garrulous p.
1-person stretcher
2-person stretcher
pertinent negative
pertrochanteric fracture
pertussis
    diphtheria, tetanus, p. (DTP)
pesticide
    p. ingestion
    p. poisoning
    p. toxicity

petechial rash
petit
    P. ligament
    p. mal seizure
petrobasilar suture
petroclinoid ligament
petroclival suture
petrosal
    p. bone
    p. nerve
    p. vein
petrosphenobasilar suture
petrosphenoidal ligament
petrosphenoid ligament
petrosphenooccipital suture
petrosquamosal suture
petrosquamous suture
petrotympanic suture
petrous
    p. pyramid fracture
    p. temporal bone
peyote button
PFC
    persistent fetal circulation
PFT
    pulmonary function test
    pulmonary function testing
phagocytophilia
    Ehrlichia p.
phalangeal
    p. bone
    p. diaphysial fracture
    p. glenoidal ligament
    p. injury
phalanx, pl. **phalanges**
phalloides
    Amanita p.
pH alteration
phantom bone
pharmaceutic aid
pharmaceutical aid
pharmacokinetic
pharmacologist
    critical care p.
pharyngeal
    p. bursa
    p. constrictor muscle
    p. erythema
    p. laceration
    p. tracheal lumen airway (PTLA)
    p. vein
pharynges (*pl. of* pharynx)

NOTES

P

pharyngitis
pharyngopalatine muscle
pharynx, pl. pharynges
phase
    alpha p.
    hypermetabolic p.
    postictal p.
phasic muscle
phencyclidine (PCP)
    p. overdose
    p. poisoning
phenelzine
phenobarbital toxicity
phenolphthalein
phenol red
phenomenon, pl. phenomena
    Ashman p.
    Gregg p.
    no-reflow p.
    Raynaud p.
    R-on-T p.
    SCIWORA p.
    Somogyi p.
phenothiazine poisoning
phenoxybenzamine
phenylephrine
phenytoin poisoning
pheochromocytoma
Philadelphia collar
Phillips muscle
Philly
    P. Bloc-Head cervical collar
    P. one-piece cervical collar
phimosis
phlebitis
    septic p.
phlebotomy
phlegmonous abscess
phobia
    fever p.
    generalized anxiety disorder and p.
phosgene
    p. oxime
    p. oxime urticant
phosphatase
    alkaline p.
    bone alkaline p.
phosphate
    aluminum p.
    codeine p.
    dexamethasone sodium p.
phosphodiesterase inhibitor
phosphorus
    white p.
phosphorylase
    muscle p.
phosphorylation
    oxidative p.
photophobia

photoplethysmography
photosensitivity
phototoxicity
phrenic
    p. nerve
    p. vein
phrenicoabdominal nerve
phrenicocolic ligament
phrenicoesophageal ligament
phrenicolienal ligament
phrenicosplenic ligament
phrenoesophageal ligament
phrenogastric ligament
phrenosplenic ligament
physeal
    p. fracture
    p. plate fracture
physical
    p. abuse
    p. age
    p. elasticity of muscle
    p. environment
    p. exam finding
    p. examination (PE)
    p. restraint
    p. sign
    p. therapy (PT)
physician
    American College of
        Emergency P.'s (ACEP)
    Association of Emergency P.'s
    attending p.
physician-assisted suicide
physiologic
    p. adaptation
    p. anemia
    p. determinant
    p. determinants of ventilator
        dependence
    p. elasticity of muscle
physiological age
physiology
    bedrest p.
physis fracture
Phytolacca
    P. americana
    P. americana ingestion
pial vein
pia mater
PICC
    peripherally inserted central catheter
    PICC line
pickup spatula suture
PICU
    pediatric intensive care unit
    pulmonary intensive care unit
PID
    pelvic inflammatory disease

PIE
    pulmonary interstitial emphysema
Piedmont fracture
Pieris
        P. floribunda
        P. japonica
Pierre Robin syndrome
pigment
        melanotic p.
PIH
    pregnancy-induced hypertension
pill
        heart p.
        morning-after p.
        water p.
pillar fracture
pillow fracture
2-pillow orthopnea
3-pillow orthopnea
pilomotor nerve
pilon
        p. ankle fracture
        p. fracture
pilonidal
        p. abscess
        p. cyst
        p. sinus
pinched nerve
pinch-off syndrome
pine
        p. oil ingestion
        p. oil odor
ping-pong fracture
pinhole
        bone p.
pink
        p. puffer
        p. sputum
        p. twisted cotton suture
pinkeye conjunctivitis
pinna, pl. **pinnae**
pinpoint pupil
pin suture
pinworm
PIOPED
    Prospective Investigation of Pulmonary
        Embolism Diagnosis
        PIOPED study
PIP
    peak inspiratory pressure
piperacillin
pipe stem cirrhosis

Pipkin femoral fracture classification
Pipracil
pirbuterol
piriform
        p. muscle
        p. nerve
piriformis muscle
pisiform
        p. bone
        p. bursa
        p. fracture
        p. metacarpal ligament
pisohamate
        p. bone
        p. ligament
pisometacarpal ligament
pisounciform ligament
pisouncinate ligament
pituitary apoplexy
pit viper envenomation
pityriasis
        p. alba
        p. rosea
PJC
    premature junctional contraction
place
        precise p.
placebo-controlled study
placebo effect
placement
        bone graft p.
        correct tube p.
        verification of correct tube p.
placenta
        p. accreta
        p. accreta vera
        premature separation of p.
        p. previa
        retained p.
placentae
        abruptio p.
Placidyl
plafond fracture
plague
        bubonic p.
plain
        p. catgut suture
        p. collagen suture
        p. film
        p. film of pelvis
        p. gut suture
        p. sinus radiograph

NOTES

P

233

plan
    aftercare p.
    subjective, objective, assessment, p. (SOAP)
plane
    frontal p.
    horizontal p.
    midsagittal p.
    sagittal p.
    transpyloric p.
    transverse p.
planning
    disaster p.
plantar
    p. bursa
    p. calcaneocuboid ligament
    p. calcaneonavicular ligament
    p. cuboideonavicular ligament
    p. cuneocuboid ligament
    p. cuneonavicular ligament
    p. digital nerve
    p. digital vein
    p. fasciitis
    p. intercuneiform ligament
    p. interossei interosseous muscle
    p. interosseous muscle
    p. metatarsal ligament
    p. metatarsal vein
    p. quadrate muscle
    p. spring ligament
    p. tarsal ligament
    p. tarsometatarsal ligament
    p. tendon sheath of fibularis longus muscle
    p. tendon sheath of peroneus longus muscle
    p. wart
plantaris
    p. muscle
    p. tendon rupture
plant poisoning
planus
    lichen p.
plaque
    atherosclerotic p.
    p. fracture
    rupture of atherosclerotic p.
plasma
    p. bicarbonate concentration
    blood p.
    p. exchange
    p. expander
    p. filtration
    fresh frozen p. (FFP)
    p. protein fraction
plasmapheresis
plasminogen
    p. activator
    single-chain urokinase-type p.

    tissue p.
    urinary p.
Plasmodium falciparum
plaster
    p. of Paris
    p. of Paris splint
plastic
    p. bowing fracture
    p. deformation fracture
    p. suture
plasty
    tendon p.
plate
    bone p.
    cribriform p.
    epiphysial p.
    p. fracture
    muscle p.
    nail p.
    tendon p.
plateau
    end-inspiratory p.
    p. fracture
    p. tibia fracture
platelet
    p. count
    P. Glycoprotein IIb/IIIa in Unstable Angina: Receptor Suppression Using Integrilin Therapy (PURSUIT)
    hemolysis, elevated liver enzymes, low p.'s (HELLP)
    p. inhibition
    p. inhibitor
    p. plug retraction
    p. thrombosis
    p. transfusion
platysma muscle
play
    muscle p.
pleasure
    muscle p.
pledgeted
    p. Ethibond suture
    p. mattress suture
plethora
    p. of complaints
    p. of problems
plethysmography
    impedance p. (IPG)
pleura, pl. **pleurae**
    parietal p.
    visceral p.
pleural
    p. effusion
    p. fluid analysis
    p. pressure (Ppl)
    p. rub

pleurisy
    mediastinal p.
pleuritic chest pain
pleurodynia
pleuroesophageal muscle
pleuroesophageus muscle
pleuropericardial rub
plexus, pl. **plexus, plexuses**
    Kiesselbach p.
    nerve p.
plica, pl. **plicae**
    tendon p.
plicating suture
plication
    suture p.
    p. suture
plombage
    bone p.
plug
    bone femoral p.
plumbism
plus
    Suture Strip P.
PMH
    past medical history
PMI
    point of maximal impulse
    point of maximal intensity
PMR
    papillary muscle rupture
PMS
    pulse, motor function, sensation
Pmus
    pressure generated by muscle contraction
PND
    paroxysmal nocturnal dyspnea
pneumatic
    p. antishock garment (PASG)
    p. bone
    p. splint
Pneumocystis
    P. aeruginosa
    P. carinii
    P. carinii pneumonia
pneumogastric nerve
pneumomediastinum
pneumonia
    acute eosinophilic p. (AEP)
    acute interstitial p. (AIP)
    adult p.
    aspiration p.
    bacterial p.

    bronchiolitis obliterans organizing p.
    (BOOP)
    Candida p.
    community-acquired p. (CAP)
    desquamatic interstitial p. (DIP)
    giant cell interstitial p. (GIP)
    hospital-acquired p.
    immunocompromised p.
    influenza-related p.
    interstitial p. (IP)
    lymphocytic interstitial p. (LIP)
    migratory p.
    Mycoplasma p.
    nonspecific interstitial p. (NIP)
    nosocomial p.
    pediatric p.
    Pneumocystis carinii p.
    Pseudomonas p.
    usual interstitial p. (UIP)
    ventilator-associated p.
    viral p.
pneumoniae
    Chlamydia p.
    Klebsiella p.
    Mycoplasma p.
pneumonitis
    radiation p.
    traumatic p.
pneumoperitoneum
pneumophila
    Legionella p.
pneumothorax
    catamenial p.
    iatrogenic p.
    open p.
    POPS-related p.
    pressure p.
    simple p.
    spontaneous p.
    tension p.
    traumatic p.
PneuSplint
    P. splint
    STI Medical Products P.
PNGT
    per nasogastric tube
PNS
    peripheral nervous system
POC
    products of conception
pocket mask
Podophyllum peltatum

NOTES

P

poikilothermia
point
    congruent p.
    end p.
    p. of maximal impulse (PMI)
    p. of maximal intensity (PMI)
    pressure p.
3-point corner stitch
2-point discrimination
pointes
    torsade de p.
pointing
    bone p.
Poirier ligament
POISINDEX database
poison
    p. antidote
    p. control center (PCC)
    corrosive p.
    household industrial p.
    p. ivy
    narcotic p.
    p. oak
    p. sumac
    p. sumac dermatitis
poisoning
    accidental p.
    acetaminophen p.
    acetanilid p.
    acetylsalicylic acid p.
    alcohol p.
    aliphatic hydrocarbon p.
    alkaloid p.
    amnestic shellfish p.
    amphetamine p.
    anchovy p.
    anticholinergic p.
    anticoagulant rodenticide p.
    p. antidote
    antidysrhythmic drug p.
    antipsychotic p.
    arsenic p.
    aspirin p.
    bacterial food p.
    barbiturate p.
    benzene p.
    benzodiazepine p.
    beta-blocker p.
    boric acid p.
    box jellyfish p.
    bretylium p.
    bromethalin p.
    calcium channel blocker p.
    camphor p.
    carbamate p.
    carbamazepine p.
    carbon monoxide p.
    catfish p.
    chemical weapon p.

chlorohydrate p.
chlorophenoxy herbicide p.
chronic salicylate p.
ciguatera p.
clupeotoxin fish p.
cocaine p.
coelenterate p.
cone shell p.
Conium p.
coprine mushroom p.
coral p.
crotalaria p.
cyanide p.
digoxin p.
dipyridyl herbicide p.
diquat p.
ethylene glycol p.
food p.
fungicide p.
gastric decontamination p.
GHB-hydroxybutyrate p.
hallucinogen p.
heavy metal p.
hemlock p.
hydrocarbon p.
hydrogen fluoride p.
hydrogen sulfide p.
hydrogen sulfide gas p.
Hydrozoa p.
hypoglycemic agent p.
ibotenic acid mushroom p.
Indole p.
iron p.
isoniazid p.
isopropanol p.
jimson weed p.
lead p.
Lepidoptera p.
lindane p.
lithium p.
mackerel p.
man-of-war p.
meprobamate p.
mercury p.
methanol p.
mollusk p.
monoamine oxidase inhibitor p.
mushroom p.
neuroleptic p.
neurotoxic shellfish p.
nonsteroidal antiinflammatory
  drug p.
opiate p.
organophosphate p.
paregoric p.
pediatric p.
pesticide p.
phencyclidine p.
phenothiazine p.

phenytoin p.
plant p.
polychlorinated biphenyl p.
puffer fish p.
radon p.
rhubarb p.
salicylate p.
scombroid fish p.
scombroid food p.
Scyphozoa p.
sea anemone p.
sea cucumber p.
soap p.
sympathomimetic p.
tetrodotoxin fish p.
thallium p.
theophylline p.
toluene p.
tricyclic antidepressant p.
turpentine p.
poisonous plant intoxication
pokeweed ingestion
Poland epiphysial fracture classification
polarizing solution
pole
apical p.
cephalic p.
police
local p.
poliglecaprone suture
polioencephalitis
bulbar p.
pollicis longus muscle
pollutant
air p.
polyamide suture
polybutester suture
polychlorinated biphenyl poisoning
polycystic kidney disease
polycythemia
Polydek suture
polydioxanone suture (PDS)
polydipsia
polyene antibiotic
polyester fiber suture
polyethylene
p. glycol electrolyte lavage solution
p. suture
polyfascicular nerve
polyfilament suture
polyfume fever
polyglactic acid suture

polyglactin 910 suture
polyglecaprone 25 suture
polyglycolate suture
polyglycolic acid suture
polyglycol suture
polyglyconate suture
polymorphic ventricular tachycardia (PVT)
polymorphism
debrisoquine p.
polymyalgia rheumatica
polymyositis
polyneuritis
anemic p.
polyneuropathy
critical illness p.
demyelinating p.
polyp
pedunculated p.
sessile p.
polypharmacy abuse
polypropylene button suture
Polysorb suture
Polysporin Ophthalmic
polysubstance abuse
polytetrafluoroethylene
expanded p. (EPTFE)
polyuria
pond fracture
pontine
p. coma
p. hemorrhage
p. vein
pontomesencephalic vein
poor
p. judgment
p. oral hygiene
poorly explained death of infant
popliteal
p. aneurysm
p. communicating nerve
p. ligament
p. muscle
p. vein
popliteus
p. bursa
p. muscle
popoff suture
POPS
pulmonary overpressurization syndrome
pop sound
POPS-related pneumothorax

NOTES

P

237

porcelain fracture
porotic bone
porous bone
porphyria
    erythrohepatic p.
port
    catheter p.
    p. infection
    self-sealing injection p.
    side p.
portable
    p. cardiopulmonary bypass
    p. radio adaptor
    p. stretcher
    p. suction device
port-access surgery
portal
    p. hypertension
    p. vein
Posada fracture
position
    anatomical p.
    anteroposterior p.
    anterosuperior p.
    bayonet p.
    coma p.
    Fowler p.
    head-down p.
    knee-to-chest p.
    lateral recumbent p.
    left lateral recumbent p.
    morning sniff p.
    postanoxic p.
    prone p.
    recovery p.
    recumbent p.
    semi-Fowler p.
    semirecumbent p.
    shock p.
    subacromial p.
    subcoracoid p.
    supine p.
    Trendelenburg p.
    tripod p.
positive
    p. airway pressure (PAP)
    p. dromotropy
    p. end-expiratory pressure (PEEP)
    p. end-expiratory pressure effect
    p. test
positive-pressure
    p.-p. breathing (PPB)
    p.-p. ventilation
post
    status p.
postabortion sepsis
postanesthesia care unit (PACU)
postanoxic position
postauricular nerve

postaxial muscle
postcardinal vein
postcardioversion prophylaxis
postcentral vein
postcoital contraception
postconcussional headache
postconcussion syndrome
postconcussive syndrome
postengraftment infection
posterior
    p. ampullar nerve
    p. ampullary nerve
    p. antebrachial cutaneous nerve
    p. anterior jugular vein
    p. anular ligament
    p. arch fracture
    p. auricular muscle
    p. auricular nerve
    p. auricular vein
    p. brachial cutaneous nerve
    p. callosal vein
    p. cardinal vein
    p. cervical intertransverse muscle
    p. ciliary vein
    p. circumflex humeral vein
    p. column fracture
    p. communicating nerve
    p. conjunctival vein
    p. cord syndrome
    p. costotransverse ligament
    p. cricoarytenoid ligament
    p. cricoarytenoid muscle
    p. cruciate ligament
    p. cutaneous femoral nerve
    p. deltoid muscle
    p. digastric muscle
    p. displacement
    p. element fracture
    p. epistaxis
    p. ethmoidal nerve
    p. facial vein
    p. false ligament
    p. femoral cutaneous nerve
    p. fixation suture
    p. fontanelle
    p. fossa hemorrhage
    p. fracture
    p. incudal ligament
    p. inferior nasal nerve
    p. inferior tibiofibular ligament
    p. intercostal vein
    p. interosseous vein
    p. interventricular vein
    p. labial nerve
    p. labial vein
    p. leaf of broad ligament
    p. lobe of cerebellum
    p. longitudinal ligament
    p. marginal vein

p. meniscofemoral ligament
p. oblique ligament
p. occipitoaxial ligament
p. palatine nerve
p. palatine suture
p. papillary muscle
p. parotid vein
p. pericallosal vein
p. pharyngeal laceration
p. process fracture
p. rib fracture
p. ring fracture
p. sacroiliac ligament
p. sacrosciatic ligament
p. sag sign
p. scalene muscle
p. scapular nerve
p. scrotal nerve
p. scrotal vein
p. serratus muscle
p. splint
p. sternoclavicular ligament
p. superior alveolar nerve
p. superior nasal nerve
p. supraclavicular nerve
p. suspensory ligament
p. talar process fracture
p. talocalcaneal ligament
p. talofibular ligament
p. talotibial ligament
p. temporal diploic vein
p. terminal vein
p. thoracic nerve
p. tibial muscle
p. tibial nerve
p. tibial pulse
p. tibial tendon
p. tibial vein
p. tibiotalar part of deltoid ligament
p. uterosacral ligament
p. vein of septum pellucidum
p. wall fracture
posterolateral thoracotomy
posterosuperior alveolar nerve
postexposure prophylaxis (PEP)
postganglionic
p. cholinergic nerve
p. short ciliary nerve
p. sympathetic nerve

postictal
p. phase
p. state
postinflation hold
postintubation barotrauma
postirradiation fracture
postmortem fracture
postobstructive diuresis
postoperative
p. case
p. flexor tendon
p. fracture
p. ileal fistula
p. jejunal fistula
p. mediastinitis
p. synergistic abdominal gangrene
postpartum
p. adnexal infection
p. hemorrhage
postpericardiotomy syndrome
postphlebitic syndrome
postplaced suture
postreduction
p. roentgenogram
p. view
postrenal azotemia
postresuscitation diuresis
postshunt
p. encephalopathy
p. hepatorenal syndrome
postsphenoid bone
posttetanic count
posttransfusion purpura
posttransplant lymphoproliferative disease (PTLD)
posttraumatic
p. amnesia (PTA)
p. shock
p. stress disorder (PTSD)
posttussive inspiratory rhonchi
postulnar bone
postural
p. drainage
p. hypotension
p. muscle
posture
decerebrate p.
decorticate p.
potassium (K)
avoidance of p.
p. bicarbonate
p. chloride (KOH)

NOTES

P

potassium *(continued)*
    p. iodide (KI)
    p. repletion
potassium-associated acute transfusion event
potassium-sparing diuretic
potential
    brainstem auditory evoked p.
    muscle action p.
    muscle fiber action p.
    myocardial cell action p.
    nerve action p.
    nerve fiber action p.
    nerve trunk action p.
    pseudomyotonic p.
    somatosensory evoked p. (SSEP)
Pott ankle fracture
Potts-Cournand needle
pouch
    p. of Douglas
    Morison p.
    nerve root axillary p.
    perineal p.
pounds per square inch (psi)
Poupart ligament
Pouteau fracture
povidone iodine
powder
    absorption p.
    bone p.
    p. burn
    TraumaDEX p.
power
    atmospheric cooling p.
    p. grip
    p. grip technique
    p. lift technique
    p. squat technique
powerful evidence
Pozzi muscle
PPB
    positive-pressure breathing
PPE
    personal protective equipment
Ppl
    pleural pressure
practice
    cultural healing p.
    family p. (FP)
pralidoxime chloride
prazepam
PRBC
    packed red blood cell
pre-Achilles bursa
preauricular nerve
preaxial muscle
precatorius
    Abrus p.

precaution
    universal p.
Precedex injection
precentral cerebellar vein
prechiasmal optic nerve
precise place
precordial
    p. lead
    p. lift
    p. thump
    p. wound
precursor symptom
predelivery
predentinal nerve
predisposing factor
preeclampsia
    p. complication
    superimposed p.
preexcitation syndrome
prefrontal
    p. bone
    p. vein
pregnancy
    bigeminal p.
    ectopic p.
    molar p.
    ruptured ectopic p.
    spontaneous termination of p.
    suspected ectopic p.
    p. test
    trauma in p.
    tubal p.
    uncomplicated p.
    vaginal bleeding in p.
pregnancy-induced hypertension (PIH)
prehospital
    p. care
    p. care report (PCR)
    p. provider
preinterparietal bone
prelaminar optic nerve
preload
    left ventricular p.
    ventricular p.
premalleolar bursa
premature
    p. atrial contraction (PAC)
    p. closure
    p. closure of coronal suture
    p. junctional contraction (PJC)
    p. rupture of membranes
    p. senility
    p. separation of placenta
    p. ventricular contraction (PVC)
prematurely closed suture
premaxillary
    p. bone
    p. suture
premedication

PremiCron nonabsorbable suture
Premilene suture
premonitory symptom
preoxygenation
preparation
    erythromycin ophthalmic p.
preparedness
    radiation disaster p.
prepatellar bursa
preplaced suture
preputial ring
prepyloric vein
prerenal
    p. azotemia
    p. uremia
presacral nerve
preschooler
presence
    p. of flail chest
    p. of gag reflex
presentation
    breech p.
    delayed p.
    limb p.
    p. of pain
    spectrum of p.
present illness
presenting symptom
preseptal orbital cellulitis
preservation
    pulsatile perfusion p.
presphenoethmoid suture
presphenoid bone
pressing chest pain
pressoreceptor nerve
pressor nerve
pressure
    abdominal p.
    ambient oxygen p.
    arterial blood p. (ABP)
    atrial p.
    auto positive end-expiratory p.
    backward, upward, and
      rightward p. (BURP)
    p. bandage
    bilevel positive airway p. (BiPAP)
    biphasic airway p.
    blood p. (BP)
    carotid sinus p. (CSP)
    central venous p. (CVP)
    cerebral perfusion p. (CPP)
    compartmental perfusion p.

continuous positive airway p.
  (CPAP)
p. control
cricoid p.
diastolic p. (DP)
diastolic blood p. (DBP)
direct p.
end-diastolic p.
end-expiratory p.
end-systolic p.
p. fracture
p. generated by muscle contraction
  (Pmus)
p. gradient
p. gun injury
intraabdominal p. (IAP)
intracerebral p.
intracranial p. (ICP)
intrapleural p.
jugular venous p. (JVP)
left ventricular end-diastolic p.
  (LVEDP)
mean airway p. (MAP)
mean alveolar p. (MalvP)
mean arterial p. (MAP)
mean systemic p. (MSP)
no obtainable blood p.
oncotic p.
optimal positive end-expiratory p.
orthostatic blood p.
peak p.
peak inspiratory p. (PIP)
perfusion p.
pleural p. (Ppl)
p. pneumothorax
p. point
positive airway p. (PAP)
positive end-expiratory p. (PEEP)
proportional blood p.
pulmonary artery catheter wedge p.
  (PACWP)
pulmonary artery occlusion p.
pulmonary artery wedge p.
  (PAWP)
pulse p.
right atrial p. (RAP)
right ventricular p. (RV)
p. splint
p. support (PS)
p. support ventilation (PSV)
p. support ventilation titration
systolic blood p. (SBP)

NOTES

P

pressure *(continued)*
    ventricular end-diastolic p.
    p. volume (PV)
pressure-controlled inverse ratio (PCIR)
pressure-volume
    p.-v. curve
    p.-v. relationship
pressure-washing technique
presyncope
preterm labor
pretransplant to engraftment infection
prevention
    Bezafibrate Infarction P. (BIP)
    Centers for Disease Control and P.
     (CDC)
    constipation p.
Prevent Recurrence of Osteoporotic Fractures (PROOF)
previa
    placenta p.
previous
    p. abdominal surgery
    p. abruption
priapism
    arterial p.
    high-flow p.
    low-flow p.
    type 1, 2 p.
    venoocclusive p.
primary
    p. abscess
    p. assessment
    p. cardiac disease
    p. care provider
    p. closure
    p. erythromelalgia
    p. glial disorder
    p. graft dysfunction
    p. hyperthyroidism
    p. intention
    p. menorrhagia
    p. neuronal disorder
    p. pain medication
    p. survey
    p. suture
4 primary medical specialties
Primaxin
primidone
primitive
    p. bone
    p. maxillary vein
principle
    Fick p.
Pringle maneuver
Prinzmetal angina
prior
    p. to admission
    p. to arrival

privilege
    bathroom p. (BRP)
proarrhythmic effect
probability
    bone cyst fracture p.
problem
    acid-pepsin p.
    concomitant medical p.
    general medical p.
    pediatric feeding p.
    plethora of p.'s
    wound p.
procainamide
procedure
    blind p.
    bone block p.
    infection control p.
    standard operation p. (SOP)
    tendon checkrein p.
procerus muscle
process
    bone destructive p.
    disciform p.
    rehabilitation p.
    septic p.
    sphenoid p.
    xiphoid p.
prochlorperazine
proctitis
procyclidine
prodromal
    p. stage
    p. symptom
    p. syndrome
prodrome
product
    p.'s of conception (POC)
    fibrin degradation p. (FDP)
    fibrinogen degradation p.
    leukocyte-depleted blood p.
production
    bone p.
profile
    biophysical p. (BPP)
    coagulation p.
    screening hepatic p.
profound
    p. anemia
    p. debility
    p. hematuria
    p. hypothermia
    p. lactic acidosis
    p. shock
profundus
    p. artery fracture
    p. muscle
progenitor
    bone marrow-derived myogenic p.

prognosis
> expected course and p.

Prograf

program
> CISM p.
> National Asthma Education and Prevention P. (NAEPP)

progress
> failure to p.

progression
> rostrocaudal p.

progressive
> p. care unit (PCU)
> p. multifocal leukoencephalopathy

proinflammatory cytokine

project
> European Myocardial Infarction P. (EMIP)

prolactin deficiency

prolapse
> mitral valve p.
> rectal p.
> uterine p.

prolapsed umbilical cord

Prolene polypropylene suture

proliferation
> intimal p.

proliferative
> p. bronchiolitis
> p. fasciitis

prolongation
> Q-T p.

prolonged
> p. Q-T syndrome
> p. warm ischemia

prominent pulmonary vein

pronation-abduction fracture

pronation-eversion/external rotation fracture

pronation-eversion fracture

pronator
> p. quadratus muscle
> p. teres muscle

prone
> p. position
> p. ventilation

Pronova suture

PROOF
> Prevent Recurrence of Osteoporotic Fractures

propafenone

prophylactic
> antibiotic p.
> p. antibiotic
> p. platelet transfusion
> p. treatment

prophylaxis
> antitetanus p.
> endocarditis p.
> postcardioversion p.
> postexposure p. (PEP)
> rabies p.
> stress ulcer p.
> tetanus p.

propionate
> fluticasone p.

propofol

proportional
> p. assist ventilation (PAV)
> p. blood pressure

propranolol

proprioception nerve

proprioceptor
> muscle p.

Prospective Investigation of Pulmonary Embolism Diagnosis (PIOPED)

prosplint
> Med Spec p.

prostaglandin
> p. agonist
> p. E

prostate
> high-riding p.

prostatitis

prosthesis
> bone p.
> tendon p.

prosthetic
> p. fracture
> p. heart valve
> p. valve endocarditis (PVE)

protease inhibitor

protected
> p. brush specimen (PBS)
> p. specimen brush

protection
> airway p.
> Caldwell p.
> cervical spine p.

protein
> bone morphogenetic p.
> bone morphogenic p.

NOTES

P

protein *(continued)*
  P. C Worldwide Evaluation in Severe Sepsis (PROWESS)
  p. homeostasis
  muscle contractile p.
protein-losing enteropathy
protein-sparing modified fast (PSMF)
proteinuria
  hematuria and p.
proteolysis
  muscle p.
Proteus mirabilis
protocol
  accelerated diagnostic p. (ADP)
  ACLS p.
  Balke-Ware p.
  Ellestad p.
  extubation p.
  trauma p.
  trauma transport p. (TTP)
Protonix I.V.
Protopam Injection
protozoa
  flagellate p.
protracted treatment
protuberant abdomen
proud flesh
Proventil inhaler
provider
  prehospital p.
  primary care p.
provocation test
provocative
  p. diagnosis
  p. factor
  p. test
prowazekii
  Rickettsia p.
PROWESS
  Protein C Worldwide Evaluation in Severe Sepsis
  PROWESS trial
proximal
  p. end tibia fracture
  p. femoral fracture
  p. humeral fracture
  p. humeral stress fracture
  p. shaft fracture
  p. tibial metaphysial fracture
  p. vein
Proxi-Strip suture
proxy
  Münchausen syndrome by p. (MSBP)
pruritus
  p. ani
  bath p.

PS
  pressure support
    PS irritant
pseudoaneurysm
pseudocyst
  pancreatic p.
pseudoephedrine
pseudogout
pseudohyperkalemia
pseudohypertrophy
  muscle p.
pseudo-Jefferson fracture
pseudo-Jones fracture
pseudomembrane
  débridement of p.
  gingival p.
  gray-white gingival p.
Pseudomonas
  P. aeruginosa
  P. fluorescens
  P. infection
  P. pneumonia
pseudomyotonic potential
pseudoobstruction
  p. of colon
  colonic p.
  intestinal p.
pseudotumor cerebri
PSH
  past surgical history
psi
  pounds per square inch
psilocybin
PSMF
  protein-sparing modified fast
psoas
  p. major muscle
  p. minor muscle
  p. sign
psoralen plus ultraviolet A (PUVA)
psoriasis
psoriatic arthritis
PSV
  pressure support ventilation
PSVT
  paroxysmal supraventricular tachycardia
psychiatric
  p. commitment
  p. history
  p. psychosis
psychiatry
  forensic p.
psychic wound
psychogenic
  p. limp
  p. unresponsiveness
psychomotor agitation
psychopathology

psychosis
> acute p.
> bipolar p.
> ICU p.
> Korsakoff p.
> medical p.
> psychiatric p.

psychosocial stressor
psychosomatic disease
psychotropic medication
PT
> physical therapy
> pulmonary therapy
>> chest PT

PTA
> posttraumatic amnesia

PTCA
> percutaneous transluminal coronary
> angioplasty

pterygoid
> p. bone
> p. muscle
> p. nerve

pterygomandibular ligament
pterygomaxillary suture
pterygopalatine nerve
pterygospinal ligament
pterygospinous ligament
PTLA
> pharyngeal tracheal lumen airway

PTLD
> posttransplant lymphoproliferative
> disease

ptosis, pl. **ptoses**
PTSD
> posttraumatic stress disorder

PTT
> partial thromboplastin time

PTV
> percutaneous transtracheal ventilation

pubic
> p. arcuate ligament
> p. bone
> p. ramus stress fracture
> p. symphysis fracture
> p. tubercle

pubis
> mons p.
> pediculosis p.
> symphysis p.

puboanalis muscle
pubocapsular ligament

pubocervical ligament
pubococcygeal muscle
pubofemoral ligament
puboprostatic
> p. ligament
> p. muscle

puborectalis muscle
puborectal muscle
pubourethral ligament
pubovaginal muscle
pubovesical
> p. ligament
> p. muscle

pudendal
> p. block
> p. nerve
> p. vein

pudic nerve
puerperal breast abscess
puffer
> p. fish poisoning
> pink p.

pulled elbow
pulley tendon
pullout suture
pulmonale
> cor p.

pulmonary
> p. abscess
> p. angiography
> p. arteriography
> p. artery (PA)
> p. artery catheter
> p. artery catheter wedge pressure
> (PACWP)
> p. artery occlusion
> p. artery occlusion pressure
> p. artery wedge (PAW)
> p. artery wedge pressure (PAWP)
> p. aspergillosis
> p. barotrauma
> p. candidiasis
> p. compliance
> p. contusion
> p. edema
> p. effusion
> p. embolism (PE)
> p. failure
> p. fibrosis
> p. function test (PFT)
> p. function testing (PFT)
> p. hypertension

NOTES

P

pulmonary *(continued)*
 p. insufficiency
 p. intensive care unit (PICU)
 p. interstitial emphysema (PIE)
 p. lavage
 p. ligament
 p. overpressurization syndrome
  (POPS)
 p. oxygen toxicity
 p. renal syndrome
 p. resection
 p. sepsis
 p. therapy (PT)
 p. toilet
 p. vascular resistance (PVR)
 p. vascular resistance index (PVRI)
 p. vein
 p. venous return
pulmonic
 p. valve
 p. valvular stenosis
pulp
pulsatile
 p. hematoma
 p. mass
 p. perfusion preservation
pulsating vein
pulse
 absent p.
 bounding p.
 brachial p.
 carotid p.
 central p.
 p. deficit
 distal p.
 dorsalis pedis p.
 feeble p.
 femoral p.
 full p.
 gaseous p.
 irregular p.
 jugular venous p. (JVP)
 p., motor function, sensation (PMS)
 p. oximeter
 p. oximetry
 paradoxic p.
 peripheral p.
 posterior tibial p.
 p. pressure
 radial p.
 rapid p.
 regular p.
 p. rhythm
 p. strength
 strong p.
 thready p.
 weak p.

pulseless
 p. electrical activity (PEA)
 p. ventricular tachycardia
pulsus paradoxus
pulverization
Pulvertaft
 P. end-to-end suture
 P. interweave suture
 P. weave suture
pump
 intraaortic balloon p. (IABP)
punch
 bone graft p.
punched-out ulceration
punctate hemorrhage
puncture
 arterial p.
 bone marrow p.
 cricothyroid p.
 epidural p.
 p. fracture
 lumbar p. (LP)
 p. wound
puncture-proof glove
pupil
 constricted p.
 dilated p.
 p.'s equal and react to light
  (PERL)
 p.'s equal and react to light and
  accommodation (PERLA)
 p.'s equal, round, and reactive to
  light and accommodation
  (PERRLA)
 pinpoint p.
 p. size
pupillary
 p. constrictor muscle
 p. sphincter muscle
pure
 p. blowout fracture
 p. culture
 p. emphysema
purging
 bone marrow p.
Purlon suture
purple mucous membrane
purpura
 autoimmune thrombocytopenia p.
 Henoch-Schönlein p.
 idiopathic thrombocytopenic p.
  (ITP)
 infarctive p.
 mechanical p.
 posttransfusion p.
 thrombocytopenic p.
 thrombotic thrombocytopenic p.
  (TTP)

purpurea
>   *Digitalis p.*

pursed lip breathing

pursestring suture

PURSUIT
>   Platelet Glycoprotein IIb/IIIa in Unstable
>   Angina: Receptor Suppression Using
>   Integrilin Therapy

purulent
>   p. discharge
>   p. sputum

puruloid

pus
>   anchovy sauce p.
>   blue p.
>   cheesy p.
>   curdy p.
>   green p.
>   laudable p.
>   p. tube

pustular

pustule

putamen hemorrhage

PUVA
>   psoralen plus ultraviolet A

PV
>   pressure volume

PVB suture

PVC
>   premature ventricular contraction

PVE
>   prosthetic valve endocarditis

PVR
>   pulmonary vascular resistance

PVRI
>   pulmonary vascular resistance index

PVT
>   polymorphic ventricular tachycardia

P-wave amplitude

pyelogram
>   intravenous p. (IVP)
>   1-shot intravenous p.

pyelography
>   intravenous p.

pyelonephritis
>   ascending p.
>   chronic p.
>   emphysematous p.

pyemesis

pyemic abscess

pylori
>   *Helicobacter p.*

pyloric
>   p. muscle
>   p. stenosis
>   p. vein

pyogenic
>   p. abscess
>   p. fever
>   p. granuloma

pyoktanin catgut suture

pyonephrosis

pyramidal
>   p. auricular muscle
>   p. bone
>   p. fracture

pyramidalis muscle

pyrazinamide

pyretic therapy

pyrexia

pyridoxal

pyridoxamine

pyridoxine

pyrimethamine-sulfadoxine

pyrogen
>   endogenous p.

pyroglycolic acid suture

pyrosis

pyuria

NOTES

P

Q
  Q fever
  Q wave
qigong
  tendon changing q.
QRS
  electrocardiographic wave
  QRS complex tachycardia
  QRS width
QT-interval syndrome
Q-T prolongation
quadrant
  left lower q. (LLQ)
  left upper q. (LUQ)
  lower outer q. (LOQ)
  outer upper right q. (OURQ)
  right lower q. (RLQ)
  right upper q. (RUQ)
  upper left q. (ULQ)
  upper outer q. (UOQ)
quadrate
  q. ligament
  q. pronator muscle
quadratus
  q. femoris bursa
  q. muscle
quadriceps
  q. muscle
  q. tendon
quadrigeminal vein
quadrilateral bone

quadripartite bone
quadriplegia
quadrumanus
  Chiropsalmus q.
quality
  q. of pain
  respiratory q.
quantum
  bone q.
quaternary ammonia
quazepam
Quervain fracture
Quickert suture
quick urine drug screen
quiescent period
quiet breathing
quilted suture
quilting suture
Quinby pelvic fracture classification
quinidine sulfate
quinine sulfate
quinoline
quinolizidine
quinolone
quinquecirrha
  Chrysaora q.
3–quinuclidinyl benzilate
quinupristin/dalfopristin
quotient
  intelligence q. (IQ)
Q-wave myocardial infarction

RA
    rheumatoid arthritis
rabbit syndrome
rabies
    dumb r.
    r. prophylaxis
raccoon eyes
raccooning
rachitic
    r. bone
    r. chest
radial
    r. artery cannulation
    r. bone
    r. bursa
    r. carpal collateral ligament
    r. digital nerve
    r. dilator muscle
    r. extensor muscle
    r. flexor muscle
    r. head fracture
    r. head subluxation
    r. metacarpal ligament
    r. neck fracture
    r. nerve block
    r. pulse
    r. sensory nerve
    r. styloid fracture
    r. surgery
    r. vein
radiate
    r. carpal ligament
    r. sternocostal ligament
radiation
    alpha r.
    background r.
    beta r.
    bone injury r.
    r. burn
    r. colitis
    r. disaster preparedness
    r. exposure
    extraabdominal r.
    gamma r.
    heat loss by r.
    r. injury
    ionizing r.
    nonionizing r.
    r. pneumonitis
    r. wound
radical
    r. cystectomy
    r. fracture
    r. measure

    r. nephrectomy
    r. treatment
radicular vein
radio
    WR-30 digital weather/hazard r.
radiocapitate ligament
radiocarpal ligament
radiograph
    chest r.
    pelvis r.
    plain sinus r.
    sinus r.
    stress r.
    sunrise r.
radiographically occult fracture
radiographic evaluation
radiography
    chest r.
radiohumeral bursa
radioisotope
radiologist
    interventional r.
radiology backup
radiolunate ligament
radiolunotriquetral ligament
radionuclide
    r. angiography
    r. scintigraphy
radioscaphocapitate ligament
radioscaphoid ligament
radioscapholunate ligament
radiotriquetral ligament
radioulnar ligament
radon poisoning
rain
    acid r.
rale
    bibasilar r.
    crepitant r.
    sonorous r.
rambling language
ramipril
Rampart EMS clinical support tool
Ramsay
    R. Hunt syndrome
    R. sedation scale
Ramsey County pyoktanin catgut suture
ramus
    r. bone
    r. fracture
Randomized Efficacy Study of Tirofiban for Outcomes and Restenosis (RESTORE)

R

range
r. of motion (ROM)
therapeutic blood r.
ranine vein
ranitidine
Rankin suture
Ranson acute pancreatitis criteria
RAP
right atrial pressure
rapamycin
rape kit
rapid
r. breathing
R. Early Action for Coronary
Treatment (REACT)
r. gut suture
r. hemoglobin determination
r. infuser
r. infuser with warming capabilities
r. medical assessment
r. pulse
r. repolarization
r. respiration
r. sequence induction
r. sequence induction technique
r. sequence intubation (RSI)
r. sequence intubation conscious
sedation
r. tranquilization
r. transport
r. trauma assessment
Rapide wound suture
rapidity of onset
Rapidpoint 400 critical care analyzer
rapture of the deep
rarefaction
bone r.
rare rhonchi
rash
diaper r.
pediatric r.
petechial r.
road r.
rate
abnormal respiratory r.
basal metabolic r. (BMR)
bone formation r.
cardiac r.
flow r.
glomerular filtration r. (GFR)
heart r. (HR)
morbidity r.
peak expiratory flow r. (PEFR)
respiratory r.
resting metabolic r.
sedimentation r.
ratio
arterial ketone body r.
body-weight r.

bone age r.
I:E r.
inverse r. (IR)
pressure-controlled inverse r.
(PCIR)
risk r.
risk-benefit r.
rattlesnake
Mojave r.
rave
fracture en r.
r. party
raw bone
Raynaud phenomenon
RB1 suture
RBC
red blood cell
red blood count
RCM
right costal margin
RDA
recommended daily allowance
RDS
respiratory distress syndrome
reabsorbable suture
reabsorption
bone r.
REACT
Rapid Early Action for Coronary
Treatment
REACT trial
reaction
adverse drug r. (ADR)
allergic r.
anaphylactic r.
Arthus r.
blood transfusion r.
conversion r.
disulfiram r.
dystonic r.
febrile r.
febrile nonhemolytic transfusion r.
hemolytic transfusion r.
hypersensitivity r.
idiosyncratic r.
IgE-mediated allergic r.
medication-induced dystonic r.
septic r.
tendon r.
toxic skin r.
transfusion r.
reactive
r. airway disease
r. airway dysfunction syndrome
r. arthritis
r. dysfunction
r. hyperfibrinogenemia
rearfoot ligament

R

rebalancing
tendon r.
rebleeding
rebound
r. hyperglycemia
r. pain
r. tenderness
recalcitrant
r. disease
r. hemorrhage
r. patient
receptor
beta 1, 2 r.
bone cell r.
bone morphogenetic protein r.
cannabinoid r.
leukotriene r.
muscle ergo r.
muscle sensory r.
nerve growth factor r.
serotonin reuptake r.
recession
bone r.
recipient
heart transplant r.
recommended daily allowance (RDA)
reconstruction
bone r.
infrainguinal r.
ligament r.
vascular r.
record
trauma care flow r.
recovery
r. position
r. room (RR)
recrudescence of fever
recrudescent
r. abscess
r. pain
recruitment
alveolar r.
end-expiratory alveolar r.
rectal
r. dyschezia
r. foreign body
r. guaiac
r. laceration
r. nerve
r. prolapse
r. temperature
r. tonography

r. trauma
r. vein
rectococcygeal muscle
rectopexy
suture r.
rectosacral ligament
rectosigmoid vein
rectourethral muscle
rectouterine
r. ligament
r. muscle
rectovesical muscle
rectum
per r.
rectus
r. abdominis muscle
r. capitis lateralis muscle
r. capitis posterior major muscle
r. capitis posterior minor muscle
r. femoris muscle
recumbent position
recuperation
recurrence
wound r.
recurrent
r. angioedema
r. atrial fibrillation
r. hemothorax
r. laryngeal nerve
r. meningeal nerve
r. runaway
red
r. back spider
r. blood cell (RBC)
r. blood count (RBC)
r. desaturation
r. eye
r. herring
r. muscle
phenol r.
reduced
r. cardiac output
r. range of motion
reducible hernia
reducing diet
reductase
methemoglobin r.
reduction
afterload r.
air r.
closed r.
r. of fracture

NOTES

reduction *(continued)*
    fracture r.
    immediate r.
    indications for immediate r.
    open r.
    relative risk r. (RRR)
Reed
    R. classification of coma
    R. coma scale
Reeves stretcher
reexamination
refeeding syndrome
reference
    delusion of r.
referral
    orthopaedic r.
    urgent orthopaedic r.
referred pain
refill
    capillary r.
reflected inguinal ligament
reflectometry
    acoustic r.
reflex
    abdominal r.
    absence of gag r.
    bone r.
    cervicoocular r.
    corneal r.
    deep tendon r. (DTR)
    doll's eye r.
    gag r.
    gasp r.
    r. glottic closure and laryngospasm
    hyperactive r.
    r. ligament
    muscle spindle r.
    muscle stretch r.
    presence of gag r.
    r. sympathetic dystrophy
    r. sympathetic response to
      laryngoscopy (RSRL)
    r. symptom
    r. tachycardia
    tendon stretch r.
    vasopressor r.
    vasovagal r.
    vestibuloocular r.
    withdrawal r.
reflux
    r. esophagitis
    gastroesophageal r.
refractory
    r. illness
    r. period
refractured bone
regenerated bone
regeneration
    nerve r.

regimen
    3-drug r.
    WASH r.
region
    abdominal r.
    core r.
    focal r.
    hypogastric r.
    inguinal r.
    lateral abdominal r.
    molar r.
    occipital r.
    pelvic r.
    sternocleidomastoid r.
    submental r.
    temporal r.
    temporoparietal-occipital r.
    thoracoabdominal r.
    umbilical r.
regional
    r. lymphadenitis
    r. lymphadenopathy
    r. poison control center
registry
    Chest Pain Evaluation R.
      (CHEPER)
    National Emergency Airway r.
      (NEAR)
regrowth
    nerve r.
regular pulse
regurgitation
    acute mitral r.
    aortic r.
    mitral r.
rehab
    rehabilitation
rehabilitation (rehab)
    cardiac r.
    r. process
    r. specialist
rehydration
reimplantation
    r. amputation
    amputation r.
    microsurgical r.
    r. response
reinforcing suture
reinsertion
    ligament r.
reintubation
Reisseisen muscle
Reiter
    R. disease
    R. syndrome
rejection
    allograft r.
    hyperacute r.

kidney r.
transplant r.

relapse
bone marrow r.
high incidence of r.

relation
patient-provider r.

relationship
pressure-volume r.

relative
r. bradycardia
r. contraindication
r. refractory period
r. risk reduction (RRR)

relaxant
muscle r.

relaxation
muscle r.
r. suture

releasable suture

release
endogenous catecholamine r.
tendon r.

Relenza

remodeling
bone r.
fracture r.
r. of wound

removal
constricting band r.
extracorporeal CO_2 r.
extrarenal fluid r.
fishhook r.
foreign body r.
ring band r.
tick r.

remover
artificial fingernail r.

renal
r. abscess
r. afferent nerve
r. buffer
r. calculus
r. crisis
r. failure
r. injury
r. injury scale
r. loss of bicarbonate
r. stab wound
r. sympathetic nerve
r. tubular acidosis (RTA)

r. tubule acidosis
r. vein

renin-angiotensin-aldosterone system

repair
admission for operative r.
bone graft r.
fracture r.
hydrocele r.
lesion r.
operative r.
secondary r.
suture anchor shoulder r.
tendon r.

repellent
moth r.

reperfusion
cerebral r.
illusion of r.
r. injury

replacement
r. bone
bone marrow r.
catheter r.
electrolyte r.
fluid r.
glucocorticoid r.
ligament r.
Parkland formula for fluid r.
surfactant r.

replantation
limb r.

repletion
potassium r.
thiamine r.

repolarization
rapid r.
terminal r.

report
ambulance call r.
prehospital care r. (PCR)
verbal bedside r.

reporter
mandated r.
Rosetta-Lt 12-lead r.

reporting
patient care r. (PCR)

repose
angle of r.

repositioning
muscle r.

NOTES

reprocessing
    eye movement desensitization
       and r. (EMDR)
rerouted tendon
RES
    reticuloendothelial system
rescue
    r. angioplasty
    bone marrow r.
    r. breathing
resecting fracture
resection
    bone r.
    hepatic r.
    muscle r.
    pulmonary r.
    sigmoid r.
    suture rectopexy with sigmoid r.
reserpine
reserve
    alkali r.
    bone marrow r.
    contractile r.
    mechanical r.
    muscle r.
reservoir
    r. infection
    wound drainage r.
residual
    r. abscess
    r. volume (RV)
residue
    bullet wipe r.
resin
    anion exchange r.
    epoxy r.
resistance
    multidrug r.
    multiple drug r.
    natural r.
    pulmonary vascular r. (PVR)
    systemic vascular r.
resistive pressure ventilation
resolution
    metabolic abnormality r.
resolving anion gap metabolic acidosis
resonance
    osteal r.
resorcinol toxicity
resorption
    bone r.
respiration
    absent r.
    accelerated r.
    accessory muscles of r.
    agonal r.
    artificial r. (AR)
    Cheyne-Stokes r.
    deep r.

    forced r.
    grunting r.
    heat loss by r.
    Kussmaul r.
    labored r.
    mouth-to-mouth r.
    rapid r.
    shallow r.
    spontaneous r.
respirator
    artificial r.
    HEPA r.
    3M Healthcare particulate r.
respirator/ventilator
respiratory
    r. acidosis
    r. alkalosis
    r. arrest
    r. bacterial infection
    r. burn
    r. depth
    r. distress
    r. distress syndrome (RDS)
    r. effort
    r. equality
    r. failure
    r. monitoring
    r. muscle
    r. quality
    r. rate
    r. syncytial virus (RSV)
    r. system
    r. therapist
    r. tract
    r. zone
Respirgard II
responder
    R. emergency vehicle car seat
    first r.
response
    brainstem auditory evoked r.
      (BAER)
    Cushing r.
    disaster r.
    hypoxic ventilatory r. (HVR)
    inflammatory r.
    r. to light touch
    multiple-vehicle r.
    neurohormonal r.
    reimplantation r.
    Staffing for Adequate Fire and
      Emergency R. (SAFER)
    twitch r.
    unconditioned r.
    visual evoked r.
Res-Q-Vac handheld emergency suction
rest
    r. angina
    pelvic r.

R

restenosis
Randomized Efficacy Study of Tirofiban for Outcomes and R. (RESTORE)
resting metabolic rate
RESTORE
Randomized Efficacy Study of Tirofiban for Outcomes and Restenosis
RESTORE trial
restraint
hobble r.
physical r.
restricted affect
restriction
dietary r.
restrictive
r. cardiomyopathy
r. lung disease
result
diagnostic r.'s
lab r.'s
test r.'s
resurfacing
bone r.
resurrection bone
resuscitate
do not r. (DNR)
resuscitation
active compression-decompression cardiopulmonary r. (ACD-CPR)
aggressive fluid r.
brain r.
cardiopulmonary r. (CPR)
cardiorespiratory r.
cerebral r.
do not attempt r. (DNAR)
fluid r.
interposed abdominal compression-cardiopulmonary r. (IAC-CPR)
intrauterine r.
mouth-to-mouth r.
mouth-to-nose r.
mouth-to-stoma r.
neonatal r.
newborn r.
pediatric r.
terminal r.
termination of r. (TOR)
trauma r.
volume r.

resuscitator
BVM r.
manual r.
retained
r. foreign body
r. placenta
Retavase
retching
retention
carbon dioxide r.
r. suture
urinary r.
reteplase
reticulated bone
reticuloendothelial system (RES)
retina
retinacular ligament
retinal
r. artery occlusion
r. detachment
r. manifestation
r. manifestation of systemic disease
r. vein
r. vein occlusion
retracted fontanelle
retracting suture
retraction
infraclavicular r.
intercostal r.
platelet plug r.
sternal r.
supraclavicular r.
wound r.
retractor
bone r.
nerve root r.
vein r.
retraining
muscle r.
retro-Achilles bursa
retroaortic renal vein
retroauricular vein
retrocalcaneal bursa
retrodisplaced fracture
retrograde
r. intubation (RI)
r. tracheal intubation
r. urethrogram
retrohepatic vein
retrohyoid bursa
retromammary bursa
retromandibular vein

NOTES

retronuchal muscle
retroperfusion
    synchronized coronary venous r.
retroperitoneal
    r. hematoma
    r. lymphadenectomy
    r. space
    r. vein
retropharyngeal abscess
retroverted uterus
return
    pulmonary venous r.
    r. of spontaneous circulation
    (ROSC)
    r. stroke
Retzius
    R. ligament
    R. vein
revascularization
    transmyocardial laser r.
reverse
    r. Barton fracture
    r. Bennett fracture
    r. Colles fracture
    r. Monteggia fracture
    r. obliquity fracture
    r. saphenous vein
    r. Segond fracture
reversed greater saphenous vein
reversibly injured myocardium
review of systems (ROS)
Revised Trauma Score (RTS)
rewarming
    active r.
    active core r. (ACR)
    active external r. (AER)
    contact r.
    core r.
    r. hemodynamic monitoring
    invasive core r.
    passive r.
Reye syndrome
Rh
    Rhesus
        Rh antibody
        Rh blood group
        Rh factor
        Rh immunization
        Rh incompatibility
        Rh isoantigen
        Rh negative
rhabarbarum
    Rheum r.
rhabdoid suture
rhabdomyolysis
    acute recurrent r.
rhabdosphincter muscle
Rhesus (Rh)

rheumatica
    polymyalgia r.
rheumatic fever
rheumatoid
    r. arthritis (RA)
    r. scleritis
Rheum rhabarbarum
rhinion
    fracture at r.
rhinitis
    allergic r.
rhinorrhea
    CSF r.
Rhizopoda
***Rhododendron* ingestion**
rhomboid
    r. ligament
    r. major muscle
    r. minor muscle
rhomboideus major muscle
rhonchus, pl. rhonchi
    audible rhonchi
    bibasilar rhonchi
    bilateral rhonchi
    coarse rhonchi
    diffuse rhonchi
    expiratory rhonchi
    faint rhonchi
    harsh rhonchi
    high-pitched rhonchi
    inspiratory rhonchi
    marked rhonchi
    musical rhonchi
    occasional rhonchi
    posttussive inspiratory rhonchi
    rare rhonchi
    scattered rhonchi
    sibilant rhonchi
    sonorous rhonchi
    upper respiratory rhonchi
    whistling rhonchi
rhubarb
    r. leaf blade ingestion
    r. poisoning
rhus dermatitis
rhythm
    accelerated idioventricular r.
    idioventricular r.
    junctional r.
    pulse r.
RI
    retrograde intubation
rib
    bone lesion of r.
    broken r.
    false r.
    r. fracture
    true r.
ribavirin

R

ribbon
    r. gut suture
    r. muscle
ricin
Ricinus communis
rickets
    scurvy r.
Rickettsia
    R. prowazekii
    R. rickettsii
    R. typhi
    R. typhus
rickettsial infection
rickettsii
    Rickettsia r.
rider's
    r. bone
    r. bursa
    r. muscle
    r. tendon
rifampicin
rifampin
right
    r. atrial pressure (RAP)
    r. brachiocephalic vein
    r. colic vein
    r. common iliac nerve
    r. costal margin (RCM)
    r. gastric vein
    r. gastroepiploic vein
    r. gastroomental vein
    r. gonadal vein
    r. hepatic vein
    r. hypogastric nerve
    r. inferior gluteal vein
    r. inferior pulmonary vein
    r. internal jugular vein
    r. lower extremity (RLE)
    r. lower quadrant (RLQ)
    r. mainstem bronchus
    r. ovarian vein
    r. pericardiacophrenic vein
    r. phrenic vein
    r. prostatic ligament
    r. pulmonary vein
    r. recurrent laryngeal nerve
    r. subclavian vein
    r. superior intercostal vein
    r. superior pulmonary vein
    r. suprarenal vein
    r. testicular vein
    r. triangular ligament

    r. upper extremity (RUE)
    r. upper quadrant (RUQ)
    r. ventricular dysfunction
    r. ventricular ejection fraction
    r. ventricular ejection fraction
      catheter
    r. ventricular infarction
    r. ventricular pressure (RV)
right-sided cardiac output
right-to-left intracardiac shunt
rigid
    r. bronchoscopy
    r. laryngoscope
    r. splint
    r. suction catheter
rigidity
    decorticate r.
    muscle r.
    nuchal r.
rigor mortis
rimantadine
ring
    anorectal r.
    r. avulsion
    r. band removal
    cricoid r.
    r. fracture
    r. ligament
    preputial r.
    suture r.
ring-disrupting fracture
Ringer
    lactated R. (LR)
    R. solution
rinse
    dilute hydrogen peroxide r.
Riolan muscle
riot control agent
rip-cord suture
Riseborough-Radin intercondylar
    fracture classification
risk
    r. of aspiration
    assumption of r.
    r. index
    r. ratio
    r. stratification
risk-benefit
    r.-b. assessment
    r.-b. ratio
risorius muscle
Risperdal

NOTES

risperidone
RLE
    right lower extremity
RLQ
    right lower quadrant
road rash
Robert ligament
Rocephin
Rochester febrile infant criteria
Rockwood
    R. classification
    R. classification of clavicular
        fracture
Rocky Mountain spotted fever
rodding
    intramedullary r.
rodenticide
roentgen diagnosis
roentgenogram
    postreduction r.
Roferon-A
Rohypnol
rolandic vein
Rolando
    R. fracture
    R. vein
Rolando-type fracture
roll
    gauze r.
roller-type injury
roll-in stretcher
rollover
    vehicle r.
ROM
    range of motion
Romazicon
Romberg test
rongeur
R-on-T phenomenon
roof fracture
room
    cast r.
    emergency r. (ER)
    operating r.
    recovery r. (RR)
    trauma r.
root
    r. fracture
    nerve r.
rootlet
    nerve r.
ROS
    review of systems
ROSC
    return of spontaneous circulation
rosea
    pityriasis r.
Rosenthal vein
roseola infantum

Rosetta-Lt 12-lead reporter
rostral cervical nerve
rostrocaudal progression
rotation
    r. fracture
    r. injury
    suture r.
rotational burst fracture
rotator
    r. cuff injury
    r. cuff muscle
    r. cuff tendon
rotavirus
Rotor syndrome
rotten egg odor
Rouget muscle
round
    r. iliac bone
    r. muscle
    r. uterine ligament
route of entry
Rouviere ligament
Rovsing sign
RR
    recovery room
RRR
    relative risk reduction
RSI
    rapid sequence intubation
RSRL
    reflex sympathetic response to
        laryngoscopy
RSV
    respiratory syncytial virus
RTA
    renal tubular acidosis
RTS
    Revised Trauma Score
rub
    friction r.
    pericardial r.
    pleural r.
    pleuropericardial r.
    tendon friction r.
rubber
    r. cement toxicity
    r. suture
rubbing
    coin r.
rubella
rubeola
rubor
rudimentary bone
RUE
    right upper extremity
Ruedi-Allgower tibial plafond fracture
Ruedi fracture
rugal pattern
rug burn

R

rule
> r. of 3s
> r. of 9s
> Ottawa ankle r.'s
> r. out myocardial infarction

Rumack-Matthew acetaminophen poisoning nomogram

runaway
> r. pacemaker
> recurrent r.

running
> r. continuous suture
> r. intradermal suture
> r. locking suture
> r. nylon penetrating keratoplasty suture

rupture
> aneurismal r.
> aortic r.
> r. of atherosclerotic plaque
> biceps brachii r.
> bladder r.
> coracoclavicular ligament r.
> costovertebral junction r.
> diaphragm r.
> esophageal r.
> free-wall r.
> globe r.
> ligament r.
> major bronchi r.
> papillary muscle r. (PMR)
> plantaris tendon r.
> splenic r.
> stomach r.
> tendon r.
> tracheal r.
> traumatic aortic r.
> umbilical r.
> uterine r.
> vein patch r.
> ventricular septal r.

ruptured
> r. abdominal aortic aneurysm
> r. ectopic pregnancy
> r. uterus

RUQ
> right upper quadrant

Russe scaphoid fracture classification

Ruysch
> R. muscle
> R. vein

RV
> residual volume
> right ventricular pressure

NOTES

Sabreloc suture
sac
 amniotic s.
 embryonic s.
saccular nerve
sacral
 s. bone
 s. bursa
 s. fracture
 s. insufficiency fracture
 s. splanchnic nerve
 s. vein
 s. wound
sacred bone
sacrococcygeal
 s. ligament
 s. muscle
sacrodural ligament
sacrogenital ligament
sacroiliac
 s. fracture
 s. ligament
sacrospinal
 s. ligament
 s. muscle
sacrospinous ligament
sacrotuberal ligament
sacrotuberous ligament
sacrouterine ligament
sacrum fracture
saddleback fever curve
SAED
 semiautomated external defibrillator
Saenger suture
SAFER
 Staffing for Adequate Fire and
 Emergency Response
safety
 margin of s.
safety-bolt suture
SafetySure transfer gurney
**Safil synthetic absorbable surgical
 suture**
Sager
 S. Combo-Pac adult/child and
 infant splint
 S. S304 bilateral splint
 S. S300 infant bilateral splint
 S. 2301 single splint
sagittal
 s. cranial suture
 s. plane
 s. slice fracture
 s. splitting fracture

sagrada
 cascara s.
**Sakellarides calcaneal fracture
 classification**
salamander toxin
salbutamol
salicylate
 s. level
 s. overdose
 s. poisoning
 s. toxicity
salicylic acid
salient finding
saline
 hypertonic s. (HTS)
 s. laxative
 s. solution
 s. sulfate cathartic
saliva ethanol assay
salivary
 s. gland
 s. gland swelling
salivation
 decreased s.
 s., lacrimation, urination, diarrhea,
 gastric cramping, emesis
 (SLUDGE)
Salmonella
 S. infection
 S. typhi
salpingopharyngeal muscle
salt
 s. depletion heat exhaustion
 magnesium s.
 smelling s.
Salter-Harris
 S.-H. epiphysial fracture
 S.-H. epiphysial fracture
 classification
 S.-H. type I–VI fracture
salt-wasting
 cerebral s.-w.
saltwater-related wound
salvage
 blood s.
salvatella vein
SAM
 SAM OnScene patient assessment
 guide
 SAM splint
SAMPLE
 sign/symptom, allergy, medications,
 pertinent past medical history, last oral
 intake, event leading up to the injury or
 illness

S

sampling
  bone marrow s.
sandbag
sandbagging long bone fracture
Sanders fracture
Sangeorzan navicular fracture
Sanguinaria canadensis
Santorini
  S. ligament
  S. muscle
  S. vein
saphenous
  s. nerve
  s. vein
Sappey
  S. ligament
  S. vein
SAPS
  Simplified Acute Physiology Scale
sarcoidosis
  bone s.
sarcoma
  bone s.
  Ewing s.
  Kaposi s.
  muscle s.
sarcomatous bone
Sarcoptes scabiei
Sarin nerve agent
SARS
  severe acute respiratory syndrome
sartorius
  s. bursa
  s. muscle
  s. nerve
  s. tendon
satellite abscess
saturated
  s. fatty acid
  s. solution of potassium iodide
    (SSKI)
saturation
  decreased oxygen s.
  jugular venous s.
  mixed venous s.
  venous oxygen s. (SVO$_2$)
saturnine gout
saver
  Haemonetics Cell S.
Savlon
  S. antiseptic
  S. antiseptic cream
saw
  cast s.
Sawyer extractor
SBE
  subacute bacterial endocarditis

SBP
  spontaneous bacterial peritonitis
  systolic blood pressure
scabiei
  Sarcoptes s.
scabies
scald
  s. burn
  immersion s.
  spill s.
scalded skin syndrome
scale
  Abbreviated Injury S.
  abdominal visceral organ injury s.
  American Spinal Injury Association
    Impairment S.
  ASIA Impairment S.
  AVPU s.
  coma s.
  Glasgow coma s. (GCS)
  Hunt-Hess s.
  Innsbruck Coma S.
  intubation difficulty s. (IDS)
  Mallampati difficult intubation s.
  Organ Injury S.
  Ramsay sedation s.
  Reed coma s.
  renal injury s.
  sedation-agitation s.
  Simplified Acute Physiology S.
    (SAPS)
  small bowel injury s.
  vascular injury s.
  Yale Observation S. (YOS)
scalene muscle
scalenus
  s. anterior muscle
  s. medius muscle
  s. minimus muscle
  s. posterior muscle
scalloped muscle
scalloping
  bone tumor s.
scalp
  s. abnormality
  s. avulsion
  s. contusion
  s. laceration
  s. muscle
scan
  bone density s.
  bone marrow s.
  computed tomographic s.
  CT s.
  gallium s.
  HIDA s.
  longitudinal s.
  noncontrast CT s.

specialized computed
  tomographic s.
transverse s.
ventilation/perfusion lung s.
scanning
  bone marrow s.
  gallium-67 s.
  technetium 99m s.
scaphoid
  s. bone
  s. fracture
  s. hand fracture
scapholunate
  s. interosseous ligament
scaphotrapezoid interosseous ligament
scaphotriquetral ligament
scapular
  s. bone
  s. fracture
  s. ligament
  s. muscle
  s. nerve
scapularis
  Ixodes s.
scapulohumeral
  s. bursa
  s. ligament
  s. muscle
scapulothoracic
  s. bursa
  s. muscle
scar
  midline s.
scarification
scarlet
  s. bergamot
  s. fever
  S. Red dressing
Scarpa
  S. ligament
  S. nerve
scarring
  cortical s.
scattered rhonchi
SCBA
  self-contained breathing apparatus
SCCM
  Society of Critical Care Medicine
scene
  s. awareness
  surroundings at s.
  s. triage

Schiotz
  S. tonometer
  S. tonometry
schistosomiasis
schizophrenia
  chronic s.
Schlemm ligament
Schlesinger vein
sciatica
sciatic nerve
scimitar vein
scintigraphy
  bone marrow s.
  dipyridamole thallium s.
  ^{131}I-MIBG s.
  radionuclide s.
  thallium-201 s.
scissors
  iris s.
  suture wire cutting s.
SCIWORA
  spinal cord injury without radiographic
    abnormality
  SCIWORA phenomenon
sclera, pl. **sclerae**
  anicteric s.
scleral
  s. flap suture
  s. vein
scleritis
  rheumatoid s.
scleroderma
sclerosed temporal bone
sclerosis, pl. **scleroses**
  amyotrophic lateral s. (ALS)
  bone s.
  multiple s.
sclerotherapy
  injection s.
sclerotic bone
scoliosis
  fracture with s.
scombroid
  s. fish poisoning
  s. food poisoning
scoop stretcher
scopolamine
score
  age-specific pediatric trauma s.
    (ASPTS)
  Alvarado appendicitis s.
  Apgar s.

NOTES

score *(continued)*
    Champion trauma s.
    combativeness s.
    Dubowitz s.
    Glasgow coma s.
    Glasgow Outcome S.
    Glasgow Pediatric Coma S.
    Injury Severity S.
    MANTRELS acute appendicitis s.
    multiple organ dysfunction s.
      (MODS)
    New Injury Severity S. (NISS)
    Orlowski s.
    Revised Trauma S. (RTS)
    trauma s.
    Trauma Injury Severity S. (TRISS)
scoring
    Gustilo open fracture s.
    mangled extremity severity s.
      (MESS)
scorpion
    s. bite
    s. envenomation
    s. sting
scotty dog fracture
scratch
    cat s.
screen
    quick urine drug s.
    toxicologic s.
    type and s.
    urine drug s.
screening
    bone density s.
    s. hepatic profile
screw
    bone mulch s.
scroll bone
scrotal
    s. gangrene
    s. nerve
    s. vein
SCU
    special care unit
scuba diving accident
scurvy rickets
Scyphozoa **poisoning**
SDD
    selective decontamination of digestive
    tract
sea
    s. anemone poisoning
    s. cucumber poisoning
    s. snake
seabather's eruption
seat
    s. belt fracture
    s. belt injury

    child restraint s.
    Medi-Pac rescue s.
    Responder emergency vehicle
      car s.
sebaceous cyst
Sebileau muscle
seborrhea
seborrheic dermatitis
Seckel syndrome
second
    s. cuneiform bone
    forced expiratory volume in 1 s.
      (FEV_1)
    s. gas effect
    s. impact syndrome
    s. intention
    S. Leicester Intravenous Magnesium
      Intervention Trial (LIMIT-2)
    s. tibial muscle
secondary
    s. abscess
    s. angioedema
    s. assessment
    s. closure
    s. closure of wound
    s. fracture
    s. hypothyroidism
    s. intention
    s. repair
    s. survey
    s. suture
second-degree
    s.-d. atrioventricular block
    s.-d. AV block
    s.-d. burn
    s.-d. hyperthermia
    s.-d. laceration
secretin
secretion
    antidiuretic hormone s.
    inability to handle s.'s
    inappropriate antidiuretic
      hormone s.
    syndrome of inappropriate
      antidiuretic hormone s.
secretomotor nerve
secretory nerve
section
    cesarean s.
    emergency cesarean s.
    perimortem cesarean s.
security
    hospital s.
sedation
    conscious s.
    intramuscular conscious s.
    intravenous conscious s.
    oral conscious s.

rapid sequence intubation
   conscious s.
   systemic anesthetic conscious s.
sedation-agitation scale
sedative
sedative-hypnotic
   s.-h. overdose
   s.-h. withdrawal syndrome
sedimentation rate
seeker needle
seesaw breathing
segment
   flail s.
segmental
   s. fracture
   s. vein
segmentation
   boxcar s.
Segond tibial avulsion fracture
Seinsheimer femoral fracture
   classification
seizure
   absence s.
   adult s.
   alcoholic withdrawal s.
   atonic s.
   cocaine-induced s.
   epileptic s.
   febrile s.
   s. free
   grand mal s.
   impact s.
   morning-after s.
   pediatric s.
   petit mal s.
   tonic-clonic s.
   veriginous s.
SELEC-3 IV set
SELEC-3+NIS set
selection
   bone plate s.
selective decontamination of digestive
   tract (SDD)
self-adherent bandage
self-contained breathing apparatus
   (SCBA)
self-inflicted
   s.-i. gunshot wound
   s.-i. stab wound
self-sealing injection port

Sellick maneuver
semiautomated external defibrillator
   (SAED)
semi-Fowler position
semilunar
   s. bone
   s. valve
semimembranosus muscle
semimembranous bursa
seminal vesicle
semipennate muscle
semirecumbent position
semispinal muscle
semitendinous muscle
sempervirens
   Gelsemium s.
Sengstaken-Blakemore tube
senile subcapital fracture
senility
   premature s.
sensation
   pulse, motor function, s. (PMS)
sense
   muscle s.
sensibility
   bone s.
sensitivity
   culture and s. (C&S)
sensorimotor nerve
sensory
   s. adaptation
   s. function
   s. loss
   s. nerve
sentinel
   s. spinous process fracture
   s. vein
separation
   acromioclavicular s.
   fracture fragment s.
   laryngotracheal s.
   suture s.
separator
   nerve s.
sepsis
   biliary s.
   cryptogenic s.
   hyperdynamic s.
   intestinal s.
   intraabdominal s.
   line s.
   neonatal s.

S

NOTES

sepsis *(continued)*
    postabortion s.
    Protein C Worldwide Evaluation in Severe S. (PROWESS)
    pulmonary s.
    s. syndrome
    wound s.
sepsis-related organ failure assessment (SOFA)
septa (*pl. of* septum)
septal
    s. bone
    s. fracture
    s. papillary muscle
    s. vein
septic
    s. abortion
    s. arthritis
    s. bursitis
    s. effusion
    s. embolism
    s. encephalopathy
    s. pelvic vein thrombophlebitis
    s. phlebitis
    s. process
    s. reaction
    s. shock
    s. wound
septicemia
    anthrax s.
    catheter-related s.
septicemic abscess
septum, pl. **septa**
    interatrial s.
    nasal s.
sequela, pl. **sequelae**
    without major s.
sequence
    muscle patterning s.
sequential
    s. multiple analyzer (SMA)
    s. multiple analyzer plus computer (SMAC)
    s. single-lung transplantation
sequestration
sequestrum
    bone s.
sera (*pl. of* serum)
Serax
serial
    s. calculation
    s. charcoal therapy
series
    acute abdominal s. (AAS)
    skeletal s.
serious noncompliance
SER-IV fracture
serofibrinous pericarditis
serologic testing

serology
    diagnostic s.
seroma
    wound s.
seromuscular Lembert suture
seropurulent exudate
seropus
serosa
serosanguineous fluid
serotonin
    s. reuptake receptor
    s. syndrome
serous
    s. abscess
    s. ligament
SERRALNYL suture
SERRALSILK suture
serrated suture
Serratia marcescens
serratus
    s. anterior muscle
    s. posterior muscle
serum, pl. **sera**
    s. amylase
    antirabies s.
    antisnakebite s.
    antitetanic s.
    s. diagnosis
    s. electrolyte
    s. ethanol concentration
    s. glucose
    s. hCG
    s. lipase
    muscle s.
    s. osmolality
    s. pregnancy test
    s. sickness
Servelle vein
service
    ambulance s.
    American Hospital Formulary S. (AHFS)
    s. benefit
    emergency call s.
    emergency medical s. (EMS)
    emergency medical radio s. (EMRS)
Serzone toxicity
sesamoid
    s. bone
    s. fracture
    s. ligament
sesamophalangeal ligament
sessile polyp
set
    SELEC-3 IV s.
    SELEC-3+NIS s.
setback suture

seton
  s. suture
  s. wound
setting
  bone s.
setup parameter
seventh nerve palsy
severe
  s. acute respiratory syndrome (SARS)
  s. dehydration
  s. head injury
  s. hemorrhage
  s. hypovolemia
severity of injury
sexual
  s. abuse
  s. asphyxia
  s. assault
  s. intercourse
sexually
  s. active female
  s. active male
  s. transmitted disease (STD)
  s. transmitted infection (STI)
shaft
  bone s.
  s. forearm fracture
shagreen patch
shaken
  s. baby syndrome
  s. impact syndrome
shallow
  s. breathing
  s. laceration
  s. respiration
shampoo toxicity
shank bone
sharing
  nerve s.
shark bite
Sharpoint ophthalmic microsurgical suture
sharp pain
shawl muscle
shear fracture
shearing
  s. fracture
  s. injury
sheath
  Cook peel-away s.
  fascial s.

  fenestrated s.
  s. ligament
  muscle s.
  nerve root s.
  synovial s.
  tendon s.
Sheehan syndrome
sheet
  draw s.
  trip s.
shellfish
shelter
  Unifold s.
Shenton line
Shepherd fracture
shift
  antigenic s.
  mediastinal s.
  midline s.
  migration of pain, anorexia, nausea, tenderness in right lower quadrant, rebound, elevated temperature, leukocytosis, s. (MANTRELS)
  tracheal s.
shifter
  suture shape s.
shift-related hyperkalemia
Shigella
  S. dysenteriae
  S. infection
shinbone
shin bone
shingles
Shirodkar suture
shiver
Shoch suture
shock
  adrenal s.
  anaphylactic s.
  s. bowel syndrome
  cardiogenic s.
  container failure s.
  electric s.
  extracardiac obstructive s.
  hemorrhagic s.
  hypervolemic s.
  hypoglycemic s.
  hypovolemic s.
  insulin s.
  irreversible s.
  neurogenic s.

S

NOTES

shock *(continued)*
    obstructive s.
    oligemic s.
    s. position
    posttraumatic s.
    profound s.
    septic s.
    stacked s.'s
    warm s.
shock-advisory defibrillator
shocklike appearance
shocky appearance
shoelace suture
shoe polish odor
shored exit wound
short
    s. abductor muscle
    s. adductor muscle
    s. anconeus muscle
    s. backboard
    s. bowel syndrome
    s. calcaneocuboid ligament
    s. ciliary nerve
    s. extensor muscle
    s. fibular muscle
    s. flexor muscle
    s. gastric vein
    s. hepatic vein
    s. levator muscle
    s. metacarpal bone
    s. oblique fracture
    s. palmar muscle
    s. peroneal muscle
    s. plantar ligament
    s. radial extensor muscle
    s. radiolunate ligament
    s. rotator muscle
    s. saphenous nerve
    s. saphenous vein
    s. wooden backboard
shortened psoas muscle
shortening
    tendon s.
shortness of breath (SOB)
shotgun wound
1-shot intravenous pyelogram
shotted suture
shoulder
    s. bone
    dislocated s.
    s. dislocation
    s. dystocia
    floating s.
    s. girdle
    s. muscle
show
    bloody s.
shower
    Hot Tap portable hot s.

SH popoff suture
shrapnel
shunt
    cerebrospinal fluid s.
    s. gas analysis
    s. infection
    intracardiac s.
    intrahepatic s.
    intrapulmonary s.
    left-to-right intracardiac s.
    s. muscle
    peritoneovenous s.
    right-to-left intracardiac s.
    splenorenal s.
    transjugular intrahepatic
        portosystemic s.
    ventricular peritoneal s.
    Warren s.
SI
    stroke index
SIADH
    syndrome of inappropriate antidiuretic
        hormone
sialoadenitis
sialoprotein
    bone s.
sibilant rhonchi
Sibson muscle
sicca syndrome
sickening
    double s.
sickle
    s. cell anemia
    s. cell disease
    s. cell thalassemia
sickness
    chronic mountain s.
    decompression s.
    high-altitude s.
    Jamaican vomiting s.
    mountain s.
    serum s.
sick sinus syndrome
SICU
    surgical intensive care unit
side
    s. effect
    s. port
sideroblastic anemia
sidestream capnometer
sideswipe elbow fracture
SIDS
    sudden infant death syndrome
    near-miss SIDS
Siemens PTCA open heart suture
sieve bone
sigmoid
    s. colon
    s. resection

S

stool in s.
s. vein

sign

Aaron s.
absent bow-tie s.
accessory s.
antecedent s.
anterior drawer s.
balance s.
Ballance s.
barrel hoop s.
Battle s.
bone bruise s.
bow-tie s.
Branham s.
Carvallo s.
cerebellar s.
chandelier s.
Chvostek s.
coffee-bean s.
Corrigan s.
crescent s.
Cullen s.
Dance s.
De Musset s.
Duroziez s.
fallen lung s.
flail chest s.
fleck s.
Grey Turner s.
hanging drop s.
Kehr s.
Kernig s.
Kussmaul s.
Lhermitte s.
Ludloff s.
McBurney s.
Murphy s.
neuropsychiatric s.
Nikolsky s.
normal vital s.'s
objective s.
obturator s.
Pastia s.
peritoneal s.
physical s.
posterior sag s.
psoas s.
Rovsing s.
soft s.
steeple s.
s. and symptom

Terry Thomas s.
Trousseau s.
vein s.
vital s.'s
Westermark s.

signal

nerve s.
s. symptom
universal distress s.

sign/symptom, allergy, medications, pertinent past medical history, last oral intake, event leading up to the injury or illness (SAMPLE)
silicone-treated

s.-t. surgical silk suture
s.-t. wound

silicosis
silk

s. braided suture
s. Mersilene suture
s. nonabsorbable suture
s. popoff suture
s. retention suture
s. stay suture
s. traction suture

silkworm gut suture
Silky Polydek suture
silo filler's disease
silver

s. fork fracture
s. nitrate
s. sulfadiazine
s. sulfadiazine cream
s. wire suture

silverized catgut suture
Simonart ligament
simple

s. abscess
s. access
s. flaring suture
s. fracture
s. pneumothorax
s. running suture
s. skull fracture
s. triage and rapid treatment (START)
s. triage and rapid treatment system

simplex

herpes s.

Simplified Acute Physiology Scale (SAPS)

NOTES

Sims suture
simultaneous pancreas/kidney
   transplantation
SIMV
   synchronized intermittent mandatory
   ventilation
sinensis
   Wisteria s.
singer's nodule
single
   s. fracture
   s. lung transplantation (SLT)
   s. running suture
single-armed suture
single-chain urokinase-type plasminogen
single-column fracture
single-layer closure
single-photon emission computed
   tomography (SPECT)
singultus
sinoatrial
   s. conduction block
   s. node
sinocarotid nerve
sinovertebral nerve
sinus
   s. bradycardia
   cavernous s.
   ethmoid s.
   frontal s.
   maxillary s.
   s. nerve
   pilonidal s.
   s. radiograph
   sphenoid s.
   s. tachycardia
sinusitis
   chronic s.
   frontal s.
sinuvertebral nerve
Sirocco evacuation chair
sirolimus
SIRS
   systemic inflammatory response
   syndrome
site
   fracture s.
   injection s.
   needleless injection s. (NIS)
   nerve entrapment s.
   wound s.
situ
   carcinoma in s. (CIS)
situation
   multiple casualty s. (MCS)
   tenuous s.
size
   pupil s.
Sjögren syndrome

SkBF
   skin blood flow
Skelaxin
skeletal
   s. age
   s. muscle
   s. series
skeleton
   appendicular s.
   axial s.
skeletonized
skew
   s. deviation
   s. distribution
skid
   bone s.
skier's fracture
skill
   life-saving s.
skilled
   s. nursing care
   s. nursing facility (SNF)
Skillern fracture
skin
   s. abscess
   s. blanching
   s. blood flow (SkBF)
   s. cancer
   clammy s.
   cool s.
   s. deficit wound
   s. dimpling
   s. discoloration
   dry s.
   flushed s.
   s. glue
   jaundiced s.
   s. ligament
   s. lightener ingestion
   s. staple
   s. suture
   s. tension line
   tenting of s.
   s. testing
   yellow s.
skull
   s. base suture
   s. fracture
   s. fracture base
   sutures of s.
slab
   s. avalanche formation
   stirrup s.
SLE
   systemic lupus erythematosus
sleep apnea
sleeve
   s. fracture
   nerve root s.

slice fracture
slide
    muscle s.
sling
    s. immobilization
    muscle s.
    suture s.
    s. suture
    tendon s.
slip
    central s.
    extensor tendon central s.
slipped
    s. capital femoral epiphysis
    s. tendon
slit lamp
slit-lamp examination
sliver
    bone s.
slot fracture
slough
sloughing
slow
    s. channel blocker
    s. muscle
slow-reacting substance of anaphylaxis
  (SRSA)
slow-twitch muscle
SLT
    single lung transplantation
SLUDGE
    salivation, lacrimation, urination,
    diarrhea, gastric cramping, emesis
slurred speech
slurry
    bone s.
SMA
    sequential multiple analyzer
SMAC
    sequential multiple analyzer plus
    computer
small
    s. bowel bacterial infection
    s. bowel injury
    s. bowel injury scale
    s. bowel obstruction
    s. cardiac vein
    s. fracture
    s. intestine obstruction
    s. maxillary bone
    s. saphenous vein
    s. vessel arteritis

smaller
    s. pectoral muscle
    s. psoas muscle
smallest
    s. cardiac vein
    s. scalene muscle
small-particle aerosol generator
smallpox
small-volume nebulizer
smart
    S. Tag triage tag
    S. Triage Pac
smear
    buccal s.
    KOH s.
smelling salt
Smith ankle fracture
Smith-Lemli-Opitz syndrome
smoke inhalation
smooth muscle
smothering chest pain
snake
    s. bite
    brown s.
    coral s.
    s. envenomation
    s. identification
    sea s.
snakebite antivenom
snapping
    tendon s.
    s. tendon
snap sound
Snellen suture
Sneppen talar fracture
SNF
    skilled nursing facility
SNOMED
    Standard Nomenclature of Medicine
snoring
snowboarder's fracture
snowflake cataract
SOAP
    subjective, objective, assessment, plan
soap
    antibacterial s.
    s. exposure
    s. poisoning
SOB
    shortness of breath
sober
    clinically s.

S

NOTES

social
    s. history
    s. stressor
Society of Critical Care Medicine (SCCM)
soda
    bicarbonate of s.
sodium
    azlocillin s.
    s. bicarbonate
    calcium edetate s.
    s. carbonate
    s. channel blocker
    s. channel blocker toxicity
    s. chloride
    cromolyn s.
    dantrolene s.
    s. depletion
    fractional excretion of s. (FENa)
    s. hypochlorite
    s. nitroprusside
    s. thiopental
    s. thiosulfate
sodomy
Soemmerring
    S. ligament
    S. muscle
SOFA
    sepsis-related organ failure assessment
Sofsilk
    S. coated and braided suture
    S. nonabsorbable silk suture
soft
    s. catheter
    s. cervical collar
    s. palate
    S. Sack IV fluid warmer
    s. sign
    s. tissue
    s. tissue abscess
    s. tissue hand injury
    s. tissue infection
    s. tissue loss
Softgut surgical chromic catgut suture
Solanum dulcamara
soleal vein
soleus muscle
solid
    s. bone
    s. organ
    s. organ injury
    s. viscus injury
solubility
    lipid s.
Solu-Medrol
solution
    balanced electrolyte s. (BES)
    balanced salt s. (BSS)
    buffered saline s. (BSS)

    crystalloid s.
    Hibiclens antiseptic s.
    hypertonic saline s.
    lactated Ringer s. (LRS)
    LET s.
    polarizing s.
    polyethylene glycol electrolyte lavage s.
    Ringer s.
    saline s.
Soman nerve agent
somatic
    s. complaint
    s. muscle
    s. nerve
    s. nerve transmitted pain
    s. nervous system
somatosensory evoked potential (SSEP)
somatostatin
somnolence
    irritable s.
Somogyi phenomenon
Sonoclot coagulation and platelet function analyzer
sonography
    focused abdominal s.
sonorous
    s. rale
    s. rhonchi
SOP
    standard operation procedure
Sorbie calcaneal fracture classification
sorbitol
sore
    canker s.
sotalol
sound
    abnormal breath s.
    absent bowel s.
    adventitious breath s.
    aortic second s. (A2)
    bowel s. (BS)
    breath s.
    decreased bowel s.
    equal bilateral breath s.'s (EBBS)
    grunting breath s.
    gurgling bowel s.
    gurgling breath s.
    harsh breath s.
    heart s.
    high-pitched breath s.
    Korotkoff s.
    muscle s.
    pop s.
    snap s.
    vesicular breath s.
    wheezing breath s.
source
    oxygen s.

space
- anatomic dead s.
- danger s.
- dead s.
- Fowler dead s.
- intercostal s.
- intersphincteric s.
- ischiorectal s.
- joint s.
- retroperitoneal s.
- supralevator s.

space-occupying lesion

spacer
- bone s.
- suture s.

Spanish blue virgin silk suture

spasm
- infantile s.
- intestinal muscularis fiber s.
- laryngeal s.
- muscle s.

spasmodic
- s. croup
- s. stricture

spastic
- s. dysuria
- s. muscle

spatial disorientation

spatula
- nerve separator s.
- suture pickup s.

special care unit (SCU)

specialist
- critical care s.
- orthopaedic s.
- rehabilitation s.
- trauma s.

specialized computed tomographic scan

specialty
- 4 primary medical s.'s
- s. referral center

species
- Cicuta s.

specific
- s. organ injury
- s. therapy

specimen
- protected brush s. (PBS)

speck
- floating black s.

SPECT
- single-photon emission computed tomography

spectinomycin

spectroscopy
- mass s.
- near infrared s.
- nuclear magnetic resonance s.

spectrum
- antimicrobial s.
- s. of presentation

speech
- slurred s.
- tremulous s.

spell
- apneic s.
- breath-holding s.

spermatic
- s. nerve
- s. vein

spermatocele

sphenoethmoidal suture

sphenofrontal suture

sphenoid
- s. bone
- s. bone fracture
- s. emissary vein
- s. process
- s. sinus

sphenomalar suture

sphenomandibular ligament

sphenomaxillary suture

sphenooccipital suture

sphenoorbital suture

sphenopalatine nerve

sphenoparietal suture

sphenopetrosal suture

sphenosquamous suture

sphenotemporal suture

sphenovomerine suture

sphenozygomatic suture

sphincter
- internal s.
- s. muscle

sphincteral achalasia

sphincteralgia

sphygmomanometer

spica splint

spiculation
- bone s.

spicule
- bone s.

S

NOTES

spider
  s. angioma
  banana s.
  s. banana
  black varicosity
  black widow s.
  brown recluse s.
  funnel web s.
  red back s.
  s. telangiectasia
  s. vein
  widow s.
spigelian vein
spike
  pacer s.
  temperature s.
spill scald
spinal
  s. accessory nerve
  s. anesthesia
  s. column
  s. compression fracture
  s. cord concussion
  s. cord infection
  s. cord injury
  s. cord injury without radiographic
    abnormality (SCIWORA)
  s. cord laceration
  s. cord motor activity
  s. cord subluxation
  s. cord syndrome
  s. dislocation
  s. fracture
  s. immobilization
  s. muscle
  s. posterior ligament
  s. transverse ligament
  s. trauma
  s. vein
spindle
  muscle s.
  tendon s.
spindle-shaped muscle
spine
  anterior inferior iliac s. (AIIS)
  axial s.
  bamboo s.
  s. board
  cervical s.
  distraction of s.
  s. distraction
  s. fracture
  thoracolumbar s.
spinoglenoid ligament
spinothalamic tract injury
spinous
  s. process fracture
  s. tarsus ligament

spiral
  s. CT
  s. fracture
  s. oblique fracture
  s. oblique retinacular ligament
  s. tibial fracture
  s. vein
  s. wound
spirochetal bacterial infection
spirometry
  incentive s.
splanchnic
  s. nerve
  s. vein
splash
  lightning s.
splayed
  s. cranial suture
  s. facial nerve
spleen
  autotransplantation s.
  s. laceration
splenectomy
splenic
  s. artery aneurysm
  s. artery embolization
  s. bed drainage
  s. injury
  s. laceration
  s. rupture
  s. vein
  s. wrapping
splenocolic ligament
splenomegaly
  hemolytic s.
splenopancreatic ligament
splenorenal
  s. ligament
  s. shunt
splenosis
splint
  abduction finger s.
  abduction thumb s.
  adjustable s.
  air pressure s.
  Alumafoam s.
  ankle s.
  arm s.
  bipolar traction s.
  buddy s.
  fiberglass s.
  finger s.
  fracture s.
  gutter s.
  knee s.
  metal s.
  plaster of Paris s.
  pneumatic s.
  PneuSplint s.

posterior s.
pressure s.
rigid s.
Sager Combo-Pac adult/child and infant s.
Sager S304 bilateral s.
Sager S300 infant bilateral s.
Sager 2301 single s.
SAM s.
spica s.
thumb spica s.
traction s.
vacuum s.
volar plaster s.
wrist s.

splintered
s. bone
s. fracture

splinting
dynamic s.
s. of joint
s. technique

split
s. anterior tibial tendon
s. compression fracture

split-heel fracture
split-lung function study
splitting
s. fracture
muscle s.

spoke bone
spondylitis
ankylosing s.
juvenile ankylosing s. (JAS)

spondylolisthesis
spondylolysis
spondylosis
spongy bone
spontaneous
s. abortion
s. augmented low-volume ventilation
s. bacterial peritonitis (SBP)
s. breech delivery
s. combustion
s. fracture
s. involvement
s. miscarriage
s. ovulation
s. pneumothorax
s. respiration
s. termination of pregnancy

spontaneously bleeding gums
Sporanox
spore
Sporothrix
sporotrichosis
spot
cherry red s.
Tardieu s.
s. test

spotted bone
spousal abuse
spouse abuse
sprain
acute cervical traumatic s. (ACTS)
ankle s.
s. fracture
ligament rupture s.

spray
Cetacaine s.
ethyl chloride s.
Hurricaine s.

spread suture
Springer fracture
spring ligament
sprinter's fracture
sprouting
nerve s.

sprue
tropical s.

spur
bone s.

spurt muscle
sputum, pl. **sputa**
bloody s.
brownish-yellow s.
carbonaceous s.
s. culture
s. examination
frothy s.
s. Gram stain
green s.
pink s.
purulent s.
thick green s.
yellow s.

squamomastoid suture
squamooccipital bone
squamoparietal suture
squamosal suture
squamosomastoid suture
squamosoparietal suture
squamososphenoid suture

S

NOTES

squamous
- s. bone
- s. cell carcinoma
- s. suture

square muscle

squeeze
- ear s.
- lung s.
- middle ear s.
- s. test

squeezing chest pain

SRSA
- slow-reacting substance of anaphylaxis

S-SCORT VX-2 suction unit

SSEP
- somatosensory evoked potential

SSKI
- saturated solution of potassium iodide

SSSS
- staphylococcal scalded skin syndrome

SS suture

stability of fracture

stabilization
- airway s.
- cervical spine s.
- fracture s.
- initial s.
- maternal s.
- surgical s.

stabilizer
- kneecap s.

stabilizing
- s. ligament
- myocardial membrane s.

stable
- s. angina
- s. burst fracture
- hemodynamically s.
- s. patient
- s. for transfer
- vital signs s. (VSS)

STA-BLOCK head immobilizer

stab wound

stacked shocks

Staffing for Adequate Fire and Emergency Response (SAFER)

stage
- aural s.
- cicatrization s.
- defervescent s.
- prodromal s.

stain
- corneal rust s.
- Gram s.
- sputum Gram s.

staining
- bone marrow s.

stainless steel wire suture

stair chair

stairstep fracture

Stallard-Liegard suture

standard
- s. of care
- S. Nomenclature of Medicine (SNOMED)
- s. operation procedure (SOP)

standing
- no prolonged s.

Stanley cervical ligament

stapedius muscle

stapes bone

staphylococcal
- s. enterotoxin B
- s. exotoxin
- s. prosthetic valve endocarditis
- s. scalded skin syndrome (SSSS)

staphylococcus
- coagulase-negative s.

Staphylococcus aureus

staple
- skin s.
- surgical s.
- s. suture

START
- simple triage and rapid treatment

starvation

stasis
- zone of s.

Statak suture

state
- bone marrow failure s.
- hypercoagulable s.
- hyperosmolar s.
- hypnotic s.
- low flow s.
- postictal s.

statement of caregiver

static
- s. muscle
- s. symptom

station
- base s.
- gait and s.

statoacoustic nerve

status
- altered mental s. (AMS)
- change in mental s.
- s. epilepticus
- mental s.
- myoclonic s.
- neurologic s.
- nutrition s.
- s. post
- unexplained altered mental s.

stavudine

stay
- hospital s.
- ICU s.

intensive care unit s.
s. suture

STD
sexually transmitted disease
steatorrhea
steatosis
StediSpine collar
Steele intraarticular fracture type I–III classification
steel mesh suture
steeple sign
ST-elevation myocardial infarction (STEMI)
stellate
s. abscess
s. fracture
s. ligament
s. nail bed laceration
s. skull fracture
s. undepressed fracture
s. vein
stem
s. cell harvest
s. cell infusion
STEMI
ST-elevation myocardial infarction
stenosed
stenosis, pl. stenoses
aortic valve s.
graft s.
hypertrophic pyloric s.
idiopathic hypertrophic subaortic s.
mitral s.
pulmonic valvular s.
pyloric s.
subaortic s.
tendon sheath s.
tricuspid s.
vein graft s.
Stensen vein
stent
balloon-expandable tracheal s.
intracoronary s.
nonfunctioning s.
transjugular intrahepatic portosystemic shunt s. (TIPSS)
stenting
esophageal s.
stent-shunt
transjugular intrahepatic portosystemic s.-s.

step
unassisted s.
stepoff
s. of fracture
orbital s.
stercoral appendicitis
stercoralis
Strongyloides s.
stereoscopic
sterile
s. abscess
s. dressing
s. gauze dressing
s. pyuria-dysuria syndrome
sterilization
voluntary s.
Steri-Strip
steri-stripped
Sterna-Band self-locking suture
sternal
s. fracture
s. muscle
s. retraction
s. wire suture
sternochondroscapular muscle
sternoclavicular
s. joint injury
s. ligament
s. muscle
sternocleidomastoid
s. muscle
s. region
s. vein
sternocostal ligament
sternohyoid muscle
sternomastoid muscle
sternopericardial ligament
sternothyroid muscle
sternotomy
median s.
s. wound
sternum fracture
steroid
anabolic s.
s. myopathy
stethoscope
binaural s.
Cammann s.
differential s.
electronic s.
Stevens-Johnson syndrome

S

NOTES

STI
sexually transmitted infection
STI Medical Products PneuSplint
stick
needle s.
Stieda fracture
stiffness
endotracheal tube cuff s.
muscle s.
stigma
stillbirth
Stimson technique
stimulant
general s.
s. laxative
stimulation
adrenocorticotropic hormone s.
caloric s.
nerve root s.
stimulator
bone growth s.
nerve s.
stimulus
train-of-4 s.
sting
ant s.
arthropod s.
bee s.
fire ant s.
Hymenoptera s.
insect s.
marine organism s.
scorpion s.
wasp s.
stingray envenomation
stippling
basophilic s.
bone s.
stirrup
s. bone
s. slab
stitch
s. abscess
horizontal mattress s.
imbricated s.
interrupted s.
Kessler s.
3-point corner s.
St. John's Wort
stock
bone s.
stockinette
stocking
compression s.
graduated compression s. (GCS)
stockinglike burn
Stokes basket

stoma
loop s.
tracheal s.
stomach
herniated s.
perforated s.
s. rupture
stomatitis
Coxsackie s.
gangrenous s.
stone
s. fish antivenom
vein s.
stool
currant jelly s.
mahogany s.
melenic s.
s. in sigmoid
stopcock
3-way s.
store
carbon dioxide s.
storm
thyroid s.
stove-in chest
strabismus
comitant s.
straddle
s. fracture
s. injury
straight blade
strain
adductor muscle s.
cervical s.
s. fracture
medial collateral ligament s.
muscle s.
strait
dire s.
stramonium
Datura s.
strangulation
bowel s.
neck injury by s.
s. neuropathy
strap
ischial s.
s. muscle
nylon s.
torso s.
Velcro s.
strategy
wait-and-see s.
stratification
risk s.
strawberry cervix
street drug
strength
bone s.

double s. (DS)
muscle s.
pulse s.
wound tensile s.

strenuous activity
streptococcal
s. disease
s. toxic shock syndrome
Streptococcus
group A beta-hemolytic S.
streptokinase
streptomycin sulfate
stress
caregiver s.
causative s.
s. echocardiography
s. fracture
s. gastric ulceration
inversion s.
s. radiograph
s. test
s. testing
s. ulcer prophylaxis
stressor
environmental s.
personal s.
psychosocial s.
social s.
stress-related erosive syndrome
stretched out ligament
stretcher
basket s.
flexible s.
orthopaedic s.
1-person s.
2-person s.
portable s.
Reeves s.
roll-in s.
scoop s.
wheeled s.
stretching
nerve s.
striated muscle
striate vein
stricture
spasmodic s.
stridor
strip
Suture S.
stripe
anechoic s.

striped muscle
stripper
tendon s.
vein s.
stripping
vein s.
stroke
acidosis, epilepsy, insulin, overdose,
uremia, tumor, infection,
psychosis, and s. (AEIOU TIPS)
alcohol intoxication, epilepsy,
insulin, overdose, uremia, trauma,
infection, psychosis, and s.
(AEIOU TIPS)
dive-related s.
embolic s.
exertional heart s.
hemorrhagic s.
s. index (SI)
ischemic s.
lacunar s.
lightning s.
mini s.
return s.
thrombotic s.
s. volume (SV)
stroma, pl. **stromata**
nerve s.
strong pulse
Strongyloides stercoralis
structure
anechoic s.
strut
bone s.
s. fracture
Struthers ligament
strychnine toxicity
study
ancillary s.
Bezafibrate Infarction Prevention s.
blood chemistry s.
bone densitometry s.
bone density s.
bone length s.
bone mineral content s.
bone mineral density s.
CHEPER s.
s. of choice
coagulation s.
dose-ranging s.
double-blind s.
Framingham Heart S.

S

NOTES

study *(continued)*
    gastric emptying s.
    GRAPE pilot s.
    imaging s.
    IMPACT-II s.
    limited s.
    National Acute Spinal Cord
      Injury S. (NASCIS)
    National Emergency X-Radiography
      Utilization S. (NEXUS)
    nerve conduction velocity s.
    OPALS s.
    PIOPED s.
    placebo-controlled s.
    split-lung function s.
stuffy nose syndrome
stump
    s. of bone
    nerve s.
stunning
    atrial s.
    myocardial s.
stupor
    benign s.
    catatonic s.
    depressive s.
stuporous
    s. catatonia
    s. depression
Sturmdorf hemostatic suture
stye
stylet, stylette
    endotracheal s.
    lighted s.
styloauricular muscle
styloglossus muscle
stylohyoid
    s. ligament
    s. muscle
    s. nerve
styloid
    s. bone
    s. fracture
stylomandibular ligament
stylomastoid vein
stylomaxillary ligament
stylopharyngeal
    s. muscle
    s. nerve
Stylus cardiovascular suture
subacromial
    s. bursa
    s. position
subacromial-subdeltoid bursa
subacute
    s. abscess
    s. bacterial endocarditis (SBE)
subannular mattress suture

subaortic
    s. muscle
    s. stenosis
subaponeurotic abscess
subarachnoid
    s. coma
    s. hemorrhage
subcapital
    s. fracture
    s. hip fracture
subcardinal vein
subchondral
    s. bone
    s. fracture
subclavian
    s. muscle
    s. nerve
    s. vein
subcondylar fracture
subconscious
subcoracoid
    s. bone
    s. bursa
    s. position
subcostal
    s. muscle
    s. nerve
    s. vein
subcrural muscle
subcutaneous
    s. acromial bursa
    s. air
    s. calcaneal bursa
    s. emphysema
    s. fracture
    s. infrapatellar bursa
    s. olecranon bursa
    s. patellar bursa
    s. prepatellar bursa
    s. suture
    s. synovial bursa
    s. temporal nerve
    s. tissue
    s. trochanteric bursa
    s. vein
    s. wound
subcuticular
    s. continuous suture
    s. layer
subdeltoid bursa
subdiaphragmatic abscess
subdural
    s. hematoma
    s. infection
subependymal vein
subfascial
    s. abscess
    s. gauze pack
    s. prepatellar bursa

subhyoid bursa
subitum
 exanthema s.
subjective
 s., objective, assessment, plan
 (SOAP)
 s. symptom
Sublimaze
sublingual
 s. bursa
 s. medication
 s. nerve
 s. nitroglycerin
 s. vein
sublobular vein
subluxated tooth
subluxation
 atlantoaxial s.
 radial head s.
 spinal cord s.
 tendon s.
subluxation-dislocation
 arytenoid s.-d.
subluxed radial head
submandibular nerve
submaxillary nerve
submental
 s. region
 s. vein
submersion injury
submucosal
 s. vaginal muscle
 s. wound
subnitrate
 bismuth s.
suboccipital
 s. muscle
 s. nerve
subpectoral abscess
subperichondrial hematoma
subperiosteal
 s. bone
 s. fracture
subperitoneal appendicitis
subpleural air cyst
subquadricipital muscle
subsalicylate
 bismuth s.
subscapular
 s. abscess
 s. bursa
 s. muscle

 s. nerve
 s. vein
substance
 s. abuse
 s. abuse history
 bone s.
 caustic s.
 H s.
 s. intoxication
 s. misuse
 volatile s.
substernal chest pain
substitute
 Biobrane skin s.
 blood s.
 bone graft s.
substitution
 s. bone
 tendon s.
subtalar interosseous ligament
subtendinous
 s. bursa
 s. bursae of gastrocnemius muscle
subtentorial lesion
subtrochanteric
 s. femoral fracture
 s. fracture
subungual hematoma
subvertebral muscle
succinylcholine
sucking
 s. chest wound
 s. muscle
sucralfate
suction
 s. embolectomy
 s. machine
 nasogastric s.
 Res-Q-Vac handheld emergency s.
 wound incision and s.
suctioning
 deep tracheal s.
 orotracheal s.
Sudafed
sudden
 s. cardiac death
 s. death
 s. death syndrome
 s. exacerbation
 s. infant death syndrome (SIDS)
sudomotor nerve
suffocation

S

NOTES

sugar
    blood s. (BS)
    high blood s.
    low blood s.
suicidal
    s. gesture
    s. ideation
suicide
    physician-assisted s.
    s. risk evaluation
sulbactam
sulfacetamide
sulfadiazine
    silver s.
sulfamethoxazole
    trimethoprim and s. (TMP-SMX)
sulfasalazine
sulfate
    aluminum s.
    amikacin s.
    amphetamine s.
    atropine s.
    magnesium s.
    morphine s. (MS)
    netilmicin s.
    quinidine s.
    quinine s.
    streptomycin s.
sulfide
    hydrogen s.
sulfonamide antibiotic
sulfoxide
    dimethyl s. (DMSO)
sulfuric acid
sulindac
sumac
    poison s.
sumatriptan
sunburn
sunken fontanelle
sunrise radiograph
sunstroke
SuperChar activated charcoal
superciliary muscle
superficial
    s. burn
    s. circumflex iliac vein
    s. dorsal sacrococcygeal ligament
    s. dorsal vein
    s. epigastric vein
    s. femoral vein
    s. medial ligament
    s. middle cerebral vein
    s. muscle
    s. palmar vein
    s. perineal vein
    s. posterior sacrococcygeal ligament
    s. suture
    s. temporal vein

    s. tibiotalar ligament
    s. transverse metacarpal ligament
    s. transverse metatarsal ligament
    s. vertebral vein
    s. wound
superimposed preeclampsia
superior
    s. anastomotic vein
    s. astragalonavicular ligament
    s. azygos vein
    s. basal vein
    s. cerebellar vein
    s. cerebral vein
    s. choroid vein
    s. costotransverse ligament
    s. epigastric vein
    s. gluteal vein
    s. hemorrhoidal vein
    s. incudal ligament
    s. intercostal vein
    s. labial vein
    s. laryngeal vein
    s. lateral genicular vein
    s. mallear ligament
    s. maxillary bone
    s. medial genicular vein
    s. mesenteric vein
    s. nasal vein
    s. ophthalmic vein
    s. palpebral vein
    s. phrenic vein
    s. pubic ligament
    s. pulmonary vein
    s. recess of omental bursa
    s. rectal vein
    s. temporal vein
    s. thalamostriate vein
    s. thyroid vein
    s. transverse scapular ligament
    s. vena cava syndrome (SVCS)
supernumerary
    s. sesamoid bone
    s. tendon
superomedial calcaneonavicular ligament
superoxide dismutase
supination-adduction fracture
supination-eversion fracture
supination-external rotation fracture
supinator muscle
supine position
Supolene suture
supplemental oxygen
support
    advanced cardiac life s. (ACLS)
    advanced cardiovascular life s.
    advanced life s. (ALS)
    advanced trauma life s. (ATLS)
    base of s.
    basic cardiac life s. (BCLS)

basic life s. (BLS)
extracorporeal life s. (ECLS)
initial airway s.
life s.
mechanical s.
Ontario Prehospital Advanced
Life S. (OPALS)
pediatric advanced life s. (PALS)
pressure s. (PS)
supporting bone
supportive
s. care
s. measure
suppository
suppression
ACTH s.
adrenocortical s.
bone marrow s.
suppurativa
hidradenitis s.
suppurative
s. appendicitis
s. pericarditis
s. thrombophlebitis
supracardinal vein
supraclavicular
s. cannulation
s. muscle
s. nerve
s. retraction
supracondylar
s. femoral fracture
s. fracture
s. humeral fracture
s. Y-shaped fracture
suprahyoid muscle
supralevator
s. abscess
s. space
supramediastinal muscle
Supramid
S. bridle collagen suture
S. Extra suture
S. lens implant suture
supraoccipital bone
supraorbital
s. fracture
s. nerve
s. vein
suprapatellar bursa
supraperiosteal dental nerve block
suprapharyngeal bone

suprapubic
s. bladder aspiration
s. catheter
s. cystostomy
s. stab wound
suprarenal
s. aneurysm
s. vein
suprascapular
s. ligament
s. nerve
s. vein
suprasellar vein
supraspinal ligament
supraspinatus
s. muscle
s. nerve
s. tendon
supraspinous
s. ligament
s. muscle
suprasternal
s. bone
s. indrawing
s. notch
suprasyndesmotic fracture
supratentorial lesion
supratrochlear
s. nerve
s. vein
supraumbilical location
supraventricular
s. tachyarrhythmia
s. tachycardia (SVT)
supreme
s. cardiac nerve
s. intercostal vein
s. turbinate bone
Supreno EC one tough nitrile glove
sural
s. nerve
s. nerve block
surface
bone s.
s. of orbital zygomatic bone
s. thalamic vein
surfactant
s. laxative
s. replacement
s. therapy
Surgaloy metallic suture

S

NOTES

surgery
> ambulatory s.
> cardiothoracic s.
> cardiovascular s. (CVS)
> conservative s.
> exploratory s.
> fracture computer-aided s. (FRACAS)
> general s. (GS)
> major s.
> muscle s.
> orthopaedic s.
> palliative s.
> port-access s.
> previous abdominal s.
> radial s.
> thoracic s.
> video-assisted thoracic s.

surgical
> s. adhesive
> s. chromic suture
> s. erysipelas
> s. gastrostomy
> s. gut suture
> s. history
> s. intensive care unit (SICU)
> s. intervention
> s. jejunostomy
> s. linen suture
> s. neck fracture
> s. silk suture
> s. stabilization
> s. staple
> s. steel suture
> s. tape
> s. team
> s. treatment
> s. wound

Surgicraft suture
Surgidac suture
Surgidev suture
Surgigut suture
Surgilar suture
Surgilene blue monofilament polypropylene suture
Surgiloid suture
Surgilon
> S. braided nylon suture
> S. monofilament polypropylene suture

Surgilope suture
Surgilube
SurgiMed suture
Surgipro suture
Surgiset suture
surroundings at scene
surveillance colonoscopy
survey
> bone s.

primary s.
secondary s.

survival
> chain of s.
> nerve cell s.
> Third International Study of Infarct S. (ISIS-3)

susceptibility to high-altitude pulmonary edema (HAPE-S)
suspected
> s. ectopic pregnancy
> s. gestational thromboblastic disease

suspending suture
suspension
> oral s.
> s. suture

suspensory
> s. ligament
> s. muscle

suspicion
> s. of appendicitis
> s. of bowel ischemia
> high index of s.

suspicious
> s. burn
> s. history
> s. location

sustained conjugate upward gaze
sustentaculum tali fracture
Sutupak suture
sutural
> s. bone
> s. ligament

suture
> s. abscess
> absorbable s.
> Acier stainless steel s.
> Acufex bioabsorbable Suretac s.
> Acutrol s.
> adjustable external s.
> s. adjustment
> Albert s.
> Albert-Lembert s.
> Alcon s.
> already-threaded s.
> alternating s.
> aluminum-bronze wire s.
> American silk s.
> s. anastomosis
> anastomotic s.
> Ancap braided silk s.
> s. anchor
> anchor s.
> anchoring s.
> s. anchor shoulder repair
> s. anchor technique
> angiocatheter with looped polypropylene s.
> angle s.

anterior palatine s.
antibody-coated s.
antitorque s.
apical s.
Appolito s.
apposition of skull s.
approximation s.
Arroyo encircling s.
Arruga encircling s.
arterial silk s.
S. Assistant instrument
Atraloc s.
atraumatic braided silk s.
atraumatic chromic s.
Aureomycin s.
Auto S.
autoplastic s.
back wall s.
Barraquer silk s.
basal bunching s.
baseball s.
basilar s.
bastard s.
basting s.
Bell s.
bioabsorbable Dexon s.
Bio-FASTak s.
BioSorb s.
Biosyn synthetic monofilament s.
biparietal s.
16-bite nylon s.
black braided nylon s.
black braided silk s.
black silk s.
black silk sling s.
black twisted s.
Blalock s.
blanket s.
blue-black monofilament s.
blue twisted cotton s.
bolster s.
Bondek absorbable s.
bone wax s.
bony s.
Bozeman s.
braided Ethibond s.
braided Mersilene s.
braided Nurolon s.
braided nylon s.
braided polyamide s.
braided polyester s.
braided polyglactin s.

braided silk s.
braided Vicryl s.
braided wire s.
Bralon s.
bregmatomastoid s.
s. bridge
bridge s.
bridle s.
bronze wire s.
Brown-Sharp gauge s.
B&S gauge s.
bulb s.
bundle s.
Bunnell crisscross s.
Bunnell figure-eight s.
Bunnell wire pull-out s.
buried s.
s. button
button s.
cable wire s.
canaliculus rod and s.
capitonnage s.
Caprolactam s.
cardinal s.
Cardioflon s.
Cardionyl s.
cardiovascular Prolene s.
cardiovascular silk s.
Carrel s.
s. carrier
catgut s.
celluloid linen s.
cervical s.
chain s.
cheesewiring of s.
Chinese fingertrap s.
Chinese twisted silk s.
chloramine catgut s.
chromated catgut s.
chromic blue dyed s.
chromic catgut s.
chromic collagen s.
chromic gut s.
chromicized catgut s.
cinch s.
circular s.
circumcisional s.
s. clamp
s. clip forceps
s. closure
s. closure technique
clove-hitch s.

S

NOTES

suture *(continued)*

coated polyester s.
coated Vicryl Rapide s.
cocoon thread s.
collagen absorbable s.
compound s.
compression s.
Connell s.
continuous over-and-over s.
continuous running monofilament s.
continuous sling s.
Cooley U s.
core s.
corneoscleral s.
corner s.
coronal s.
cotton s.
cotton Deknatel s.
cotton nonabsorbable s.
cottony Dacron s.
cranial s.
cranial vault s.
CT1 s.
Cushing s.
s. cushion
Custodis s.
s. cutter
Czerny s.
Czerny-Lembert s.
Dacron bolstered s.
Dacron traction s.
Dafilon s.
Dagrofil s.
Davis-Geck s.
deep dermal s.
deep suspension s.
Deklene II cardiovascular s.
Deklene polypropylene s.
Deknatel silk s.
delayed s.
delayed closure of s.
dentate s.
denticulate s.
dermal s.
Dermalene polyethylene s.
Dermalon cuticular s.
Dexon absorbable synthetic
  polyglycolic acid s.
Dexon II s.
Dexon Plus s.
DG Softgut s.
diastasis of s.
s. diastasis
diastatic lambdoid s.
Docktor s.
dome-binding s.
Donati s.
double-armed wire s.
double right-angle s.

double-running penetrating
  keratoplasty s.
Dulox s.
Dupuytren s.
dural tack-up s.
Edinburgh s.
EEA Auto S.
elastic s.
en bloc running locking s.
Endoloop s.
end-to-end s.
end-to-side s.
epineurial s.
epiperineurial s.
epitendinous s.
epitenon s.
EPTFE vascular s.
Equisetene s.
Ethibond extra polyester s.
Ethibond polybutylate-coated
  polyester s.
Ethicon-Atraloc s.
Ethicon micropoint s.
Ethicon Sabreloc s.
Ethicon silk s.
Ethiflex retention s.
Ethilon nylon s.
ethmoidolacrimal s.
ethmoidomaxillary s.
everting mattress s.
expanded polytetrafluoroethylene s.
extrachromic s.
eyelid crease s.
Faden s.
s. failure
false s.
fascial s.
s. fatigue
fetal Y s.
figure-of-8 s.
filament s.
fine chromic s.
fine silk s.
fingertrap s.
fishmouth end-to-end s.
s. fixation
fixation s.
flat s.
Flaxedil s.
Flexitone s.
formaldehyde catgut s.
Foster s.
Fothergill s.
frontal s.
frontoethmoidal s.
frontolacrimal s.
frontomalar s.
frontomaxillary s.
frontonasal s.

frontoparietal s.
frontosphenoid s.
frontozygomatic s.
Frost s.
Furnas s.
furrier s.
Gaillard-Arlt s.
Gambee s.
gastrointestinal surgical gut s.
gastrointestinal surgical linen s.
gastrointestinal surgical silk s.
general closure s.
Giampapa s.
Gillies horizontal dermal s.
GI popoff silk s.
glue-in s.
s. of Goethe
Gore-Tex nonabsorbable s.
gossamer silk s.
Gould inverted mattress s.
s. granuloma
s. grasper forceps
grasping s.
green braided s.
green Mersilene s.
green monofilament
  polyglyconate s.
groove s.
Gruber s.
s. guide
Gussenbauer s.
gut s.
Guyton-Friedenwald s.
half-buried mattress s.
Halsted epitendinous s.
Halsted interrupted mattress s.
Halsted interrupted quilt s.
harelip s.
harmonic s.
Hatch s.
Heaney s.
heavy-gauge s.
heavy monofilament s.
heavy retention s.
heavy silk s.
heavy silk retention s.
heavy wire s.
helical s.
hemostatic s.
Herculon s.
s. holder
s. hole drill

horizontal dermal s.
horizontal mattress s.
Horsley s.
Hu-Friedy PermaSharp s.
IKI catgut s.
incisive s.
India rubber s.
infiltration s.
infraorbital s.
intercrural-septal s.
interdomal s.
interendognathic s.
interfascicular guide s.
intermaxillary s.
internal s.
internasal s.
interpalatine s.
interpalpebral s.
interparietal s.
interrupted loop mattress s.
interrupted manual mucomucosal
  absorbable s.
interrupted nylon s.
interrupted pledgeted s.
interrupted quilt s.
interrupted seromuscular s.
intracameral s.
intracuticular running s.
intradermal continuous s.
intrafascicular s.
intraluminal s.
inverted mattress s.
inverted subcuticular s.
inverting s.
Investa s.
iodine catgut s.
iodized surgical gut s.
iodochromic catgut s.
iris s.
Ivalon s.
Jobert de Lamballe s.
juxtalimbal s.
Kal-Dermic s.
kangaroo tendon s.
Kessler grasping s.
Kessler-Kleinert s.
Kessler-Tajima s.
Kirschner s.
Krackow s.
s. of Krause
Küstner s.
L-25 absorbable surgical s.

S

NOTES

suture *(continued)*

lacidem s.
lacrimoconchal s.
lacrimoethmoidal s.
lacrimomaxillary s.
lacrimoturbinal s.
lambdoid s.
lambdoidal cranial s.
lancet s.
s. lancet
Lang s.
Lapra-Ty s.
large-caliber nonabsorbable s.
lashing s.
lateral trap s.
lead s.
lead-shot tie s.
Le Dentu s.
Le Fort s.
Lembert inverting seromuscular s.
Lembert running s.
s. of lens
lens s.
Ligapak s.
s. ligated
s. ligation
s. ligature
limbal s.
limbous s.
Linatrix s.
Lindner corneoscleral s.
s. line
s. line cancer
s. line carcinoma
s. line dehiscence
linen thread s.
s. line ulceration
Linvatec meniscal BioStinger
  anchor s.
locking horizontal mattress s.
lockout s.
lock-stitch s.
S. Lok device
longitudinal s.
Look s.
looped polypropylene s.
loop mattress s.
Lukens catgut s.
lumbar s.
malar periosteum-SMAS flap
  fixation s.
malomaxillary s.
mamillary s.
Mannis s.
Marlex s.
Marshall U-stitch s.
Mason-Allen s.
mastoid s.
mastoid-conchal s.

s. material
mattress s.
Maxam s.
maxillofrontal s.
maxillojugal s.
maxillonasal s.
Maxon absorbable s.
Maxon delayed-absorbable s.
Mayo linen s.
McCannel s.
McLaughlin modification of
  Bunnell pull-out s.
McLean s.
Measuroll s.
medial crural s.
median palatine s.
Medrafil wire s.
Meigs s.
Mersilene braided nonabsorbable s.
Mersilk black silk s.
mesh s.
metal band s.
metallic s.
metopic s.
Micrins microsurgical s.
Micro-Glide corneal s.
MicroMite anchor s.
micropoint s.
middle palatine s.
mild chromic s.
Millipore s.
Miralene s.
modified Frost s.
modified Kessler s.
modified Kessler-Tajima s.
Monocryl poliglecaprone s.
monofilament absorbable s.
monofilament clear s.
monofilament green s.
monofilament nonabsorbable s.
monofilament nylon s.
monofilament polypropylene s.
monofilament skin s.
monofilament steel s.
monofilament wire s.
Monosof s.
multifilament steel s.
multistrand s.
muscle-to-bone s.
Mustardé s.
nail s.
nasal s.
nasofrontal s.
nasomaxillary s.
natural s.
Needle-Less S.
nerve s.
neurocentral s.
neurosurgical s.

Nicoladoni s.
Nissen s.
nonabsorbable mattress s.
nonabsorbable surgical s.
nonfusion of cranial s.
nonresorbable s.
Novafil s.
Nurolon s.
nylon 66 s.
nylon monofilament s.
nylon retention s.
occipital s.
occipitomastoid s.
occipitoparietal s.
occipitosphenoid s.
occipitosphenoidal s.
oiled silk s.
opaque wire s.
Ophthalon s.
over-and-over s.
overlapping s.
overriding of s.
Oyloidin s.
Pagenstecher linen thread s.
palatine s.
palatoethmoidal s.
palatomaxillary s.
Palfyn s.
s. palpation
Panacryl s.
Panalok absorbable s.
Pancoast s.
Paré s.
parietal s.
parietomastoid s.
parietooccipital s.
parietosquamous s.
parietotemporal s.
Parker-Kerr basting s.
s. passer
passing s.
patent s.
PDS II Endoloop s.
PDS Vicryl s.
Pearsall Chinese twisted s.
Pearsall silk s.
s. penile laceration
perianal s.
periareolar pursestring s.
pericostal s.
perineurial s.
Perlon s.

Perma-Hand braided silk s.
permanent mattress s.
PermaSharp PGA s.
persistent frontal s.
persistent metopic s.
petrobasilar s.
petroclival s.
petrosphenobasilar s.
petrosphenooccipital s.
petrosquamosal s.
petrosquamous s.
petrotympanic s.
s. pickup hook
s. pickup spatula
pickup spatula s.
pin s.
pink twisted cotton s.
plain catgut s.
plain collagen s.
plain gut s.
plastic s.
pledgeted Ethibond s.
pledgeted mattress s.
plicating s.
plication s.
s. plication
poliglecaprone s.
polyamide s.
polybutester s.
Polydek s.
polydioxanone s. (PDS)
polyester fiber s.
polyethylene s.
polyfilament s.
polyglactic acid s.
polyglactin 910 s.
polyglecaprone 25 s.
polyglycol s.
polyglycolate s.
polyglycolic acid s.
polyglyconate s.
polypropylene button s.
Polysorb s.
popoff s.
posterior fixation s.
posterior palatine s.
postplaced s.
premature closure of coronal s.
prematurely closed s.
premaxillary s.
PremiCron nonabsorbable s.
Premilene s.

NOTES

suture *(continued)*
    preplaced s.
    presphenoethmoid s.
    primary s.
    Prolene polypropylene s.
    Pronova s.
    Proxi-Strip s.
    pterygomaxillary s.
    pullout s.
    Pulvertaft end-to-end s.
    Pulvertaft interweave s.
    Pulvertaft weave s.
    Purlon s.
    pursestring s.
    s. pusher talofibular joint
    PVB s.
    pyoktanin catgut s.
    pyroglycolic acid s.
    Quickert s.
    quilted s.
    quilting s.
    Ramsey County pyoktanin catgut s.
    Rankin s.
    Rapide wound s.
    rapid gut s.
    RB1 s.
    reabsorbable s.
    s. rectopexy
    s. rectopexy with sigmoid resection
    reinforcing s.
    relaxation s.
    releasable s.
    retention s.
    retracting s.
    rhabdoid s.
    ribbon gut s.
    s. ring
    rip-cord s.
    s. rotation
    s. rotation technique
    rubber s.
    running continuous s.
    running intradermal s.
    running locking s.
    running nylon penetrating keratoplasty s.
    Sabreloc s.
    Saenger s.
    safety-bolt s.
    Safil synthetic absorbable surgical s.
    sagittal cranial s.
    scleral flap s.
    secondary s.
    s. separation
    seromuscular Lembert s.
    SERRALNYL s.
    SERRALSILK s.
    serrated s.

    setback s.
    seton s.
    s. shape shifter
    Sharpoint ophthalmic microsurgical s.
    Shirodkar s.
    Shoch s.
    shoelace s.
    shotted s.
    SH popoff s.
    Siemens PTCA open heart s.
    silicone-treated surgical silk s.
    silk braided s.
    silk Mersilene s.
    silk nonabsorbable s.
    silk popoff s.
    silk retention s.
    silk stay s.
    silk traction s.
    silkworm gut s.
    Silky Polydek s.
    silverized catgut s.
    silver wire s.
    simple flaring s.
    simple running s.
    Sims s.
    single-armed s.
    single running s.
    skin s.
    s.'s of skull
    skull base s.
    sling s.
    s. sling
    Snellen s.
    Sofsilk coated and braided s.
    Sofsilk nonabsorbable silk s.
    Softgut surgical chromic catgut s.
    s. spacer
    Spanish blue virgin silk s.
    sphenoethmoidal s.
    sphenofrontal s.
    sphenomalar s.
    sphenomaxillary s.
    sphenooccipital s.
    sphenoorbital s.
    sphenoparietal s.
    sphenopetrosal s.
    sphenosquamous s.
    sphenotemporal s.
    sphenovomerine s.
    sphenozygomatic s.
    splayed cranial s.
    spread s.
    squamomastoid s.
    squamoparietal s.
    squamosal s.
    squamosomastoid s.
    squamosoparietal s.
    squamososphenoid s.

squamous s.
SS s.
stainless steel wire s.
Stallard-Liegard s.
staple s.
Statak s.
stay s.
steel mesh s.
Sterna-Band self-locking s.
sternal wire s.
S. Strip
S. Strip Plus
s. Strip Plus wound closure
Sturmdorf hemostatic s.
Stylus cardiovascular s.
subannular mattress s.
subcutaneous s.
subcuticular continuous s.
superficial s.
Supolene s.
Supramid bridle collagen s.
Supramid Extra s.
Supramid lens implant s.
Surgaloy metallic s.
surgical chromic s.
surgical gut s.
surgical linen s.
surgical silk s.
surgical steel s.
Surgicraft s.
Surgidac s.
Surgidev s.
Surgigut s.
Surgilar s.
Surgilene blue monofilament
  polypropylene s.
Surgiloid s.
Surgilon braided nylon s.
Surgilon monofilament
  polypropylene s.
Surgilope s.
SurgiMed s.
Surgipro s.
Surgiset s.
suspending s.
suspension s.
Sutupak s.
swaged s.
swaged-on s.
Swedgeon s.
Swiss blue virgin silk s.
synthetic absorbable s.

Synthofil s.
s. system
tacking s.
tag s.
s. tag forceps
Tajima modified Kessler s.
tantalum wire monofilament s.
Tapercut s.
tarsal s.
Techstar percutaneous s.
Teflon-coated Dacron s.
Teflon-pledgeted s.
temporal s.
temporomalar s.
temporozygomatic s.
tendon s.
tension s.
tension-requiring s.
tentalum wire tension s.
Tevdek pledgeted s.
Thermo-Flex s.
Thiersch s.
thread s.
through-and-through continuous s.
through-and-through reabsorbable s.
through-the-wall mattress s.
Ti-Cron s.
tiger gut s.
Tinel s.
tip-refining s.
Tom Jones s.
tongue suspension s.
traction s.
transdomal s.
transfixation s.
transfixion s.
transition s.
transosseous s.
transscleral s.
transverse palatal s.
transverse palatine s.
true s.
twisted cotton s.
twisted dermal s.
twisted linen s.
twisted virgin silk s.
tympanomastoid s.
tympanosquamosal s.
tympanosquamous s.
Tyrrell-Gray s.
U s.
s. ulcer

NOTES

S

suture *(continued)*
UltraFix MicroMite anchor s.
umbilical tape s.
unabsorbable s.
undyed s.
uninterrupted s.
USP#2 s.
uteroparietal s.
vascular silk s.
Verhoeff s.
vertical mattress s.
vertical plication s.
Vicryl popoff s.
Vicryl Rapide s.
Vicryl SH s.
Vienna wire s.
virgin silk s.
Viro-Tec s.
wedge-and-groove s.
white braided silk s.
white nylon s.
white twisted s.
wide cranial s.
wing s.
s. wire
s. wire cutting scissors
wire Zytor s.
Worst s.
Y s.
Z s.
ZF s.
zygomatic s.
zygomaticofrontal s.
zygomaticomaxillary s.
zygomaticosphenoid s.
zygomaticotemporal s.
suxamethonium
SV
stroke volume
SVCS
superior vena cava syndrome
SVO$_2$
venous oxygen saturation
SVRI
systemic vascular resistance index
SVT
supraventricular tachycardia
swab
wound s.
swaged-on suture
swaged suture
swallow
Gastrografin s.
Swan-Ganz catheter
sweat
thermal s.
Swedgeon suture
sweep
finger s.

swelling
deformity, contusion, abrasion,
puncture/penetrating wound, burn,
tenderness, laceration, s. (DCAP-
BTLS)
oropharyngeal s.
salivary gland s.
testicular s.
swinging flashlight test
Swiss blue virgin silk suture
sylvian vein
Symadine
Syme amputation
Symmetrel
symmetrical chest expansion
symmetric chest wall rise and fall
symmetry
facial s.
sympathetic
s. nerve
s. ophthalmia
s. symptom
sympathoadrenal axis
sympathomimetic
s. intoxication
s. poisoning
s. syndrome
symphysial fracture
symphysis pubis
symptom
acute on chronic s.'s
s. of alcohol withdrawal
cardinal s.
characteristic s.
concomitant s.
consecutive s.
constellation of s.'s
constitutional s.
dearth of s.'s
equivocal s.
general s.
GI s.
induced s.
local s.
localizing s.
objective s.
pathognomonic s.
precursor s.
premonitory s.
presenting s.
prodromal s.
reflex s.
sign and s.
signal s.
static s.
subjective s.
sympathetic s.
systemic s.
Uhthoff s.

urinary s.'s
withdrawal s.'s

symptomatic
s. treatment
s. vasospasm

symptomatology
depressive s.

synchondritic fracture

synchronized
s. atrial fibrillation
s. atrial flutter
s. coronary venous retroperfusion
s. intermittent mandatory ventilation
(SIMV)
s. supraventricular tachycardia

syncopal episode

syncope
neurocardiogenic s.

syndesmotic ligament

syndrome
abdominal compartment s.
acquired immunodeficiency s.
(AIDS)
acute coronary s. (ACS)
acute respiratory distress s.
(ARDS)
acute tumor lysis s.
adult respiratory distress s. (ARDS)
air leak s.
alcohol withdrawal s.
Alice in Wonderland s.
anterior spinal artery s.
anticholinergic s.
aspiration s.
battered child s.
battered spouse s.
Beckwith-Wiedemann s.
Boerhaave s.
Brown s.
Brown-Séquard s.
Budd-Chiari s.
burning hands s.
carcinoid s.
Carney s.
carpal tunnel s.
cauda equina s.
central cord s. (CCS)
central herniation s.
cerebral hyperperfusion s.
cerebro-oculo-facio-skeletal s.
Chinese restaurant s.
Churg-Strauss s.

compartment s.
compensatory antiinflammatory
response s.
complex regional pain s. type 1
(CRPS-1)
conus medullaris s.
cord hemisection s.
Cornelia de Lange s.
CREST s.
crush s.
crush injury s.
Cushing s.
Dandy-Walker s.
de Lange s.
dialysis disequilibrium s.
DiGeorge s.
distal intestinal obstruction s.
disulfiram-alcohol s.
Down s.
Dressler s.
drug-induced acute coronary s.
Dubin-Johnson s.
Eaton-Lambert s.
Ehlers-Danlos s.
Eisenmenger s.
embolic s.
fat embolism s. (FES)
fetal alcohol s. (FAS)
fibrinogen-fibrin conversion s.
Fitz-Hugh-Curtis s.
Goldenhar s.
Goodpasture s.
Guillain-Barré s.
Hantavirus cardiopulmonary s.
HELLP s.
hemolytic uremic s. (HUS)
hemophagocytic s.
hemorrhagic fever with renal s.
(HFRS)
hepatorenal s.
herniation s.
high T_4 s.
Horner s.
HSE s.
Hurler s.
hyperkinetic s.
hyperosmolar s.
hyperparathyroid s.
hyperventilation s.
hyperviscosity s. (HVS)
ileocecal s.
impingement s.

S

NOTES

syndrome *(continued)*
s. of inappropriate antidiuretic hormone (SIADH)
s. of inappropriate antidiuretic hormone secretion
intestinal obstruction s.
irritable bowel s. (IBS)
Kawasaki s.
Klippel-Feil s.
Korsakoff s.
Lambert-Eaton myasthenic s.
Landry-Guillain-Barré s.
lateral pressure s.
locked-in s.
lupuslike s.
Mallory-Weiss s.
marasmus s.
Marfan s.
massive transfusion s.
metal oxide fume s.
milk-alkali s.
multiorgan dysfunction s.
multiple organ dysfunction s. (MODS)
Münchausen s.
nephritic s.
nephronic s.
nephrotic s.
nerve compression s.
nerve compression-degeneration s.
nerve entrapment s.
nerve root s.
neuroleptic malignant s. (NMS)
Noonan s.
Ogilvie s.
Osler-Weber-Rendu s.
Parinaud s.
penetration s.
Pierre Robin s.
pinch-off s.
postconcussion s.
postconcussive s.
posterior cord s.
postpericardiotomy s.
postphlebitic s.
postshunt hepatorenal s.
preexcitation s.
prodromal s.
prolonged Q-T s.
pulmonary overpressurization s. (POPS)
pulmonary renal s.
QT-interval s.
rabbit s.
Ramsay Hunt s.
reactive airway dysfunction s.
refeeding s.
Reiter s.
respiratory distress s. (RDS)

Reye s.
Rotor s.
scalded skin s.
Seckel s.
second impact s.
sedative-hypnotic withdrawal s.
sepsis s.
serotonin s.
severe acute respiratory s. (SARS)
shaken baby s.
shaken impact s.
Sheehan s.
shock bowel s.
short bowel s.
sicca s.
sick sinus s.
Sjögren s.
Smith-Lemli-Opitz s.
spinal cord s.
staphylococcal scalded skin s. (SSSS)
sterile pyuria-dysuria s.
Stevens-Johnson s.
streptococcal toxic shock s.
stress-related erosive s.
stuffy nose s.
sudden death s.
sudden infant death s. (SIDS)
superior vena cava s. (SVCS)
sympathomimetic s.
systemic inflammatory response s. (SIRS)
tachycardia-bradycardia s.
temporomandibular joint s.
thoracic outlet s.
toxic s.
toxic shock s. (TSS)
Treacher Collins s.
tumor compression s.
tumor lysis s.
Turner s.
washout s.
Waterhouse-Friderichsen s.
Wellen s.
withdrawal s.
Wolff-Parkinson-White s.
WPW s.
Zollinger-Ellison s.

Synercid
synergic muscle
synergistic
s. gangrene
s. muscle
s. necrotizing cellulitis
synergy
synovial
s. bursa
s. ligament

s. sheath
s. trochlear bursa
synovitis
toxic s.
synovium
joint s.
Synthaderm foam
synthesis, pl. **syntheses**
muscle protein s.
synthetic
s. absorbable suture
s. bone
Synthofil suture
syphilis
bone s.
syphilitic aneurysm
syringe
bulb s.
Luer-type s.
syrup
ipecac s.
s. of ipecac
system
autonomic nervous s.
basolateral membrane transport s.
Bentley autotransfusion s.
bicarbonate buffer s.
Broselow-Hinkle pediatric
emergency s.
Broselow-Luten s.
cardiac conduction s.
cardiovascular s. (CVS)
central nervous s. (CNS)
chloracne grading s.
electronic patient care reporting s.
electronic PCR s.
emergency medical service s.
(EMSS)
fracture computer-aided surgery s.
gastrointestinal s. (GIS)
genitourinary s. (GUS)
incident command s.
incident management s. (IMS)

integumentary s.
Lauge-Hansen s.
Mapleson D breathing s.
MESS s.
muscle tone inhibitor s.
Oxygen Tank Lift S.'s
Oxylator positive pressure
resuscitation and inhalation s.
peripheral nervous s. (PNS)
renin-angiotensin-aldosterone s.
respiratory s.
reticuloendothelial s. (RES)
review of s.'s (ROS)
simple triage and rapid
treatment s.
somatic nervous s.
suture s.
Therapeutic Intervention Scoring S.
(TISS)
Toxic Exposure Surveillance S.
(TESS)
trauma care s.
vein s.
voluntary nervous s.
Wound Stick measuring s.
systemic
s. anesthetic conscious sedation
s. disease
s. effect
s. inflammatory manifestation
s. inflammatory response syndrome
(SIRS)
s. involvement
s. lupus erythematosus (SLE)
s. mastocytosis
s. perfusion
s. symptom
s. vascular resistance
s. vascular resistance index (SVRI)
s. vein
systolic
s. blood pressure (SBP)
s. hypertension

S

NOTES

297

T

T condylar fracture
T fracture
T wave
T-2 mycotoxin
TAB
threatened abortion
tabacum
Nicotiana t.
table
fracture t.
tablet
fixed-dose oral contraceptive t.
oral disintegrating t. (ODT)
Tabun nerve agent
TAC
tetracaine, adrenaline, cocaine
TAC anesthesia
tachyarrhythmia
supraventricular t.
wide-complex t.
tachycardia
antidromic atrioventricular
reentrant t.
atrial t.
chaotic atrial t.
ectopic atrial t. (EAT)
incessant atrial t.
intraatrial reentrant t.
multifocal atrial t. (MAT)
nodal t.
nonparoxysmal atrioventricular
junctional t.
nonsustained ventricular t.
orthodromic t.
pacemaker-mediated t.
paroxysmal atrial t. (PAT)
paroxysmal reentrant
supraventricular t.
paroxysmal supraventricular t.
(PSVT)
polymorphic ventricular t. (PVT)
pulseless ventricular t.
QRS complex t.
reflex t.
sinus t.
supraventricular t. (SVT)
synchronized supraventricular t.
ventricular t. (VT)
wide-complex sinus t.
tachycardia-bradycardia syndrome
tachydysrhythmia
tachypnea
tacking suture
Tacrolimus

tactile
t. fever
t. fremitus
tag
Smart Tag triage t.
t. suture
triage t.
TAH
total artificial heart
tail bone
tailor's muscle
Tajima modified Kessler suture
Takayasu arteritis
talar
t. avulsion fracture
t. dome fracture
t. neck fracture
t. osteochondral fracture
t. tendon
t. tilt
talc ingestion
talocalcaneal interosseous ligament
talocalcaneonavicular ligament
talofibular ligament
talonavicular
t. bone
t. ligament
talus
t. body fracture
t. bone
Tambocor
Tamiflu
tamoxifen
tamponade
balloon t.
cardiac t.
nasal balloon t.
neoplastic pericardial t.
pericardial t.
tangential wound
tangle of hemorrhoidal veins
tannic
t. acid
t. acid toxicity
tantalum wire monofilament suture
tape
Broselow emergency t.
Broselow pediatric resuscitative t.
buddy t.
surgical t.
Tapercut suture
tapeworm infestation
taping
buddy t.
tarantula bite

T

Tardieu spot
tardive dyskinesia
target bone
tarsal
  t. bone
  t. bone fracture
  t. injury
  t. interosseous ligament
  t. laceration
  t. muscle
  t. suture
  t. tunneld
tarsometatarsal ligament
taste nerve
tattoo hole
Taxus
  T. canadensis
  T. cuspidata
Tazicef
Tazidime
Tazocin
TB
  tuberculosis
TBB
  transbronchial biopsy
TBI
  traumatic brain injury
T-boned
TBSA
  total body surface area
TC
  traffic collision
TCD
  transcranial Doppler
TCIE
  transient cerebral ischemic episode
TCP
  transcutaneous cardiac pacing
teacup fracture
team
  critical care t.
  disaster medical assistance t.
    (DMAT)
  flight t.
  HazMat t.
  operative t.
  surgical t.
  trauma response t.
  treating t.
  ventilator management t.
tear
  artificial t.'s
  bladder t.
  t. gas
  intimal t.
  ligament t.
  Mallory-Weiss t.
  tendon t.

  tracheobronchial t.
  traumatic aortic t.
teardrop burst fracture
teardrop-shaped flexion-compression
    fracture
technetium
  t. 99m isonitrile
  t. 99m scanning
technician
  cardiac care t.
  cardiac rescue t.
  emergency medical t. (EMT)
  National Registry of Emergency
    Medical T.'s (NREMT)
technician–advanced
  emergency medical t.-a. (EMT-A)
technician–basic
  emergency medical t.-b. (EMT-B)
technician–intermediate
  emergency medical t.-i. (EMT-I)
technician–paramedic
  emergency medical t.-p. (EMT-P)
technique
  bag-valve-mask t.
  bandaging t.
  bent-arm drag t.
  blanket drag t.
  bone marrow stimulating t.
  bone transport t.
  clothing drag t.
  crossed-finger t.
  direct carry t.
  direct ground lift t.
  Ellis t.
  enzyme multiplied immunoassay t.
    (EMIT)
  esophageal obturator intubation t.
  extremity lift t.
  Fick t.
  finger sweep t.
  forced-air t.
  log roll t.
  muscle mobilizing t.
  nerve stimulator anesthetic t.
  nerve suture t.
  power grip t.
  power lift t.
  power squat t.
  pressure-washing t.
  rapid sequence induction t.
  splinting t.
  Stimson t.
  suture anchor t.
  suture closure t.
  suture rotation t.
  2 thumb-encircling hands t.
technology
  Adaptiv biphasic t.
Techstar percutaneous suture

tectoral ligament
TEE
  transesophageal echocardiography
teeth (*pl. of* tooth)
Teflon-coated Dacron suture
Teflon-pledgeted suture
Tegaderm dressing
Tegasorb dressing
teichoic acid antibody
teicoplanin
telangiectasia
  calcinosis, Raynaud syndrome,
    esophageal dysmotility,
    scleroderma, and t. (CREST)
  spider t.
telecanthus
telencephalic vein
telescoping septal fracture
temperature
  ambient t.
  axillary t.
  basal body t.
  body t.
  core body t.
  maximum t.
  minimum t.
  oral t.
  rectal t.
  t. spike
temporal
  t. arteritis
  t. bone
  t. bone fracture
  t. contusion
  t. diploic vein
  t. muscle
  t. nerve
  t. region
  t. suture
temporalis muscle
temporary pacemaker
temporizing measure
temporomalar
  t. nerve
  t. suture
temporomandibular
  t. joint (TMJ)
  t. joint injury
  t. joint syndrome
  t. ligament
  t. nerve
temporomaxillary vein

temporoparietal muscle
temporoparietal-occipital region
temporozygomatic suture
TEN
  toxic epidermal necrolysis
tender eye
tenderness
  abdominal t.
  bony t.
  cervical motion t.
  costovertebral angle t. (CVAT)
  nonspecific t.
  palpable t.
  rebound t.
tendinitis, tendonitis
  bicipital t.
tendinotrochanteric ligament
tendinum
  juncturae t.
tendon
  abductor digiti quinti t.
  abductor hallucis t.
  abductor pollicis brevis t.
  abductor pollicis longus t.
  accessory communicating t.
  Achilles t.
  adductor hallucis t.
  adductor magnus t.
  adductor pollicis brevis t.
  adherent profundus t.
  t. adhesion
  t. advancement
  anchoring t.
  anterior tibial t.
  anterior tibialis t.
  t. aponeurosis
  t. attenuation
  biceps brachii t.
  biceps femoris t.
  bicipital t.
  bifid biceps t.
  boomerang t.
  t. bowing
  brachial plexus t.
  Brown t.
  t. bundle
  calcaneal t.
  canthal t.
  t. carrier
  t. cartilage
  t. cell
  central t.

NOTES

T

tendon *(continued)*

t. centralization
central perineal t.
t. changing qigong
t. checkrein procedure
common anular t.
common extensor t.
communis t.
conjoined t.
coronary t.
t. corpuscle
cricoesophageal t.
deep flexor t.
digital extensor t.
digital flexor t.
t. dislocation
t. disorder
t. displacement
elbow extensor t.
t. entrapment
t. excursion
extensor t.
false t.
flexor t.
t. friction rub
Gerlach anular t.
Golgi t.
t. grabber
gracilis t.
t. graft
t. grafting
hamstring t.
Hector t.
heel t.
iliopsoas t.
t. implant
t. inflammation
infrapatellar t.
infraspinatus t.
t. injury
t. insertion
intermediate t.
interosseous t.
t. interposition arthroplasty
t. irregularity
t. jerk
lacerated t.
t. laceration
lateral canthal t.
lateral rectus t.
t. leader
t. lengthening
Lockwood t.
long abductor t.
long head biceps t.
longitudinal split biceps t.
lumbrical t.
masseter t.
medial canthal t.

membranaceous t.
midpatellar t.
t. necrosis
t. needle
t. nodularity
t. nodule
oblique t.
ocular t.
palmaris brevis t.
palmaris longus t.
t. palpation
t. passer
patellar t.
pectoralis minor t.
t. plasty
t. plate
t. plica
posterior tibial t.
postoperative flexor t.
t. prosthesis
pulley t.
quadriceps t.
t. reaction
t. rebalancing
t. release
t. repair
rerouted t.
rider's t.
rotator cuff t.
t. rupture
sartorius t.
t. sheath
t. sheath irrigation
t. sheath space infection
t. sheath stenosis
t. sheath thickening
t. shortening
t. sling
slipped t.
t. snapping
snapping t.
t. spindle
split anterior tibial t.
t. stretch reflex
t. stripper
t. subluxation
t. substitution
supernumerary t.
supraspinatus t.
t. suture
talar t.
t. tear
thumb extensor t.
thumb flexor t.
tibial t.
t. tissue
Todaro t.
toe extensor t.
t. transfer

t. transplantation
t. transposition
t. trapping
trefoil t.
triceps t.
trifoliate central t.
t. tucker
t. tunneler
t. unction
wing t.
wrist extensor t.
t. xanthoma
Zinn t.
t. Z-lengthening
tendonitis (*var. of* tendinitis)
tennis fracture
tenodesis
tenosynovitis
de Quervain stenosing t.
flexor t.
tense joint effusion
tension
alveolar oxygen t.
t. fracture
t. headache
muscle t.
oxygen pressure t.
t. pneumothorax
t. suture
wound t.
tension-requiring suture
tentalum wire tension suture
tented T wave
tenting of skin
tentorial
t. laceration
t. nerve
tenuous situation
Tequin
terbutaline therapy
teres
t. major muscle
t. minor muscle
terminal
t. nerve
t. repolarization
t. resuscitation
t. vein
termination of resuscitation (TOR)
terpene
Terry Thomas sign
tertiary care

TESS
Toxic Exposure Surveillance System
test
Allen t.
Apley t.
arterial blood gas t.
Bárány t.
battery of t.'s
breath t.
Breathalyzer t.
D–dimer t.
deferoxamine challenge t.
dipstick t.
dithionite urine t.
double-blind edrophonium t.
ferric chloride t.
fistula t.
forced duction t.
Fudaka stepping t.
glucagon stimulation t.
glucose tolerance t. (GTT)
Heaf tuberculosis t.
Hennebert pressure t.
hypoxemia t.
ice water caloric t.
immunoassay t.
intranasal palpation t.
Kleihauer-Betke t.
Lee-Jones t.
long ACTH stimulation t.
McMurray t.
Monospot t.
mucin clot t.
muscle enzyme t.
nerve compression t.
nerve conduction velocity t.
nerve excitability t.
positive t.
pregnancy t.
provocation t.
provocative t.
pulmonary function t. (PFT)
t. results
Romberg t.
serum pregnancy t.
spot t.
squeeze t.
stress t.
swinging flashlight t.
thyroid function t. (TFT)
transillumination t.

T

NOTES

test *(continued)*
  urine pregnancy t.
  whiff t.
testes *(pl. of* testis)
testicular
  t. pain
  t. swelling
  t. torsion
  t. vein
testing
  cardiac t.
  ligament stress t.
  muscle strength t.
  nerve involvement t.
  pulmonary function t. (PFT)
  serologic t.
  skin t.
  stress t.
testis, pl. **testes**
  t. fracture
  high-riding t.
  transverse lie of t.
tetani
  Clostridium t.
tetanus
  t. antitoxin
  diphtheria, pertussis, t. (DPT)
  t. immune globulin
  local t.
  t. prophylaxis
  t. toxoid booster
tetracaine
  t., adrenaline, cocaine (TAC)
  lidocaine, epinephrine, t. (LET)
tetrachloride
  carbon t.
tetracycline antibiotic
9-tetrahydrocannabinol
tetralogy
  Fallot t.
  t. of Fallot
tetranitrate
  erythrityl t.
tetrodotoxin fish poisoning
Teutleben ligament
Tevdek pledgeted suture
TFT
  thyroid function test
THA
  total hip arthroplasty
thalamic
  t. fracture
  t. hemorrhage
  t. vein
thalamostriate vein
thalassemia
  sickle cell t.
thallium-201 scintigraphy
thallium poisoning

thebesian vein
The Center for Pediatric Emergency Medicine (CPEM)
Theile muscle
thenar muscle
theophylline
  t. intoxication
  t. poisoning
theory
  3-column spinal stability t.
therapeutic
  t. abortion
  t. alliance
  t. blood range
  t. efficacy
  t. intervention
  T. Intervention Scoring System (TISS)
  t. paralysis
  t. plasma concentration
  t. plasma exchange
therapist
  respiratory t.
therapy
  adenosine t.
  adjuvant t.
  aerosol t.
  alkalinization t.
  alpha-adrenergic t.
  aminocaproic acid t.
  aminoglycoside t.
  amphotericin t.
  ancillary t.
  antiarrhythmic t.
  antidiarrheal t.
  anti-digoxin Fab t.
  antihypertensive t.
  antioxidant t.
  antiparasitic t.
  antiplatelet t.
  antipyretic t.
  antivenin t.
  antiviral t.
  arginine t.
  aspirin t.
  benzylpenicillin t.
  beta lactam t.
  bicarbonate t.
  bland-aerosol t.
  calcium salt t.
  cardiac reperfusion t.
  cathartic t.
  cerebral reperfusion t.
  chelation t.
  chest physical t.
  colloid fluid t.
  compression t.
  conservative t.
  continuous renal replacement t.

cryoprecipitate t.
deferoxamine chelation t.
dextrose t.
diazoxide t.
didanosine t.
digitalis glycoside t.
digoxin-specific antibody
  fragment t.
dilution t.
diphenylhydantoin t.
dobutamine t.
empiric t.
enzymatic t.
epinephrine t.
ergonovine t.
ergotamine t.
extracorporeal renal replacement t.
factor IX replacement t.
factor VIII replacement t.
fluid t.
gentamicin t.
glucagon t.
haloperidol t.
HBO t.
helium-oxygen t.
heparin t.
hyperbaric oxygen t.
initial t.
injection t.
inotropic t.
Integrilin t.
intracoronary laser t.
isoproterenol t.
Kayexalate t.
magnesium t.
milieu t.
multiple t.
muscle t.
neoadjuvant t.
nitroprusside t.
operative t.
outpatient t.
palliative t.
physical t. (PT)
Platelet Glycoprotein IIb/IIIa in
  Unstable Angina: Receptor
  Suppression Using Integrilin T.
  (PURSUIT)
pulmonary t. (PT)
pyretic t.
serial charcoal t.
specific t.

surfactant t.
terbutaline t.
thrombolytic t.
trauma t.
vitamin K t.
thermal
  t. burn
  t. sweat
thermocoagulation
thermodilution cardiac output
Thermo-Flex suture
thermogenesis
  nonshivering t.
thermometer
  Celsius t.
  centigrade t.
thermoregulation
thiamine repletion
thiazide diuretic
thickening
  nerve t.
  tendon sheath t.
  wall t.
thick green sputum
Thiersch suture
thigh
  t. bone
  t. muscle
thinking
  coherent stream of t.
thiopental
  sodium t.
thioridazine
thiosulfate
  sodium t.
thiotepa
thiothixene
thiourea
  ethylene t.
third
  t. cuneiform bone
  t. fibular muscle
  t. intention
  T. International Study of Infarct
    Survival (ISIS-3)
  t. peroneal muscle
third-degree
  t.-d. atrioventricular block
  t.-d. AV block
  t.-d. burn
  t.-d. hyperthermia
  t.-d. laceration

NOTES

Thomas endotracheal tube holder
Thompson-Epstein femoral fracture
    classification
Thompson ligament
thoracentesis
    needle t.
thoraces (*pl. of* thorax)
thoracic
    t. aorta
    t. aorta aneurysm
    t. aortic dissection
    t. bone
    t. cardiac branch of vagus nerve
    t. computed tomography
    t. empyema
    t. great vessel injury
    t. impedance cardiography
    t. interspinal muscle
    t. intertransverse muscle
    t. longissimus muscle
    t. outlet syndrome
    t. rotator muscle
    t. spinal nerve
    t. spine fracture
    t. spine injury
    t. splanchnic nerve
    t. surgery
    t. valvular disease
    t. vein
thoracoabdominal
    t. collateral vein
    t. gunshot wound
    t. incision
    t. nerve
    t. region
thoracoacromial vein
thoracoappendicular muscle
thoracodorsal nerve
thoracoepigastric vein
thoracolumbar
    t. burst fracture
    t. junction fracture
    t. spine
    t. spine fracture
    t. sympathetic nerve
thoracoscopy
thoracostomy
    chest tube t.
    needle t.
    tube t.
thoracotomy
    anterolateral t.
    clamshell t.
    posterolateral t.
thorax, pl. thoraces
thought disorder
thread suture
thready pulse

threat
    t. to abandon
    t. to institutionalize
threatened
    t. abortion (TAB)
    t. pathologic fracture
threshold
    bone conduction t.
    t. of discomfort
    fracture t.
    let-go t.
    pain t.
thrive
    failure to t.
throat
    ear, nose, t. (ENT)
    eyes, ears, nose, t. (EENT)
    head, eyes, ears, nose, t. (HEENT)
throbbing
thrombectomy
thrombi (*pl. of* thrombus)
thromboblastic disease
thrombocyte
thrombocytopathy
thrombocytopenia
    autoimmune t.
    essential t.
thrombocytopenic purpura
thromboelastogram
thromboelastograph
thromboembolism
    deep venous t.
    venous t.
thrombolytic
    t. agent
    t. therapy
thrombophlebitis
    septic pelvic vein t.
    suppurative t.
thromboplastin generation accelerator
thrombosed
    t. hemorrhoid
    t. thick-walled vein
thrombosis
    catheter-induced venous t.
    cavernous sinus t.
    deep vein t. (DVT)
    deep venous t. (DVT)
    graft t.
    platelet t.
    vein graft t.
    venous t.
Thrombosis-II
    Integrilin to Minimize Platelet
        Aggregation and Coronary T.-II
        (IMPACT-II)
thrombotic
    t. microangiopathy

t. stroke
t. thrombocytopenic purpura (TTP)
thrombus, pl. **thrombi**
mural t.
vein tumor t.
through-and-through
t.-a.-t. continuous suture
t.-a.-t. fracture
t.-a.-t. laceration
t.-a.-t. reabsorbable suture
through-the-catheter culture (TTC)
through-the-wall mattress suture
thrower's fracture
thrust
abdominal t.
chest t.
jaw t.
modified jaw t.
thumb
t. extensor tendon
t. flexor tendon
t. fracture
gamekeeper's t.
t. spica splint
2 thumb-encircling hands technique
thump
precordial t.
thunder
blood and t.
thunderclap headache
Thurston Holland fracture
thymic vein
thyroarytenoid muscle
thyroepiglottic
t. ligament
t. muscle
thyrohyoid
t. ligament
t. muscle
thyroid
t. bone
t. disease
t. function test (TFT)
t. gland
t. hormone
t. muscle
t. storm
t. vein
thyropharyngeal muscle
thyrotoxicosis
Ti
inspiratory time

TIA
transient ischemic attack
TIBC
total iron-binding capacity
tibia bone
tibia-fibula fracture
tibial
t. bending fracture
t. collateral ligament
t. collateral ligament bursa
t. communicating nerve
t. condyle fracture
t. cortical bone
t. diaphysial fracture
t. footprint
t. intertendinous bursa
t. lateral ligament
t. muscle
t. nerve block
t. open fracture
t. pilon fracture
t. plafond fracture
t. plateau fracture
t. plateau injury
t. sesamoid bone
t. sesamoid ligament
t. shaft fracture
t. stress fracture
t. tendon
t. triplane fracture
t. tuberosity
t. tuberosity fracture
t. vein
tibial-fibular shaft fracture
tibialis
t. anterior muscle
t. posterior muscle
tibiocalcaneal ligament
tibiofibular
t. fracture
t. ligament
tibionavicular ligament
ticarcillin-clavulanate
tic douloureux
tick
Dermacentor t.
t. paralysis
t. removal
ticlopidine
Ti-Cron suture
tidal
t. ventilation

T

NOTES

tidal *(continued)*
>t. volume
>t. volume control

TIE
>transient ischemic episode

Tiedemann nerve
tiger gut suture
tightness
>chest t.

Tillaux
>fracture of T.
>T. fracture

Tillaux-Chaput fracture
Tillaux-Kleiger fracture
tilt
>talar t.

time
>activated clotting t. (ACT)
>activated partial thromboplastin t. (aPTT)
>bleeding t.
>clotting t.
>dead t.
>door-to-balloon inflation t.
>door-to-drug t.
>t. of exposure
>inspiratory t. (Ti)
>t. of onset of pain
>onset, provocation, quality, region/radiation, severity, t. (OPQRST)
>partial thromboplastin t. (PTT)
>turnaround t.

time-cycled ventilator
timed
>forced expired volume t. (FEVT)

tincture
tinea
>t. capitis
>t. corporis
>t. cruris
>t. cutaneous infection
>t. pedis
>t. unguium
>t. versicolor

Tinel suture
tinnitus
>transitory t.

tip
>Yankauer suction t.

tip-refining suture
TIPSS
>transjugular intrahepatic portosystemic shunt stent

tirofiban
TISS
>Therapeutic Intervention Scoring System

tissue
>adipose t.
>bone t.
>cryptic tonsil t.
>t. glue
>granulation t.
>t. healing
>t. hypoxia
>t. ischemia
>muscle t.
>nerve t.
>nonnecrotic t.
>t. plasminogen
>t. plasminogen activator (TPA, t-PA)
>soft t.
>subcutaneous t.
>tendon t.

titratable
>t. acid
>t. acidity

titration
>pressure support ventilation t.

TKA
>total knee arthroplasty

TLC
>total lung capacity

TMJ
>temporomandibular joint

TMP-SMX
>trimethoprim-sulfamethoxazole
>trimethoprim and sulfamethoxazole

toad
>bufo t.
>t. toxin

toast
>bananas, rice cereal, applesauce, t. (BRAT)

tobacco abuse
tocainide hydrochloride
tocolysis
Todaro tendon
Todd
>T. muscle
>T. paralysis

toddler's fracture
toe
>t. bone
>t. extensor muscle
>t. extensor tendon
>t. flexor muscle
>muscle t.

toenail
>ingrown t.

toilet
>pulmonary t.

tolazoline
Toldt ligament
tolerance
>decreased exercise t.

drug t.
exercise t.
tolerating oral fluids well
tolmetin
toluene poisoning
Tom Jones suture
tomography
axial t.
computed t. (CT)
computed axial t. (CAT)
computerized axial t. (CAT)
conventional t.
single-photon emission computed t. (SPECT)
thoracic computed t.
Xenon-enhanced computed t.
TON
traumatic optic neuropathy
tone
decreased fetal heart t.'s
fetal heart t.'s
muscle t.
tongue
t. bone
t. depressor
t. fracture
t. suspension suture
tongue-type intraarticular fracture
tonic-clonic
t.-c. activity
t.-c. seizure
tonicity
muscle t.
tonic muscle
tonography
rectal t.
tonometer
Goldmann t.
Schiotz t.
tonometry
applanation t.
gastric t.
Goldmann applanation t.
Schiotz t.
Tono-Pen
tonsillar herniation
tonsil-tip catheter
tonus
muscle t.

tool
clinical support t. (CST)
Rampart EMS clinical support t.
tooth, pl. **teeth**
avulsed t.
displaced t.
t. fracture
fractured t.
t. lead
subluxated t.
toothache
toothed forceps
toothpaste toxicity
topical
t. anesthesia
t. antibiotic
t. isosorbide dinitrate
t. pain management
TOR
termination of resuscitation
Torg fracture
torn meniscotibial ligament
Tornwaldt bursa
torsade de pointes
torsemide
torsion
adnexal t.
t. fracture
ovarian t.
testicular t.
torsional fracture
torso strap
torticollis
tortuosity
elongation and t.
tortuous vein
Torulopsis glabrata
torus fracture
TOSCA
Toxic Substances Control Act
total
t. artificial heart (TAH)
t. body surface area (TBSA)
t. body water
t. breech extraction
t. condylar depression fracture
t. elasticity of muscle
t. electrical alternans
t. hip arthroplasty (THA)
t. iron-binding capacity (TIBC)
t. knee arthroplasty (TKA)
t. lung capacity (TLC)

T

NOTES

total (*continued*)
t. parenteral nutrition (TPN)
t. peripheral parenteral nutrition (TPPN)
t. shoulder arthroplasty
t. talus fracture
t. upper airway obstruction
toto
in t.
touch
light t.
response to light t.
tourniquet ischemia
towel
wound t.
toxaphene
toxemia
toxic
t. appearance
t. dose
t. epidermal necrolysis (TEN)
T. Exposure Surveillance System (TESS)
t. gas inhalation
t. ingestion
t. megacolon
t. overdose
t. shock syndrome (TSS)
t. skin reaction
t. skin reaction to dibenzofurans
t. substance in automobile airbag
T. Substances Control Act (TOSCA)
t. syndrome
t. synovitis
toxicity
acute digoxin t.
albuterol t.
amphetamine t.
anabolic steroid t.
antacid t.
anticholinergic t.
anticoagulant t.
antidote t.
antidysrhythmic t.
antipsychotic t.
antithyroid agent t.
ant killer t.
aromatic halogenated hydrocarbon t.
arsenic t.
autumn crocus t.
Avon Skin So Soft t.
beta-blocker t.
beta-naphthol t.
bismuth subsalicylate t.
bone marrow t.
boric acid t.
bromide t.
butyl t.

caffeine t.
calcium channel blocker t.
camphor t.
carbamate t.
carbon monoxide t.
castor bean t.
centrally acting agent t.
ceramic glaze t.
chalk t.
chemotherapy t.
chloral hydrate t.
chlorhexidine t.
chlorocresol t.
cholinergic t.
cigarette t.
citrate t.
clinical t.
clozapine t.
coal tar t.
cocaine t.
crayon t.
creosote t.
curare t.
cyanide t.
Daphne t.
Datura t.
delayed organ system t.
deprenyl t.
Desyrel t.
Dieffenbachia t.
digitalis t.
digoxin t.
Dilantin t.
dinitrophenol t.
dioxin t.
Effexor t.
ergotamine tartrate t.
ergot fungus t.
ethchlorvynol t.
fire-induced cyanide t.
formalin t.
foxglove t.
glue t.
hair dye t.
herbal t.
holly t.
hydrogen fluoride t.
hydrogen sulfide t.
increased risk of t.
iodine t.
iodothymol t.
iron t.
isopropyl alcohol t.
Lee-Jones test for cyanide t.
lidocaine t.
maprotiline t.
marijuana t.
mercury t.
metal casting t.

methaqualone t.
monoamine oxidase inhibitor t.
multiorgan t.
mushroom t.
naphthalene t.
nitrate t.
nitrite t.
nonsteroidal antiinflammatory t.
oral anticoagulant t.
organic bound iodide t.
oxygen t.
paraben t.
paraldehyde t.
pesticide t.
phenobarbital t.
pulmonary oxygen t.
resorcinol t.
rubber cement t.
salicylate t.
Serzone t.
shampoo t.
sodium channel blocker t.
strychnine t.
tannic acid t.
toothpaste t.
urea formaldehyde t.
vitamin A t.
vitamin B_1 t.
vitamin B_2 t.
vitamin B_6 t.
vitamin B_{12} t.
vitamin C t.
vitamin D t.
vitamin E t.
vitamin K t.
water hemlock t.
zolpidem t.
toxic-metabolic encephalopathy
toxicodendron
toxicokinetics
toxicologic screen
toxicus
    Gambierdiscus t.
toxin
    amphibian t.
    anthrax t.
    aquarium t.
    brazing t.
    cardiac t.
    Crotalus t.
    diphtheria t.
    disulfiram-like t.

t. exposure
t. exposure with suspicious history
foodborne t.
frog t.
Gyromitra t.
hemoglobin t.
t. identification
newt t.
salamander t.
toad t.
woodworking t.
toxin-specific measure
Toxoplasma gondii
toxoplasmosis
Toynbee muscle
TPA
    tissue plasminogen activator
t-PA
    tissue plasminogen activator
    I.V. t-PA
T-piece
    T-p. weaning
TPN
    total parenteral nutrition
TPPN
    total peripheral parenteral nutrition
TPT
    typhoid-paratyphoid
    TPT vaccine
trabecula
    bone t.
trabecular
    t. bone fracture
    t. vein
trabeculated bone
trabeculation
    muscle t.
tracheal
    t. carina
    t. deviation
    t. fracture
    t. intubation
    t. muscle
    t. rupture
    t. shift
    t. stoma
    t. tube
    t. vein
trachealis muscle
tracheitis
    bacterial t.
tracheloclavicular muscle

NOTES

trachelomastoid muscle
tracheobronchial
    t. tear
    t. tree injury
tracheobronchitis
tracheoinnominate fistula
tracheostomy
    t. collar
    mini t.
    percutaneous dilational t. (PDT)
    t. tube
tracheotomy
trachomatis
    Chlamydia t.
tracing
    nerve t.
Tracrium
tract
    AV bypass t.
    biliary t.
    lower respiratory t.
    nerve t.
    respiratory t.
    selective decontamination of
      digestive t. (SDD)
    upper respiratory t.
    wound t.
traction
    t. device
    t. fracture
    halo t.
    t. helmet
    t. splint
    t. suture
traffic collision (TC)
tragicus muscle
tragus muscle
train-of-4
    t.-o.-4 monitoring
    t.-o.-4 stimulus
trampoline fracture
tranexamic acid
tranquilization
    rapid t.
transaminase
    alanine t.
transbronchial biopsy (TBB)
transcaphoid fracture
transcapitate fracture
transcarpal ligament
transcerebral medullary vein
transcervical femoral fracture
transchondral talar fracture
transcondylar fracture
transcranial
    t. Doppler (TCD)
    t. Doppler ultrasonography
    t. Doppler ultrasound

transcutaneous
    t. cardiac pacing (TCP)
    t. nerve
    t. oximetry
transdomal suture
transducer
transection
    aortic t.
transepiphysial fracture
transesophageal
    t. echocardiography (TEE)
    t. fistula
transfer
    t. board
    bone t.
    Flight-for-Life t.
    muscle t.
    nerve t.
    stable for t.
    tendon t.
transfixation suture
transfixion suture
transfusion
    autologous blood t.
    blood t.
    t. complication
    cryoprecipitate t.
    early blood t.
    fetomaternal t.
    massive blood t.
    need for t.
    platelet t.
    prophylactic platelet t.
    t. reaction
transfusion-transmitted disease (TTD)
transhamate fracture
transient
    t. cerebral ischemic episode (TCIE)
    t. ischemic attack (TIA)
    t. ischemic episode (TIE)
transiliac fracture
transillumination
    t. intubation
    t. test
transitional zone
transition suture
transitory
    t. fever
    t. tinnitus
transjugular
    t. intrahepatic portosystemic shunt
    t. intrahepatic portosystemic shunt
      stent (TIPSS)
    t. intrahepatic portosystemic stent-
      shunt
translational fracture
transmediastinal penetrating wound
transmission
    airborne t.

endogenous t.
nerve t.
transmyocardial laser revascularization
transosseous suture
transpalpebral corrugator muscle
transpelvic gunshot wound
transplant
  bone marrow t.
  cadaveric renal t.
  heart t.
  heart-lung t.
  heterotopic t.
  isolated lung t.
  liver t.
  lung t.
  orthotopic heart t.
  t. rejection
transplantation
  bone marrow t.
  double-lung t. (DLT)
  heart-lung t. (HLT)
  hepatic t.
  heterotopic t.
  kidney t.
  liver t.
  multivisceral t.
  orthotopic heart t.
  orthotopic liver t. (OLTx)
  sequential single-lung t.
  simultaneous pancreas/kidney t.
  single lung t. (SLT)
  tendon t.
transport
  aeromedical t.
  air medical t.
  intestinal t.
  mucociliary t.
  rapid t.
  t. vehicle
transposition
  muscle t.
  tendon t.
transpyloric plane
transsacral fracture
transscaphoid dislocation fracture
transscleral suture
transsection
  nerve t.
transseptal ligament
transtentorial herniation
transtracheal jet ventilation (TTJV)
transtriquetral fracture

transvenous temporary pacing
transverse
  t. abdominal muscle
  t. acetabular ligament
  t. arytenoid muscle
  t. atlantal ligament
  t. atlas ligament
  t. auricular muscle
  t. carpal ligament
  t. cervical ligament
  t. cervical nerve
  t. cervical vein
  t. colli nerve
  t. colon
  t. comminuted fracture
  t. crural ligament
  t. facial fracture
  t. facial vein
  t. fracture
  t. genicular ligament
  t. humeral ligament
  t. intertarsal ligament
  t. lie
  t. lie of testis
  t. maxillary fracture
  t. metacarpal ligament
  t. metatarsal ligament
  t. myelitis
  t. palatal suture
  t. palatine suture
  t. part of iliofemoral ligament
  t. perineal ligament
  t. perineal muscle
  t. plane
  t. process fracture
  t. rectus abdominis muscle
  t. retinacular ligament
  t. scan
  t. scapular ligament
  t. spinal ligament
  t. tibiofibular ligament
transversely oriented endplate
compression fracture
transversospinal muscle
transversus abdominis muscle
tranylcypromine
trap
  finger t.
trap-door laceration
trapezial ridge fracture
trapezium fracture
trapezius muscle

T

NOTES

trapezoid
  t. bone
  t. ligament
trapping
  air t.
  Conrad-Bugg t.
  ion t.
  tendon t.
trauma
  ABCDE of t.
  abdominal t.
  anterior blunt neck t.
  A Severity Characterization of T.
    (ASCOT)
  t. assessment
  birth t.
  blunt t.
  blunt abdominal t. (BAT)
  blunt anterior neck t.
  blunt chest t.
  blunt head t.
  blunt neck t.
  blunt thoracic t.
  cardiac t.
  t. care flow record
  t. care system
  t. center
  chest t.
  closed head t.
  colon t.
  dental t.
  dentoalveolar t.
  diaphragmatic t.
  duodenal t.
  esophageal t.
  extremity t.
  facial t.
  focused abdominal sonography
    for t. (FAST)
  genitourinary t.
  head t.
  history of t.
  insertion t.
  kidney t.
  laryngotracheal t.
  liver t.
  lower genitourinary t.
  major t.
  massive facial t.
  neck t.
  otologic t.
  pancreatic t.
  pediatric t.
  pelvic t.
  penetrating abdominal t.
  penetrating anterior neck t.
  penetrating cardiac t.
  penetrating chest t.
  penetrating extremity t.

  penetrating head t.
  t. in pregnancy
  t. protocol
  rectal t.
  t. response team
  t. resuscitation
  t. room
  t. room evaluation
  t. score
  t. specialist
  spinal t.
  t. surgical intensive care unit
  t. therapy
  t. transport protocol (TTP)
  upper genitourinary t.
  urethral t.
  uterine t.
  victim of multiple t.
TraumaDEX powder
traumatic
  t. abruption
  t. abscess
  t. amnesia
  t. amputation
  t. aortic rupture
  t. aortic tear
  t. asphyxia
  t. axonal shear injury
  t. brain injury (TBI)
  t. deafness
  t. disruption of aorta
  t. fracture
  t. headache
  t. hemoperitoneum
  t. ischemia
  t. optic neuropathy (TON)
  t. pneumonitis
  t. pneumothorax
traumatism
traumatized ligament
traversing the fracture
trazodone
Treacher Collins syndrome
treat
  needed to t.
treating team
treatment
  aforementioned t.
  aggressive t.
  antibiotic t.
  bone cyst t.
  breathing t.
  chiropractic t.
  conservative t.
  t. course
  drug t.
  empiric t.
  expectant t.
  t. failure

hemoductal surgical t.
holding room t.
ICU t.
isopropyl alcohol t.
nebulization t.
operative t.
outpatient t.
palliative t.
prophylactic t.
protracted t.
radical t.
Rapid Early Action for
   Coronary T. (REACT)
simple triage and rapid t.
   (START)
surgical t.
symptomatic t.

tree
ingestion of golden chain t.

trefoil tendon

Treitz
T. ligament
T. muscle

tremens
delirium t. (DT)

tremor
arsenic t.
dystonic t.

tremulous speech

trench foot

Trendelenburg position

trephine
bone t.

Treponema
T. pallidum
T. pallidum infection

triad
acute compression t.
Beck t.
t. model interview
Virchow stasis t.
Waddell t.

triage
field t.
hospital t.
t. intervention
scene t.
t. tag

trial
Brain Resuscitation Clinical T.
   (BRCT)
CAPTURE t.

Enlimomab Acute Stroke T.
   (EAST)
ESSENCE t.
Fracture Intervention T.
FRISC t.
IMPACT-AMI t.
ISIS-3 t.
PROWESS t.
REACT t.
RESTORE t.
Second Leicester Intravenous
   Magnesium Intervention T.
   (LIMIT-2)
Veterans Affairs High-Density
   Lipoprotein Intervention T. (VA-
   HIT)

triamterene

triangular
t. area
t. bandage
t. deltoid ligament
t. ligament of liver
t. muscle
t. wrist bone

triceps
t. brachii muscle
t. bursa
t. coxae muscle
t. surae muscle
t. tendon

trichinosis

trichiura
Trichuris t.

trichloroacetic acid

trichloroethanol

trichomonad

Trichomonas hominis

trichomoniasis

Trichosporon

Trichuris trichiura

tricipital muscle

Tricor

tricuspid
t. insufficiency
t. stenosis
t. valve

tricyclic
t. antidepressant
t. antidepressant intoxication
t. antidepressant poisoning

**triethanolamine polypeptide oleate-
condensate**

NOTES

T

315

trifacial nerve
trifoliate central tendon
trigeminal
  t. nerve
  t. neuralgia
trigger
  allergic t.
  avoidance of t.
  known t.
trigonal muscle
trigone muscle
Trilafon
trimalar fracture
trimalleolar ankle fracture
trimester
  first t.
trimethoprim-sulfamethoxazole (TMP-SMX)
trimethoprim and sulfamethoxazole (TMP-SMX)
trimming
  muscle t.
trinitrate
  glyceryl t. (GTN)
Tri-Pak
  Zithromax T.-P.
tripartite bone
triphosphatase
  adenosine t. (ATPase)
triplane
  t. fracture
  t. tibial fracture
triple acid base disorder
tripod
  t. fracture
  t. position
trip sheet
triquetral fracture
triquetrohamate ligament
triquetroscaphoid ligament
triquetrum bone
TRISS
  Trauma Injury Severity Score
trocar wound
trochanter
  greater t.
trochanteric bursa
troche
  clotrimazole t.
trochlear
  t. muscle
  t. nerve
  t. synovial bursa
Trolard vein
Tronzo intertrochanteric fracture
  classification
tropane
trophic fracture

tropicalis
  Candida t.
tropical sprue
troponin
trough
  bone t.
trousers
  military antishock t. (MAST)
Trousseau sign
true
  t. aneurysm
  t. collateral ligament
  t. muscle
  t. rib
  t. suture
trumpet
  nasal t.
trunk
  t. muscle
  nerve t.
trypanosomiasis
  American t.
tryptamine
L-tryptophan
T-shaped fracture
TSS
  toxic shock syndrome
TTC
  through-the-catheter culture
TTD
  transfusion-transmitted disease
TTJV
  transtracheal jet ventilation
TTP
  thrombotic thrombocytopenic purpura
  trauma transport protocol
T-tube
tubal pregnancy
tube
  bag-valve device to tracheostomy t.
  Blakemore-Sengstaken t.
  bronchial t.
  t. condensation
  t. drainage
  endotracheal t. (ETT)
  Endotrol tracheal t.
  Ewald t.
  fallopian t.
  feeding t.
  t. feeding
  t. fogging
  French nasogastric t.
  gastric t. (GT)
  gastrostomy t. (G-tube)
  intubation t.
  nasogastric t. (NGT)
  nasotracheal t.
  neural t.
  NG t.

orogastric feeding t.
orotracheal t.
PEG t.
per nasogastric t. (PNGT)
pus t.
Sengstaken-Blakemore t.
t. thoracostomy
tracheal t.
tracheostomy t.
ventilatory support t.
tubercle
pubic t.
tuberculoma
bone t.
tuberculosis (TB)
bone and joint t.
Mycobacterium t.
tuberculous bone
tuberosity
t. avulsion fracture
t. fracture
ischial t.
tibial t.
tubocurarine
tuboovarian abscess
tubular
t. bone
t. necrosis
tucker
tendon t.
Tuffier inferior ligament
tuft fracture
tularemia
tumescent
tumor
anal canal t.
Aniridia-Wilms t.
t. bone
bone marrow t.
central nervous system t.
cerebellar t.
t. compression syndrome
encased t.
exuberant t.
fibroid t.
t. lysis syndrome
t. necrosis factor
t. necrosis factor alpha
nerve cell t.
nerve root t.
nerve sheath malignant t.
Wilms t.

tumor-bearing bone
tunnel
graft t.
tarsal t.
tunneled catheter
tunneler
tendon t.
turbid fluid
turbidity
turbinate
t. bone
nasal t.
turbulent flow
turnaround time
Turner syndrome
turnout gear
turnover
bone t.
turpentine
t. ingestion
t. poisoning
twig
nerve t.
twin
discordant t.
Twinrix
twisted
t. cotton suture
t. dermal suture
t. linen suture
t. virgin silk suture
twisting force
twitch
muscle t.
t. muscle
t. response
tympanic
t. abscess
t. bone
t. membrane perforation
t. muscle
t. nerve
t. vein
tympanocentesis
tympanomastoid suture
tympanosquamosal suture
tympanosquamous suture
type
t. A, B hemophilia
blood t.
t. and crossmatch
t. and crossmatch blood

T

NOTES

type *(continued)*
    muscle fiber t.
    t. 1, 2 priapism
    t. and screen
type-specific blood
typhi
    Rickettsia t.
    Salmonella t.

typhoid fever
typhoid-paratyphoid (TPT)
typhus
    Rickettsia t.
typing
    blood t.
tyramine oxidase
Tyrrell-Gray suture

UA
    urinalysis
Uhthoff symptom
UIP
    usual interstitial pneumonia
ulcer
        aphthous u.
        u. base
        chancroid u.
        decubitus u.
        indolent u.
        painless u.
        peptic u.
        perforated u.
        suture u.
ulceration
        corneal u.
        punched-out u.
        stress gastric u.
        suture line u.
ulcerative
        u. colitis
        u. keratitis
ULN
    upper limits of normal
ulnar
        u. artery aneurysm
        u. bursa
        u. carpal collateral ligament
        u. flexor muscle
        u. nerve
        u. nerve block
        u. sesamoid bone
        u. styloid bone
        u. styloid fracture
        u. vein
ulnocarpal ligament
ulnolunate ligament
ulnotriquetral ligament
ULQ
    upper left quadrant
ultrafiltration
UltraFix MicroMite anchor suture
ultrasonic nebulizer
ultrasonography
        abdominal u.
        Doppler u.
        transcranial Doppler u.
ultrasound (US)
        A-mode u.
        duplex u.
        u. intercom
        pelvic u.

        transcranial Doppler u.
        vaginal u.
ultraviolet (UV)
        u. keratitis
        psoralen plus u. A (PUVA)
umbilical
        u. cord
        u. ligament
        u. region
        u. rupture
        u. tape suture
        u. vein
unabsorbable suture
unassisted step
Unasyn
uncal herniation
unciform
        u. bone
        u. fracture
uncinate
        u. bone
        u. process fracture
uncommon fracture
uncompensated metabolic acidosis
uncomplicated
        u. delivery
        u. pregnancy
unconditioned response
unction
        tendon u.
undepressed skull fracture
underlying
        u. cause
        u. cause of death
        u. chest muscle
        u. disease
        u. disorder
        u. rib fracture
undisplaced fracture
undulating fever
undyed suture
unexplained
        u. altered mental status
        u. apnea
        u. burn
        u. death of infant
        u. fracture
        u. injury
unguium
        tinea u.
unicondylar fracture
Unifold shelter
unilateral
        u. condylar fracture

U

unilateral *(continued)*
  u. hemianopia
  u. hypoplastic pectoral muscle
unimalleolar fracture
uninjured brain
uninterrupted suture
unipennate muscle
unit
  alcohol and drug dependency u.
    (ADDU)
  antitoxic u.
  bag-valve u.
  Bair-Hugger convective warming u.
  body cooling u. (BCU)
  bone marrow transplant u.
  bone metabolic u.
  bone structural u.
  burn u. (BU)
  cardiac care u. (CCU)
  cardiac intensive care u. (CICU)
  cardiology intensive care u. (CICU)
  chemical dependency u. (CDU)
  chest pain observation u. (CPOU)
  coronary care u. (CCU)
  coronary intensive care u. (CICU)
  critical care u. (CCU)
  emergency department
    observation u. (EDOU)
  fixed suction u.
  higher trauma u.
  inpatient u. (IPU)
  intensive care u. (ICU)
  intensive coronary care u. (ICCU)
  Life SoftPac AED companion
    oxygen u.
  medical intensive care u. (MICU)
  mobile response u.
  neonatal intensive care u. (NICU)
  neurological intensive care u.
    (NICU)
  pediatric intensive care u. (PICU)
  postanesthesia care u. (PACU)
  progressive care u. (PCU)
  pulmonary intensive care u. (PICU)
  special care u. (SCU)
  S-SCORT VX-2 suction u.
  surgical intensive care u. (SICU)
  trauma surgical intensive care u.
Uni-Vent Eagle portable ventilator
universal
  u. distress signal
  u. dressing
  u. precaution
unloading
  bone u.
unmyelinated nerve
unreactive mydriasis

unresponsive
  alert, verbal stimuli, painful
    stimuli, u. (AVPU)
unresponsiveness
  psychogenic u.
unsaturated fatty acid
unstable
  u. angina
  u. fracture
  u. injury
  u. patient
  u. tibial shaft fracture
  u. zygomatic complex fracture
unstriated muscle
unstriped muscle
untoward effect
ununited fracture
UOQ
  upper outer quadrant
upper
  u. airway
  u. airway obstruction
  u. cervical nerve
  u. extremity aneurysm
  u. gastrointestinal bleeding
  u. genitourinary trauma
  u. jaw bone
  u. left quadrant (ULQ)
  u. limits of normal (ULN)
  u. outer quadrant (UOQ)
  u. respiratory infection (URI)
  u. respiratory rhonchi
  u. respiratory tract
  u. respiratory tract infection
    (URTI)
  u. subscapular nerve
  u. thoracic spine fracture
  u. thoracic splanchnic nerve
  u. trapezius muscle
UPPP
  uvulopalatopharyngoplasty
upright
  KUB and u.
upstroke
  expiratory u.
uptake
  bone mineral u.
  muscle u.
uptight muscle
upward gaze
urachal ligament
urea formaldehyde toxicity
urealyticum
  Ureaplasma u.
Ureaplasma
  U. urealyticum
  U. urealyticum infection
uremia
  prerenal u.

uremic encephalopathy
ureter
    dilated u.
ureteral obstruction
urethra
urethral
    u. discharge
    u. trauma
    u. vein
urethritis
    chlamydial u.
    gonococcal u.
urethrogram
    retrograde u.
urethrography
urethropelvic ligament
urgency
urgent
    u. orthopaedic referral
    u. synchronized cardioversion
URI
    upper respiratory infection
urinalysis (UA)
urinary
    u. antimuscarinic
    u. bladder
    u. diversion
    u. incontinence
    u. plasminogen
    u. retention
    u. symptoms
    u. tract fistula
    u. tract infection (UTI)
    u. tract obstruction
urine
    u. anion gap
    blue u.
    brown-black u.
    u. color
    u. drug panel
    u. drug screen
    u. electrolyte
    u. odor
    u. osmolal gap
    u. pregnancy test
urogenital
    u. injury
    u. sphincter muscle
urography
    intravenous u.
urokinase
urosepsis

urostomy
    ileal loop u.
URTI
    upper respiratory tract infection
urticant
    phosgene oxime u.
urticaria
    chronic u.
US
    ultrasound
usage
    heroin u.
    ventilator u.
use
    accessory muscle u.
    intravenous drug u. (IVDU)
user
    cannabis u.
U-shaped arch
USP#2 suture
usual interstitial pneumonia (UIP)
U suture
uteri (*pl. of* uterus)
uterine
    u. ligament
    u. massage
    u. muscle
    u. prolapse
    u. rupture
    u. tocographic monitoring
    u. trauma
    u. vein
uteroovarian ligament
uteroparietal suture
uteropelvic ligament
uterosacral ligament
uterovesical ligament
uterus, pl. **uteri**
    anteverted u.
    bifid u.
    boggy u.
    retroverted u.
    ruptured u.
UTI
    urinary tract infection
utilization
    oxygen u.
utricular nerve
utriculoampullar nerve
UV
    ultraviolet

U

NOTES

uveitis
    anterior u.
uvula, pl. **uvuli**
    bifid u.

uvular muscle
uvulopalatopharyngoplasty (UPPP)

vaccinate
vaccine, vaccination
DPT v.
Fermi v.
TPT v.
vacuum splint
VAD
ventricular assist device
vagal
v. antiarrhythmic maneuver
v. effect
v. preganglionic cardiomotor neuron
vaginal
v. bacterial infection
v. bleeding
v. bleeding in pregnancy
v. candidiasis
v. discharge
v. foreign body
v. hand ligament
v. laceration
v. muscle
v. nerve
v. ultrasound
vaginitis
nonspecific v.
vaginosis
bacterial v.
vague explanation
vagus nerve
VA-HIT
Veterans Affairs High-Density
Lipoprotein Intervention Trial
Valentin nerve
valerian
valgus
v. deformity
v. fracture
Valium
vallecula
valproate
valproic
v. acid
v. acid intoxication
Valsalva
V. ligament
V. maneuver
V. muscle
value
flow rate v.
valve
aortic v.
atrioventricular v.
bicuspid v.
heart v.

mitral v.
prosthetic heart v.
pulmonic v.
semilunar v.
tricuspid v.
valvulae conniventes
valvular heart disease
Vanceril
vancomycin
vapor inhalation
variability
baseline v.
beat-to-beat v.
fetal beat-to-beat v.
heart rate v.
variant
migraine v.
v. nerve
variceal
v. bleeding
v. hemorrhage
varicella
v. encephalitis
v. zoster
varicella-zoster virus
varices (pl. of varix)
varicose vein
varicosity
spider v.
varix, pl. varices
varus deviation
varying degrees of erythema
vascular
v. access
v. access infection
v. anastomosis
v. catastrophe
v. deficit
v. headache
v. injury
v. injury scale
v. laceration
v. metaphysial bone
v. nerve
v. occlusion
v. reconstruction
v. silk suture
v. smooth muscle
vasculitis
cerebral v.
mesenteric v.
necrotizing v.
vasculopathy
cardiac allograft v.
vasoactive medication

V

vasoconstriction
    hypocapnia-induced v.
    hypoxic pulmonary v. (HPV)
vasoconstrictor
    v. agent
    v. nerve
vasodilation
    passive v.
vasodilator
    v. nerve
    nitro v.
    peripheral v.
vasogenic edema
vasomotor
    v. manifestation
    v. nephropathy
    v. nerve
vasopressin
    arginine v.
    1-desamino-8-didanosine-arginine v.
    (DDAVP)
    glycine v.
vasopressor
    v. agent
    v. reflex
vasosensory nerve
vasospasm
    arterial v.
    cerebral v.
    coronary artery v.
    symptomatic v.
vasotropic drug
vasovagal
    v. collapse
    v. reflex
vastus
    v. intermedius muscle
    v. lateralis muscle
    v. medialis muscle
Vater
    ampulla of V.
VC
    vital capacity
vecuronium
vehicle
    v. rollover
    transport v.
vein
    aberrant obturator v.
    abscessed v.
    absent peripheral v.
    accessory cephalic v.
    accessory hemiazygos v.
    accessory hepatic v.
    accessory saphenous v.
    accessory venous v.
    accessory vertebral v.
    accompanying v.
    adrenal v.

afferent v.
anal v.
anastomotic v.
aneurysmal v.
angular v.
anomalous pulmonary v.
anonymous v.
antebrachial v.
antecubital v.
anterior auricular v.
anterior basal v.
anterior cardiac v.
anterior cardinal v.
anterior cerebral v.
anterior ciliary v.
anterior circumflex humeral v.
anterior condylar v.
anterior conjunctival v.
anterior facial v.
anterior intercostal v.
anterior internal vertebral v.
anterior interosseous v.
anterior jugular v.
anterior labial v.
anterior pontomesencephalic v.
anterior scrotal v.
anterior temporal diploic v.
anterior terminal v.
anterior tibial v.
apical v.
apicoposterior v.
appendicular v.
aqueous v.
arciform v.
arcuate v.
arterial v.
arterialized leptomeningeal v.
ascending lumbar v.
Ascher v.
auditory v.
auricular v.
autogenous v.
autologous internal jugular v.
axillary v.
azygos v.
basal v.
basilic v.
basivertebral v.
Baumgarten v.
bladder v.
Boyd communicating perforation v.
Boyd perforating v.
brachial v.
brachiocephalic v.
brain bridging v.
Breschet v.
bridging v.
broken v.
bronchial v.

Browning v.
buccal v.
Burow v.
cannulated central v.
capacious v.
capillary v.
cardiac v.
cardinal v.
carotid v.
caudate v.
cavernous v.
central v.
cephalic v.
cerebellar v.
cerebral v.
cervical v.
choroid v.
ciliary v.
cilioretinal v.
circumflex v.
cochlear v.
Cockett communicating
  perforating v.
colic v.
collateral v.
collecting v.
common anterior facial v.
common basal v.
common cardinal v.
common femoral v.
common iliac v.
common modiolar v.
communicating v.
companion v.
v. compression
condylar emissary v.
v. confluence
conjunctival v.
coronary v.
cortical v.
costoaxillary v.
cremasteric v.
crural v.
cryopreserved v.
cubital v.
v. cuff
cutaneous v.
cystic v.
v. decompression
deep cerebral v.
deep cervical v.
deep circumflex iliac v.

deep dorsal v.
deep epigastric v.
deep facial v.
deep femoral v.
deep inferior epigastric v.
deep lingual v.
deep middle cerebral v.
deep temporal v.
descending genicular v.
diencephalic v.
digital v.
dilated v.
v. dilation
v. dilator
diploic v.
direct lateral v.
distended v.
Dodd perforating v.
dorsal callosal v.
dorsalis pedis v.
dorsal lingual v.
dorsal metacarpal v.
dorsal metatarsal v.
dorsal penile v.
dorsal scapular v.
dorsispinal v.
draining v.
duodenal v.
embryonic umbilical v.
emissary v.
engorged v.
epigastric v.
epigastric inferior v.
episcleral v.
esophageal v.
ethmoidal v.
external carotid v.
external iliac v.
external jugular v.
external mammary v.
external nasal v.
external palatine v.
external pterygoid v.
external pudendal v.
external pudic v.
external radial v.
external spermatic v.
extrahepatic portal v.
facial v.
familial varicose v.
feeder v.
femoral v.

V

NOTES

vein *(continued)*

femoropopliteal v.
fetal intrahepatic v.
fibular v.
v. flap
flat neck v.
frontal v.
frontal diploic v.
Galen v.
gastric v.
gastroepiploic v.
genicular v.
gluteal v.
gonadal v.
v. graft
grafting v.
v. graft occlusion
v. graft patency
v. graft stenosis
v. graft thrombosis
greater saphenous v.
gubernacular v.
harvested v.
hemiazygos v.
hemispheric v.
hemorrhoidal v.
hepatic v.
hepatic portal v.
highest intercostal v.
human umbilical v.
hypogastric v.
hypophyseoportal v.
ileal v.
ileocolic v.
ileofemoral v.
iliac v.
iliofemoral v.
ilioinguinal v.
iliolumbar v.
inferior adrenal v.
inferior alveolar v.
inferior anastomotic v.
inferior basal v.
inferior cardiac v.
inferior cerebellar v.
inferior cerebral v.
inferior choroid v.
inferior epigastric v.
inferior gluteal v.
inferior hemiazygos v.
inferior hemorrhoidal v.
inferior labial v.
inferior laryngeal v.
inferior mesenteric v.
inferior nasal v.
inferior ophthalmic v.
inferior palpebral v.
inferior phrenic v.
inferior pulmonary v.

inferior radicular v.
inferior rectal v.
inferior temporal v.
inferior thalamostriate v.
inferior thyroid v.
inferior ventricular v.
v. inflammation
infradiaphragmatic v.
infraorbital v.
infrasegmental v.
innominate cardiac v.
insular v.
intercapital v.
intercapitular v.
intercostal v.
interlobar v.
intermediate antebrachial v.
intermediate basilic v.
intermediate cephalic v.
intermediate cubital v.
intermediate hepatic v.
intermetatarsal v.
internal auditory v.
internal cerebral v.
internal iliac v.
internal jugular v.
internal maxillary v.
internal pudendal v.
internal thoracic v.
interosseous v.
interventricular v.
intervertebral v.
intestinal v.
intradural draining v.
intraforaminal v.
intrahepatic umbilical v.
intraportal v.
intrarenal v.
v. intussusception
jugular v. (JV)
jugulocephalic v.
juxtahepatic v.
key v.
Kohlrausch v.
Krukenberg v.
Kuhnt postcentral v.
labial v.
labyrinthine v.
lacrimal v.
large saphenous v.
laryngeal v.
Latarjet v.
lateral atrial v.
lateral circumflex femoral v.
lateral direct v.
lateral mammary v.
lateral plantar v.
lateral sacral v.
lateral thoracic v.

leaking v.
left brachiocephalic v.
left colic v.
left coronary v.
left gastric v.
left gastroepiploic v.
left gastroomental v.
left gonadal v.
left hepatic v.
left inferior pulmonary v.
left internal jugular v.
left marginal v.
left median v.
left ovarian v.
left pericardiacophrenic v.
left phrenic v.
left pulmonary v.
left retroaortic renal v.
left subclavian v.
left superior gluteal v.
left superior intercostal v.
left superior pulmonary v.
left suprarenal v.
left testicular v.
left umbilical v.
left vertical v.
lesser ovarian v.
lesser saphenous v.
levoatriocardinal v.
lienal v.
lingual v.
lingular v.
linguofacial v.
long saphenous v.
long thoracic v.
lumbar v.
v. lumen
main renal v.
mammary v.
marginal v.
Marshall v.
masseteric v.
mastoid emissary v.
maternal cortical v.
maxillary v.
Mayo v.
medial atrial v.
medial circumflex femoral v.
medial genicular v.
medial plantar v.
median antebrachial v.
median basilic v.

median cephalic v.
median cubital v.
median sacral v.
mediastinal v.
medium v.
medullary v.
meningeal v.
meningorachidian v.
mesencephalic v.
mesenteric superior v.
metacarpal v.
middle cardiac v.
middle colic v.
middle genicular v.
middle hemorrhoidal v.
middle hepatic v.
middle lobe v.
middle meningeal v.
middle rectal v.
middle sacral v.
middle temporal v.
middle thyroid v.
nasal v.
nasofrontal v.
native portal v.
neck v.
v. nicking
nodularity v.
v. nodularity
oblique v.
obliterated v.
v. obstruction
obturator v.
occipital cerebral v.
occipital diploic v.
occipital emissary v.
omental v.
omphalomesenteric v.
ophthalmic v.
ophthalmomeningeal v.
opticociliary shunt v.
orbital varix ophthalmic v.
v. orifice
oscillating v.
ovarian v.
palatal v.
palatine v.
palisade-type v.
palmar cutaneous v.
palmar digital v.
palmar metacarpal v.
v. palpation

V

NOTES

327

vein *(continued)*

palpebral v.
pampiniform v.
pancreatic v.
pancreaticoduodenal v.
paraesophageal collateral v.
parathyroid v.
paratonsillar v.
paraumbilical v.
paraventricular v.
parent v.
parietal emissary v.
parotid v.
partial anomalous pulmonary v.'s
v. patch
v. patch angioplasty
v. patch rupture
patent portal v.
pectoral v.
peduncular v.
penile v.
percutaneous femoral v.
perforating v.
pericallosal v.
pericardiac v.
pericardiacophrenic v.
pericardial v.
periesophageal collateral v.
peripancreatic v.
peripheral acinar v.
perithyroid v.
peritoneal v.
peritumoral v.
periurethral v.
peroneal v.
persistent right umbilical v.
petrosal v.
pharyngeal v.
phrenic v.
pial v.
plantar digital v.
plantar metatarsal v.
pontine v.
pontomesencephalic v.
popliteal v.
portal v.
postcardinal v.
postcentral v.
posterior anterior jugular v.
posterior auricular v.
posterior callosal v.
posterior cardinal v.
posterior ciliary v.
posterior circumflex humeral v.
posterior conjunctival v.
posterior facial v.
posterior intercostal v.
posterior interosseous v.
posterior interventricular v.

posterior labial v.
posterior marginal v.
posterior parotid v.
posterior pericallosal v.
posterior scrotal v.
posterior temporal diploic v.
posterior terminal v.
posterior tibial v.
precentral cerebellar v.
prefrontal v.
prepyloric v.
primitive maxillary v.
prominent pulmonary v.
proximal v.
pudendal v.
pulmonary v.
pulsating v.
pyloric v.
quadrigeminal v.
radial v.
radicular v.
ranine v.
rectal v.
rectosigmoid v.
renal v.
retinal v.
v. retractor
retroaortic renal v.
retroauricular v.
retrohepatic v.
retromandibular v.
retroperitoneal v.
Retzius v.
reversed greater saphenous v.
reverse saphenous v.
right brachiocephalic v.
right colic v.
right gastric v.
right gastroepiploic v.
right gastroomental v.
right gonadal v.
right hepatic v.
right inferior gluteal v.
right inferior pulmonary v.
right internal jugular v.
right ovarian v.
right pericardiacophrenic v.
right phrenic v.
right pulmonary v.
right subclavian v.
right superior intercostal v.
right superior pulmonary v.
right suprarenal v.
right testicular v.
rolandic v.
Rolando v.
Rosenthal v.
Ruysch v.
sacral v.

salvatella v.
Santorini v.
saphenous v.
Sappey v.
Schlesinger v.
scimitar v.
scleral v.
scrotal v.
segmental v.
sentinel v.
septal v.
Servelle v.
short gastric v.
short hepatic v.
short saphenous v.
sigmoid v.
v. sign
small cardiac v.
smallest cardiac v.
small saphenous v.
soleal v.
spermatic v.
sphenoid emissary v.
spider v.
spigelian v.
spinal v.
spiral v.
splanchnic v.
splenic v.
stellate v.
Stensen v.
sternocleidomastoid v.
v. stone
striate v.
v. stripper
v. stripping
stylomastoid v.
subcardinal v.
subclavian v.
subcostal v.
subcutaneous v.
subependymal v.
sublingual v.
sublobular v.
submental v.
subscapular v.
superficial circumflex iliac v.
superficial dorsal v.
superficial epigastric v.
superficial femoral v.
superficial middle cerebral v.
superficial palmar v.

superficial perineal v.
superficial temporal v.
superficial vertebral v.
superior anastomotic v.
superior azygos v.
superior basal v.
superior cerebellar v.
superior cerebral v.
superior choroid v.
superior epigastric v.
superior gluteal v.
superior hemorrhoidal v.
superior intercostal v.
superior labial v.
superior laryngeal v.
superior lateral genicular v.
superior medial genicular v.
superior mesenteric v.
superior nasal v.
superior ophthalmic v.
superior palpebral v.
superior phrenic v.
superior pulmonary v.
superior rectal v.
superior temporal v.
superior thalamostriate v.
superior thyroid v.
supracardinal v.
supraorbital v.
suprarenal v.
suprascapular v.
suprasellar v.
supratrochlear v.
supreme intercostal v.
surface thalamic v.
sylvian v.
v. system
systemic v.
tangle of hemorrhoidal v.'s
telencephalic v.
temporal diploic v.
temporomaxillary v.
terminal v.
testicular v.
thalamic v.
thalamostriate v.
thebesian v.
thoracic v.
thoracoabdominal collateral v.
thoracoacromial v.
thoracoepigastric v.
thrombosed thick-walled v.

V

NOTES

vein *(continued)*
    thymic v.
    thyroid v.
    tibial v.
    tortuous v.
    trabecular v.
    tracheal v.
    transcerebral medullary v.
    transverse cervical v.
    transverse facial v.
    Trolard v.
    v. tumor thrombus
    tympanic v.
    ulnar v.
    umbilical v.
    urethral v.
    uterine v.
    v. valve wrapping
    varicose v.
    ventricular v.
    vermian v.
    vertebral v.
    vertical v.
    vesalian v.
    Vesalius v.
    vesical v.
    vestibular v.
    vidian v.
    Vieussens v.
    vitelline v.
    vortex v.
    vorticose v.
    v. wall
Velcro strap
velocity
    bone quantitative ultrasound v.
    muscle fiber conduction v.
    muzzle v.
    nerve conduction v.
vena caval filter
venenosus
    Zygadenus v.
venereum
    lymphogranuloma v.
Venezuelan equine encephalitis
venlafaxine
venomous
    v. caterpillar
    v. moth
venoocclusive
    v. disease
    v. disease of liver
    v. priapism
venous
    v. air embolism
    v. air embolization
    v. bleeding
    v. catheter
    v. cutdown

    v. insufficiency
    v. ligament
    v. oximetry
    v. oxygen saturation (SVO_2)
    v. saturation monitoring
    v. smooth muscle
    v. thromboembolism
    v. thrombosis
venovenous
    v. extracorporeal membrane oxygenation
    v. hemodialysis
ventilation
    adequate v.
    airway pressure release v. (APRV)
    alternate mode of mechanical v.
    alveolar v.
    artificial v.
    assist control v. (ACV)
    bag v.
    bag-and-mask v.
    bag-valve-mask v.
    conventional mechanical v. (CMV)
    dead-space v.
    demand-valve v.
    flow-restricted oxygen powered v.
    gas v.
    high-frequency v. (HFV)
    high-frequency jet v. (HFJV)
    high-frequency oscillatory v. (HFOV)
    hyperbaric saline v.
    independent lung v. (ILV)
    intermittent v.
    intermittent mandatory v. (IMV)
    inverse ratio v. (IRV)
    liquid v.
    low-frequency positive pressure v. (LFPPV)
    mandatory minute v. (MMV)
    mask v.
    maximal voluntary v. (MVV)
    mechanical v.
    mouth-to-mask v.
    needle-catheter cricothyroid v.
    nocturnal v.
    noninvasive nocturnal v.
    noninvasive positive pressure v. (NPPV)
    optimum v.
    partial liquid v.
    PCIR v.
    percutaneous transtracheal v. (PTV)
    positive-pressure v.
    pressure support v. (PSV)
    prone v.
    proportional assist v. (PAV)
    resistive pressure v.

spontaneous augmented low-volume v.
synchronized intermittent mandatory v. (SIMV)
tidal v.
transtracheal jet v. (TTJV)
ventilation/perfusion (V/Q)
v./p. lung scan
v./p. mismatch
ventilator
automatic transport v. (ATV)
v. circuit change
v. dependence
flow-cycled v.
jet v.
v. management team
manual jet v.
time-cycled v.
Uni-Vent Eagle portable v.
v. usage
volume-cycled v.
v. weaning
ventilator-associated pneumonia
ventilator-induced lung injury
ventilatory
v. failure
v. support tube
Venti mask
Ventolin
ventral
v. aspect
v. cavity
v. sacrococcygeal ligament
v. sacrococcygeal muscle
v. sacroiliac ligament
ventricle
air trapping in v.
ventricular
v. afterload
v. aneurysm
v. assist device (VAD)
v. asystole
v. defibrillation
v. dysrhythmia
v. ectopy
v. ejection fraction
v. elasticity
v. end-diastolic pressure
v. end-diastolic volume
v. fibrillation (VF)
v. flutter
v. independence

v. interdependence
v. ligament
v. peritoneal shunt
v. preload
v. septal rupture
v. tachycardia (VT)
v. vein
ventriculitis
nosocomial v.
ventriculography
ECG-gated v.
Venturi mask
vera
placenta accreta v.
verapamil
Veratrum viride
verbal bedside report
Verelan
verge
anal v.
Verhoeff suture
verification of correct tube placement
vermian vein
vermicide
vermicularis
Enterobius v.
vermicular movement
vermiform appendix
verminous
v. abscess
v. appendicitis
Versed
versenate
calcium disodium v.
versicolor
tinea v.
vertebra, pl. **vertebrae**
lumbar v.
v. plana fracture
vertebral
v. artery dissection
v. body fracture
v. column muscle
v. compression fracture
v. nerve
v. stable burst fracture
v. vein
v. wedge compression fracture
vertebrobasilar atherothrombotic disease
vertebropelvic ligament
vertical
v. length

NOTES

V

vertical *(continued)*
- v. mattress suture
- v. muscle
- v. oblique pattern fracture
- v. plication suture
- v. shear fracture
- v. tooth fracture
- v. vein

vertiginous seizure

vertigo
- alternobaric v.
- benign positional v. (BPV)
- central v.
- epidemic v.
- peripheral v.

vesalian
- v. bone
- v. vein

Vesalius vein

vesical
- v. ligament
- v. vein

vesicant

vesicle
- v. formation
- seminal v.

vesicosacral ligament

vesicoumbilical ligament

vesicouterine ligament

vesicular breath sound

vesnarinone

vessel
- major v.

vestibular
- v. apparatus
- v. ligament
- v. nerve
- v. neuronitis
- v. vein

vestibulocochlear nerve

vestibuloocular reflex

vest-type
- v.-t. backboard
- v.-t. extrication device

Veterans Affairs High-Density Lipoprotein Intervention Trial (VA-HIT)

VF
- ventricular fibrillation

V flap

viability of fetus

viable alternative

Viagra

Vibrio cholerae

Vicryl
- V. popoff suture
- V. Rapide suture
- V. SH suture

victim
- v. dependency
- v. of multiple trauma

video-assisted thoracic surgery

vidian
- v. nerve
- v. vein

Vienna wire suture

Vietnam catheter

Vieussens vein

view
- abdominal v.
- anteroposterior v.
- apical and subcostal four-chambered v.
- AP supine portable v.
- axial v.
- frontal v.
- jug-handle v.
- oblique v.
- occipital v.
- OMO v.
- parasternal short axis v.
- postreduction v.

vinegar odor

vinyl shower curtain odor

violence
- domestic v.
- v. history
- intimate partner v. (IPV)
- management of v.

violet
- aniline gentian v.
- gentian v.
- v. odor

viral
- v. exanthema
- v. hemorrhagic fever
- v. infection
- v. meningitis
- v. meningoencephalitis
- v. pneumonia

Virchow stasis triad

Virginia creeper

virgin silk suture

viride
- *Veratrum v.*

Viro-Tec suture

virus
- Hantaan v.
- hepatitis A v. (HAV)
- hepatitis B v. (HBV)
- hepatitis C v. (HBC)
- hepatitis D v. (HDV)
- herpes simplex v. (HSV)
- human immunodeficiency v. (HIV)
- influenza v.
- respiratory syncytial v. (RSV)
- varicella-zoster v.

West Nile v.
wound tumor v.
viscera (*pl. of* viscus)
visceral
v. aneurysm
v. distention
v. ischemia
v. ischemic obstruction
v. muscle
v. nerve
v. pain
v. pleura
viscerocutaneous loxoscelism
visceromegaly
viscid
viscosity
blood v.
viscous
v. distention
v. lidocaine
viscus, pl. **viscera**
perforated v.
viselike chest pain
vision
blurred v.
Vistide
visual
v. acuity
v. change
v. deficit
v. disturbance
v. evoked response
v. hallucination
v. loss
vital
v. capacity (VC)
v. signs
v. signs stable (VSS)
vitamin
v. A toxicity
v. B_{12} deficiency
v. B_1 toxicity
v. B_2 toxicity
v. B_6 toxicity
v. B_{12} toxicity
v. C toxicity
v. D toxicity
v. E toxicity
v. K
v. K therapy
v. K toxicity
vitelline vein

vitiligo
vitreous
v. hemorrhage
v. hemorrhage facet
v. humor
vivid dream
vivo
in v.
vocal
v. cord avulsion
v. ligament
v. muscle
volar
v. beak ligament
v. carpal ligament
v. interosseous nerve
v. plaster splint
v. radiocarpal ligament
v. radiotriquetral ligament
v. rim distal radial fracture
v. shear fracture
volatile substance
Volkmann fracture
volume
cerebral blood v.
corpuscular v.
v. depletion
expiratory reserve v. (ERV)
forced expiratory v.
increased plasma v.
intravascular v.
minute v.
pressure v. (PV)
residual v. (RV)
v. resuscitation
stroke v. (SV)
tidal v.
ventricular end-diastolic v.
volume-cycled ventilator
voluntary
v. muscle
v. nervous system
v. sterilization
volvulus
cecal v.
vomer bone
vomeronasal nerve
vomit
coffee-grounds v.
vomiting
adult v.
cerebral v.

V

NOTES

vomiting *(continued)*
    nausea and v.
    pediatric v.
vomitus
    bilious v.
    bloody v.
von
    v. Recklinghausen disease of bone
    v. Willebrand disease
    v. Willebrand factor
vortex vein
vorticose vein
Voshell bursa
Vostal radial fracture classification
V/Q
    ventilation/perfusion
    V/Q mismatch

V-shaped fracture
VSS
    vital signs stable
V-suture
    Marshall V-s.
VT
    ventricular tachycardia
vulgaris
    acne v.
vulvar irritation
vulvovaginitis
V-Y advancement flap

Waddell triad
wagon wheel fracture
Wagstaffe fracture
Wagstaffe-Le Fort fracture
waist fracture
wait-and-see strategy
Waldeyer preurethral ligament
wall
    chest w. (CW)
    paradoxical movement of chest w.
    w. thickening
    vein w.
wallet card identifier
Walther
    W. fracture
    W. oblique ligament
wand
    light w.
wandering atrial pacemaker
waned
    waxed and w.
warfarin skin necrosis
warm
    w. shock
    w. water, analgesic, stool softener, high-fiber diet (WASH)
warmer
    Soft Sack IV fluid w.
Warren shunt
wart
    genital w.
    plantar w.
WASH
    warm water, analgesic, stool softener, high-fiber diet
    WASH regimen
washout syndrome
wasp sting
Wassermann antibody
wasting
    muscle w.
    muscle fiber w.
water
    body w.
    w. brash
    w. depletion heat exhaustion
    dextrose in w. (D/W)
    extravascular lung w.
    w. hemlock toxicity
    w. homeostasis
    intracellular w.
    w. pill
    total body w.
water-bottle appearance
Waterhouse-Friderichsen syndrome

watershed infarction
Watson-Jones
    W.-J. navicular fracture
    W.-J. tibial tubercle avulsion fracture classification
wave
    coved T w.
    electrocardiographic w. (QRS)
    non-Q w.
    peaked T w.
    Q w.
    T w.
    tented T w.
waxed and waned
3-way stopcock
WBC
    white blood cell
WBI
    whole bowel irrigation
WCC
    white cell count
weakness
    ligamentous w.
    muscle w.
weak pulse
weaning
    w. outcome
    T-piece w.
    ventilator w.
weapon
    bone w.
Weathertech EMS 3-in-1 systems jacket
Weber (B, C) fracture
web ligament
wedge
    w. bone
    bone w.
    w. compression fracture
    w. flexion-compression fracture
    pulmonary artery w. (PAW)
wedge-and-groove suture
wedge-shaped uncomminuted tibial plateau fracture
weed
    jimson w.
week
    day of the w.
Weigert ligament
weight
    birth w. (BW)
    body w.
weightbearing
    avoid w.
    w. bone
    painful w.

W

Weitbrecht ligament
welfare agency
well
    tolerating oral fluids w.
Wellen syndrome
well-localized pain
Wenckebach block
Wernicke encephalopathy
Westermark sign
western boot in open fracture
West Nile virus
wet drowning
wheal
wheeled stretcher
wheeze
    expiratory w.
wheezing
    audible w.
    w. breath sound
whettle bone
whiff test
whistle-tip catheter
whistling rhonchi
white
    w. blood cell (WBC)
    w. blood cell count
    w. braided silk suture
    w. cell count (WCC)
    w. middle-aged female
    w. middle-aged male
    w. muscle
    w. nylon suture
    w. phosphorus
    w. twisted suture
whitlow
    herpetic w.
Whitnall ligament
whole
    w. blood
    w. bowel irrigation (WBI)
wide-complex
    w.-c. arrhythmia
    w.-c. sinus tachycardia
    w.-c. tachyarrhythmia
wide cranial suture
widened mediastinum
widening
    mediastinal w.
widow spider
width
    QRS w.
Wieger ligament
Wilkins radial fracture classification
will
    living w.
Willis nerve
willow fracture
Wilms tumor

Wilson
    W. fracture
    W. muscle
wind-chill factor
window
    acoustic w.
    bone w.
    pericardial w.
windpipe
wing
    w. suture
    w. tendon
Winquist-Hansen femoral fracture
  classification
Winslow ligament
wintergreen odor
wipe
    bullet w.
wire
    suture w.
    w. Zytor suture
Wisconsin blade
Wisteria sinensis
withdrawal
    alcohol w.
    alpha-2 receptor w.
    amphetamine w.
    concurrent alcohol w.
    drug w.
    neonatal w.
    opiate w.
    w. reflex
    symptom of alcohol w.
    w. symptoms
    w. syndrome
withdrawn
without major sequela
Witness
    Jehovah's W.
WOB
    work of breathing
Wolff-Parkinson-White (WPW)
    W.-P.-W. syndrome
wood
    w. alcohol
    W. light
Woods corkscrew maneuver
Woodward operation wound
woodworking toxin
Word catheter
work of breathing (WOB)
working alliance
workstation
    GEMS CAREpoint EMS w.
workup
    further w.
worm
    helminthic w.
wormian bone

Worst suture
Wort
St. John's W.
worth
comparable w.
wound
abdominal gunshot w.
abraded w.
w. abscess
acute w.
anal w.
anterior w.
w. approximation
aseptic w.
avulsed w.
back gunshot w.
w. ballistics
w. bed
w. biopsy
blowing w.
w. botulism
w. breakdown
bullet w.
burn w.
w. care
w. cavity
central hepatic gunshot w.
chest w.
w. cleanser
w. cleansing
w. clip
closed w.
w. closure
collagen hemostatic material
  for w.'s
w. complication
w. contraction
contused w.
w. covering
crease w.
crepitant w.
w. culture
w. débridement
w. dehiscence
w. discharge
w. disruption
w. drain
w. drainage
w. drainage collector
w. drainage reservoir
w. dressing
w. dressing emulsion

w. entrance
entrance w.
w. eversion
w. excision
exit w.
factitious w.
w. failure
w. fever
w. fibroblast
fishmouth w.
flank gunshot w.
w. fluid
foot puncture w.
w. forceps
fragment w.
fresh w.
full-jacketed bullet w.
fungating w.
w. gape
gaping w.
w. gel
glancing w.
w. 1-6 grading
gun w.
gunshot w. (GSW)
Gustilo classification of
  puncture w.
gutter w.
w. healing
w. healing disorder
w. hematoma
hepatic gunshot w.
w. hernia
high-energy gunshot w.
high-velocity gunshot w.
w. hypoxia
incised w.
w. incision and suction
w. infection
intrabuccal w.
w. irrigation
w. ischemia
joint w.
knife w.
lacerated w.
lacerating w.
laparoscopic trocar w.
lateral w.
w. margin
w. margin biopsy
w. matrix contraction
w. measuring guide

NOTES

W

wound *(continued)*
    missile w.
    missile-caused w.
    Mohs w.
    multiple fragment w.
    multiple stab w.'s
    mutilating w.
    w. myiasis
    w. necrosis
    nonhealing w.
    nonpenetrating w.
    open w.
    open-sky cataract w.
    w. packing
    penetrating neck w.
    perforating w.
    precordial w.
    w. problem
    psychic w.
    puncture w.
    radiation w.
    w. recurrence
    remodeling of w.
    renal stab w.
    w. retraction
    sacral w.
    saltwater-related w.
    secondary closure of w.
    self-inflicted gunshot w.
    self-inflicted stab w.
    w. sepsis
    septic w.
    w. seroma
    seton w.
    shored exit w.
    shotgun w.
    silicone-treated w.
    w. site
    skin deficit w.
    spiral w.
    stab w.
    sternotomy w.
    W. Stick measuring system

    subcutaneous w.
    submucosal w.
    sucking chest w.
    superficial w.
    suprapubic stab w.
    surgical w.
    w. swab
    tangential w.
    w. tensile strength
    w. tension
    thoracoabdominal gunshot w.
    w. towel
    w. tract
    transmediastinal penetrating w.
    transpelvic gunshot w.
    trocar w.
    w. tumor virus
    Woodward operation w.
    zone of antemortem w.
    3 zones of a burn w.
woven bone
WPW
    Wolff-Parkinson-White
    WPW syndrome
WR-30 digital weather/hazard radio
wrapping
    nerve w.
    splenic w.
    vein valve w.
wringer-type injury
wrinkler muscle
Wrisberg
    W. ligament
    W. nerve
wrist
    w. arthrocentesis
    w. disarticulation
    w. extensor tendon
    w. splint
    w. triquetrum bone
writhing with pain
written consent

xanthogranuloma
  bone x.
xanthoma
  tendon x.
xenogeneic bone
xenograft
Xenon-enhanced computed tomography
xenotransplantation
Xigris
xiphicostal ligament

xiphoid
  x. bone
  x. ligament
  x. process
Xpouch emergency kit
x-ray
  chest x-r. (CXR)
  x-r. dosimetry
Xyrem

X

Y
 Y fracture
 Y suture
Yale Observation Scale (YOS)
Yankauer
 Y. suction tip
 Y. tonsil-tip suction catheter
yaw
 bullet y.
yeast
 brewer's y.
yellow
 y. fever

 y. ligament
 y. skin
 y. sputum
yohimbine
yoke bone
yoked muscle
YOS
 Yale Observation Scale
yo-yo dieting
Y-shaped
 Y-s. fracture
 Y-s. ligament
Y-T fracture

Y

Zaglas ligament
zalcitabine
zanamavir
Zavanelli maneuver
Zemuron
Zenapax
Zenotech
    Z. biomaterial-synthetic ligament
    Z. synthetic ligament
Zephiran antiseptic
zero-order kinetics
ZF suture
Zickel fracture
zigzag laceration
Zingg type A1 zygomatic arch fracture
Zinn
    Z. ligament
    Z. tendon
zipper injury
Zithromax
    Z. Tri-Pak
    Z. Z-Pak
Z-lengthening
    tendon Z-l.
ZMC fracture
Zofran ODT
Zoll
    Z. M Series Critical Care transport defibrillator
    Z. M Series defibrillator monitor pacemaker
Zollinger-Ellison syndrome
zolpidem toxicity
zomepirac
zone
    z. of antemortem wound
    z. of coagulation
    cold z.
    comfort z.
    fracture z.
    z. of hyperemia
    Looser z.
    respiratory z.

    z. of stasis
    transitional z.
3 zones of a burn wound
zoning
zoster
    herpes z.
    varicella z.
Zovirax
Z-Pak
    Zithromax Z-P.
Z suture
Zygadenus
    Z. paniculatis
    Z. venenosus
zygoma fracture
zygomatic
    z. arch
    z. arch fracture
    z. body fracture
    z. bone
    z. complex fracture
    z. fracture
    z. maxillary complex fracture
    z. muscle
    z. nerve
    z. osteocutaneous ligament
    z. retaining ligament
    z. suture
zygomaticofacial nerve
zygomaticofrontal suture
zygomaticomalar complex fracture
zygomaticomaxillary
    z. complex fracture
    z. suture
zygomaticosphenoid suture
zygomaticotemporal
    z. nerve
    z. suture
zygomaticus
    z. major muscle
    z. minor muscle
Zyvox

Z

Appendix 1

Anatomical Illustrations

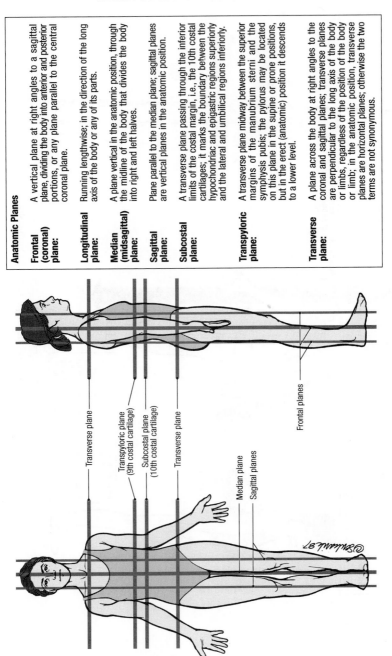

Anatomic Planes

Frontal (coronal) plane: A vertical plane at right angles to a sagittal plane, dividing the body into anterior and posterior portions, or any plane parallel to the central coronal plane.

Longitudinal plane: Running lengthwise; in the direction of the long axis of the body or any of its parts.

Median (midsagittal) plane: A plane vertical in the anatomic position, through the midline of the body that divides the body into right and left halves.

Sagittal plane: Plane parallel to the median plane; sagittal planes are vertical planes in the anatomic position.

Subcostal plane: A transverse plane passing through the inferior limits of the costal margin, i.e., the 10th costal cartilages; it marks the boundary between the hypochondriac and epigastric regions superiorly and the lateral and umbilical regions inferiorly.

Transpyloric plane: A transverse plane midway between the superior margins of the manubrium sterni and the symphysis pubis; the pylorus may be located on this plane in the supine or prone positions, but in the erect (anatomic) position it descends to a lower level.

Transverse plane: A plane across the body at right angles to the coronal and sagittal planes; transverse planes are perpendicular to the long axis of the body or limbs, regardless of the position of the body or limb; in the anatomic position, transverse planes are horizontal planes; otherwise the two terms are not synonymous.

Figure 1. Terms of relationship. Anatomic planes.

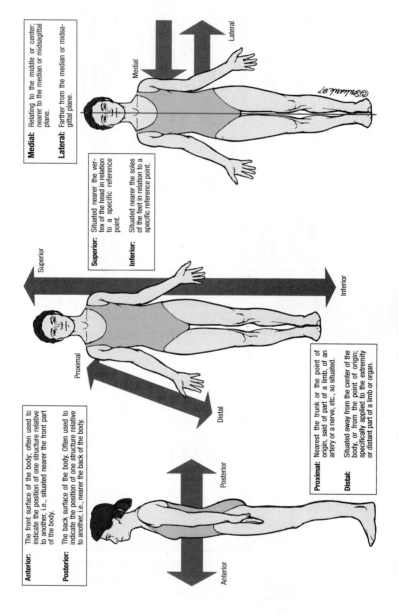

Figure 2. Terms of relationship. Body part terminology.

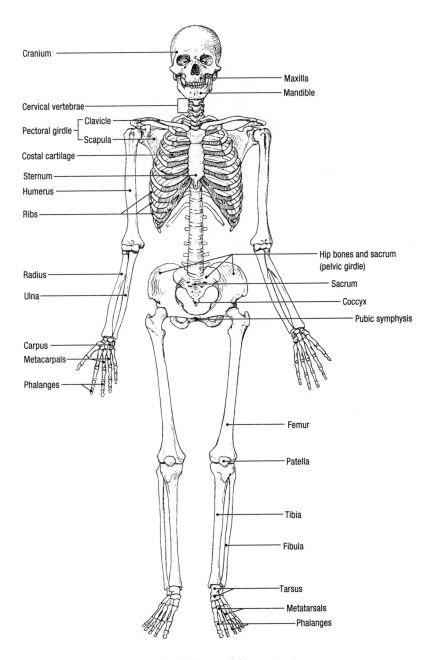

Figure 3. Skeleton, adult, anterior view.

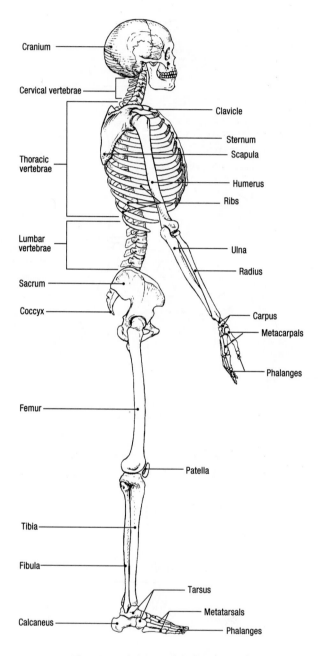

Figure 4. Skeleton, adult, lateral view.

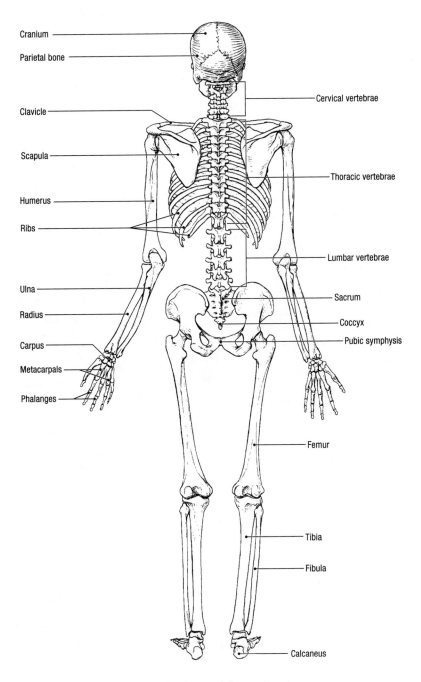

Cranium

Parietal bone

Cervical vertebrae

Clavicle

Scapula

Thoracic vertebrae

Humerus

Ribs

Lumbar vertebrae

Ulna

Sacrum

Radius

Coccyx

Pubic symphysis

Carpus

Metacarpals

Phalanges

Femur

Tibia

Fibula

Calcaneus

Figure 5. Skeleton, adult, posterior view.

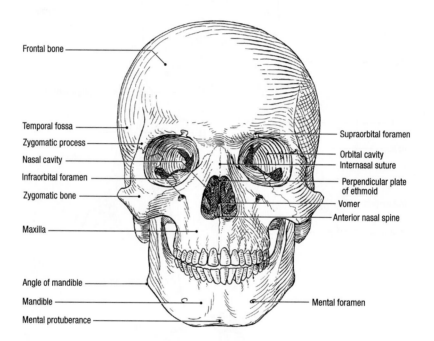

Figure 6. Skull, frontal view.

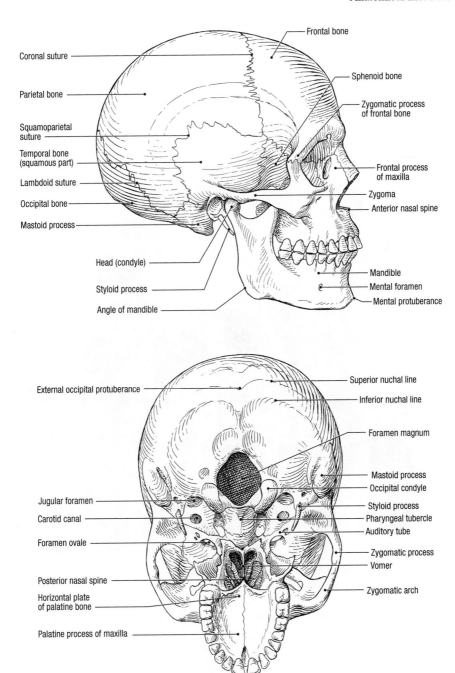

Figure 7. Skull. Lateral view (top), inferior view (bottom).

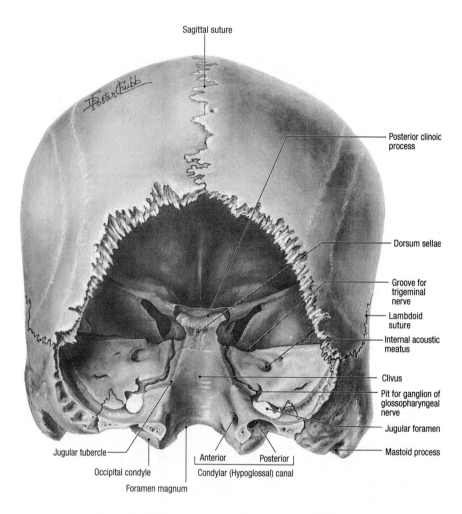

Figure 8. Skull. Bony features of posterior cranial fossa.

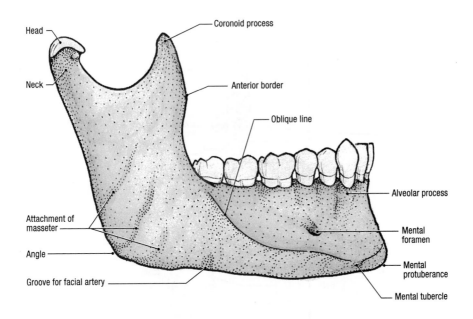

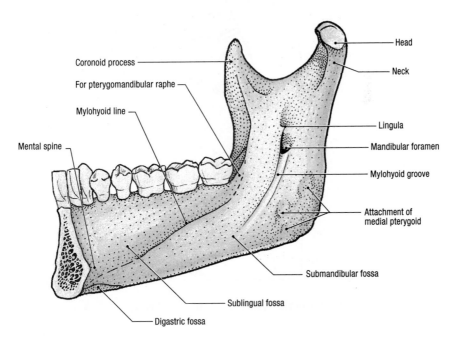

Figure 9. Mandible. External surface, lateral view (top) and internal surface, medial view (bottom).

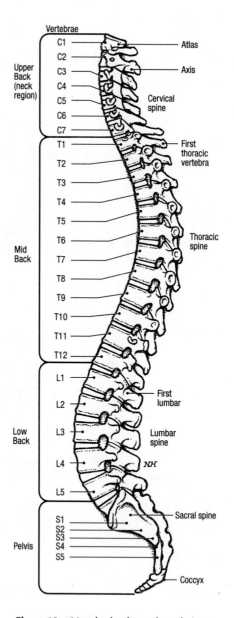

Figure 10. Vertebral column, lateral view.

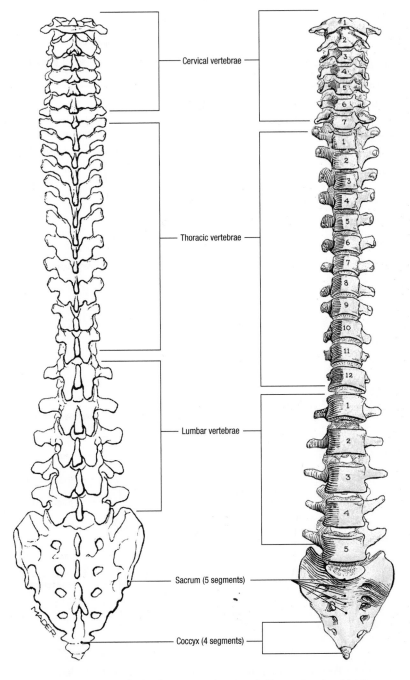

Figure 11. Vertebral column, posterior view (left), anterior view (right).

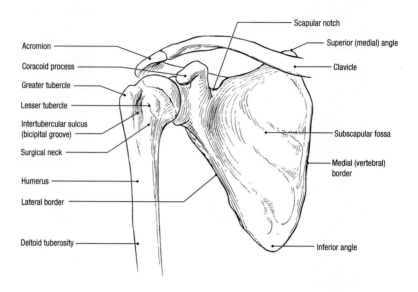

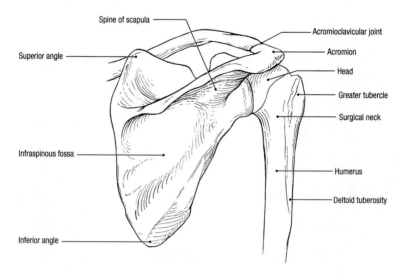

Figure 12. Pectoral girdle and humerus. Anterior view (top), posterior view (bottom).

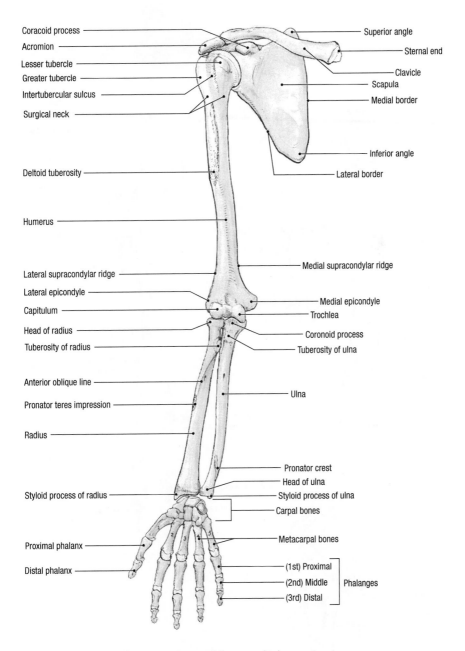

Coracoid process
Acromion
Lesser tubercle
Greater tubercle
Intertubercular sulcus
Surgical neck
Deltoid tuberosity
Humerus
Lateral supracondylar ridge
Lateral epicondyle
Capitulum
Head of radius
Tuberosity of radius
Anterior oblique line
Pronator teres impression
Radius
Styloid process of radius
Proximal phalanx
Distal phalanx

Superior angle
Sternal end
Clavicle
Scapula
Medial border
Inferior angle
Lateral border
Medial supracondylar ridge
Medial epicondyle
Trochlea
Coronoid process
Tuberosity of ulna
Ulna
Pronator crest
Head of ulna
Styloid process of ulna
Carpal bones
Metacarpal bones
(1st) Proximal
(2nd) Middle   Phalanges
(3rd) Distal

Figure 13. Bones of the upper limb, anterior view.

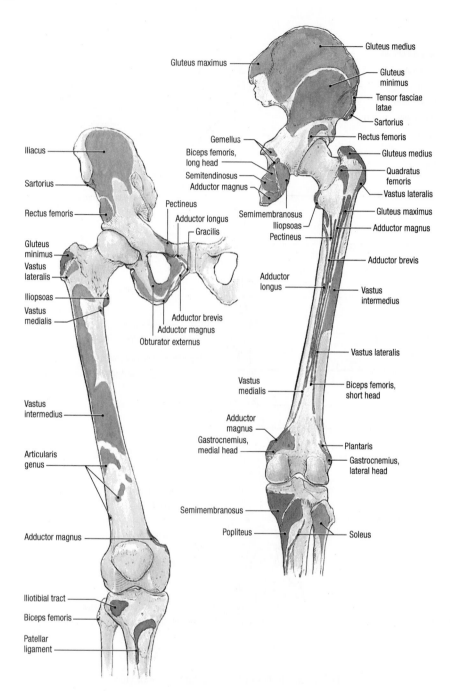

Figure 14. Bones of the lower limbs showing muscle attachments. Anterior view (left), posterior view (right).

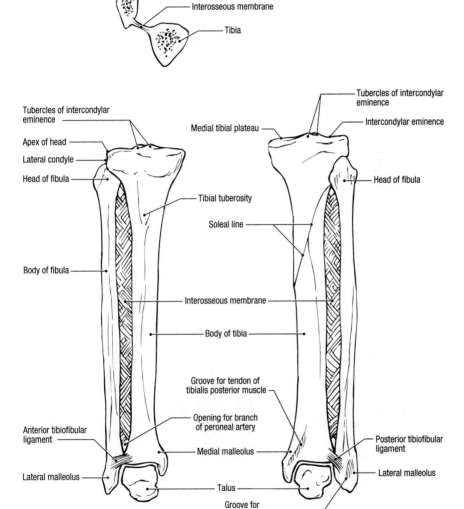

Figure 15. Bones of the lower leg. Anterior view (left), posterior view (right), cross-section (top).

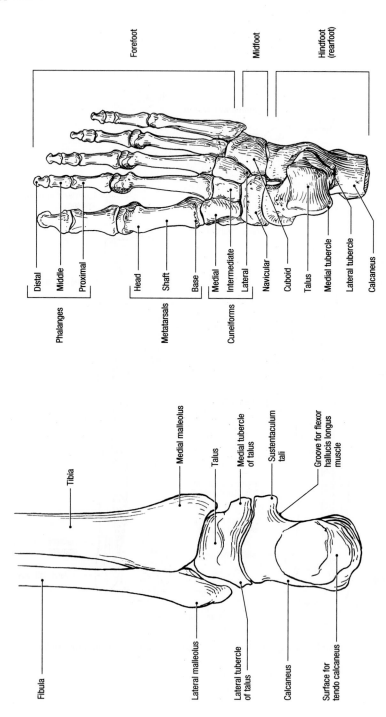

Figure 16. Bones of the ankle and foot. Posterior view (left), dorsal view (right).

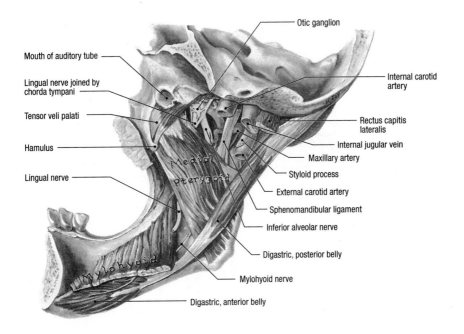

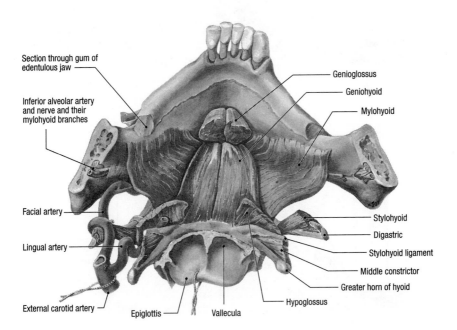

Figure 17. Muscles and vessels of the mandible and base of skull, medial view (top). Muscles of the floor of the mouth, superior view (bottom).

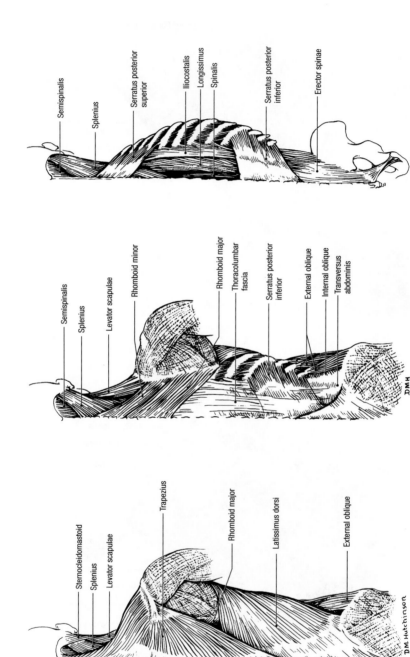

Figure 18. Extrinsic and intrinsic muscles of the back.

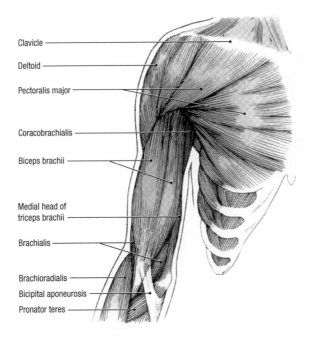

Clavicle

Deltoid

Pectoralis major

Coracobrachialis

Biceps brachii

Medial head of triceps brachii

Brachialis

Brachioradialis

Bicipital aponeurosis

Pronator teres

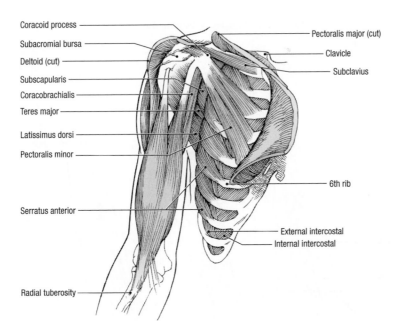

Coracoid process

Subacromial bursa

Deltoid (cut)

Subscapularis

Coracobrachialis

Teres major

Latissimus dorsi

Pectoralis minor

Serratus anterior

Radial tuberosity

Pectoralis major (cut)

Clavicle

Subclavius

6th rib

External intercostal

Internal intercostal

Figure 19. Superficial (top) and deep (bottom) muscles of the shoulder and chest.

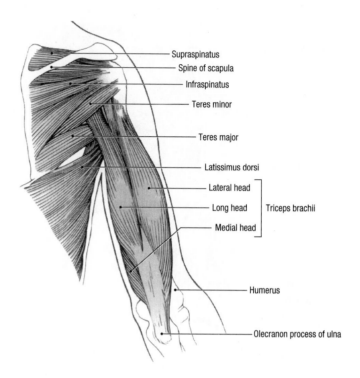

Figure 20. Muscles of the arm, posterior view.

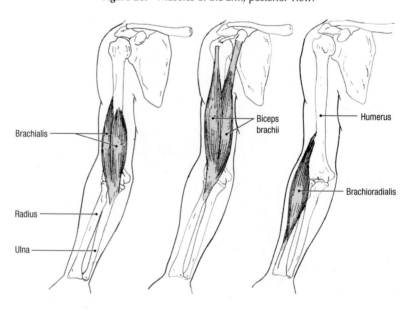

Figure 21. Muscles of the arm, anterior view.

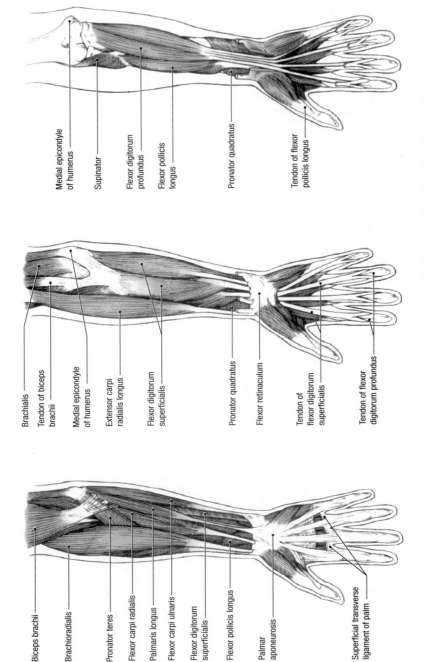

Figure 22. Muscles of the wrist and hand, anterior view. Superficial (left), midlevel (middle), deep (right).

Medial epicondyle of humerus

Supinator

Flexor digitorum profundus

Flexor pollicis longus

Pronator quadratus

Tendon of flexor pollicis longus

Brachialis

Tendon of biceps brachii

Medial epicondyle of humerus

Extensor carpi radialis longus

Flexor digitorum superficialis

Pronator quadratus

Flexor retinaculum

Tendon of flexor digitorum superficialis

Tendon of flexor digitorum profundus

Biceps brachii

Brachioradialis

Pronator teres

Flexor carpi radialis

Palmaris longus

Flexor carpi ulnaris

Flexor digitorum superficialis

Flexor pollicis longus

Palmar aponeurosis

Superficial transverse ligament of palm

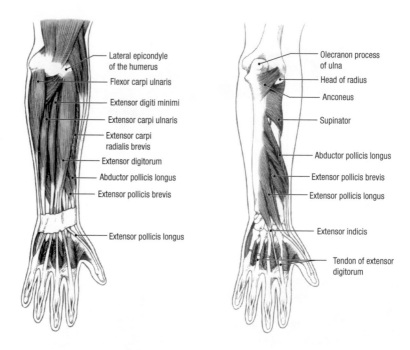

Figure 23. Muscles of the wrist and hand, posterior view. Superficial (left), deep (right).

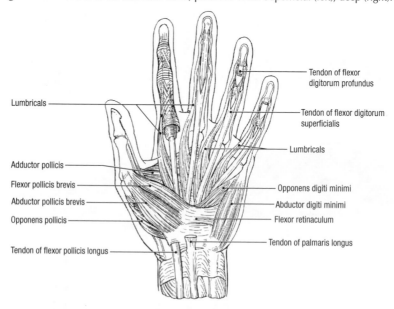

Figure 24. Muscles of the hand, anterior (palmar) view.

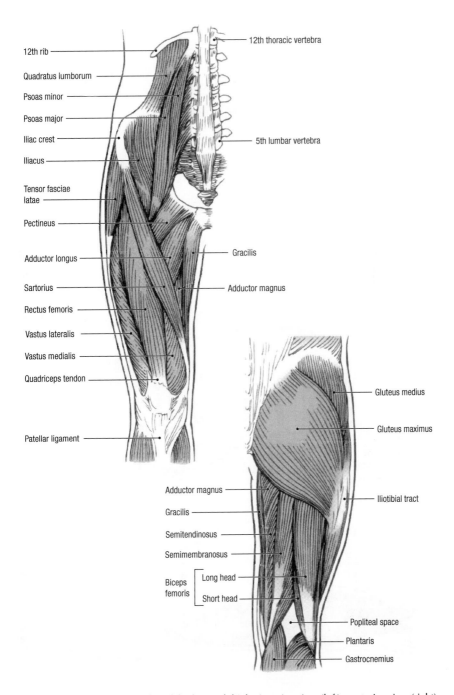

Figure 25. Superficial muscles of the hip and thigh. Anterior view (left), posterior view (right).

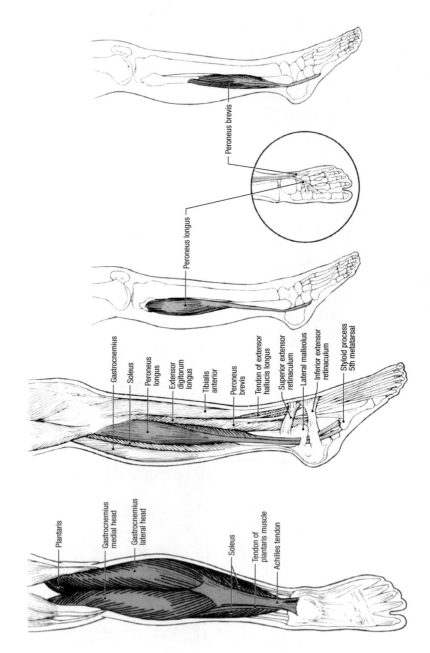

Figure 26. Muscles of the lower leg. Superficial compartment, posterior view (left), lateral compartment (middle and right).

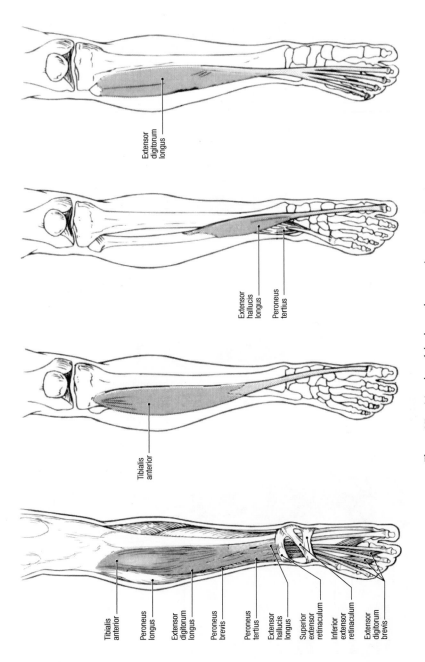

Figure 27. Muscles of the lower leg, anterior compartment.

Extensor
digitorum
longus

Extensor
hallucis
longus

Peroneus
tertius

Tibialis
anterior

Tibialis
anterior

Peroneus
longus

Extensor
digitorum
longus

Peroneus
brevis

Peroneus
tertius

Extensor
hallucis
longus

Superior
extensor
retinaculum

Inferior
extensor
retinaculum

Extensor
digitorum
brevis

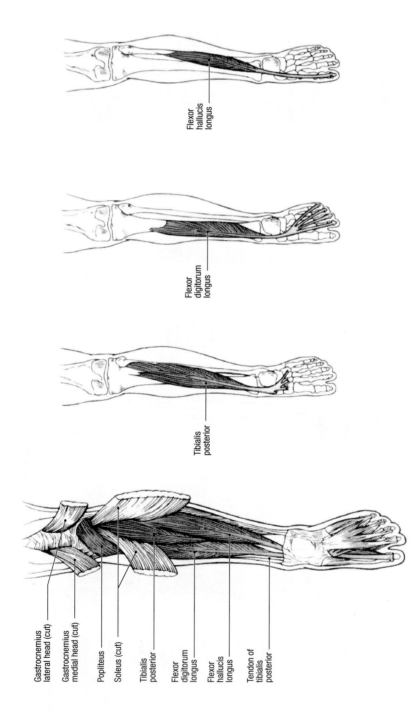

Figure 28. Muscles of the lower leg, deep compartment, anterior view.

Flexor hallucis longus

Flexor digitorum longus

Tibialis posterior

Gastrocnemius lateral head (cut)

Gastrocnemius medial head (cut)

Popliteus

Soleus (cut)

Tibialis posterior

Flexor digitorum longus

Flexor hallucis longus

Tendon of tibialis posterior

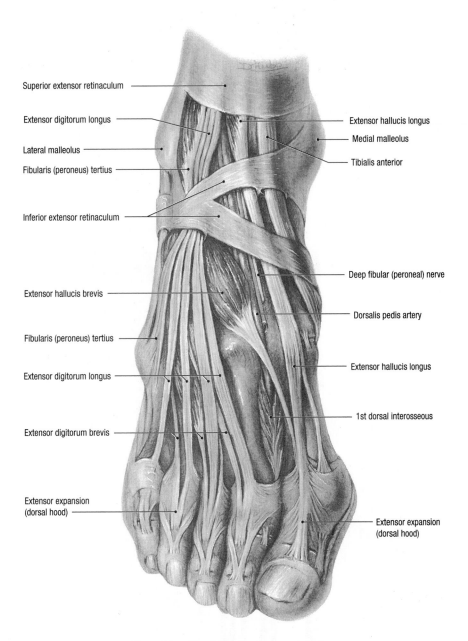

Superior extensor retinaculum

Extensor digitorum longus

Lateral malleolus

Fibularis (peroneus) tertius

Inferior extensor retinaculum

Extensor hallucis brevis

Fibularis (peroneus) tertius

Extensor digitorum longus

Extensor digitorum brevis

Extensor expansion
(dorsal hood)

Extensor hallucis longus

Medial malleolus

Tibialis anterior

Deep fibular (peroneal) nerve

Dorsalis pedis artery

Extensor hallucis longus

1st dorsal interosseous

Extensor expansion
(dorsal hood)

Figure 29. Muscles of the dorsum of the foot.

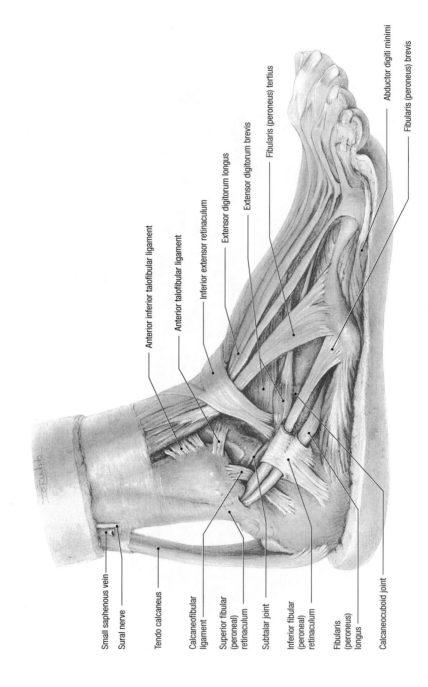

Figure 30. Tendons of the ankle, lateral view.

Small saphenous vein

Sural nerve

Tendo calcaneus

Calcaneofibular ligament

Superior fibular (peroneal) retinaculum

Subtalar joint

Inferior fibular (peroneal) retinaculum

Fibularis (peroneus) longus

Calcaneocuboid joint

Anterior inferior talofibular ligament

Anterior talofibular ligament

Inferior extensor retinaculum

Extensor digitorum longus

Extensor digitorum brevis

Fibularis (peroneus) tertius

Abductor digiti minimi

Fibularis (peroneus) brevis

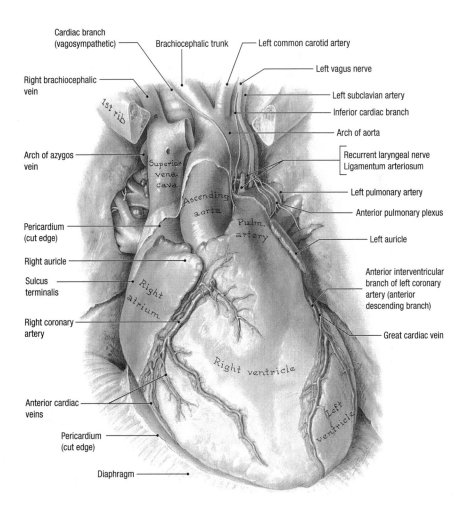

Figure 31. Sternocostal (anterior) surface of the heart and great vessels in situ.

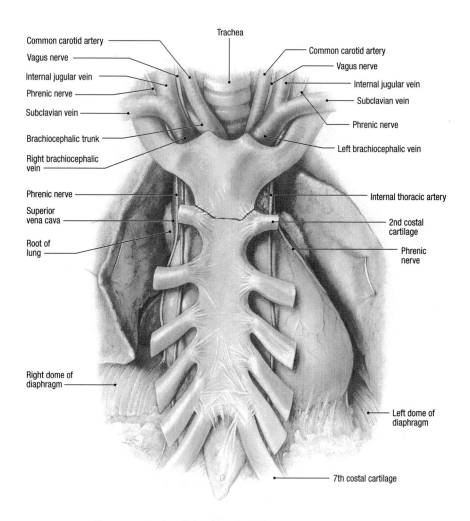

Figure 32. Pericardial sac in relation to sternum, anterior view.

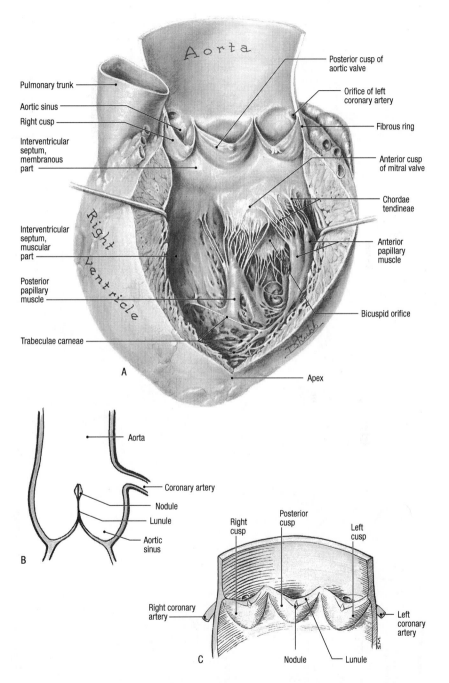

Figure 33. Left ventricle. (A) Interior of left ventricle. (B) Closed aortic valve, cross-section. (C) Spread out aortic valve.

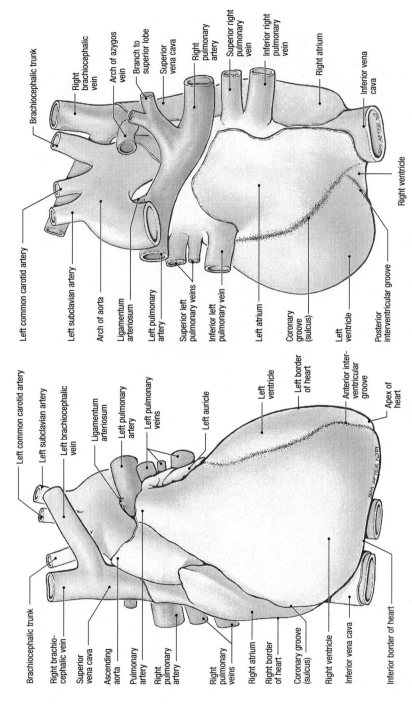

Figure 35. Heart and great vessels, posterior view.

Figure 34. Heart and great vessels, anterior view.

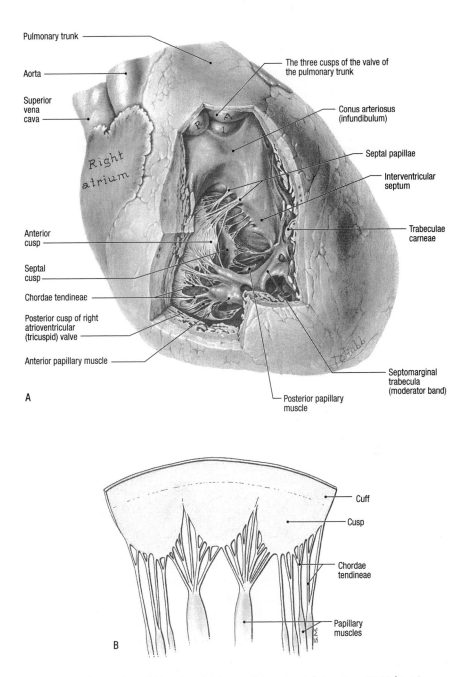

Pulmonary trunk

Aorta

Superior vena cava

Right atrium

Anterior cusp

Septal cusp

Chordae tendineae

Posterior cusp of right atrioventricular (tricuspid) valve

Anterior papillary muscle

A

The three cusps of the valve of the pulmonary trunk

Conus arteriosus (infundibulum)

Septal papillae

Interventricular septum

Trabeculae carneae

Septomarginal trabecula (moderator band)

Posterior papillary muscle

Cuff

Cusp

Chordae tendineae

Papillary muscles

B

Figure 36. Right ventricle. (A) Interior of right ventricle, anteroinferior view. (B) Right atrioventricular (tricuspid) valve spread out.

A33

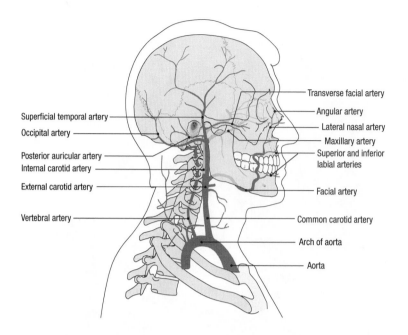

Figure 37. Arteries of the head and neck.

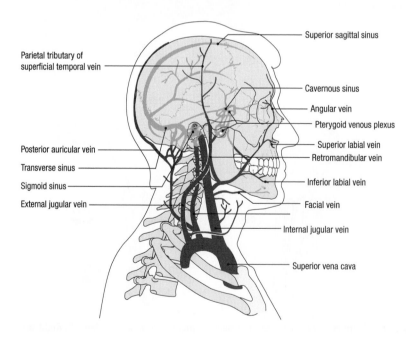

Figure 38. Veins of the head and neck.

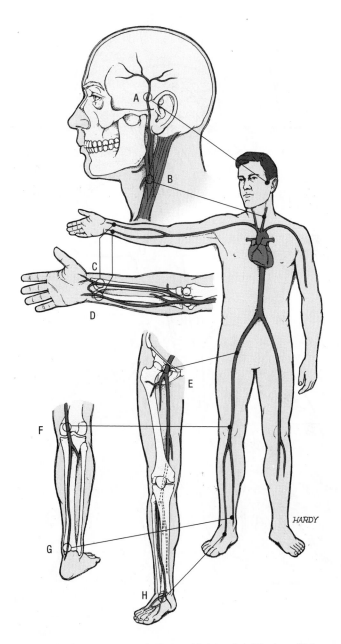

Figure 39. Peripheral pulses. (A) temporal, (B) carotid, (c) radial, (D) ulnar, (E) femoral, (F) popliteal, (G) posterior tibial, (H) dorsalis pedis.

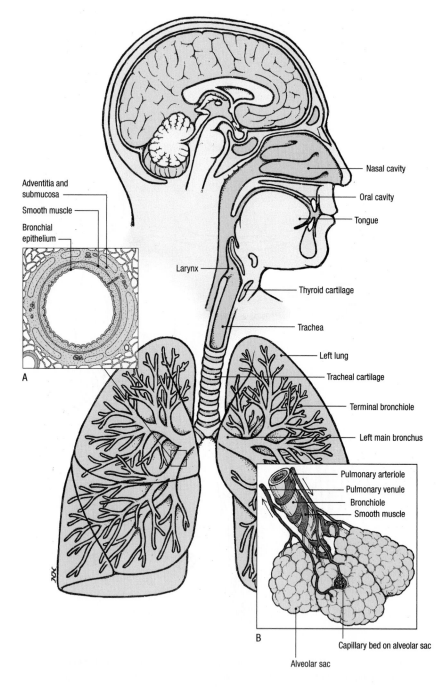

Figure 40. Lungs and respiratory anatomy. (A) intrapulmonary bronchus, (B) pulmonary alveolus.

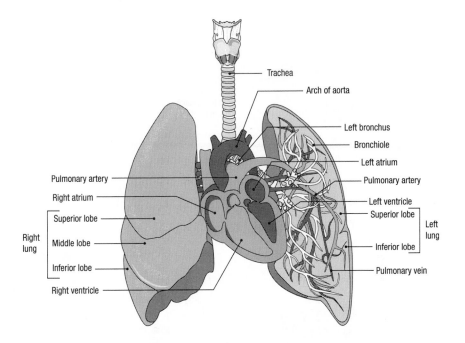

Figure 41. Cardiopulmonary system shown with cutaway of heart and left lung revealing internal anatomy.

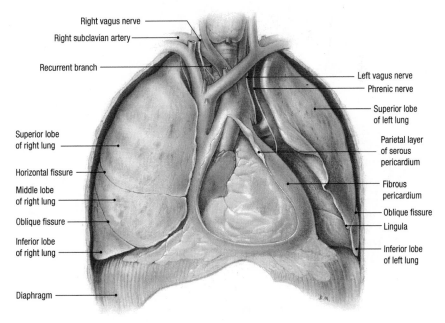

Figure 42. Thoracic contents in situ, anterior view.

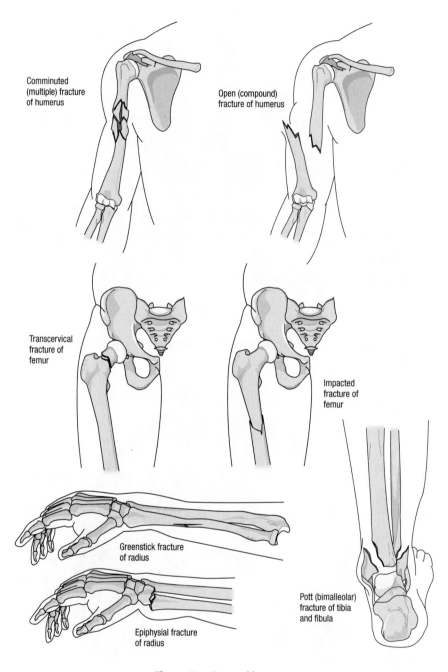

Figure 43. Types of fractures.

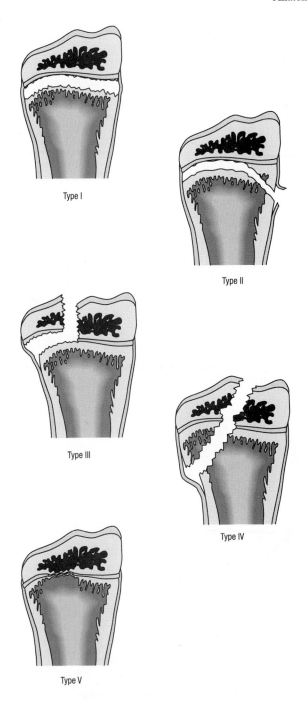

Type I

Type II

Type III

Type IV

Type V

Figure 44. Five groups of the Salter-Harris classification of epiphysial plate injuries.

Direction of Fracture Lines

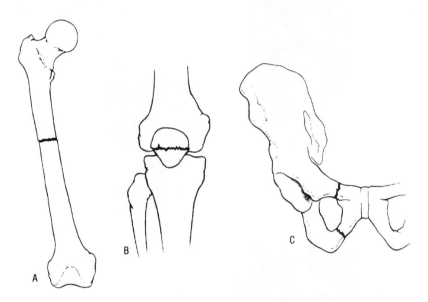

Figure 45. Transverse fractures. (A) Transverse fracture of the middle third of the femur. (B) Transverse fracture of the midpatella. (C) Transverse fracture of the superior and inferior pubic rami.

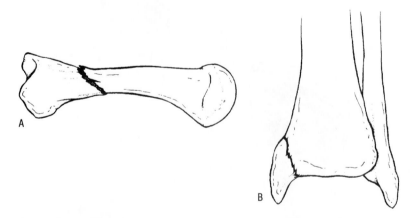

Figure 46. Oblique fractures. (A) Oblique fracture of the proximal third of metacarpal. (B) Oblique fracture of the medial malleolus.

Spinal Fractures

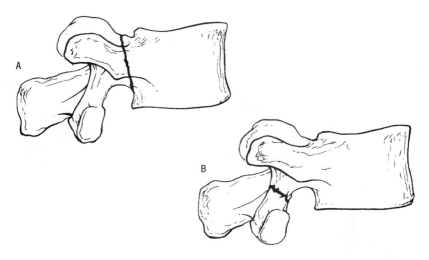

Figure 47. (A) Fracture through the pedicle. (B) Fracture through the pars interartricularis.

Shoulder Fractures

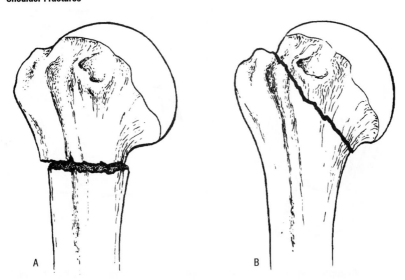

Figure 48. (A) Transverse fracture of the surgical neck of the humerus. (B) Fracture of the anatomic neck of the humerus.

Elbow Fractures

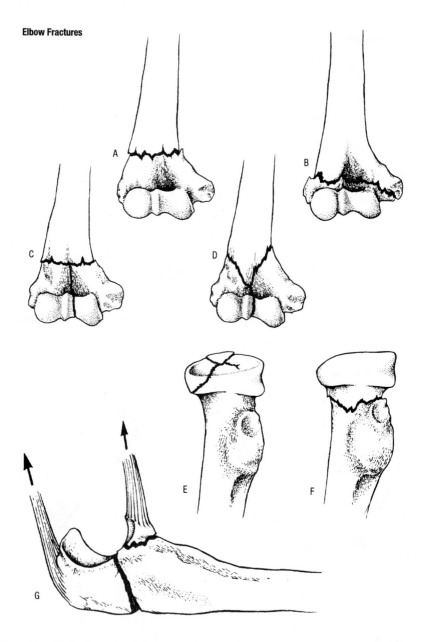

Figure 49. (A) Supracondylar fractures are fractures that occur above the level of the condyles. (B) Transcondylar fracture. Note that the fracture extends through both condyles. Comminuted intraarticular fractures of the distal humerus. (C) T-shaped fracture. (D) Y-shaped fracture. (E) Comminuted fracture of the head of the radius. (F) Transverse nondisplaced fracture of the neck of the radius. (G) Fracture of the olecranon and coronoid process. Muscle contraction can cause distraction of fracture fragments.

Pelvic Fractures

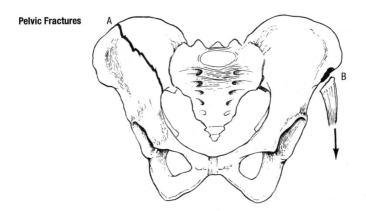

Figure 50. Fractures of the ilium. (A) Oblique fracture through the wind of the ilium. (B) Avulsion fracture of the anteroinferior iliac spine.

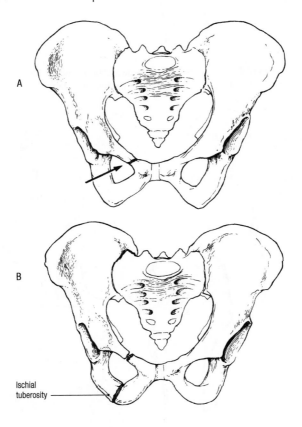

Ischial
tuberosity

Figure 51. (A) Oblique fracture of the superior pubic ramus. (B) Transverse fractures of the inferior ischial ramus and superior pubic ramus.

Hip Fractures

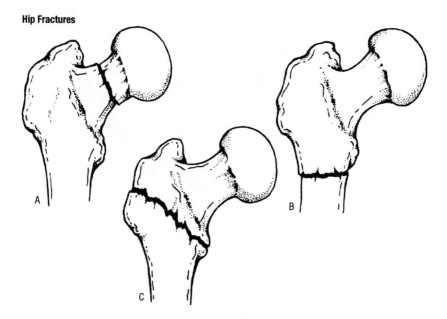

Figure 52. Fractures of the hip are described by the location in which they occur. (A) Transverse intracapsular fracture. (B) Oblique intertrochanteric fracture. (C) Transverse subtrochanteric fracture.

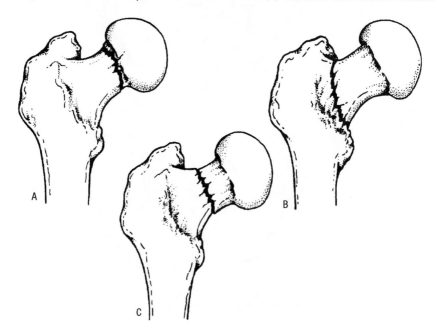

Figure 53. Subclassification of intracapsular fractures. (A) Subcapital fracture. (B) Transcervical fracture. (C) Base of neck fracture.

Knee Fractures

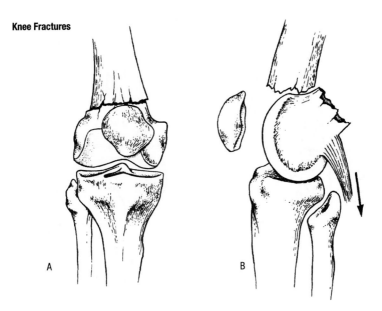

A

B

Figure 54. Supracondylar fracture. Transverse supracondylar fracture of the femur. Note the pull of the gastrocnemius muscle, causing the distal fragment to be rotated posteriorly.

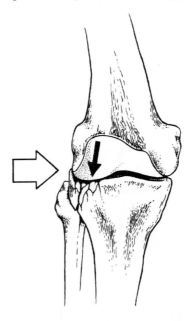

Figure 55. A valgus force applied to the knee causes the hard femoral condyle to be driven into the softer tibial plateau, resulting in depression of the tibial plateau.

A45

Ankle Fractures

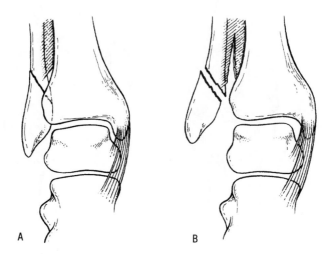

Figure 56. (A) Fracture of the lateral malleolus occurring above its articular surface; thus, the ankle mortise is not involved. (B) Similar fracture as in A, above the articular surface with disturbance of the mortise is due to separation of the syndesmosis.

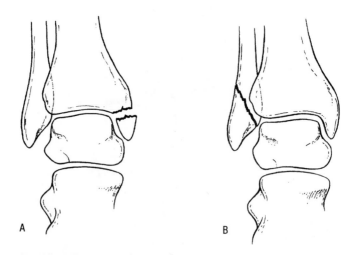

Figure 57. Fractures of the malleoli. (A) Transverse fracture of the medial malleolus. (B) Oblique fracture of the lateral malleolus.

Ankle Fractures

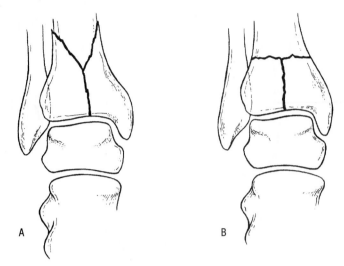

Figure 58. (A) Y-shaped comminuted intraarticular fracture of the distal tibia. (B) T-shaped comminuted intraarticular fracture of the distal tibia.

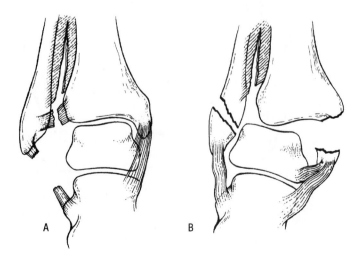

Figure 59. Separation of the distal tibiofibular syndesmosis. (A) Separation of the tibiofibular syndesmosis without an accompanying fracture. (B) Separation of the syndesmosis associated with fracture of the medial and lateral malleoli.

Leg Fractures

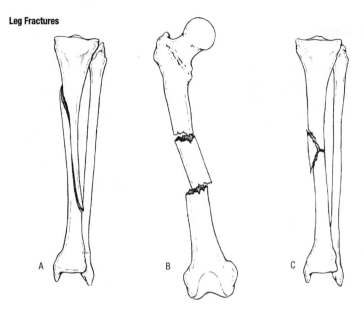

Figure 60.　(A) Spiral fractures of the middle third of the tibia. (B) Segmental fracture of the femur. (C) Butterfly fragment.

Leg Fractures

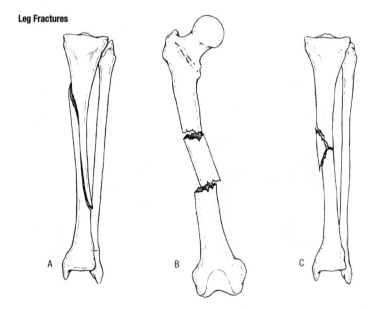

Figure 61.　(A) Compound fracture caused by an inside-out injury. The skin defect is caused, following the fracture, by the bone perforating the skin from within. (B) Outside-in compound fracture. In this injury, the skin defect is produced by the fracturing agent entering from without.

Ankle Fractures

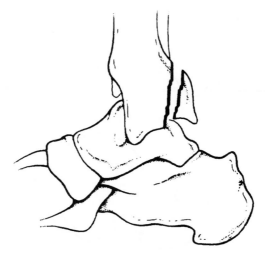

Figure 62. Fracture of the posterior malleolus.

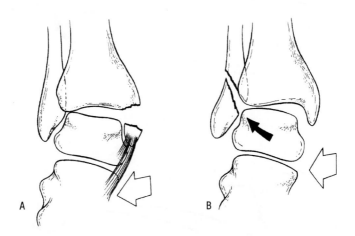

A

B

Figure 63. (A) Avulsion fracture of the medial malleolus. (B) Oblique fracture of the lateral malleolus.

Appendix 1

Foot Fractures

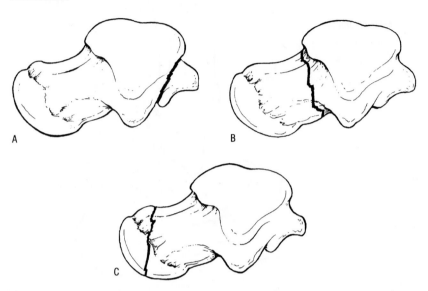

Figure 64. Fractures of the talus can be described by the anatomic area involved. (A) Fracture of the posterior process. (B) Fracture of the body. (C) Fracture of the head.

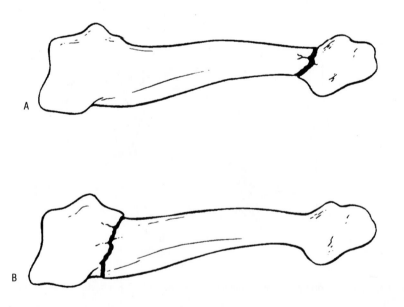

Figure 65. (A) Fracture of the head of a metatarsal. (B) Fracture of the base of a metatarsal.

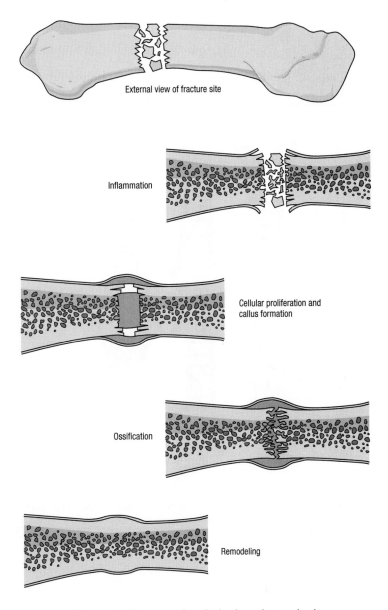

External view of fracture site

Inflammation

Cellular proliferation and
callus formation

Ossification

Remodeling

Figure 66. The process by which a bone fracture heals.

Appendix 1

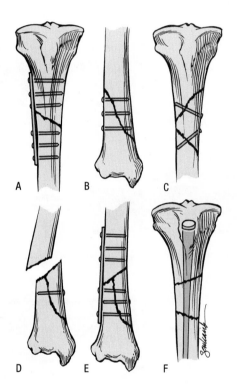

Figure 67. Internal fixation. (A) Plate and six screws for a transverse or short oblique fracture. (B) Screws for a long oblique or spiral fracture. (C) Screws for a long butterfly fragment. (D), (E) Plate and six screws for a short butterfly fragment. (F) Medullary nail for a segmental fracture.

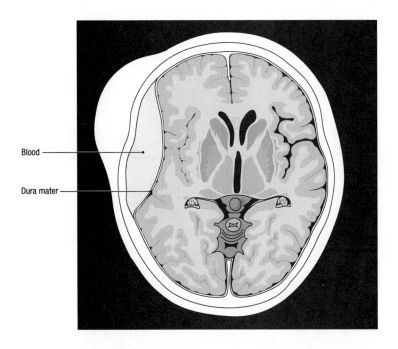

Blood ——

Dura mater ——

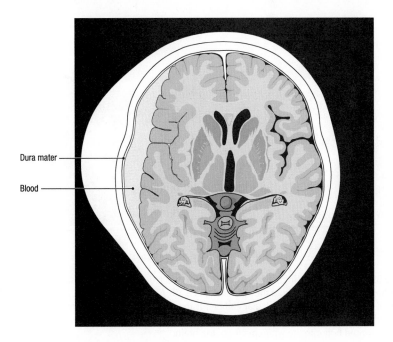

Dura mater ——

Blood ——

Figure 68. Epidural hematoma (top), subdural hematoma (bottom).

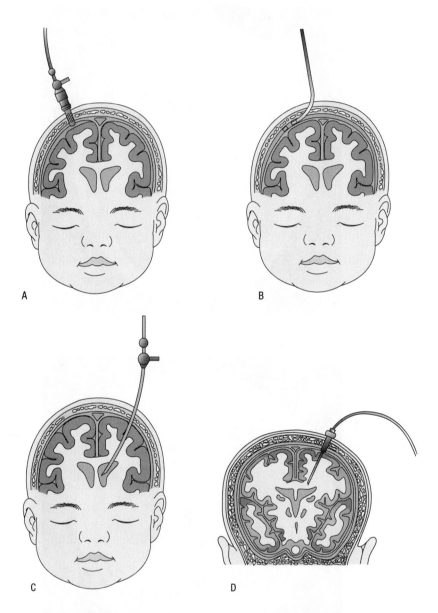

Figure 69. Placement of intracranial pressure monitor. (A) A subarachnoid screw passes through a bur hole in the skull ending in the epidural space. (B) A fiberoptic sensor is implanted into the epidural space. (C) An intraventricular catheter is inserted through the anterior fontanelle and threaded into the lateral ventricle. (D) A fiberoptic transducer-tipped catheter is inserted through a subarachnoid bolt into the white matter of the brain.

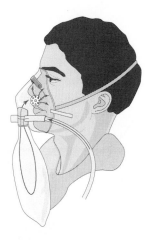

Figure 70. Bag-valve-mask unit.

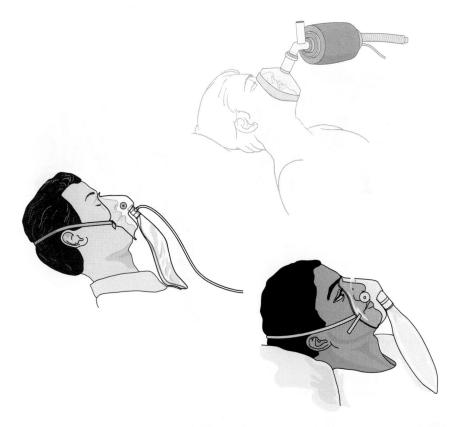

Figure 71. Types of nonrebreathing masks.

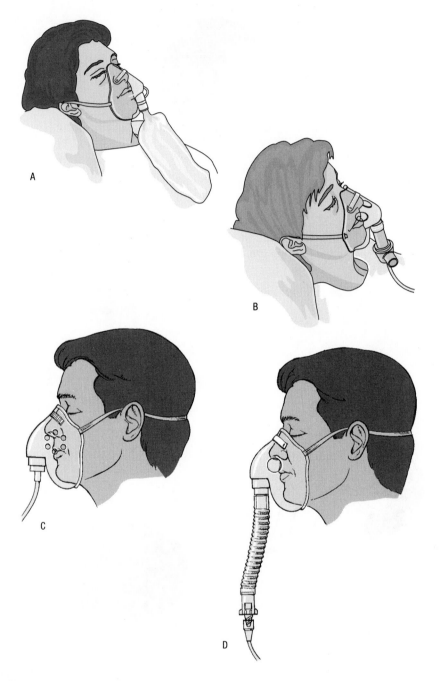

Figure 72. (A) Partial rebreathing oxygen mask. (B) Venturi oxygen mask. (C) Simple face mask. (D) Mask with heated nebulizer.

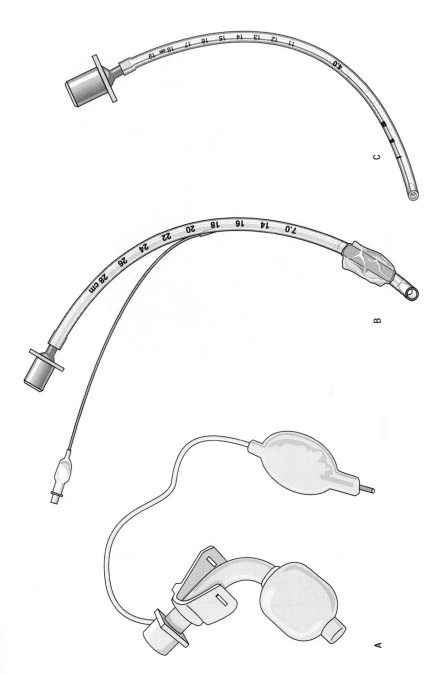

Figure 73. Endotracheal tubes. (A) single-lumen, (B) cuffed, (C) uncuffed.

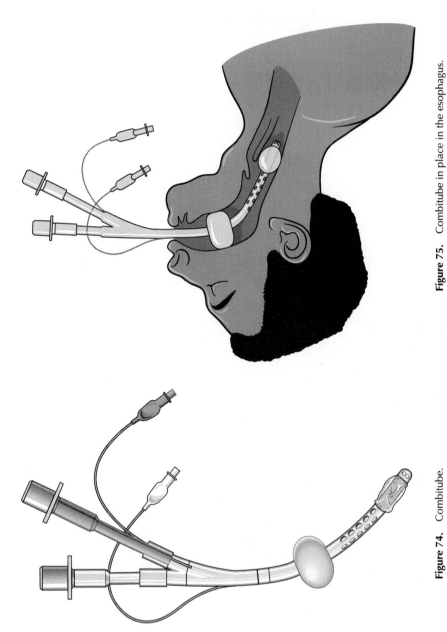

Figure 75. Combitube in place in the esophagus.

Figure 74. Combitube.

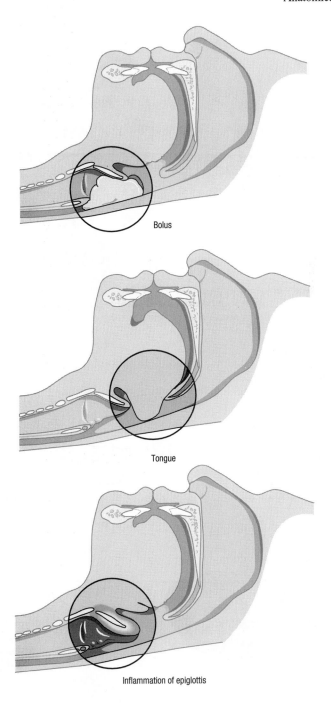

Bolus

Tongue

Inflammation of epiglottis

Figure 76. Types of airway obstruction.

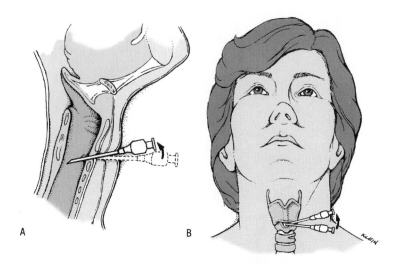

Figure 77. Cricothyroidotomy technique. Two views of a cricothyroid membrane puncture. (A) Sagittal view of neck region with needle inserted just above upper part of cricoid cartilage. (B) Anterior view of head, with needle inserted below thyroid cartilage.

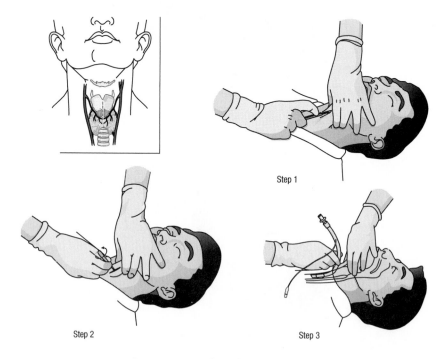

Step 1

Step 2

Step 3

Figure 78. Cricothyroidotomy technique.

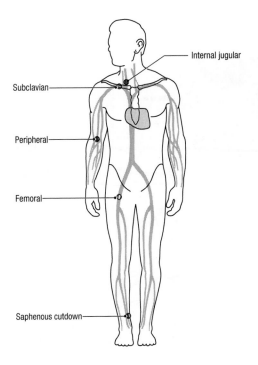

Figure 79. Adult IV sites.

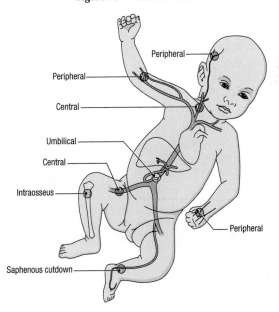

Figure 80. Pediatric IV sites.

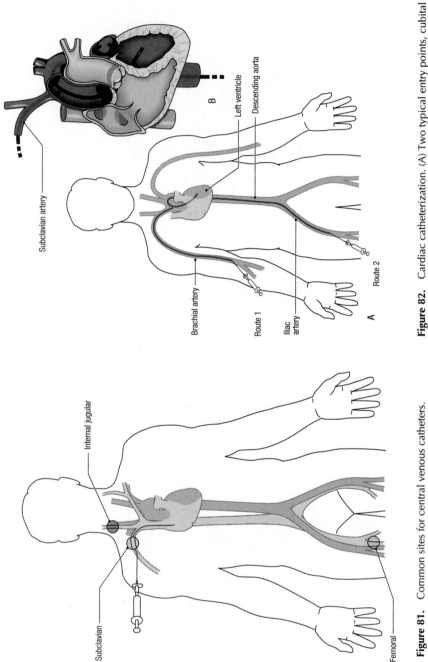

Figure 82. Cardiac catheterization. (A) Two typical entry points, cubital (route 1) and femoral (route 2). (B) Routes entering the heart via the descending aorta and subclavian artery.

Figure 81. Common sites for central venous catheters.

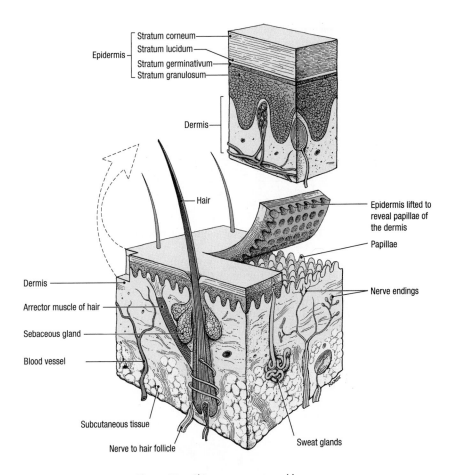

Figure 83. Skin components and layers.

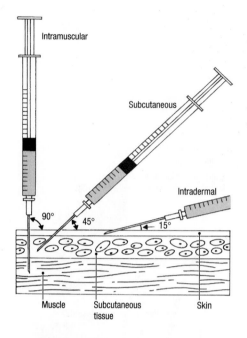

Figure 84. Angles of insertion of injection.

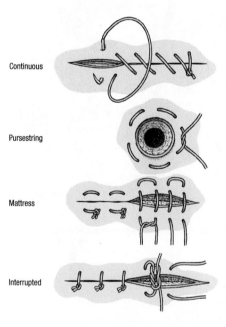

Figure 85. Surgical sutures.

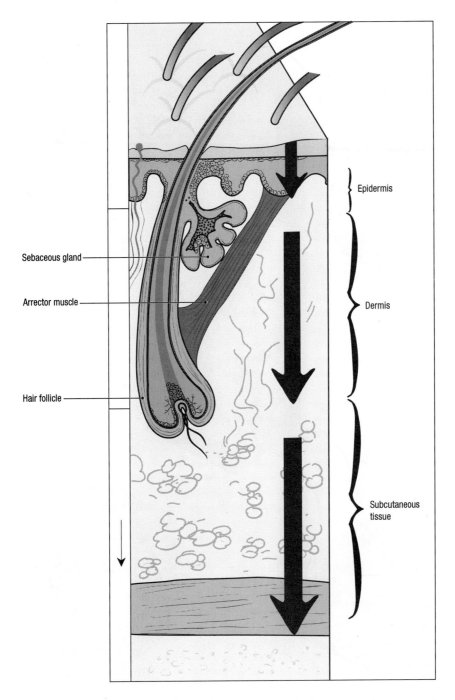

Figure 86. Cross-section of skin layers, muscle and bone, with corresponding classification of burn depths.

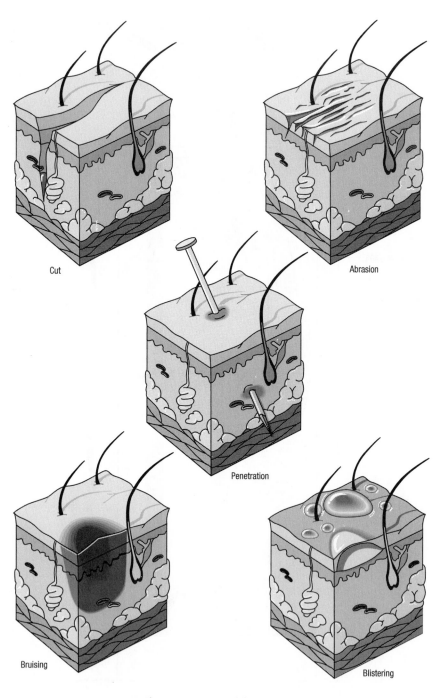

Figure 87. Types of skin injuries.

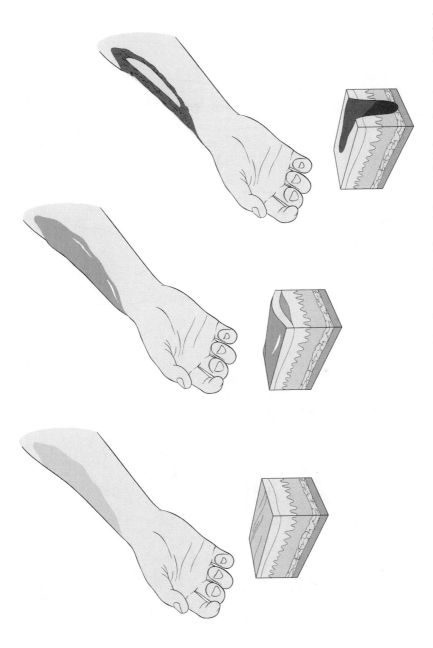

Figure 88. Three types of burns shown on arm and in cross-section of the skin. Superficial burn (left). Partial-thickness burn (center). Full-thickness burn (right).

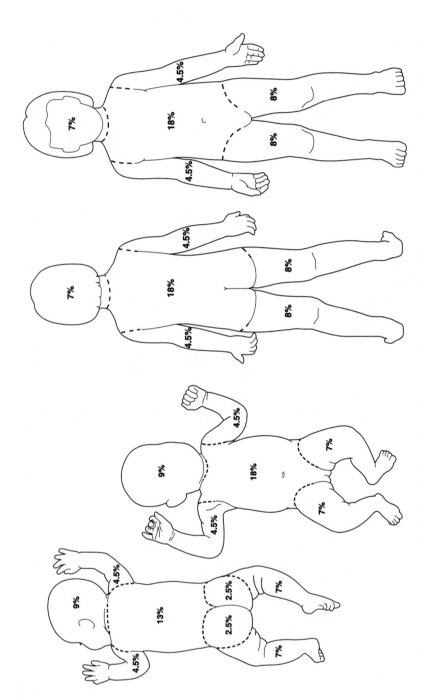

Figure 89. Rule of nines (infant). Outline of infant's body with areas and percentages indicated to calculate total burn surface area.

Figure 90. Rule of nines (child, 5–9 years). Outline of child's body with areas and percentages indicated to calculate total burn surface area.

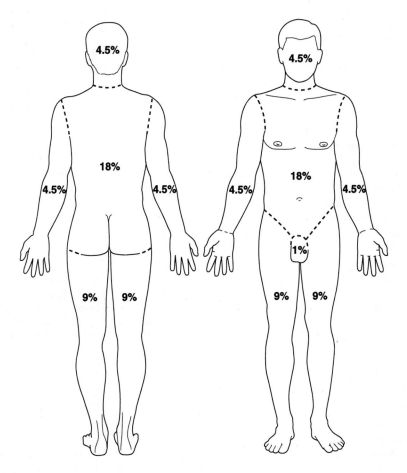

Figure 91. Rule of nines (adult). Outline of adult's body with areas and percentages indicated to calculate total burn surface area.

Normal Lab Values

Tests	Conventional Units	SI Units
Acetaminophen, serum or plasma (Hep or EDTA)		
Therapeutic	10–30 μg/mL	66–199 μmol/L
Toxic	>200 μg/ml	>1324 μmol/L
Acetone		
Serum		
Qualitative	Negative	Negative
Quantitative	0.3–2.0 mg/dL	0.05–0.34 mmol/L
Urine		
Qualitative	Negative	Negative
Acid hemolysis test (Ham)	<5% lysis	<0.05 lysed fraction
Adrenocorticotropin (ACTH), plasma		
8 a.m.	<120 pg/mL	<26 pmol/L
Midnight (supine)	<10 pg/mL	<2.2 pmol/L
Alanine aminotransferase* (ALT, SGPT), serum		
Male	13–40 U/L (37° C)	0.22–0.68 μkat/L (37° C)
Female	10–28 U/L (37° C)	0.17–0.48 μkat/L (37° C)
Albumin		
Serum		
Adult	3.5–5.2 g/dL	35–52 g/L
>60 y	3.2–4.6 g/dL	32–46 g/L
	Avg. of 0.3 g/dL higher in upright individuals	Avg. of 3 g/dL higher in upright individuals
Urine		
Qualitative	Negative	Negative
Quantitative	50–80 mg/24 h	50–80 mg/24 h
CSF	10–30 mg/dL	100–300 mg/dL
Aldolase, serum*	1.0–7.5 U/L (30° C)	0.02–0.13 μkat/L (30° C)
Aldosterone		
Serum		
Supine	3–16 ng/dL	0.08–0.44 nmol/L
Standing	7–30 ng/dL	0.19–0.83 nmol/L
Urine	3–19 μg/24 h	8–51 nmol/24 h
Amikacin, serum or plasma (EDTA)		
Therapeutic		
Peak	25–35 μg/mL	43–60 μmol/L
Trough		
Less severe infection	1–4 μg/mL	1.7–6.8 μmol/L
Life-threatening infection	4–8 μg/mL	6.8–13.7 μmol/L

(continued)

Tests	Conventional Units	SI Units
Toxic		
Peak	>35–40 μg/mL	>60–68 μmol/L
Trough	>10–15 μg/mL	>17–26 μmol/L
∂-Aminolevulinic acid, urine	1.3–7.0 mg/24 h	10–53 μmol/24 h
Amitriptyline, serum or plasma (Hep or EDTA); trough (≥12 h after dose)		
Therapeutic	80–250 ng/mL	289–903 nmol/L
Toxic	>500 ng/mL	>1805 nmol/L
Ammonia		
Plasma (Hep)	9–33 μmol/L	9–33 μmol/L
Amylase*		
Serum	27–131 U/L	0.46–2.23 μkat/L
Urine	1–17 U/h	0.017–0.29 μkat/h
Amylase/creatine clearance ratio	1–4%	0.01–0.04
Androstenedione, serum		
Male	75–205 ng/dL	2.6–7.2 nmol/L
Female	85–275 ng/dL	3.0–9.6 nmol/L
Anion gap		
$(Na - (Cl + HCO_3))$	7–16 mEq/L	7–16 mmol/L
$((Na + K) - (Cl + HCO_3))$	10–20 mEq/L	10–20 mmol/L
α_1-Antitrypsin, serum	78–200 mg/dL	0.78–2.00 g/L
Apolipoprotein A-1		
Male	94–178 mg/dL	0.94–1.78 g/L
Female	101–199 mg/dL	1.01–1.99 g/L
Apolipoprotein B		
Male	63–133 mg/dL	0.63–1.33 g/L
Female	60–126 mg/dL	0.60–1.26 g/L
Arsenic		
Whole blood (Hep)	0.2–2.3 μg/dL	0.03–0.31 μmol/L
Chronic poisoning	10–50 μg/dL	1.33–6.65 μmol/L
Acute poisoning	60–930 μg/dL	7.98–124 μmol/L
Urine, 24 h	5–50 μg/d	0.07–0.67 μmol/d
Ascorbic acid, plasma (Ox, Hep, EDTA)	0.4–1.5 mg/dL	23–85 μmol/L
Aspartate aminotransferase* (AST, SGOT), serum	10–59 U/L (37°C)	0.17–1.00 –2 to +3 kat/L (37°C)
Base excess, blood (Hep)	−2 to +3 mmol/L	−2 to +3 mmol/L
Bicarbonate, serum (venous)	22–29 mmol/L	22–29 mmol/L

(continued)

Appendix 2

Tests	Conventional Units	SI Units
Bilirubin*		
Serum		
Adult		
Conjugated	0.0–0.3 mg/dL	0–5 μmol/L
Unconjugated	0.1–1.1 mg/dL	1.7–19 μmol/L
Delta	0–0.2 mg/dL	0–3 μmol/L
Total	0.2–1.3 mg/L	3–22 μmol/L
Neonate		
Conjugated	0–0.6 mg/dL	0–10 μmol/L
Unconjugated	0.6–10.5 mg/dL	10–180 μmol/L
Total	1.5–12 mg/dL	1.7–180 μmol/L
Urine, qualitative	Negative	Negative
Bone marrow, differential cell count		
Adult		
Undifferentiated cells	0–1%	0–0.01
Myeloblast	0–2%	0–0.02
Promyelocyte	0–4%	0–0.04
Myelocytes		
Neutrophilic	5–20%	0.05–0.20
Eosinophilic	0–3%	0–0.03
Basophilic	0–1%	0–0.01
Metamyelocytes and bands		
Neutrophilic	5–35%	0.05–0.35
Eosinophilic	0–5%	0–0.05
Basophilic	0–1%	0–0.01
Segmented neutrophils	5–15%	0.05–0.15
Pronormoblast	0–1.5%	0–0.015
Basophilic normoblast	0–5%	0–0.05
Polychromatophilic normoblast	5–30%	0.05–0.30
Orthochromatic normoblast	5–10%	0.05–0.10
Lymphocytes	10–20%	0.10–0.20
Plasma cells	0–2%	0–0.02
Monocytes	0–5%	0–0.05
CA15-3, serum	<30 U/mL	<30 kU/L
CA19-9, serum	<37 U/mL	<37 kU/L
CA125, serum	<35 U/mL	<35 kU/L
Cadmium, whole blood (Hep)	0.1–0.5 μg/dL	8.9–44.5 nmol/L
Toxic	10–300 μg/dL	0.89–26.70 μmol/L
Cadmium, urine, 24 h	<15 μg/d	<0.13 μmol/d
Calcitonin, serum or plasma		
Male	=100 pg/mL	=100 ng/L
Female	=30 pg/mL	=30 ng/L
Calcium, serum	8.6–10.0 mg/dL (Slightly higher in children)	2.15–2.50 mmol/L (Slightly higher in children)

(continued)

Tests	Conventional Units	SI Units
Calcium, ionized, serum	4.64–5.28 mg/dl	1.16–1.32 mmol/L
Calcium, urine		
Low calcium diet	50–150 mg/24 h	1.25–3.75 mmol/24 h
Usual diet; trough	100–300 mg/24 h	2.50–7.50 mmol/24 h
Carbamazepine, serum or plasma		
(Hep or EDTA); trough		
Therapeutic	4–12 μg/mL	17–51 μmol/L
Toxic	>15 μg/mL	>63 μmol/L
Carbon dioxide, total		
serum/plasma (Hep)	22–28 mmol/L	22–28 mmol/L
Carbon dioxide (P_{CO2}),	Male 35–48 mmHg	4.66–6.38 kPa
blood arterial	Female 32–45 mmHg	4.26–5.99 kPa
Carbon monoxide as		
carboxyhemoglobin (HbCO),		
whole blood (EDTA)		
Nonsmokers	0.5–1.5% total Hb	0.005–0.015 HbCO fraction
Smokers		
1–2 packs/d	4–5% total Hb	0.04–0.05 HbCO fraction
>2 packs/d	8–9% total Hb	0.08–0.09 HbCO fraction
Toxic	>20% total Hb	>0.20 HbCO fraction
Lethal	>50% total Hb	>0.50 HbCO fraction
Carotene, serum	10–85 μg/dL	0.19–1.58 μmol/L
Catecholamines, plasma (EDTA)		
Dopamine	<30 pg/mL	<196 pmol/L
Epinephrine	<140 pg/mL	<764 pmol/L
Norepinephrine	<1700 pg/mL	<10,047 pmol/L
Catecholamines, urine		
Dopamine	65–400 μg/24 h	425–2610 nmol/24 h
Epinephrine	0–20 μg/24 h	0–109 nmol/24 h
Norepinephrine	15–80 μg/24 h	89–473 nmol/24 h
CEA, serum		
Nonsmokers	<5.0 ng/mL	<5.0 μg/L

Cell counts, adult*
RBC

		Conventional Units	SI Units
Male		$4.7–6.1 \times 10^6/\mu L$	$4.7–6.1 \times 10^{12}/L$
Female		$4.2–5.4 \times 10^6/\mu L$	$4.2–5.4 \times 10^{12}/L$
Leukocytes			
Total		$4.8–10.8 \times 10^3/\mu L$	$4.8–10.8 \times 10^6/L$
Differential	Percentage	Absolute	Absolute (SI)
Myelocytes	0	0/μL	0/L
Neutrophils			
Bands	3–5	150–400/μL	$150–400 \times 10^6/L$
Segmented	54–62	3000–5800/μL	$3000–5800 \times 10^6/L$

(*continued*)

Tests		Conventional Units	SI Units
Lymphocytes	20.5–51.1	$1.2–3.4 \times 10^3/\mu L$	$1.2–3.4 \times 10^9/L$
Monocytes	1.7–9.3	$0.11–0.59 \times 10^3/\mu L$	$0.11–0.59 \times 10^9/L$
Granulocytes	42.2–75.2	$1.4–6.5 \times 10^3/\mu L$	$1.4–6.5 \times 10^9/L$
Eosinophils		$0.07 \times 10^3/\mu L$	$0.07 \times 10^9/L$
Basophils		$0.02 \times 10^3/\mu L$	$0.11–0.59 \times 10^9/L0.02 \times 10^9/L$
Platelets		$130–400 \times 10^3/\mu L$	$1340–400 \times 10^9/L$
Reticulocytes		0.5–1.5% red cells	0.005–0.015 of RBC
		$24,000–84.000/\mu L$	$24–84 \times 10^9/L$
Cells, CSF		0–10 lymphocytes /mm^3	0–10 lymphocytes /mm^3
		0 RBC/ mm^3	0 RBC/ mm^3
Ceruloplasmin, serum		20–60 mg/dL	0.2–6.0 g/L
Chloramphenicol, serum or plasma (Hep or EDTA); trough			
Therapeutic		10–25 μg/mL	31–77 μmol/L
Toxic		>25 μg/mL	>77 μmol/L
Chloride			
Serum or plasma		98–107 mmol/L	98–107 mmol/L
Sweat			
Normal		5–35 mmol/L	5–35 mmol/L
Cystic fibrosis		60–200 mmol/L	60–200 mmol/L
Urine, 24 h (vary greatly with Cl intake)			
Infant		2–10 mmol/24 h	2–10 mmol/24 h
Child		15–40 nmol/24 h	15–40 mmol/24 h
Adult		110–250 mmol/24 h	110–250 mmol/24 h
CSF		118–332 mmol/L (20 mmol/L higher than serum)	118–332 mmol/L (20 mmol/L higher than serum)
Cholesterol, serum			
Adult desirable		<200 mg/dL	<5.2 mmol/L
borderline		200–239 mg/dL	5.2–6.2 mmol/L
high risk		≥240 mg/dL	≥6.2 mmol/L
Cholinesterase, serum*		4.9–11.9 U/mL	4.9–11.9 kU/L
Dibucaine inhibition		79–84%	0.79–0.84
Fluoride inhibition		58–64%	0.58–0.64
Chorionic gonadotropin, intact*			
Serum or plasma (EDTA)			
Male and nonpregnant female		<5.0 mIU/mL	<5.0 IU/L
Pregnant female		Varies with gestational age	
Urine, qualitative			
Male and nonpregnant female		Negative	Negative
Pregnant female		Positive	Positive

(continued)

Tests	Conventional Units	SI Units
Clonazepam, serum or plasma (Hep or EDTA); trough		
Therapeutic	15–60 ng/mL	48–190 nmol/L
Toxic	>80 ng/mL	>254 nmol/L
Coagulation tests		
Antithrombin III (synthetic substrate)	80–120% of normal	0.8–1.2 of normal
Bleeding time (Duke)	0–6 min	0–6 min
Bleeding time (Ivy)	1–6 min	1–6 min
Bleeding time (template)	2.3–9.5 min	2.3–9.5 min
Clot retraction, qualitative	50–100% in 2 h	0.5–1.0/2 h
Coagulation time (Lee-White)	5–15 min (glass tubes)	5–15 min (glass tubes)
	19–60 min (siliconized tubes)	19–60 min (siliconized tubes)
Cold hemolysin test (Donath-Landsteiner)	No hemolysis	No hemolysis
Complement components		
Total hemolytic complement activity, plasma (EDTA)	75–160 U/mL	75–160 kU/L
Total complement decay rate (functional),	10–20%	Fraction decay rate: 0.10–0.20
plasma (EDTA)	Deficiency: >50%	>0.50
C1q, serum	14.9–22.1 mg/dL	149–221 mg/L
C1r, serum	2.5–10.0 mg/dL	25–100 mg/L
C1s (C1 esterase), serum	5.0–10.0 mg/dL	50–100 mg/L
C2, serum	1.6–3.6 mg/dL	16–36 mg/L
C3, serum	90–180 mg/dL	0.9–1.8 g/L
C4, serum	10–40 mg/dL	0.1–0.4 g/L
C5, serum	5.5–11.3 mg/dL	55–113 mg/L
C6, serum	17.9–23.9 mg/dL	179–239 mg/L
C7, serum	2.7–7.4 mg/dL	27–74 mg/L
C8, serum	4.9–10.6 mg/dL	49–106 mg/L
C9, serum	3.3–9.5 mg/dL	33–95 mg/L
Coombs test		
Direct	Negative	Negative
Indirect	Negative	Negative
Copper		
Serum		
Male	70–140 μg/dL	11–22 μmol/L
Female	80–155 μg/dL	13–24 μmol/L
Urine	3–35 μg/24 h	0.05–0.55 μmol/24 h
Corpuscular values of (Hep or EDTA)(values are for adults; in children values vary with age)		
Mean corpuscular hemoglobin (MCH)	27–31 pg	0.42–0.48 fmol

(continued)

Appendix 2

Tests	Conventional Units	SI Units
Mean corpuscular hemoglobin concentration (MCHC)	33–37 g/dL	330–370 g/L
Mean corpuscular volume (MCV)	Male 80–94 μ^3 Female 81–99 μ^3	80–94 fL 81–99 fL
Cortisol, serum		
Plasma (Hep, EDTA, Ox)		
8 AM	5–23 μg/dL	138–635 nmol/L
4 PM	3–16 μg/dL	83–441 nmol/L
10 PM	<50% of 8 AM value	<0.5 of 8 AM value
Free, urine	<50 μg/24 h	<138 mmol/24 h
Creatine kinase (CK), serum†*		
Male	15–105 U/L (30°C)	0.26–1.79 μkat/L (30°C)
Female	10–80 U/L (30°C)	0.17–1.36 μkat/L (30°C)
Note: Strenuous exercise or intramuscular injections may cause transient elevation of CK.		
Creatine kinase MB*		
isoenzyme, serum	0–7 ng/mL	0–7 μg/l
Creatinine*		
Serum or plasma, adult		
Male	0.7–1.3 mg/dL	62–115 μmol/L
Female	0.6–1.1 mg/dL	53–97 μmol/L
Urine		
Male	14–26 mg/kg body weight/24 h	124–230 μmol/kg body weight/24 h
Female	11–20 mg/kg body weight/24 h	97–177 μmol/kg body weight/24 h
Creatinine clearance, serum* or plasma and urine		
Male	94–140 mL/min/1.73 m^2	0.91–1.35 mL/s/m^2
Female	72–110 mL/min/1.73 m^2	0.69–1.06 mL/s/m^2
Cryoglobulins, serum	0	0
Cyanide		
Serum		
Nonsmokers	0.004 mg/L	0.15 μmol/L
Smokers	0.006 mg/L	0.23 μmol/L
Nitroprusside therapy	0.01–0.06 mg/L	0.38–2.30 μmol/L
Toxic	>0.1 mg/L	>3.84 μmol/L
Whole blood (Ox)		
Nonsmokers	0.016 mg/L	0.61 μmol/L
Smokers	0.041 mg/L	1.57 μmol/L
Nitroprusside therapy	0.05–0.5 mg/L	1.92–19.20 μmol/L
Toxic	>1 mg/L	>38.40 μmol/L
Cyclic AMP		
Plasma (EDTA)		
Male	4.6–8.6 ng/mL	14–26 nmol/L
Female	4.3–7.6 ng/mL	13–23 nmol/L

(continued)

Tests	Conventional Units	SI Units
Urine, 24 h	0.3–3.6 mg/d or 0.29–2.1 mg/g creatinine	100–723 μmol/d or 100–723 μmol/mol creatinine
Cystine or cysteine, urine, qualitative	Negative	Negative
C-peptide, serum*	0.78–1.89 ng/mL	0.26–0.62 nmol/L
C-reactive protein, serum	<0.5 mg/dL	<5 mg/L
Cyclosporine, whole blood‡*		
Therapeutic, trough	100–200 ng/mL	83–166 nmol/L
Dehydroepiandrosterone (DHEA), serum		
Male	180–1250 ng/dL	6.2–43.3 nmol/L
Female	130–980 ng/dL	4.5–34.0 nmol/L
Dehydroepiandrosterone sulfate (DHEAS) serum or plasma (Hep, EDTA)		
Male	59–452 μg/dL	1.6–12.2 μmol/L
Female		
Premenopausal	12–379 μg/dL	0.8–10.2 μmol/L
Postmenopausal	30–260 μg/dL	0.8–7.1 μmol/L
Desipramine, serum or plasma (Hep or EDTA); trough (12 h after dose)		
Therapeutic	75–300 ng/mL	281–1125 nmol/L
Toxic	>400 ng/mL	>1500 nmol/L
Diazepam, serum or plasma (Hep or EDTA); trough		
Therapeutic	100–1000 ng/mL	0.35–3.51 μmol/L
Toxic	>5000 ng/mL	>17.55 μmol/L
Digitoxin, serum or plasma (Hep or EDTA); 7.8 h after dose		
Therapeutic	20–35 ng/mL	26–46 nmol/L
Toxic	>45 ng/mL	>59 nmol/L
Digoxin, serum or plasma (Hep or EDTA): ≥12 h after dose		
Therapeutic		
CHF	0.8–1.5 ng/mL	1.0–1.9 nmol/L
Arrhythmias	1.5–2.0 ng/mL	1.9–2.6 nmol/L
Toxic		
Adult	>2.5 ng/mL	>3.2 nmol/L
Child	>3.0 ng/mL	>3.8 nmol/L
Disopyramide, serum or plasma (Hep or EDTA); trough		
Therapeutic arrhythmias		
Atrial	2.8–3.2 μg/mL	8.3–9.4 μmol/L
Ventricular	3.3–7.5 μg/mL	9.7–22 μmol/L
Toxic	> 7 μg/mL	20.7 μmol/L

(continued)

Tests	Conventional Units	SI Units
Doxepin, serum or plasma (Hep or EDTA); trough (≥12 h after dose)		
Therapeutic	150–250 ng/mL	537–895 nmol/L
Toxic	>500 ng/mL	>1790 nmol/L
Estradiol, serum*		
Adult		
Male	10–50 pg/mL	37–184 pmol/L
Female	Varies with menstrual cycle	
Ethanol, whole blood (Ox) or serum		
Depression of CNS	>100 mg/dL	>21.7 mmol/L
Fatalities reported	>400 mg/dL	>86.8 mmol/L
Ethosuximide, serum or plasma (Hep or EDTA): trough		
Therapeutic	40–100 μg/mL	283–708 μmol/L
Toxic	>150 μg/mL	1062 μmol/L
Euglobulin lysis	No lysis in 2 h	No lysis in 2 h
α-fetoprotein (AFP), serum	<15 ng/mL	<15 μg/L
Fat, fecal, F, 72 h		
Infant, breastfed	<1 g/d	<1 g/d
0–6 y	<2 g/d	<2 g/d
Adult	<7 g/d	<7 g/d
Adult (fat-free diet)	<4 g/d	<4 g/d
Fatty acids, total, serum§	190–240 mg/dL	7–15 mmol/L
Nonesterified, serum	8–25 mg/dL	0.28–0.89 mmol/L
Ferritin, serum		
Male	20–150 ng/mL	20–250 μg/L
Female	10–120 ng/mL	10–120 μg/L
Ferritin values of <20 ng/mL (20 μg/L) have been reported to be generally associated with depleted iron stores.		
Fibrin degradation products	<10 μg/mL	<10 mg/L
Fibrinogen, plasma (NaCit)*	200–400 mg/dL	2–4 g/L
Fluoride		
Plasma (Hep)	0.01–0.2 μg/mL	0.5–10.5 μmol/L
Urine	0.2–3.2 μg/mL	10.5–168 μmol/L
Urine, occupational exposure	<8 μg/mL	<421 μmol/L
Folate, serum*	3–20 ng/mL	7–45 nmol/L
Erythrocytes	140–628 ng/mL RBC	317–1422 nmol/L
RBC		
Follicle-stimulating hormone (FSH), serum and plasma (Hep)		
Male	1.4–15.4 mIU/mL	1.4–15.4 IU/L

(continued)

Tests	Conventional Units	SI Units
Female		
Follicular phase	1–10 mIU/mL	1–10 IU/L
Mid cycle	6–17 mIU/mL	6–17 IU/L
Luteal phase	1–9 mIU/mL	1–9 IU/L
Postmenopausal	19–100 mIU/mL	19–100 IU/L
Free thyroxine index (FTI), serum*	4.2–13	4.2–13
Gastrin, serum	<100 pg/mL	<100 ng/L
Gentamicin, serum or plasma (EDTA)		
Therapeutic		
Peak		
Less severe infection	5–8 μg/mL	10.4–16.7 μmol/L
Severe infection	8–10 μg/mL	16.7–20.9 μmol/L
Trough		
Less severe infection	<1μg/mL	<2.1 μmol/L
Moderate infection	<2 μg/mL	<4.2 μmol/L
Severe infection	<2–4 μg/mL	<4.2–8.4 μmol/L
Toxic		
Peak	>10–12 μg/mL	>21–25 μmol/L
Trough	>2–4 μg/mL	>4.2–8.4 μmol/L
Glucose (fasting)		
Blood	65–95 mg/dL	3.5–5.3 mmol/L
Plasma or serum	74–106 mg/dL	4.1–5.9 mmol/L
Glucose, 2 h postprandial, serum	<120 mg/dL	<6.7 mmol/L
Glucose, urine		
Quantitative	<500 mg/24 h	<2.8 mmol/24 h
Qualitative	Negative	Negative
Glucose, CSF	40–70 mg/dL	2.2–3.9 mmol/L
Glucose-6-phosphate*	12.1 ± 2.1 U/g Hb (SD)	0.78 ± 0.13 mU/mol Hb
dehydrogenase	351 ± 60.6 U/10^{12} RBC	0.35 ± 0.06 nU/RBC
(G-6-PD) in erythrocytes, whole blood (ACD, EDTA, or Hep)	4.11 ± 0.71 U/mL RBC	4.11 ± 0.71 kU/L RBC
γ-Glutamyltransferase (GGT), serum		
Males	2–30 U/L (37° C)	0.03–0.51 μkat/L (37° C)
Females	1–24 U/L (37° C)	0.02–0.41 μkat/L (37° C)
Glutethimide, serum		
Therapeutic	2–6 μg/mL	9–28 μmol/L
Toxic	>5 μg/mL	>23 μmol/L
Glycated hemoglobin (Hemoglobin A1c), whole blood (EDTA)	4.2%–5.9%	0.042–0.059

(*continued*)

Tests	Conventional Units	SI Units
Growth hormone, serum		
Male	<5 ng/mL	<5 μg/L
Female	<10 ng/mL	<10 μg/L
Haptoglobin, serum	30–200 mg/dL	0.3–2.0 g/L
HDL-cholesterol (HDL-C), serum		
or plasma (EDTA)		
Adult		
desirable	>40 mg/dL	>1.04 mmol/L
borderline	35–40 mg/dL	0.78–1.04 mmol/L
high risk	<35 mg/dL	<0.78 mmol/L
Hematocrit		
Males	42–52%	0.42–0.52
Females	37–47%	0.37–0.47
Newborns	53–65%	0.53–0.65
Children (varies with age)	30–43%	0.30–0.43
Hemoglobin (Hb)		
Males	14.0–18.0 g/dL	2.17–2.79 mmol/L
Females	12.0–16.0 g/dL	1.86–2.48 mmol/L
Newborn	17.0–23.0 g/dL	2.64–3.57 mmol/L
Children (varies with age)	11.2–16.5 g/dL	1.74–2.56 mmol/L
Hemoglobin, fetal	≥1 y old: <2% of total Hb	≥1 y old: <0.02% of total Hb
Hemoglobin, plasma	<3 mg/dL	<0.47 μmol/L
Hemoglobin and myoglobin, urine, qualitative	Negative	Negative
Hemoglobin electrophoresis, whole blood (EDTA, Cit, or Hep)		
HbA	>95%	>0.95 Hb fraction
HbA$_2$	1.5–3.7%	0.015–0.37 Hb fraction
HbF	<2%	<0.02 Hb fraction
Homogentisic acid, urine, qualitative	Negative	Negative
β-hydroxybutyric acids, serum, plasma	0.21–2.81 mg/dL	20–270 μmol/L
17-Hydroxycorticosteroids		
Urine		
Males	3–10 mg/24 h	8.3–27.6 μmol/24 h (as cortisol)
Females	2–8 mg/24 h	5.5–22 μmol/24 h (as cortisol)
5-hydroxyindoleacetic acid, urine		
Qualitative	Negative	Negative
Quantitative	2–7 mg/24 h	10–4–36.6 μmol/24 h

(*continued*)

Tests	Conventional Units	SI Units
Imipramine, serum or plasma (Hep or EDTA); trough (≥12 h after dose)		
Therapeutic	150–250 ng/mL	536–893 nmol/L
Toxic	>500 ng/mL	>1785 nmol/L
Immunoglobulins, serum		
IgG	700–1600 mg/dL	7–16 g/L
IgA	70–400 mg/dL	0.7–4.0 g/L
IgM	40–230 mg/dL	0.42.3 g/L
IgD	0–8 mg/dL	0–80 mg/L
IgE	3–423 mg/dL	3–423 kIU/L
Immunoglobulin G (IgG), CSF	0.5–6.1 mg/dL	0.5–6.1 g/L
Insulin, plasma (fasting)	2–25 μU/mL	13–174 pmol/L
Iron, serum*		
Males	65–175 μg/dL	11.6–31.3 μmol/L
Females	50–170 μg/dL	9.0–30.4 μmol/L
Iron binding capacity, serum total (TIBC)	250–425 μg/dL	44.8–71.6 μmol/L
Iron saturation, serum		
Male	20–50%	0.2–0.5
Female	15–50%	0.15–0.5
17-ketosteroids, urine		
Males	10–25 mg/24 h	38–87 μmol/24 h
Females	6–14 mg/24 h (decreases with age)	21–52 μmol/24 h (decreases with age)
L-lactate		
Plasma (NaF)		
Venous	4.5–19.8 mg/dL	0.5–2.2 mmol/L
Arterial	4.5–14.4 mg/dL	0.5–1.6 mmol/L
Whole blood (Hep), at bedrest		
Venous	8.1–15.3 mg/dL	0.9–1.7 mmol/L
Arterial	<11.3 mg/dL	<1.3 mmol/L
Urine, 24 h	496–1982 mg/d	5.5–22 mmol/d
CSF	10–22 mg/dL	1.1–2.4 mmol/L
Lactate dehydrogenase (LDH)*		
Total (L P), 37°C, serum		
Newborn	290–775 U/L	4.9–13.2 μkat/L
Neonate	545–2000 U/L	9.3–34 μkat/L
Infant	180–430 U/L	3.1–7.3 μkat/L
Child	110–295 U/L	1.9–5 μkat/L
Adult	100–190 U/L	1.7–3.2 μkat/L
>60 y	110–210 U/L	1.9–3.6 μkat/L

(continued)

Tests	Conventional Units	SI Units
Isoenzymes, serum by agarose gel* electrophoresis		
Fraction 1	14–26% of total	0.14–0.26 fraction of total
Fraction 2	29–39% of total	0.29–0.39 fraction of total
Fraction 3	20–26% of total	0.20–0.26 fraction of total
Fraction 4	8–16% of total	0.08–0.16 fraction of total
Fraction 5	6–16% of total	0.06–0.16 fraction of total
Lactate dehydrogenase, CSF*	10% of serum value	0.10 fraction of serum value
LDL-cholesterol (LDL-C), serum or plasma (EDTA)		
Adult desirable	<130 mg/dL	<3.37 mmol/L
borderline	130–159 mg/dL	3.37–4.12 mmol/L
high risk	≥ 160 mg/dL	≥ 4.13 mmol/L
Lead		
Whole blood (Hep)	<25 μg/dL	<1.2 μmol/L
Urine, 24 h	<80 μg/d	<0.39μmol/d
Lecithin-sphingomyelin (L/S) ratio, amniotic fluid	2.0–5.0 indicates probable fetal lung maturity; >3.5 in diabetics	2.0–5.0 indicates probable fetal lung maturity; >3.5 in diabetics
Lidocaine, serum or plasma (Hep or EDTA); 45 min. after bolus dose		
Therapeutic	1.5–6.0 μg/mL	6.4–26 μmol/L
Toxic		
CNS, cardiovascular depression	6–8 μg/mL	26–34.2 μmol/L
Seizures, obtundation, decreased cardiac output	>8 μg/mL	>34.2μmol/L
Lipase, serum*	23–300 U/L (37°C)	0.39–5.1 μkat/L (37°C)
Lithium, serum or plasma (Hep or EDTA); 12 h after last dose		
Therapeutic	0.6–1.2 mmol/L	0.6–1.2 mmol/L
Toxic	>2 mmol/L	>2 mmol/L
Lorazepam, serum or plasma (Hep or EDTA), therapeutic	50–240 ng/mL	156–746 nmol/L
Luteinizing hormone (LH), serum or plasma (Hep)*		
Male	1.24–7.8 mIU/mL	1.24–7/8 IU/l
Female		
Follicular phase	1.68–15.0 mIU/mL	1.68–15.0 IU/L
Midcycle peak	21.9–56.6 mIU/mL	21.9–56.6 IU/L
Luteal phase	0.61–16.3 mIU/mL	0.61–16.3 IU/L
Postmenopausal	14.2–52.5 mIU/mL	14.2–52.3 IU/L

(*continued*)

Tests	Conventional Units	SI Units
Magnesium		
Serum	1.3–2.1 mEq/L	0.65–1.07 mmol/L
	1.6–2.6 mg/dL	16–26 mg/L
Urine	6.0–10.0 mEq/24 h	3.0–5.0 mmol/24 h
Mercury		
Whole blood (EDTA)	0.6–59 μg/L	<0.29 μmol/L
Urine, 24 h	<20 μg/d	<0.01 μmol/d
Toxic	>150 μg/d	>0.75 μmol/d
Metanephrine, total, urine	0.1–1.6 mg/24 h	0.5–8.1 μmol/24 h
Methemoglobin, (MetHb, hemoglobin), whole blood (EDTA), Hep or ACD)	0.06–0.24 g/dL or 0.78 ± 0.37% of total Hb (SD)	9.3–37.2 μmol/L or mass fraction of total Hb: 0.008 ± 0.0037 (SD)
Methotrexate, serum or plasma (Hep or EDTA)		
Therapeutic	Variable	Variable
Toxic		
1–2 wk after low dose therapy	≥0.02 μmol/L	≥0.02 μmol/L
post-IV infusion 24 h	≥5 μmol/L	≥5 μmol/L
48 h	≥0.5 μmol/L	≥0.5 μmol/L
72 h	≥0.05 μmol/L	≥0.05 μmol/L
Myelin basic protein, CSF	<2.5 ng/mL	<2.5 μg/L
Myoglobin, serum	<85 ng/mL	<85 μg/L
Nortriptyline, serum or plasma (Hep or EDTA); trough (≥12 h after dose)		
Therapeutic	50–150 ng/mL	190–570 nmol/L
Toxic	>500 ng/mL	>1900 nmol/L
5′-Nucleotidase, serum*	2–17 U/L	0.034–0.29 μkat/L
N-acetylprocainamide, serum or plasma (Hep or EDTA); trough		
Therapeutic	5–30 μg/mL	18–108 μmol/L
Toxic	>40 μg/mL	>144 μmol/L
Occult blood, feces, random	Negative (<2 mL blood/150 g stool/d)	Negative (<13.3 mL blood/kg stool/d)
Qualitative, urine, random	Negative	Negative
Osmolality		
Serum	275–295 mOsm/kg serum water	275–295 mmol/kg serum water
Urine	50–1200 mOsm/kg water	50–1200 mmol/kg water
Ratio, urine/serum	1.0–3.0, 3.0–4.7 after 12 h fluid restriction	1.0–3.0, 3.0–4.7 after 12 h fluid restriction

(continued)

Appendix 2

Tests	Conventional Units	SI Units
Osmotic fragility of erythrocytes	Begins in 0.45–0.39% NaCl Complete in 0.33–0.30% NaCl	Begins in 77–67 mmol/L NaCl Complete in 56–51 mmol/L NaCl
Oxazepam, serum or plasma (Hep or EDTA), therapeutic	0.2–1.4 µg/mL	0.70–4.9 µmol/L
Oxygen, blood		
Capacity	16–24 vol% (varies with hemoglobin)	7.14–10.7 mmol/L (varies with hemoglobin)
Content		
Arterial	15–23 vol%	6.69–10.3 mmol/L
Venous	10–16 vol%	4.46–7.14 mmol/L
Saturation		
Arterial and capillary	95–98% of capacity	0.95–0.98 of capacity
Venous	60–85% of capacity	0.60–0.85 of capacity
Tension		
PO_2 arterial and capillary	83–108 mmHg	11.1–14.4 kPa
Venous	35–45 mmHg	4.6–6.0 kPa
P50, blood	25–29 mmHg (adjusted to pH 7.4)	3.33–3.86 kPa
Partial thromboplastin time activated (APTT)	<35 sec	<35 sec
Pentobarbital, serum or plasma (Hep or EDTA); trough		
Therapeutic		
Hypnotic	1.5 µg/mL	4–22 µmol/L
Therapeutic coma	20–50 µg/mL	88–221 µmol/L
Toxic	>10 µg/mL	>44 µmol/L
pH		
Blood, arterial	7.35–7.45	7.35–7.45
Urine	4.6–8.0 (depends on diet)	Same
Phenacetin, plasma (EDTA)		
Therapeutic	1.30 µg/mL	6–167 µmol/L
Toxic	50–250 µg/mL	279–1395 µmol/L
Phenobarbital, serum or plasma (Hep or EDTA); trough		
Therapeutic	15–40 µg/mL	65–172 µmol/L
Toxic		
Slowness, ataxia, nystagmus	35–80 µg/mL	151–345 µmol/L
Coma with reflexes	65–117 µg/mL	280–504 µmol/L
Coma without reflexes	>100 µg/mL	>430 µmol/L
Phenolsulfonphthalein excretion (PSP), urine	28–51% in 15 min 13–24% in 30 min 9–17% in 60 min	0.28–0.51 in 15 min 0.13–0.24 in 30 min 0.09–0.17 in 60 min

(continued)

A84

Tests	Conventional Units	SI Units
	3–10% in 2 h (After injection of 1 mL PSP intravenously)	0.03–0.10 in 2 h (After injection of 1 mL PSP intravenously)
Phenylalanine, serum	0.8–1.8 mg/dL	48–109 μmol/L
Phenytoin, serum or plasma (Hep or EDTA); trough		
Therapeutic	10–20 μg/mL	40–79 μmol/L
Toxic	>20 μg/mL	>79 μmol/L
Phosphatase, acid, prostatic, serum RIA*	<3.0 ng/mL	<3.0 μg/L
Phosphatase, alkaline, total, serum*	38–126 U/L (37°C)	0.65–2.14 μkat/L
Phosphate, inorganic, serum		
Adults	2.7–4.5 mg/dL	0.87–1.45 mmol/L
Children	4.5–5.5 mg/dL	1.45–1.78 mmol/L
Phosphatidylglycerol (PG), amniotic fluid		
Fetal lung immaturity	Absent	Same
Fetal lung maturity	Present	Same
Phospholipids, serum	125–275 mg/dL	1.25–2.75 g/L
Phosphorus, urine	0.4–1.3 g/24 h	12.9–42 mmol/24 h
Porphobilinogen, urine		
Qualitative	Negative	Negative
Quantitative	<2.0 mg/24 h	<9 μmol/24 h
Porphyrins, urine		
Coproporphyrin	34–230 μg/24 h	52–351 nmol/ 24 h
Uroporphyrin	27–52 μg/24 h	32–63 nmol/ 24 h
Potassium, plasma (Hep)		
Males	3.5–4.5 mmol/L	3.5–4.5 mmol/L
Females	3.4–4.4 mmol/L	3.4–4.4 mmol/L
Potassium		
Serum		
Premature		
Cord	5.0–10.2 mmol/L	5.0–10.2 mmol/L
48 h	3.0–6.0 mmol/L	3.0–6.0 mmol/L
Newborn cord	5.6–12.0 mmol/L	5.6–12.0 mmol/L
Newborn	3.7–5.9 mmol/L	3.7–5.9 mmol/L
Infant	4.1–5.3 mmol/L	4.1–5.3 mmol/L
Child	3.4–4.7 mmol/L	3.4–4.7 mmol/L
Adult	3.5–5.1 mmol/L	3.5–5.1 mmol/L
Urine, 24 h	25–125 mmol/d; varies with diet	25–125 mmol/d; varies with diet

(*continued*)

Tests	Conventional Units	SI Units
CSF	70% of plasma level or 2.5–3.2 mmol/L; rises with plasma hyper-osmolality	0.70 of plasma level; rises with plasma hyperosmolality
Prealbumin (Transthyretin), serum	10–40 mg/dL	100–400 mg/L
Primidone, serum or plasma (Hep or EDTA); trough		
Therapeutic	5–12 μg/mL	23–55 μmol/L
Toxic	>15 μg/mL	>69 μmol/L
Procainamide, serum or plasma (Hep or EDTA); trough		
Therapeutic	4–10 μg/mL	17–42 μmol/L
Toxic (also consider effect of metabolite [NAPA])	>10–12 μg/mL	>42–51 μmol/L
Progesterone, serum*		
Adult		
Male	13–97 ng/dL	0.4–3.1 nmol/L
Female		
Follicular phase	15–70 ng/dL	0.5–2.2 nmol/L
Luteal phase	200–2500 ng/dL	6.4–79.5 nmol/L
Pregnancy	Varies with gestational week	
Prolactin, serum*		
Males	2.5–15.0 ng/mL	2.5–15.0 μg/L
Females	2.5–19.0 ng/mL	2.5–19.0 μg/L
Propoxyphene, plasma (EDTA)		
Therapeutic	0.1–0.4 μg/mL	0.3–1.2 μmol/L
Toxic	>0.5 μg/mL	>1.5 μmol/L
Propranolol, serum or plasma (Hep or EDTA); trough		
Therapeutic	50–100 ng/mL	193–386 nmol/L
Prostate-specific antigen (PSA), serum*		
Male	<4.0 ng/mL	<4.0 μg/L
Protein, serum*		
Total	6.4–8.3 g/dL	64–83 g/L
Albumin	3.9–5.1 g/dL	39–51 g/L
Globulin		
α_1	0.2–0.4 g/dL	2–4 g/L
α_2	0.4–0.8 g/dL	4–8 g/L
β	0.5–1.0 g/dL	5–10 g/L
γ	0.6–1.3 g/dL	6–13 g/L
Urine		
Qualitative	Negative	Negative
Quantitative	50–80 mg/24 h (at rest)	50–80 mg/24 h (at rest)
CSF, total	8–32 mg/dL	80–320 mg/dL

(continued)

Tests	Conventional Units	SI Units
Prothrombin, consumption	>20 sec	>20 sec
Prothrombin time (PT)*	12–14 sec	12–14 sec
Protoporphyrin, total, WB	<60 μg/dL	<600 μg/L
Pyruvate, blood	0.3–0.9 mg/dL	34–103 μmol/L
Quinidine, serum or plasma (Hep or EDTA); trough		
Therapeutic	2–5 μg/mL	6–15 μmol/L
Toxic	>6 μg/mL	>18 μmol/L
Salicylates, serum or plasma (Hep or EDTA); trough		
Therapeutic	150–300 μg/mL	1.09–2.17 mmol/L
Toxic	>500 μg/mL	>3.62 mmol/L
Sedimentation rate		
Wintrobe		
Males	0–10 mm in 1 h	0–10 mm/h
Females	0–20 mm in 1 h	0–20 mm/h
Westergren		
Males (<50 yr)	0–15 mm in 1 h	0–15 mm/h
Females (<50 yr)	0–20 mm in 1 h	0–20 mm/h
Sodium		
serum or plasma (Hep)		
Premature		
Cord	116–140 mmol/L	116–140 mmol/L
48 h	128–148 mmol/L	128–148 mmol/L
Newborn, cord	126–166 mmol/L	126–166 mmol/L
Newborn	133–146 mmol/L	133–146 mmol/L
Infant	139–146 mmol/L	139–146 mmol/L
Child	138–145 mmol/L	138–145 mmol/L
Adult	136–145 mmol/L	136–145 mmol/L
Urine, 24 h	40–220 mEq/d (diet dependent)	40–220 mmol/d (diet dependent)
Sweat		
Normal	10–40 mmol/L	10–40 mmol/L
Cystic fibrosis	70–190 mmol/L	70–190 mmol/L
Specific gravity, urine	1.002–1.030	1.002–1.030
Testosterone, serum*		
Male	280–1100 ng/dL	0.52–38.17 nmol/L
Female	15–70 ng/dL	0.52–2.43 nmol/L
Pregnancy	3–4 × normal	3–4 × normal
Postmenopausal	8–35 ng/dL	0.28–1.22 nmol/L
Theophylline, serum or plasma (Hep or EDTA)		
Therapeutic		
Bronchodilator	8–20 μg/mL	44–111 μmol/L
Prem. apnea	6–13 μg/mL	33–72 μmol/L
Toxic	>20 μg/mL	>110 μmol/L

(*continued*)

Tests	Conventional Units	SI Units
Thiocyanate, serum or plasma (EDTA)		
Nonsmoker	1–4 µg/mL	17–69 µmol/L
Smoker	3–12 µg/mL	52–206 µmol/L
Therapeutic after nitroprusside infusion	6–29 µg/mL	103–499 µmol/L
Urine		
Nonsmoker	1–4 mg/d	17–69 µmol/d
Smoker	7–17 mg/d	120–292 µmol/d
Thiopental, serum or plasma (Hep or EDTA); trough		
Hypnotic	1.0–5-0 µg/mL	4.1–20.7 µmol/L
Coma	30–100 µg/mL	124–413 µmol/L
Anesthesia	7–130 µg/mL	29–536 µmol/L
Toxic concentration	>10 µg/mL	>41 µmol/L
Thyroid-stimulating hormone (TSH), serum*	0.4–4.2 µU/mL	0.4–4.2 µU/L
Thyroxine (T$_4$) serum	5–12 µg/dL (varies with age, higher in children and pregnant women)	65–155 nmol/L (varies with age, higher in children and pregnant women)
Thyroxine, free, serum*	0.8–2.7 ng/dL	10.3–35 pmol/L
Thyroxine binding globulin (TBG), serum	1.2–3.0 mg/dL	12–30 mg/L
Tobramycin, serum or plasma (Hep or EDTA)		
Therapeutic		
Peak		
Less severe infection	5–8 µg/mL	11–17 µmol/L
Severe infection	8–10 µg/mL	17–21 µmol/L
Trough		
Less severe infection	<1 µg/mL	<2 µmol/L
Moderate infection	<2 µg/mL	<4 µmol/L
Severe infection	<2–4 µg/mL	<4–9 µmol/L
Toxic		
Peak	>10–12 µg/mL	>21–26 µmol/L
Trough	>2–4 µg/mL	>4–9 µmol/L
Transferrin, serum		
Newborn	130–275 mg/dL	1.30–2.75 g/L
Adult	212–360 mg/dL	2.12–3.60 g/L
>60 yr	190–375 mg/dL	1.9–3.75 g/L
Triglycerides, serum, fasting		
Desirable	<250 mg/dL	<2.83 mmol/L
Borderline high	250–500 mg/dL	2.83–5.67 mmol/L
Hypertriglyceridemic	>500 mg/dL	>5.65 mmol/L

(continued)

Tests	Conventional Units	SI Units
Triiodothyronine, total (T_3) serum*	100–200 ng/dL	1.54–3.8 nmol/L
Troponin-I, cardiac, serum*	undetectable	undetectable
Troponin-T, cardiac, serum	undetectable	undetectable
Urea nitrogen, serum	6–20 mg/dL	2.1–7.1 mmol Urea/L
Urea nitrogen/creatinine ratio, serum	12:1 to 20:1	48–80 urea/creatinine mole ratio
Uric acid* Serum, enzymatic		
Male	4.5–8.0 mg/dL	0.27–0.47 mmol/L
Female	2.5–6.2 mg/dL	0.15–0.37 mmol/L
Child	2.0–5.5 mg/dL	0.12–0.32 mmol/L
Urine	250–750 mg/24 h (with normal diet)	1.48–4.43 mmol/24 h (with normal diet)
Urobilinogen, urine	0.1–0.8 Ehrlich unit/2 h 0.5–4.0 EU/d	0.1–0.8 EU/2 h 0.5–4.0 EU/d
Valproic acid, serum or plasma (Hep or EDTA); trough Therapeutic	50–100 µg/mL	347–693 µmol/L
Toxic	>100 µg/mL	>693 µmol/L
Vancomycin, serum or plasma (Hep or EDTA) Therapeutic		
Peak	20–40 µg/mL	14–28 µmol/L
Trough	5–10 µg/mL	3–7 µmol/L
Toxic	>80–100 µg/mL	>55–69 µmol/L
Vanillylmandelic acid (VMA), urine (4-hydroxy-3-methoxymandelic acid)	1.4–6.5 mg/24h	7–33 µmol/d
Viscosity, serum	1.00–1.24 cP	1.00–1.24 cP
Vitamin A, serum	30–80 µg/dL	1.05–2.8 µmol/L
Vitamin B_{12}, serum	110–800 pg/mL	81–590 pmol/L
Vitamin E, serum Normal	5–18 µg/mL	12–42 µmol/L
Therapeutic	30–50 µg/mL	69.6–116 µmol/L
Zinc, serum	70–120 µg/dL	10.7–18.4 µmol/L

* Test values are method dependent.
† Test values are race dependent.
‡ Actual therapeutic range should be adjusted for individual patient.
§ "Fatty acids" include a mixture of different aliphatic acids of varying molecular weight; a mean molecular weight of 284 daltons has been assumed.

Appendix 3
Drugs by Indication

ABORTION
Antiprogestin
  Mifeprex® [US]
  mifepristone
Electrolyte Supplement, Oral
  sodium chloride
Oxytocic Agent
  oxytocin
  Pitocin® [US/Can]
Prostaglandin
  carboprost tromethamine
  Cervidil® Vaginal Insert [US/Can]
  dinoprostone
  Hemabate™ [US/Can]
  Prepidil® Vaginal Gel [US/Can]

ACETAMINOPHEN POISONING
Mucolytic Agent
  acetylcysteine
  Acys-5® [US]
  Mucomyst® [US/Can]
  Parvolex® [Can]

ACHALASIA
Adrenergic Agonist Agent
  Brethine® [US]
  Bricanyl® [Can]
  terbutaline
Calcium Channel Blocker
  Adalat® CC [US]
  Adalat® XL® [Can]
  Apo®-Nifed [Can]
  Apo®-Nifed PA [Can]
  Nifedical™ XL [US]
  nifedipine
  Novo-Nifedin [Can]
  Nu-Nifed [Can]
  Procardia® [US/Can]
  Procardia XL® [US]

Vasodilator
  Apo®-ISDN [Can]
  Cedocard®-SR [Can]
  Dilatrate®-SR [US]
  Isordil® [US]
  isosorbide dinitrate
  Minitran™ [US/Can]
  Nitrek® [US]
  Nitro-Bid® Ointment [US]
  Nitro-Dur® [US/Can]
  Nitrogard® [US]
  nitroglycerin
  Nitrolingual® [US]
  Nitrol® [US/Can]
  Nitrong® SR [Can]
  NitroQuick® [US]
  Nitrostat® [US/Can]
  Nitro-Tab® [US]
  NitroTime® [US]
  Transderm-Nitro® [Can]

ACIDOSIS (METABOLIC)
Alkalinizing Agent
  Neut® [US]
  Polycitra®-K [US]
  potassium citrate and citric acid
  sodium acetate
  sodium bicarbonate
  sodium lactate
  THAM® [US]
  tromethamine
Electrolyte Supplement, Oral
  sodium phosphates

ACUTE CORONARY SYNDROME
Antiplatelet Agent
  Aggrastat® [US/Can]
  eptifibatide
  Integrilin® [US/Can]
  tirofiban

ADAMS-STOKES SYNDROME
Adrenergic Agonist Agent
Adrenalin® Chloride [US/Can]
epinephrine
isoproterenol
Isuprel® [US]

ADDISON DISEASE
Adrenal Corticosteroid
A-HydroCort® [US/Can]
Betaject™ [Can]
betamethasone (systemic)
Betnesol® [Can]
Celestone® Phosphate [US]
Celestone® Soluspan® [US/Can]
Celestone® [US]
Cel-U-Jec® [US]
Cortef® [US/Can]
cortisone acetate
Cortone® [Can]
hydrocortisone (systemic)
Hydrocortone® Acetate [US]
Solu-Cortef® [US/Can]
Adrenal Corticosteroid
    (Mineralocorticoid)
Florinef® Acetate [US/Can]
fludrocortisone
Diagnostic Agent
Cortrosyn® [US/Can]
cosyntropin

ADRENOCORTICAL FUNCTION ABNORMALITY
Adrenal Corticosteroid
Acthar® [US]
A-HydroCort® [US/Can]
Alti-Dexamethasone [Can]
A-methaPred® [US]
Apo®-Prednisone [Can]
Aristocort® Forte Injection [US]
Aristocort® Intralesional
    Injection [US]

Aristocort® Tablet [US/Can]
Aristospan® Intra-articular Injection
    [US/Can]
Aristospan® Intralesional Injection
    [US/Can]
Betaject™ [Can]
betamethasone (systemic)
Betnesol® [Can]
Celestone® Phosphate [US]
Celestone® Soluspan® [US/Can]
Celestone® [US]
Cel-U-Jec® [US]
Cortef® [US/Can]
corticotropin
cortisone acetate
Cortone® [Can]
Decadron®-LA [US]
Decadron® [US/Can]
Decaject-LA® [US]
Decaject® [US]
Delta-Cortef® [US]
Deltasone® [US]
Depo-Medrol® [US/Can]
Depopred® [US]
dexamethasone (systemic)
Dexasone® L.A. [US]
Dexasone® [US/Can]
Dexone® LA [US]
Dexone® [US]
Hexadrol® [US/Can]
H.P. Acthar® Gel [US]
hydrocortisone (systemic)
Hydrocortone® Acetate [US]
Kenalog® Injection [US/Can]
Key-Pred-SP® [US]
Key-Pred® [US]
Medrol® Tablet [US/Can]
methylprednisolone
Meticorten® [US]
Orapred™ [US]
Pediapred® [US/Can]
PMS-Dexamethasone [Can]
Prednicot® [US]

prednisolone (systemic)
Prednisol® TBA [US]
prednisone
Prelone® [US]
Solu-Cortef® [US/Can]
Solu-Medrol® [US/Can]
Solurex L.A.® [US]
Sterapred® DS [US]
Sterapred® [US]
Tac™-3 Injection [US]
Triam-A® Injection [US]
triamcinolone (systemic)
Triam Forte® Injection [US]
Winpred™ [Can]
Adrenal Corticosteroid
    (Mineralocorticoid)
Florinef® Acetate [US/Can]
fludrocortisone

ALCOHOL WITHDRAWAL (TREATMENT)

Alpha-Adrenergic Agonist
Apo®-Clonidine [Can]
clonidine
Duraclon™ [US]
Anticonvulsant
paraldehyde
Paral® [US]
Antihistamine
ANX® [US]
Apo®-Hydroxyzine [Can]
Atarax® [US/Can]
hydroxyzine
Hyzine-50® [US]
Novo-Hydroxyzin [Can]
PMS-Hydroxyzine [Can]
Restall® [US]
Vistacot® [US]
Vistaril® [US/Can]
Benzodiazepine
alprazolam
Alprazolam Intensol® [US]

Alti-Alprazolam [Can]
Apo®-Alpraz [Can]
Apo®-Chlordiazepoxide [Can]
Apo®-Clorazepate [Can]
Apo®-Diazepam [Can]
Apo®-Oxazepam [Can]
chlordiazepoxide
clorazepate
Diastat® [US/Can]
Diazemuls® [Can]
diazepam
Diazepam Intensol® [US]
Gen-Alprazolam [Can]
Librium® [US]
Novo-Alprazol [Can]
Novo-Clopate [Can]
Nu-Alprax [Can]
oxazepam
Serax® [US]
Tranxene® [US/Can]
Valium® [US/Can]
Xana TS™ [Can]
Xanax® [US/Can]
Beta-Adrenergic Blocker
Apo®-Atenol [Can]
Apo®-Propranolol [Can]
atenolol
Gen-Atenolol [Can]
Inderal® LA [US/Can]
Inderal® [US/Can]
Novo-Atenol [Can]
Nu-Atenol
Nu-Propranolol [Can]
PMS-Atenolol [Can]
propranolol
Rhoxal-atenolol [Can]
Tenolin [Can]
Tenormin® [US/Can]
Phenothiazine Derivative
Apo®-Thioridazine [Can]
Mellaril® [US/Can]
thioridazine

ALKALOSIS
Electrolyte Supplement, Oral
  ammonium chloride
Vitamin, Water Soluble
  Cenolate® [US]
  sodium ascorbate

ALLERGIC DISORDER (NASAL)
Corticosteroid, Topical
  Nasacort® AQ [US/Can]
  Nasacort® [US/Can]
  triamcinolone (inhalation, nasal)
  Trinasal® [Can]
Mast Cell Stabilizer
  Apo®-Cromolyn [Can]
  cromolyn sodium
  Nalcrom® [Can]
  Nasalcrom® [US-OTC]

ALLERGIC DISORDER (OPHTHALMIC)
Adrenal Corticosteroid
  HMS Liquifilm® [US]
  medrysone

ALLERGIC RHINITIS
Antihistamine
  azelastine
  Optivar™ [US]

ALOPECIA
Antiandrogen
  finasteride
  Propecia® [US/Can]
Progestin
  hydroxyprogesterone caproate
  Hylutin® [US]
  Prodrox® [US]
Topical Skin Product
  Apo®-Gain [Can]
  Minox [Can]
  minoxidil

Rogaine® [Can]
Rogaine® Extra Strength for Men
  [US-OTC]
Rogaine® for Men [US-OTC]
Rogaine® for Women [US-OTC]

ALTITUDE SICKNESS
Carbonic Anhydrase Inhibitor
  acetazolamide
  Apo®-Acetazolamide [Can]
  Diamox Sequels® [US]
  Diamox® [US/Can]

ALZHEIMER DISEASE
Acetylcholinesterase Inhibitor
  Aricept® [US/Can]
  Cognex® [US]
  donepezil
  Exelon® [US/Can]
  rivastigmine
  tacrine
Acetylcholinesterase Inhibitor (Central)
  galantamine
  Reminyl® [US]
Cholinergic Agent
  Exelon® [US/Can]
  rivastigmine
Ergot Alkaloid and Derivative
  ergoloid mesylates
  Germinal® [US]
  Hydergine® LC [US]
  Hydergine® [US/Can]

AMEBIASIS
Amebicide
  Apo®-Metronidazole [Can]
  Diodoquin® [Can]
  Diquinol® [US]
  Flagyl ER® [US]
  Flagyl® [US/Can]
  Humatin® [US/Can]
  iodoquinol
  MetroLotion® [US]

metronidazole
Nidagel™ [Can]
Noritate™ [US/Can]
Novo-Nidazol [Can]
paromomycin
Yodoxin® [US]
Aminoquinoline (Antimalarial)
Aralen® Phosphate [US/Can]
chloroquine phosphate

AMENORRHEA

Ergot Alkaloid and Derivative
Apo® Bromocriptine [Can]
bromocriptine
Parlodel® [US/Can]
PMS-Bromocriptine [Can]
Gonadotropin
Factrel® [US]
gonadorelin
Lutrepulse™ [Can]
Progestin
Alti-MPA [Can]
Aygestin® [US]
Crinone® [US/Can]
Depo-Provera® [US/Can]
Gen-Medroxy [Can]
hydroxyprogesterone caproate
Hylutin® [US]
medroxyprogesterone acetate
Micronor® [US/Can]
norethindrone
Norlutate® [Can]
Nor-QD® [US]
Novo-Medrone [Can]
Prodrox® [US]
Progestasert® [US]
progesterone
Prometrium® [US/Can]
Provera® [US/Can]

AMMONIA INTOXICATION

Ammonium Detoxicant
Acilac [Can]
Cholac® [US]

Constilac® [US]
Constulose® [US]
Enulose® [US]
Generlac® [US]
Kristalose™ [US]
lactulose
Laxilose [Can]
PMS-Lactulose [Can]

AMYOTROPHIC LATERAL SCLEROSIS (ALS)

Anticholinergic Agent
atropine
Atropine-Care® [US]
Atropisol® [US/Can]
Isopto® Atropine [US/Can]
Sal-Tropine™ [US]
Cholinergic Agent
Mestinon®-SR [Can]
Mestinon® Timespan® [US]
Mestinon® [US/Can]
pyridostigmine
Regonol® [US]
Dopaminergic Agent (Anti-Parkinson)
levodopa
Miscellaneous Product
Rilutek® [US]
riluzole
Skeletal Muscle Relaxant
Apo®-Baclofen [Can]
baclofen
Gen-Baclofen [Can]
Lioresal® [US/Can]
Liotec [Can]
Nu-Baclo [Can]
PMS-Baclofen [Can]

ANAPHYLACTIC SHOCK

Adrenergic Agonist Agent
Adrenalin® Chloride [US/Can]
epinephrine

ANESTHESIA (LOCAL)

Local Anesthetic
Alcaine® [US/Can]

Americaine® Anesthetic Lubricant [US]
Americaine® [US-OTC]
Ametop™ [Can]
Anbesol® Baby [US/Can]
Anbesol® Maximum Strength [US-OTC]
Anbesol® [US-OTC]
Anestacon® [US]
Anusol® [US-OTC]
Babee® Teething® [US-OTC]
benzocaine
benzocaine, butyl aminobenzoate, tetracaine, and benzalkonium chloride
benzocaine, gelatin, pectin, and sodium carboxymethylcellulose
Benzodent® [US-OTC]
bupivacaine
Carbocaine® [US/Can]
Cēpacol® Anesthetic Troches [US-OTC]
Cēpacol® Mouthwash/Gargle [US-OTC]
Cetacaine® [US]
cetylpyridinium
cetylpyridinium and benzocaine
Chiggerex® [US-OTC]
Chiggertox® [US-OTC]
chloroprocaine
Citanest® Forte [Can]
Citanest® Plain [US/Can]
cocaine
Cylex® [US-OTC]
Dermaflex® Gel [US]
Detane® [US-OTC]
dibucaine
Diocaine® [Can]
Duranest® [US/Can]
Dyclone® [US]
dyclonine
ELA-Max® [US-OTC]
ethyl chloride

ethyl chloride and dichlorotetrafluoroethane
etidocaine
Fleet® Pain Relief [US-OTC]
Fluoracaine® [US]
Fluro-Ethyl® Aerosol [US]
Foille® Medicated First Aid [US-OTC]
Foille® Plus [US-OTC]
Foille® [US-OTC]
HDA® Toothache [US-OTC]
hexylresorcinol
Hurricaine® [US]
Isocaine® HCl [US]
Itch-X® [US-OTC]
lidocaine
lidocaine and epinephrine
Lidodan™ [Can]
Lidoderm® [US/Can]
LidoPen® Auto-Injector [US]
Marcaine® Spinal [US]
Marcaine® [US/Can]
mepivacaine
Mycinettes® [US-OTC]
Naropin™ [US/Can]
Nesacaine®-CE [Can]
Nesacaine®-MPF [US]
Nesacaine® [US]
Novocain® [US/Can]
Nupercainal® [US-OTC]
Ophthetic® [US]
Orabase®-B [US-OTC]
Orabase® With Benzocaine [US-OTC]
Orajel® Baby Nighttime [US-OTC]
Orajel® Baby [US-OTC]
Orajel® Maximum Strength [US-OTC]
Orajel® [US-OTC]
Orasol® [US-OTC]
Parcaine® [US]
Phicon® [US-OTC]
Polocaine® [US/Can]

Pontocaine® [US/Can]
Pontocaine® With Dextrose [US]
PrameGel® [US-OTC]
pramoxine
Prax® [US-OTC]
prilocaine
procaine
ProctoFoam® NS [US-OTC]
proparacaine
proparacaine and fluorescein
ropivacaine
Sensorcaine®-MPF [US]
Sensorcaine® [US/Can]
Solarcaine® Aloe Extra Burn Relief
    [US-OTC]
Solarcaine® [US-OTC]
Sucrets® Sore Throat [US-OTC]
Sucrets® [US-OTC]
tetracaine
tetracaine and dextrose
Trocaine® [US-OTC]
Tronolane® [US-OTC]
Tronothane® [US-OTC]
Xylocaine® [US/Can]
Xylocaine® With Epinephrine
    [US/Can]
Xylocard® [Can]
Zilactin® Baby [US/Can]
Zilactin®-B [US/Can]
Zilactin® [Can]
Zilactin-L® [US-OTC]
Local Anesthetic, Amide Derivative
    Chirocaine® [US/Can]
    levobupivacaine
Local Anesthetic, Injectable
    Chirocaine® [US/Can]
    levobupivacaine

ANESTHESIA (OPHTHALMIC)

Local Anesthetic
    Fluoracaine® [US]
    proparacaine and fluorescein

ANGINA PECTORIS

Beta-Adrenergic Blocker
    acebutolol
    Alti-Nadolol [Can]
    Apo-Acebutolol [Can]
    Apo®-Atenol [Can]
    Apo®-Metoprolol [Can]
    Apo®-Nadol [Can]
    Apo®-Propranolol [Can]
    atenolol
    Betaloc® [Can]
    Betaloc® Durules®
    carvedilol
    Coreg® [US/Can]
    Corgard® [US/Can]
    Gen-Acebutolol [Can]
    Gen-Atenolol [Can]
    Gen-Metoprolol [Can]
    Inderal® LA [US/Can]
    Inderal® [US/Can]
    Lopressor® [US/Can]
    metoprolol
    Monitan® [Can]
    nadolol
    Novo-Acebutolol [Can]
    Novo-Atenol [Can]
    Novo-Metoprolol [Can]
    Novo-Nadolol [Can]
    Nu-Acebutolol [Can]
    Nu-Atenol
    Nu-Metop [Can]
    Nu-Propranolol [Can]
    PMS-Atenolol [Can]
    PMS-Metoprolol [Can]
    propranolol
    Rhotral [Can]
    Rhoxal-atenolol [Can]
    Sectral® [US/Can]
    Tenolin [Can]
    Tenormin® [US/Can]
    Toprol-XL® [US/Can]
Calcium Channel Blocker
    Adalat® CC [US]

Adalat® XL® [Can]
Alti-Diltiazem [Can]
Alti-Diltiazem CD [Can]
Alti-Verapamil [Can]
amlodipine
Apo®-Diltiaz [Can]
Apo®-Diltiaz CD [Can]
Apo®-Diltiaz SR [Can]
Apo®-Nifed [Can]
Apo®-Nifed PA [Can]
Apo®-Verap [Can]
bepridil
Calan® SR [US]
Calan® [US/Can]
Cardene® I.V. [US]
Cardene® SR [US]
Cardene® [US]
Cardizem® CD [US/Can]
Cardizem® SR [US/Can]
Cardizem® [US/Can]
Cartia® XT [US]
Chronovera® [Can]
Covera® [Can]
Covera-HS® [US]
Dilacor® XR [US]
Diltia® XT [US]
diltiazem
felodipine
Gen-Diltiazem [Can]
Gen-Verapamil [Can]
Gen-Verapamil SR [Can]
Isoptin® SR [US/Can]
Isoptin® [US/Can]
nicardipine
Nifedical™ XL [US]
nifedipine
Norvasc® [US/Can]
Novo-Diltazem [Can]
Novo-Diltazem SR [Can]
Novo-Nifedin [Can]
Novo-Veramil [Can]
Novo-Veramil SR [Can]
Nu-Diltiaz [Can]

Nu-Diltiaz-CD [Can]
Nu-Nifed [Can]
Nu-Verap [Can]
Plendil® [US/Can]
Procardia® [US/Can]
Procardia XL® [US]
Renedil® [Can]
Rhoxal-diltiazem SR [Can]
Syn-Diltiazem® [Can]
Tiazac® [US/Can]
Vascor® [US/Can]
verapamil
Verelan® PM [US]
Verelan® [US]
Vasodilator
amyl nitrite
Apo®-Dipyridamole FC [Can]
Apo®-ISDN [Can]
Cedocard®-SR [Can]
Dilatrate®-SR [US]
dipyridamole
Imdur® [US/Can]
Ismo® [US]
Isordil® [US]
isosorbide dinitrate
isosorbide mononitrate
Minitran™ [US/Can]
Monoket® [US]
Nitrek® [US]
Nitro-Bid® Ointment [US]
Nitro-Dur® [US/Can]
Nitrogard® [US]
nitroglycerin
Nitrolingual® [US]
Nitrol® [US/Can]
Nitrong® SR [Can]
NitroQuick® [US]
Nitrostat® [US/Can]
Nitro-Tab® [US]
NitroTime® [US]
Novo-Dipiradol [Can]
Persantine® [US/Can]
Transderm-Nitro® [Can]

ANTHRAX
Penicillin
  amoxicillin
  Amoxicot® [US]
  Amoxil® [US/Can]
  Apo®-Amoxi [Can]
  Gen-Amoxicillin [Can]
  Lin-Amox [Can]
  Moxilin® [US]
  Novamoxin® [Can]
  Nu-Amoxi [Can]
  penicillin G (parenteral/aqueous)
  penicillin G procaine
  Pfizerpen® [US/Can]
  Trimox® [US]
  Wycillin® [US/Can]
  Wymox® [US]
Quinolone
  ciprofloxacin
  Cipro® [US/Can]
Tetracycline Derivative
  Adoxa™ [US]
  Alti-Minocycline [Can]
  Apo®-Doxy [Can]
  Apo®-Doxy Tabs [Can]
  Apo®-Minocycline [Can]
  Apo®-Tetra [Can]
  Brodspec® [US]
  Declomycin® [US/Can]
  demeclocycline
  Doryx® [US]
  Doxy-100™ [US]
  Doxycin [Can]
  doxycycline
  Doxytec [Can]
  Dynacin® [US]
  EmTet® [US]
  Gen-Minocycline [Can]
  Minocin® [US/Can]
  minocycline
  Monodox® [US]
  Novo-Doxylin [Can]
  Novo-Minocycline [Can]
  Novo-Tetra [Can]
  Nu-Doxycycline [Can]
  Nu-Tetra [Can]
  oxytetracycline
  Rhoxal-Minocycline [Can]
  Sumycin® [US]
  Terramycin® I.M. [US/Can]
  tetracycline
  Vibramycin® [US]
  Vibra-Tabs® [US/Can]
  Wesmycin® [US]
Vaccine
  anthrax vaccine, adsorbed
  BioThrax™ [US]

ANTICHOLINERGIC DRUG POISONING
Cholinesterase Inhibitor
  physostigmine

ANTIFREEZE POISONING
Antidote
  Antizol® [US]
  fomepizole

ANXIETY
Antianxiety Agent
  Apo®-Buspirone [Can]
  BuSpar® [US/Can]
  Buspirex [Can]
  buspirone
  Gen-Buspirone [Can]
  Lin-Buspirone [Can]
  Novo-Buspirone [Can]
  Nu-Buspirone [Can]
  PMS-Buspirone [Can]
Antianxiety Agent, Miscellaneous
  Apo®-Meprobamate [Can]
  meprobamate
  Miltown® [US]
Antidepressant/Phenothiazine
  amitriptyline and perphenazine
  Etrafon® [US/Can]
  Triavil® [US/Can]

Antidepressant, Tetracyclic
  Ludiomil® [US/Can]
  maprotiline
Antidepressant, Tricyclic (Secondary
    Amine)
  amoxapine
Antidepressant, Tricyclic (Tertiary
    Amine)
  Alti-Doxepin [Can]
  amitriptyline and chlordiazepoxide
  Apo®-Doxepin [Can]
  doxepin
  Limbitrol® DS [US]
  Limbitrol® [US/Can]
  Novo-Doxepin [Can]
  Sinequan® [US/Can]
  Zonalon® Cream [US/Can]
Antihistamine
  Acot-Tussin® Allergy [US-OTC]
  Alercap® [US-OTC]
  Aler-Dryl® [US-OTC]
  Alertab® [US-OTC]
  Allerdryl® [Can]
  Allermax® [US-OTC]
  Allernix [Can]
  Altaryl® [US-OTC]
  Anti-Hist® [US-OTC]
  ANX® [US]
  Apo®-Hydroxyzine [Can]
  Atarax® [US/Can]
  Banaril® [US-OTC]
  Banophen® [US-OTC]
  Benadryl® [US/Can]
  Compoz® Nighttime Sleep Aid [US-
    OTC]
  Dermamycin® [US-OTC]
  Derma-Pax® [US-OTC]
  Diphendryl® [US-OTC]
  Diphenhist® [US-OTC]
  diphenhydramine
  Diphen® [US-OTC]
  Diphenyl® [US-OTC]
  Dormin® Sleep Aid [US-OTC]

Dytuss® [US-OTC]
Genahist® [US-OTC]
Geridryl® [US-OTC]
Hydramine® [US-OTC]
hydroxyzine
Hyrexin® [US-OTC]
Hyzine-50® [US]
Mediphedryl® [US-OTC]
Miles® Nervine [US-OTC]
Novo-Hydroxyzin [Can]
Nytol™ [Can]
Nytol™ Extra Strength [Can]
Nytol® Quickcaps® [US-OTC]
PMS-Diphenhydramine [Can]
PMS-Hydroxyzine [Can]
Polydryl® [US-OTC]
Q-Dryl® [US-OTC]
Quenalin® [US-OTC]
Restall® [US]
Siladryl® Allerfy® [US-OTC]
Silphen® [US-OTC]
Simply Sleep® [US-OTC]
Sleepinal® [US-OTC]
Sleep® Tabs [US-OTC]
Sominex® [US-OTC]
Truxadryl® [US-OTC]
Tusstat® [US-OTC]
Twilite® [US-OTC]
Unison® Sleepgels® Maximum
  Strength [US-OTC]
Vistacot® [US]
Vistaril® [US/Can]
Barbiturate
  butabarbital sodium
  butalbital compound and codeine
  Butisol Sodium® [US]
  Fiorinal®-C 1/2 [Can]
  Fiorinal®-C 1/4 [Can]
  Fiorinal® With Codeine [US]
  Tecnal C 1/2 [Can]
  Tecnal C 1/4 [Can]
Benzodiazepine
  alprazolam

Alprazolam Intensol® [US]
Alti-Alprazolam [Can]
Alti-Bromazepam [Can]
Apo®-Alpraz [Can]
Apo®-Bromazepam [Can]
Apo®-Chlordiazepoxide [Can]
Apo®-Clorazepate [Can]
Apo®-Diazepam [Can]
Apo®-Lorazepam [Can]
Apo®-Oxazepam [Can]
Apo®-Temazepam [Can]
Ativan® [US/Can]
bromazepam (Canada only)
chlordiazepoxide
clorazepate
Diastat® [US/Can]
Diazemuls® [Can]
diazepam
Diazepam Intensol® [US]
Gen-Alprazolam [Can]
Gen-Bromazepam [Can]
Gen-Temazepam [Can]
halazepam
Lectopam® [Can]
Librium® [US]
lorazepam
Novo-Alprazol [Can]
Novo-Bromazepam [Can]
Novo-Clopate [Can]
Novo-Lorazem® [Can]
Novo-Temazepam [Can]
Nu-Alprax [Can]
Nu-Bromazepam [Can]
Nu-Loraz [Can]
Nu-Temazepam [Can]
oxazepam
Paxipam® [US/Can]
PMS-Temazepam [Can]
Restoril® [US/Can]
Riva-Lorazepam [Can]
Serax® [US]
temazepam
Tranxene® [US/Can]

Valium® [US/Can]
Xana TS™ [Can]
Xanax® [US/Can]
General Anesthetic
    Actiq® [US/Can]
    Duragesic® [US/Can]
    fentanyl
    Sublimaze® [US]
Neuroleptic Agent
    Apo®-Methoprazine [Can]
    methotrimeprazine (Canada only)
    Novo-Meprazine [Can]
    Nozinan® [Can]
Phenothiazine Derivative
    Apo®-Trifluoperazine [Can]
    Stelazine® [US]
    trifluoperazine
Sedative
    Alti-Bromazepam [Can]
    Apo®-Bromazepam [Can]
    bromazepam (Canada only)
    Gen-Bromazepam [Can]
    Lectopam® [Can]
    Novo-Bromazepam [Can]
    Nu-Bromazepam [Can]

APNEA (NEONATAL IDIOPATHIC)
Theophylline Derivative
    Aerolate III® [US]
    Aerolate JR® [US]
    Aerolate SR® [US]
    aminophylline
    Apo®-Theo LA [Can]
    Elixophyllin® [US]
    Novo-Theophyl SR [Can]
    Phyllocontin®-350 [Can]
    Phyllocontin® [Can]
    Quibron®-T/SR [US/Can]
    Quibron®-T [US]
    Slo-Phyllin® [US]
    Theo-24® [US]
    Theochron® [US]

Theo-Dur® [US/Can]
Theolair™ [US/Can]
theophylline
T-Phyl® [US]
Uniphyl® [US/Can]

APNEA OF PREMATURITY
Respiratory Stimulant
Cafcit® [US/Can]
caffeine (citrated)

ARRHYTHMIA
Adrenergic Agonist Agent
isoproterenol
Isuprel® [US]
phenylephrine
Antiarrhythmic Agent, Class I
Ethmozine® [US/Can]
moricizine
Antiarrhythmic Agent, Class I-A
Apo®-Procainamide [Can]
Apo®-Quinidine [Can]
disopyramide
Norpace® CR [US]
Norpace® [US/Can]
procainamide
Procanbid® [US]
Procan™ SR [Can]
Pronestyl-SR® [US/Can]
Pronestyl® [US/Can]
Quinaglute® Dura-Tabs® [US]
Quinidex® Extentabs® [US]
quinidine
Rythmodan® [Can]
Rythmodan®-LA [Can]
Antiarrhythmic Agent, Class I-B
lidocaine
mexiletine
Mexitil® [US/Can]
Novo-Mexiletine [Can]
phenytoin
tocainide
Tonocard® [US]
Xylocaine® [US/Can]

Xylocard® [Can]
Antiarrhythmic Agent, Class I-C
flecainide
propafenone
Rythmol® [US/Can]
Tambocor™ [US/Can]
Antiarrhythmic Agent, Class II
acebutolol
Alti-Sotalol [Can]
Apo-Acebutolol [Can]
Apo®-Propranolol [Can]
Apo®-Sotalol [Can]
Betapace AF™ [US/Can]
Betapace® [US]
Brevibloc® [US/Can]
esmolol
Gen-Acebutolol [Can]
Gen-Sotalol [Can]
Inderal® LA [US/Can]
Inderal® [US/Can]
Monitan® [Can]
Novo-Acebutolol [Can]
Novo-Sotalol [Can]
Nu-Acebutolol [Can]
Nu-Propranolol [Can]
Nu-Sotalol [Can]
PMS-Sotalol [Can]
propranolol
Rho®-Sotalol [Can]
Rhotral [Can]
Sectral® [US/Can]
Sorine™ [US]
Sotacor®
sotalol
Antiarrhythmic Agent, Class III
Alti-Amiodarone [Can]
Alti-Sotalol [Can]
amiodarone
Apo®-Sotalol [Can]
Betapace AF™ [US/Can]
Betapace® [US]
bretylium
Cordarone® [US/Can]

Corvert® [US]
dofetilide
Gen-Amiodarone [Can]
Gen-Sotalol [Can]
ibutilide
Novo-Amiodarone [Can]
Novo-Sotalol [Can]
Nu-Sotalol [Can]
Pacerone® [US]
PMS-Sotalol [Can]
Rho®-Sotalol [Can]
Sorine™ [US]
Sotacor®
sotalol
Tikosyn™ [US/Can]
Antiarrhythmic Agent, Class IV
Alti-Verapamil [Can]
Apo®-Verap [Can]
Calan® SR [US]
Calan® [US/Can]
Chronovera® [Can]
Covera® [Can]
Covera-HS® [US]
Gen-Verapamil [Can]
Gen-Verapamil SR [Can]
Isoptin® SR [US/Can]
Isoptin® [US/Can]
Novo-Veramil [Can]
Novo-Veramil SR [Can]
Nu-Verap [Can]
verapamil
Verelan® PM [US]
Verelan® [US]
Antiarrhythmic Agent,
    Miscellaneous
Adenocard® [US/Can]
Adenoscan® [US]
adenosine
Digitek® [US]
digoxin
Lanoxicaps® [US/Can]
Lanoxin® Pediatric [US]
Lanoxin® [US/Can]

Anticholinergic Agent
atropine
Calcium Channel Blocker
Alti-Diltiazem [Can]
Alti-Diltiazem CD [Can]
Apo®-Diltiaz [Can]
Apo®-Diltiaz CD [Can]
Apo®-Diltiaz SR [Can]
Cardizem® CD [US/Can]
Cardizem® SR [US/Can]
Cardizem® [US/Can]
Cartia® XT [US]
Dilacor® XR [US]
Diltia® XT [US]
diltiazem
Gen-Diltiazem [Can]
Novo-Diltazem [Can]
Novo-Diltazem SR [Can]
Nu-Diltiaz [Can]
Nu-Diltiaz-CD [Can]
Rhoxal-diltiazem SR [Can]
Syn-Diltiazem® [Can]
Tiazac® [US/Can]
Cholinergic Agent
edrophonium
Enlon® [US/Can]
Reversol® [US]
Tensilon® [US]
Theophylline Derivative
aminophylline
Phyllocontin®-350 [Can]
Phyllocontin® [Can]

ARSENIC POISONING
Chelating Agent
BAL in Oil® [US]
dimercaprol

ASCITES
Diuretic, Loop
Apo®-Furosemide [Can]
bumetanide
Bumex® [US/Can]
Burinex® [Can]

Demadex® [US]
Edecrin® [US/Can]
ethacrynic acid
Furocot® [US]
furosemide
Lasix® Special [Can]
Lasix® [US/Can]
torsemide
Diuretic, Miscellaneous
Apo®-Chlorthalidone [Can]
Apo®-Indapamide [Can]
chlorthalidone
Gen-Indapamide [Can]
indapamide
Lozide® [Can]
Lozol® [US/Can]
metolazone
Mykrox® [US/Can]
Novo-Indapamide [Can]
Nu-Indapamide [Can]
PMS-Indapamide [Can]
Thalitone® [US]
Zaroxolyn® [US/Can]
Diuretic, Potassium Sparing
Aldactone® [US/Can]
Novo-Spiroton [Can]
spironolactone
Diuretic, Thiazide
Apo®-Hydro [Can]
Aquacot® [US]
Aquatensen® [US/Can]
Aquazide H® [US]
bendroflumethiazide
chlorothiazide
Diuril® [US/Can]
Enduron® [US/Can]
Ezide® [US]
hydrochlorothiazide
Hydrocot® [US]
HydroDIURIL® [US/Can]
Metatensin® [Can]
methyclothiazide
Microzide™ [US]

Naqua® [US/Can]
Naturetin® [US]
Oretic® [US]
polythiazide
Renese® [US]
Trichlorex® [Can]
trichlormethiazide
Zide® [US]

ASPERGILLOSIS
Antifungal Agent
Abelcet® [US/Can]
Amphocin® [US]
Amphotec® [US]
amphotericin B cholesteryl sulfate
    complex
amphotericin B (conventional)
amphotericin B lipid complex
Ancobon® [US/Can]
flucytosine
Fungizone® [US/Can]
VFEND® [US]
voriconazole
Antifungal Agent, Systemic
AmBisome® [US/Can]
amphotericin B liposomal
Cancidas® [US]
caspofungin

ASTHMA
Adrenal Corticosteroid
Alti-Beclomethasone [Can]
Alti-Dexamethasone [Can]
Apo®-Beclomethasone [Can]
Azmacort® [US]
beclomethasone
Decadron®-LA [US]
Decadron® [US/Can]
Decaject-LA® [US]
Decaject® [US]
dexamethasone (systemic)
Dexasone® L.A. [US]
Dexasone® [US/Can]
Dexone® LA [US]

Dexone® [US]
Flovent® Rotadisk® [US]
Flovent® [US]
fluticasone (oral inhalation)
Gen-Beclo [Can]
Hexadrol® [US/Can]
Nu-Beclomethasone [Can]
PMS-Dexamethasone [Can]
Propaderm® [Can]
QVAR™ [US/Can]
Rivanase AQ [Can]
triamcinolone (inhalation, oral)
Vanceril® [US/Can]
Adrenergic Agonist Agent
AccuNeb™ [US]
Adrenalin® Chloride [US/Can]
albuterol
Alti-Salbutamol [Can]
Alupent® [US]
Apo®-Salvent [Can]
bitolterol
Brethine® [US]
Bricanyl® [Can]
Bronchial Mist® [US]
ephedrine
epinephrine
isoetharine
isoproterenol
Isuprel® [US]
Levophed® [US/Can]
Maxair™ Autohaler™ [US]
Maxair™ [US]
metaproterenol
norepinephrine
Novo-Salmol [Can]
pirbuterol
Pretz-D® [US-OTC]
Primatene® Mist [US-OTC]
Proventil® HFA [US]
Proventil® Repetabs® [US]
Proventil® [US]
salmeterol
Serevent® Diskus® [US]

Serevent® [US/Can]
terbutaline
Tornalate® [US/Can]
Vaponefrin® [Can]
Ventolin® HFA [US]
Ventolin® [US]
Volmax® [US]
Anticholinergic Agent
Alti-Ipratropium [Can]
Apo®-Ipravent [Can]
Atrovent® [US/Can]
Gen-Ipratropium [Can]
ipratropium
Novo-Ipramide [Can]
Nu-Ipratropium [Can]
PMS-Ipratropium [Can]
Beta2-Adrenergic Agonist Agent
Advair™ Diskus® [US/Can]
Berotec® [Can]
fenoterol (Canada only)
fluticasone and salmeterol
Foradil® Aerolizer™ [US/Can]
formoterol
Corticosteroid, Inhalant
Advair™ Diskus® [US/Can]
fluticasone and salmeterol
Leukotriene Receptor Antagonist
Accolate® [US/Can]
montelukast
Singulair® [US/Can]
zafirlukast
5-Lipoxygenase Inhibitor
zileuton
Zyflo™ [US]
Mast Cell Stabilizer
Apo®-Cromolyn [Can]
cromolyn sodium
Intal® [US/Can]
nedocromil (inhalation)
Nu-Cromolyn [Can]
Tilade® [US/Can]
Theophylline Derivative
Aerolate III® [US]

Aerolate JR® [US]
Aerolate SR® [US]
aminophylline
Apo®-Theo LA [Can]
Choledyl SA® [US]
Dilor® [US/Can]
dyphylline
Elixophyllin® GG [US]
Elixophyllin® [US]
Lufyllin® [US/Can]
Neoasma® [US]
Novo-Theophyl SR [Can]
oxtriphylline
Phyllocontin®-350 [Can]
Phyllocontin® [Can]
Quibron®-T/SR [US/Can]
Quibron®-T [US]
Quibron® [US]
Slo-Phyllin® [US]
Theo-24® [US]
Theochron® [US]
Theocon® [US]
Theo-Dur® [US/Can]
Theolair™ [US/Can]
Theolate® [US]
Theomar® GG [US]
theophylline
theophylline and guaifenesin
T-Phyl® [US]
Uniphyl® [US/Can]

ASTHMA (CORTICOSTEROID-DEPENDENT)
Macrolide (Antibiotic)
  Tao® [US]
  troleandomycin

ASTHMA (DIAGNOSTIC)
Diagnostic Agent
  methacholine
  Provocholine® [US/Can]

ATELECTASIS
Expectorant
  potassium iodide
  SSKI® [US]
Mucolytic Agent
  acetylcysteine
  Acys-5® [US]
  Mucomyst® [US/Can]
  Parvolex® [Can]

ATOPIC DERMATITIS
Immunosuppressant Agent
  Elidel® [US]
  pimecrolimus
Topical Skin Product
  Elidel® [US]
  pimecrolimus

ATTENTION-DEFICIT/HYPERACTIVITY DISORDER (ADHD)
Amphetamine
  Adderall® [US]
  Adderall XR™ [US]
  Desoxyn® Gradumet® [US]
  Desoxyn® [US/Can]
  Dexedrine® Spansule® [US/Can]
  Dexedrine® Tablet [US/Can]
  dextroamphetamine
  dextroamphetamine and amphetamine
  Dextrostat® [US]
  methamphetamine
Central Nervous System Stimulant, Nonamphetamine
  Concerta™ [US]
  Cylert® [US]
  dexmethylphenidate
  Focalin™ [US]
  Metadate® CD [US]
  Metadate™ ER [US]
  Methylin™ ER [US]
  Methylin™ [US]

methylphenidate
PemADD CT® [US]
PemADD® [US]
pemoline
PMS-Methylphenidate [Can]
Riphenidate [Can]
Ritalin® LA [US]
Ritalin-SR® [US/Can]
Ritalin® [US/Can]

BACK PAIN (LOW)

Analgesic, Narcotic
codeine
Analgesic, Nonnarcotic
Apo®-ASA [Can]
Arthropan® [US-OTC]
Asaphen [Can]
Asaphen E.C. [Can]
Ascriptin® Arthritis Pain [US-OTC]
Ascriptin® Enteric [US-OTC]
Ascriptin® Extra Strength [US-OTC]
Ascriptin® [US-OTC]
Aspercin Extra [US-OTC]
Aspercin [US-OTC]
aspirin
Bayer® Aspirin Extra Strength [US-OTC]
Bayer® Aspirin Regimen Children's [US-OTC]
Bayer® Aspirin Regimen Regular Strength [US-OTC]
Bayer® Aspirin [US-OTC]
Bayer® Plus Extra Strength [US-OTC]
Bufferin® Arthritis Strength [US-OTC]
Bufferin® Extra Strength [US-OTC]
Bufferin® [US-OTC]
choline salicylate
Easprin® [US]
Ecotrin® Maximum Strength [US-OTC]
Ecotrin® [US-OTC]
Entrophen® [Can]

Halfprin® [US-OTC]
Novasen [Can]
St. Joseph® Pain Reliever [US-OTC]
Sureprin 81™ [US-OTC]
Teejel® [Can]
ZORprin® [US]
Benzodiazepine
Apo®-Diazepam [Can]
diazepam
Diazepam Intensol® [US]
Valium® [US/Can]
Nonsteroidal Antiinflammatory Drug (NSAID)
Backache Pain Relief Extra Strength [US]
Doan's® Original [US-OTC]
Extra Strength Doan's® [US-OTC]
Keygesic-10® [US]
magnesium salicylate
Mobidin® [US]
Momentum® [US-OTC]
Skeletal Muscle Relaxant
Aspirin® Backache [Can]
methocarbamol
methocarbamol and aspirin
Methoxisal [Can]
Methoxisal-C [Can]
Robaxin® [US/Can]
Robaxisal® Extra Strength [Can]
Robaxisal® [US/Can]

BARBITURATE POISONING

Antidote
Actidose-Aqua® [US-OTC]
Actidose® [US-OTC]
Charcadole® Aqueous [Can]
Charcadole® [Can]
Charcadole® TFS [Can]
charcoal
Liqui-Char® [US/Can]

BEHÇET SYNDROME

Immunosuppressant Agent
Alti-Azathioprine [Can]

azathioprine
cyclosporine
Gen-Azathioprine [Can]
Gengraf™ [US]
Imuran® [US/Can]
Neoral® [US/Can]
Sandimmune® [US/Can]

BENIGN PROSTATIC HYPERPLASIA (BPH)

Alpha-Adrenergic Blocking Agent
Alti-Prazosin [Can]
Alti-Terazosin [Can]
Apo®-Doxazosin [Can]
Apo®-Prazo [Can]
Apo®-Terazosin [Can]
Cardura® [US/Can]
doxazosin
Flomax® [US/Can]
Gen-Doxazosin [Can]
Hytrin® [US/Can]
Minipress® [US/Can]
Novo-Doxazosin [Can]
Novo-Prazin [Can]
Novo-Terazosin [Can]
Nu-Prazo [Can]
Nu-Terazosin [Can]
prazosin
tamsulosin
terazosin
Antiandrogen
finasteride
Propecia® [US/Can]
Proscar® [US/Can]
Antineoplastic Agent, Anthracenedione
Avodart™ [US]
dutasteride

BENZODIAZEPINE OVERDOSE

Antidote
Anexate® [Can]
flumazenil
Romazicon® [US/Can]

BIPOLAR DEPRESSION DISORDER

Anticonvulsant
Alti-Divalproex [Can]
Apo®-Divalproex [Can]
Depacon® [US]
Depakene® [US/Can]
Depakote® Delayed Release [US]
Depakote® ER [US]
Depakote® Sprinkle® [US]
Epival® I.V. [Can]
Gen-Divalproex [Can]
Novo-Divalproex [Can]
Nu-Divalproex [Can]
PMS-Valproic Acid [Can]
PMS-Valproic Acid E.C. [Can]
Rhoxal-valproic [Can]
valproic acid and derivatives
Antimanic Agent
Carbolith™ [Can]
Duralith® [Can]
Eskalith CR® [US]
Eskalith® [US]
Lithane™ [Can]
lithium
Lithobid® [US]
PMS-Lithium Carbonate [Can]
PMS-Lithium Citrate [Can]
Antipsychotic Agent
Clopixol-Acuphase® [Can]
Clopixol® [Can]
Clopixol® Depot [Can]
zuclopenthixol (Canada only)

BIRTH CONTROL

Contraceptive
estradiol cypionate and medroxyprogesterone acetate
ethinyl estradiol and drospirenone
ethinyl estradiol and etonogestrel
ethinyl estradiol and norelgestromin
Lunelle™ [US]
NuvaRing® [US]

Ortho Evra™ [US]
Yasmin® [US]
Contraceptive, Implant (Progestin)
levonorgestrel
Mirena® [US]
Norplant® Implant [Can]
Plan B™ [US/Can]
Contraceptive, Oral
Alesse® [US/Can]
Apri® [US]
Aviane™ [US]
Brevicon® [US]
Cryselle™ [US]
Cyclessa® [US]
Demulen® 30 [Can]
Demulen® [US]
Desogen® [US]
Enpresse™ [US]
Estrostep® Fe [US]
ethinyl estradiol and desogestrel
ethinyl estradiol and ethynodiol diac-
etate
ethinyl estradiol and levonorgestrel
ethinyl estradiol and norethindrone
ethinyl estradiol and norgestimate
ethinyl estradiol and norgestrel
femhrt® [US/Can]
Jenest™-28 [US]
Kariva™ [US]
Lessina™ [US]
Levlen® [US]
Levlite™ [US]
Levora® [US]
Loestrin® Fe [US]
Loestrin® [US/Can]
Lo/Ovral® [US]
Low-Ogestrel® [US]
Marvelon® [Can]
mestranol and norethindrone
Microgestin™ Fe [US]
Minestrin™ 1/20 [Can]
Min-Ovral® [Can]
Mircette® [US]

Modicon® [US]
Necon® 0.5/35 [US]
Necon® 1/35 [US]
Necon® 1/50 [US]
Necon® 10/11 [US]
Nordette® [US]
Norinyl® 1+35 [US]
Norinyl® 1+50 [US]
Nortrel™ [US]
Ogestrel®
Ortho-Cept® [US/Can]
Ortho-Cyclen® [US/Can]
Ortho-Novum® 1/50 [US/Can]
Ortho-Novum® [US]
Ortho-Tri-Cyclen® Lo [US]
Ortho Tri-Cyclen® [US/Can]
Ovcon® [US]
Ovral® [US/Can]
Portia™ [US]
PREVEN™ [US]
Select™ 1/35 [Can]
Synphasic® [Can]
Tri-Levlen® [US]
Tri-Norinyl® [US]
Triphasil® [US/Can]
Triquilar® [Can]
Trivora® [US]
Zovia™ [US]
Contraceptive, Progestin Only
Alti-MPA [Can]
Aygestin® [US]
Depo-Provera® [US/Can]
Gen-Medroxy [Can]
levonorgestrel
medroxyprogesterone acetate
Micronor® [US/Can]
Mirena® [US]
norethindrone
norgestrel
Norlutate® [Can]
Norplant® Implant [Can]
Nor-QD® [US]
Novo-Medrone [Can]

Ovrette® [US/Can]
Plan B™ [US/Can]
Provera® [US/Can]
Estrogen and Progestin Combination
    ethinyl estradiol and etonogestrel
    ethinyl estradiol and
        norelgestromin
    NuvaRing® [US]
    Ortho Evra™ [US]
Spermicide
    Advantage 24™ [Can]
    Advantage-S™ [US-OTC]
    Aqua Lube Plus [US-OTC]
    Conceptrol® [US-OTC]
    Delfen® [US-OTC]
    Emko® [US-OTC]
    Encare® [US-OTC]
    Gynol II® [US-OTC]
    nonoxynol 9
    Semicid® [US-OTC]
    Shur-Seal® [US-OTC]
    VCF™ [US-OTC]

BITES (INSECT)

Adrenergic Agonist Agent
    Adrenalin® Chloride [US/Can]
    epinephrine
    EpiPen® Jr [US/Can]
    EpiPen® [US/Can]
Analgesic, Topical
    Anestacon® [US]
    Dermaflex® Gel [US]
    ELA-Max® [US-OTC]
    lidocaine
    Lidodan™ [Can]
    Lidoderm® [US/Can]
    LidoPen® Auto-Injector [US]
    Solarcaine® Aloe Extra Burn Relief
        [US-OTC]
    Xylocaine® [US/Can]
    Xylocard® [Can]
    Zilactin® [Can]
    Zilactin-L® [US-OTC]

Antidote
    Ana-Kit® [US]
    insect sting kit
Antihistamine
    Alercap® [US-OTC]
    Aler-Dryl® [US-OTC]
    Alertab® [US-OTC]
    Allerdryl® [Can]
    Allermax® [US-OTC]
    Allernix [Can]
    Altaryl® [US-OTC]
    Anti-Hist® [US-OTC]
    Banaril® [US-OTC]
    Banophen® [US-OTC]
    Benadryl® [US/Can]
    Dermamycin® [US-OTC]
    Derma-Pax® [US-OTC]
    Diphendryl® [US-OTC]
    Diphenhist® [US-OTC]
    diphenhydramine
    Diphen® [US-OTC]
    Diphenyl® [US-OTC]
    Genahist® [US-OTC]
    Geridryl® [US-OTC]
    Hydramine® [US-OTC]
    Hyrexin® [US-OTC]
    Mediphedryl® [US-OTC]
    PMS-Diphenhydramine [Can]
    Polydryl® [US-OTC]
    Q-Dryl® [US-OTC]
    Quenalin® [US-OTC]
    Siladryl® Allerfy® [US-OTC]
    Silphen® [US-OTC]
Corticosteroid, Topical
    Aclovate® [US]
    Acticort® [US]
    Aeroseb-HC® [US]
    Ala-Cort® [US]
    Ala-Scalp® [US]
    alclometasone
    amcinonide
    Aquacort® [Can]
    Aristocort® A Topical [US]

Aristocort® Topical [US/Can]
Bactine® Hydrocortisone [US-OTC]
CaldeCORT® Anti-Itch Spray [US]
CaldeCORT® [US-OTC]
Capex™ [US/Can]
Carmol-HC® [US]
Cetacort®
clobetasol
Clocort® Maximum Strength
 [US-OTC]
clocortolone
Cloderm® [US/Can]
Cordran® SP [US]
Cordran® [US/Can]
Cormax® [US]
CortaGel® [US-OTC]
Cortaid® Maximum Strength [US-OTC]
Cortaid® with Aloe [US-OTC]
Cort-Dome® [US]
Cortizone®-5 [US-OTC]
Cortizone®-10 [US-OTC]
Cortoderm [Can]
Cutivate™ [US]
Cyclocort® [US/Can]
Delcort® [US]
Dermacort® [US]
Dermarest Dricort® [US]
Derma-Smoothe/FS® [US/Can]
Dermatop® [US]
Dermolate® [US-OTC]
Dermovate® [Can]
Dermtex® HC with Aloe [US-OTC]
Desocort® [Can]
desonide
DesOwen® [US]
desoximetasone
diflorasone
Eldecort® [US]
Elocon® [US/Can]
fluocinolone
fluocinonide
Fluoderm [Can]
flurandrenolide

fluticasone (topical)
Gen-Clobetasol [Can]
Gynecort® [US-OTC]
halcinonide
halobetasol
Halog®-E [US]
Halog® [US/Can]
Hi-Cor-1.0® [US]
Hi-Cor-2.5® [US]
Hyderm [Can]
hydrocortisone (topical)
Hydrocort® [US]
Hydro-Tex® [US-OTC]
Hytone® [US]
Kenalog® Topical [US/Can]
LactiCare-HC® [US]
Lidemol® [Can]
Lidex-E® [US]
Lidex® [US/Can]
Locoid® [US/Can]
Lyderm® [Can]
Lydonide [Can]
Maxiflor® [US]
mometasone furoate
Novo-Clobetasol [Can]
Nutracort® [US]
Olux™ [US]
Orabase® HCA [US]
Penecort® [US]
prednicarbate
Prevex® HC [Can]
Psorcon™ E [US]
Psorcon™ [US/Can]
Sarna® HC [Can]
S-T Cort® [US]
Synacort® [US]
Synalar® [US/Can]
Taro-Desoximetasone [Can]
Tegrin®-HC [US-OTC]
Temovate® [US]
Texacort® [US]
Tiamol® [Can]
Ti-U-Lac® H [Can]
Topicort®-LP [US]

Topicort® [US/Can]
Topsyn® [Can]
Triacet™ Topical [US] Oracort [Can]
Triaderm [Can]
triamcinolone (topical)
Tridesilon® [US]
U-Cort™ [US]
Ultravate™ [US/Can]
urea and hydrocortisone
Uremol® HC [Can]
Westcort® [US/Can]
Local Anesthetic
Ametop™ [Can]
Fleet® Pain Relief [US-OTC]
Itch-X® [US-OTC]
Phicon® [US-OTC]
Pontocaine® [US/Can]
PrameGel® [US-OTC]
pramoxine
tetracaine

BITES (SNAKE)

Antivenin
antivenin (Crotalidae) polyvalent
antivenin (Micrurus fulvius)
Antivenin Polyvalent [Equine] [US]
CroFab™ [Ovine] [US]

BITES (SPIDER)

Antivenin
antivenin (Latrodectus mactans)
Electrolyte Supplement, Oral
calcium gluconate
Skeletal Muscle Relaxant
methocarbamol
Robaxin® [US/Can]

BLADDER IRRIGATION

Antibacterial, Topical
acetic acid

BLASTOMYCOSIS

Antifungal Agent
Apo®-Ketoconazole [Can]
itraconazole

ketoconazole
Nizoral® [US/Can]
Novo-Ketoconazole [Can]
Sporanox® [US/Can]

BLEPHARITIS

Antifungal Agent
Natacyn® [US/Can]
natamycin

BLEPHAROSPASM

Ophthalmic Agent, Toxin
Botox® [US/Can]
botulinum toxin type A

BOWEL CLEANSING

Laxative
castor oil
Citro-Mag® [Can]
Colyte® [US/Can]
Emulsoil® [US-OTC]
Fleet® Enema [US/Can]
Fleet® Phospho®-Soda [US/Can]
GoLYTELY® [US]
Klean-Prep® [Can]
Lyteprep™ [Can]
magnesium citrate
MiraLax™ [US]
Neoloid® [US-OTC]
NuLytely® [US]
OCL® [US]
PegLyte® [Can]
polyethylene glycol-electrolyte
    solution
Purge® [US-OTC]
sodium phosphates
Visicol™ [US]

BREAST ENGORGEMENT (POSTPARTUM)

Androgen
fluoxymesterone
Halotestin® [US]
Estrogen and Androgen Combination
Climacteron® [Can]

Depo-Testadiol® [US]
estradiol and testosterone
Valertest No. 1® [US]
Estrogen Derivative
Alora® [US]
Cenestin™ [US/Can]
Climara® [US/Can]
Congest [Can]
Delestrogen® [US/Can]
Depo®-Estradiol [US/Can]
Esclim® [US]
Estrace® [US/Can]
Estraderm® [US/Can]
estradiol
Estring® [US/Can]
Estrogel® [Can]
estrogens (conjugated A/synthetic)
estrogens (conjugated/equine)
Gynodiol™ [US]
Oesclim® [Can]
PMS-Conjugated Estrogens [Can]
Premarin® [US/Can]
Vagifem® [US/Can]
Vivelle-Dot® [US]
Vivelle® [US/Can]

BRONCHIECTASIS

Adrenergic Agonist Agent
AccuNeb™ [US]
Adrenalin® Chloride [US/Can]
albuterol
Alti-Salbutamol [Can]
Alupent® [US]
Apo®-Salvent [Can]
Brethine® [US]
Bricanyl® [Can]
Bronchial Mist® [US]
ephedrine
epinephrine
isoproterenol
Isuprel® [US]
metaproterenol
Novo-Salmol [Can]

Pretz-D® [US-OTC]
Primatene® Mist [US-OTC]
Proventil® HFA [US]
Proventil® Repetabs® [US]
Proventil® [US]
terbutaline
Vaponefrin® [Can]
Ventolin® HFA [US]
Ventolin® [US]
Volmax® [US]
Mucolytic Agent
acetylcysteine
Acys-5® [US]
Mucomyst® [US/Can]
Parvolex® [Can]

BRONCHIOLITIS

Antiviral Agent
Rebetol® [US]
ribavirin
Virazole® [US/Can]

BRONCHITIS

Adrenergic Agonist Agent
AccuNeb™ [US]
Adrenalin® Chloride [US/Can]
albuterol
Alti-Salbutamol [Can]
Apo®-Salvent [Can]
bitolterol
Bronchial Mist® [US]
ephedrine
epinephrine
isoetharine
isoproterenol
Isuprel® [US]
Novo-Salmol [Can]
Primatene® Mist [US-OTC]
Proventil® HFA [US]
Proventil® Repetabs® [US]
Proventil® [US]
Tornalate® [US/Can]
Vaponefrin® [Can]
Ventolin® HFA [US]

Ventolin® [US]
Volmax® [US]
Antibiotic, Cephalosporin
  cefditoren
  Spectracef™ [US]
Antibiotic, Quinolone
  ABC Pack™ (Avelox®) [US]
  Avelox® [US/Can]
  moxifloxacin
  trovafloxacin
  Trovan® [US/Can]
Cephalosporin (Third Generation)
  cefdinir
  Omnicef® [US/Can]
Mucolytic Agent
  acetylcysteine
  Acys-5® [US]
  Mucomyst® [US/Can]
  Parvolex® [Can]
Theophylline Derivative
  Aerolate III® [US]
  Aerolate JR® [US]
  Aerolate SR® [US]
  aminophylline
  Apo®-Theo LA [Can]
  Choledyl SA® [US]
  Dilor® [US/Can]
  dyphylline
  Elixophyllin® GG [US]
  Elixophyllin® [US]
  Lufyllin® [US/Can]
  Neoasma® [US]
  Novo-Theophyl SR [Can]
  oxtriphylline
  Phyllocontin®-350 [Can]
  Phyllocontin® [Can]
  Quibron®-T/SR [US/Can]
  Quibron®-T [US]
  Quibron® [US]
  Slo-Phyllin® [US]
  Theo-24® [US]
  Theochron® [US]
  Theocon® [US]

Theo-Dur® [US/Can]
Theolair™ [US/Can]
Theolate® [US]
Theomar® GG [US]
theophylline
theophylline and guaifenesin
T-Phyl® [US]
Uniphyl® [US/Can]

BRONCHOSPASM

Adrenergic Agonist Agent
  AccuNeb™ [US]
  Adrenalin® Chloride [US/Can]
  albuterol
  Alti-Salbutamol [Can]
  Alupent® [US]
  Apo®-Salvent [Can]
  bitolterol
  Brethine® [US]
  Bricanyl® [Can]
  Bronchial Mist® [US]
  ephedrine
  epinephrine
  isoetharine
  isoproterenol
  Isuprel® [US]
  levalbuterol
  Maxair™ Autohaler™ [US]
  Maxair™ [US]
  metaproterenol
  Novo-Salmol [Can]
  pirbuterol
  Pretz-D® [US-OTC]
  Primatene® Mist [US-OTC]
  Proventil® HFA [US]
  Proventil® Repetabs® [US]
  Proventil® [US]
  salmeterol
  Serevent® Diskus® [US]
  Serevent® [US/Can]
  terbutaline
  Tornalate® [US/Can]
  Vaponefrin® [Can]

Ventolin® HFA [US]
Ventolin® [US]
Volmax® [US]
Xopenex™ [US/Can]
Anticholinergic Agent
  atropine
Beta2-Adrenergic Agonist Agent
  Foradil® Aerolizer™ [US/Can]
  formoterol
  levalbuterol
  Xopenex™ [US/Can]
Bronchodilator
  levalbuterol
  Xopenex™ [US/Can]
Mast Cell Stabilizer
  Apo®-Cromolyn [Can]
  cromolyn sodium
  Intal® [US/Can]
  Nu-Cromolyn [Can]

BURN

Antibacterial, Topical
  Dermazin™ [Can]
  Flamazine® [Can]
  mafenide
  nitrofurazone
  Silvadene® [US]
  silver sulfadiazine
  SSD® AF [US]
  SSD® Cream [US/Can]
  Sulfamylon® [US]
  Thermazene® [US]
Protectant, Topical
  A and D™ Ointment [US-OTC]
  Desitin® [US-OTC]
  vitamin A and vitamin D
  zinc oxide, cod liver oil, and talc

BURSITIS

Nonsteroidal Antiinflammatory Drug
    (NSAID)
  Advil® Children's [US-OTC]
  Advil® Infants' Concentrated Drops
    [US-OTC]

Advil® Junior [US-OTC]
Advil® [US/Can]
Aleve® [US-OTC]
Anaprox® DS [US/Can]
Anaprox® [US/Can]
Apo®-ASA [Can]
Apo®-Ibuprofen [Can]
Apo®-Indomethacin [Can]
Apo®-Napro-Na [Can]
Apo®-Napro-Na DS [Can]
Apo®-Naproxen [Can]
Apo®-Naproxen SR [Can]
Arthropan® [US-OTC]
Asaphen [Can]
Asaphen E.C. [Can]
Ascriptin® Arthritis Pain [US-OTC]
Ascriptin® Enteric [US-OTC]
Ascriptin® Extra Strength
    [US-OTC]
Ascriptin® [US-OTC]
Aspercin Extra [US-OTC]
Aspercin [US-OTC]
aspirin
Bayer® Aspirin Extra Strength [US-
    OTC]
Bayer® Aspirin Regimen Children's
    [US-OTC]
Bayer® Aspirin Regimen Regular
    Strength [US-OTC]
Bayer® Aspirin [US-OTC]
Bayer® Plus Extra Strength [US-
    OTC]
Bufferin® Arthritis Strength [US-
    OTC]
Bufferin® Extra Strength [US-OTC]
Bufferin® [US-OTC]
choline magnesium trisalicylate
choline salicylate
Easprin® [US]
EC-Naprosyn® [US]
Ecotrin® Maximum Strength [US-
    OTC]
Ecotrin® [US-OTC]

Entrophen® [Can]
Gen-Naproxen EC [Can]
Genpril® [US-OTC]
Haltran® [US-OTC]
ibuprofen
Ibu-Tab® [US]
Indocid® [Can]
Indocid® P.D.A. [Can]
Indocin® SR [US]
Indocin® [US]
Indo-Lemmon [Can]
indomethacin
Indotec [Can]
I-Prin [US-OTC]
Menadol® [US-OTC]
Motrin® Children's [US/Can]
Motrin® IB [US/Can]
Motrin® [US/Can]
Naprelan® [US]
Naprosyn® [US/Can]
naproxen
Naxen® [Can]
Novasen [Can]
Novo-Methacin [Can]
Novo-Naprox [Can]
Novo-Naprox Sodium [Can]
Novo-Naprox Sodium DS [Can]
Novo-Naprox SR [Can]
Novo-Profen® [Can]
Nu-Ibuprofen [Can]
Nu-Indo [Can]
Nu-Naprox [Can]
Rhodacine® [Can]
Riva-Naproxen [Can]
St. Joseph® Pain Reliever
  [US-OTC]
Sureprin 81™ [US-OTC]
Synflex® [Can]
Synflex® DS [Can]
Teejel® [Can]
Tricosal® [US]
Trilisate® [US/Can]
ZORprin® [US]

CACHEXIA
Progestin
  Apo®-Megestrol [Can]
  Lin-Megestrol [Can]
  Megace® OS
  Megace® [US/Can]
  megestrol acetate
  Nu-Megestrol [Can]

CALCIUM CHANNEL BLOCKER TOXICITY
Electrolyte Supplement, Oral
  calcium gluceptate
  calcium gluconate
  Calfort® [US]
  Cal-G® [US]

CANDIDIASIS
Antifungal Agent
  Abelcet® [US/Can]
  Absorbine Jr.® Antifungal [US-OTC]
  Aftate® for Athlete's Foot [US-OTC]
  Aftate® for Jock Itch [US-OTC]
  Aloe Vesta® 2-n-1 Antifungal [US-OTC]
  Amphocin® [US]
  Amphotec® [US]
  amphotericin B cholesteryl sulfate complex
  amphotericin B (conventional)
  amphotericin B lipid complex
  Ancobon® [US/Can]
  Apo®-Fluconazole [Can]
  Apo®-Ketoconazole [Can]
  AVC™ [US/Can]
  Baza® Antifungal [US-OTC]
  Bio-Statin® [US]
  butoconazole
  Candistatin® [Can]
  Carrington Antifungal [US-OTC]
  ciclopirox
  Clotrimaderm [Can]
  clotrimazole

A115

Cruex® [US-OTC]
1-Day™ [US-OTC]
Diflucan® [US/Can]
econazole
Ecostatin® [Can]
Exelderm® [US/Can]
Femstat® One [Can]
fluconazole
flucytosine
Fungizone® [US/Can]
Fungoid® Tincture [US-OTC]
Genaspor® [US-OTC]
Gynazole-1™ [US]
GyneCure™ [Can]
Gynix® [US-OTC]
itraconazole
ketoconazole
Micatin® [US/Can]
miconazole
Micozole [Can]
naftifine
Naftin® [US]
Nilstat [Can]
Nizoral® [US/Can]
Novo-Ketoconazole [Can]
Nyaderm [Can]
nystatin
Nystat-Rx® [US]
Nystop® [US]
oxiconazole
Oxistat® [US/Can]
Oxizole® [Can]
Penlac™ [US/Can]
Pitrex [Can]
PMS-Nystatin [Can]
Quinsana Plus® [US-OTC]
Spectazole™ [US/Can]
Sporanox® [US/Can]
sulconazole
sulfanilamide
terbinafine (topical)
terconazole
Ting® [US-OTC]

tioconazole
tolnaftate
Trosyd™ AF [Can]
Trosyd™ J [Can]
Vagistat®-1 [US-OTC]
Antifungal Agent, Systemic
 AmBisome® [US/Can]
 amphotericin B liposomal
Antifungal/Corticosteroid
 Mycolog®-II [US]
 Mytrex® [US]
 nystatin and triamcinolone

CANKER SORE
Antiinfective Agent, Oral
 carbamide peroxide
 Gly-Oxide® Oral [US-OTC]
 Orajel® Perioseptic® [US-OTC]
 Proxigel® Oral [US-OTC]
Antiinflammatory Agent, Locally
  Applied
 amlexanox
 Aphthasol™ [US]
Local Anesthetic
 Anbesol® Baby [US/Can]
 Anbesol® Maximum Strength [US-OTC]
 Anbesol® [US-OTC]
 Babee® Teething® [US-OTC]
 benzocaine
 Benzodent® [US-OTC]
 Orabase®-B [US-OTC]
 Orajel® Baby Nighttime [US-OTC]
 Orajel® Baby [US-OTC]
 Orajel® Maximum Strength [US-OTC]
 Orajel® [US-OTC]
 Orasol® [US-OTC]
 Zilactin® Baby [US/Can]
 Zilactin®-B [US/Can]
Protectant, Topical
 gelatin, pectin, and methylcellulose
 Orabase® Plain [US-OTC]

CARDIOGENIC SHOCK

Adrenergic Agonist Agent
  dobutamine
  Dobutrex® [US/Can]
  dopamine
  Intropin® [Can]
Cardiac Glycoside
  Digitek® [US]
  digoxin
  Lanoxicaps® [US/Can]
  Lanoxin® Pediatric [US]
  Lanoxin® [US/Can]

CARDIOMYOPATHY

Cardiovascular Agent, Other
  dexrazoxane
  Zinecard® [US/Can]

CELIAC DISEASE

Electrolyte Supplement, Oral
  Alka-Mints® [US-OTC]
  Amitone® [US-OTC]
  Apo®-Cal [Can]
  Apo®-Ferrous Gluconate [Can]
  Apo®-Ferrous Sulfate [Can]
  Calbon® [US]
  Cal Carb-HD® [US-OTC]
  Calci-Chew™ [US-OTC]
  Calci-Mix™ [US-OTC]
  Calcionate® [US-OTC]
  Calciquid® [US-OTC]
  Cal-Citrate® 250 [US-OTC]
  calcium carbonate
  calcium citrate
  calcium glubionate
  calcium lactate
  Cal-Lac® [US]
  Caltrate® 600 [US/Can]
  Chooz® [US-OTC]
  Citracal® [US-OTC]
  Fe-40® [US-OTC]
  Femiron® [US-OTC]
  Feosol® [US-OTC]
  Feostat® [US-OTC]
  Feratab® [US-OTC]
  Fergon® [US-OTC]
  Fer-In-Sol® Drops [US/Can]
  Fer-Iron® [US-OTC]
  Ferodan™ [Can]
  Feronate® [US-OTC]
  Ferro-Sequels® [US-OTC]
  ferrous fumarate
  ferrous gluconate
  ferrous sulfate
  Florical® [US-OTC]
  Hemocyte® [US-OTC]
  Ircon® [US-OTC]
  Mallamint® [US-OTC]
  Nephro-Calci® [US-OTC]
  Nephro-Fer™ [US-OTC]
  Os-Cal® 500 [US/Can]
  Oyst-Cal 500 [US-OTC]
  Oystercal® 500 [US]
  Palafer® [Can]
  Ridactate® [US]
  Rolaids® Calcium Rich
    [US-OTC]
  Slow FE® [US-OTC]
  Tums® E-X Extra Strength Tablet
    [US-OTC]
  Tums® Ultra [US-OTC]
  Tums® [US-OTC]
Vitamin
  Fero-Grad 500® [US-OTC]
  ferrous sulfate and ascorbic acid
  ferrous sulfate, ascorbic acid, and vit-
    amin B-complex
  ferrous sulfate, ascorbic acid, vitamin
    B-complex, and folic acid
  Iberet-Folic-500® [US]
  Iberet®-Liquid 500 [US-OTC]
  Iberet®-Liquid [US-OTC]
Vitamin, Fat Soluble
  AquaMEPHYTON® [US/Can]
  Mephyton® [US/Can]
  phytonadione

CEREBROVASCULAR ACCIDENT (CVA)
Antiplatelet Agent
  Alti-Ticlopidine [Can]
  Apo®-ASA [Can]
  Apo®-Ticlopidine [Can]
  Asaphen [Can]
  Asaphen E.C. [Can]
  aspirin
  Bayer® Aspirin Regimen Adult Low
    Strength [US-OTC]
  Bayer® Aspirin Regimen Adult Low
    Strength with Calcium [US-OTC]
  Ecotrin® Low Adult Strength [US-
    OTC]
  Entrophen® [Can]
  Gen-Ticlopidine [Can]
  Halfprin® [US-OTC]
  Novasen [Can]
  Nu-Ticlopidine [Can]
  Rhoxal-ticlopidine [Can]
  Ticlid® [US/Can]
  ticlopidine
Fibrinolytic Agent
  Activase® rt-PA [Can]
  Activase® [US]
  alteplase
  Cathflo™ Activase® [US]

CHICKENPOX
Antiviral Agent
  acyclovir
  Apo®-Acyclovir [Can]
  Avirax™ [Can]
  Gen-Acyclovir [Can]
  Nu-Acyclovir [Can]
  Zovirax® [US/Can]
Vaccine, Live Virus
  varicella virus vaccine
  Varivax® [US/Can]

CHOLELITHIASIS
Gallstone Dissolution Agent
  Actigall™ [US]

Moctanin® [US/Can]
monoctanoin
ursodiol
Urso® [US/Can]

CHOLESTASIS
Vitamin, Fat Soluble
  AquaMEPHYTON® [US/Can]
  Mephyton® [US/Can]
  phytonadione

CHOLINESTERASE INHIBITOR POISONING
Antidote
  pralidoxime
  Protopam® Injection [US/Can]

CHRONIC OBSTRUCTIVE PULMONARY DISEASE (COPD)
Adrenergic Agonist Agent
  AccuNeb™ [US]
  albuterol
  Alti-Salbutamol [Can]
  Alupent® [US]
  Apo®-Salvent [Can]
  isoproterenol
  Isuprel® [US]
  metaproterenol
  Novo-Salmol [Can]
  Proventil® HFA [US]
  Proventil® Repetabs® [US]
  Proventil® [US]
  Ventolin® HFA [US]
  Ventolin® [US]
  Volmax® [US]
Anticholinergic Agent
  Alti-Ipratropium [Can]
  Apo®-Ipravent [Can]
  Atrovent® [US/Can]
  Gen-Ipratropium [Can]
  ipratropium
  Novo-Ipramide [Can]
  Nu-Ipratropium [Can]
  PMS-Ipratropium [Can]

Bronchodilator
  Combivent® [US/Can]
  DuoNeb™ [US]
  ipratropium and albuterol
Expectorant
  potassium iodide
  SSKI® [US]
Theophylline Derivative
  Aerolate III® [US]
  Aerolate JR® [US]
  Aerolate SR® [US]
  aminophylline
  Apo®-Theo LA [Can]
  Dilor® [US/Can]
  dyphylline
  Elixophyllin® GG [US]
  Elixophyllin® [US]
  Lufyllin® [US/Can]
  Neoasma® [US]
  Novo-Theophyl SR [Can]
  Phyllocontin®-350 [Can]
  Phyllocontin® [Can]
  Quibron®-T/SR [US/Can]
  Quibron®-T [US]
  Quibron® [US]
  Slo-Phyllin® [US]
  Theo-24® [US]
  Theochron® [US]
  Theocon® [US]
  Theo-Dur® [US/Can]
  Theolair™ [US/Can]
  Theolate® [US]
  Theomar® GG [US]
  theophylline
  theophylline and guaifenesin
  T-Phyl® [US]
  Uniphyl® [US/Can]

CIRRHOSIS
Bile Acid Sequestrant
  cholestyramine resin
  LoCHOLEST® Light [US]
  LoCHOLEST® [US]

  Novo-Cholamine [Can]
  Novo-Cholamine Light [Can]
  PMS-Cholestyramine [Can]
  Prevalite® [US]
  Questran® Light [US/Can]
  Questran® Powder [US/Can]
Chelating Agent
  Cuprimine® [US/Can]
  Depen® [US/Can]
  penicillamine
Electrolyte Supplement, Oral
  calcium carbonate
  calcium citrate
  calcium glubionate
  calcium lactate
Immunosuppressant Agent
  Alti-Azathioprine [Can]
  azathioprine
  Gen-Azathioprine [Can]
  Imuran® [US/Can]
Vitamin D Analog
  Calciferol™ [US]
  Drisdol® [US/Can]
  ergocalciferol
  Ostoforte® [Can]
Vitamin, Fat Soluble
  AquaMEPHYTON® [US/Can]
  Aquasol A® [US]
  Mephyton® [US/Can]
  Palmitate-A® [US-OTC]
  phytonadione
  vitamin A

CISPLATIN TOXICITY
Antidote
  sodium thiosulfate

CLAUDICATION
Blood Viscosity Reducer Agent
  Albert® Pentoxifylline [Can]
  Apo®-Pentoxifylline SR [Can]
  Nu-Pentoxifylline SR [Can]
  pentoxifylline
  Trental® [US/Can]

COLITIS (ULCERATIVE)
Adrenal Corticosteroid
    Cortenema® [US/Can]
    hydrocortisone (rectal)
5-Aminosalicylic Acid Derivative
    Alti-Sulfasalazine® [Can]
    Asacol® [US/Can]
    Azulfidine® EN-tabs® [US]
    Azulfidine® Tablet [US]
    balsalazide
    Canasa™ [US]
    Colazal™ [US]
    Dipentum® [US/Can]
    mesalamine
    Mesasal® [Can]
    Novo-ASA [Can]
    olsalazine
    Pentasa® [US/Can]
    Quintasa® [Can]
    Rowasa® [US/Can]
    Salazopyrin® [Can]
    Salazopyrin En-Tabs® [Can]
    Salofalk® [Can]
    S.A.S.™ [Can]
    sulfasalazine
Antiinflammatory Agent
    balsalazide
    Colazal™ [US]

COLONIC EVACUATION
Laxative
    Alophen® [US-OTC]
    Apo®-Bisacodyl [Can]
    Bisac-Evac™ [US-OTC]
    bisacodyl
    Dulcolax® [US/Can]
    Feen-A-Mint® [US-OTC]
    Femilax™ [US-OTC]
    Fleet® Bisacodyl Enema
        [US-OTC]
    Fleet® Stimulant Laxative
        [US-OTC]
    Modane Tablets® [US-OTC]

CONDYLOMA ACUMINATUM
Antiviral Agent
    interferon alfa-2b and ribavirin combination pack
    Rebetron™ [US/Can]
Biological Response Modulator
    Alferon® N [US/Can]
    interferon alfa-2a
    interferon alfa-2b
    interferon alfa-2b and ribavirin combination pack
    interferon alfa-n3
    Intron® A [US/Can]
    Rebetron™ [US/Can]
    Roferon-A® [US/Can]
Immune Response Modifier
    Aldara™ [US/Can]
    imiquimod
Keratolytic Agent
    Condyline™ [Can]
    Condylox® [US]
    Podocon-25™ [US]
    Podofilm® [Can]
    podofilox
    podophyllum resin
    Wartec® [Can]

CONGESTIVE HEART FAILURE
Adrenergic Agonist Agent
    dopamine
    inamrinone
    Intropin® [Can]
Alpha-Adrenergic Blocking Agent
    Alti-Prazosin [Can]
    Apo®-Prazo [Can]
    Minipress® [US/Can]
    Novo-Prazin [Can]
    Nu-Prazo [Can]
    prazosin
Angiotensin-Converting Enzyme (ACE)
    Inhibitor

Accupril® [US/Can]
Altace™ [US/Can]
Alti-Captopril [Can]
Apo®-Capto [Can]
Apo®-Lisinopril [Can]
Capoten® [US/Can]
captopril
cilazapril (Canada only)
enalapril
fosinopril
Gen-Captopril [Can]
Inhibace® [Can]
lisinopril
Mavik® [US/Can]
Monopril® [US/Can]
Novo-Captopril [Can]
Nu-Capto® [Can]
PMS-Captopril® [Can]
Prinivil® [US/Can]
quinapril
ramipril
trandolapril
Vasotec® I.V. [US/Can]
Vasotec® [US/Can]
Zestril® [US/Can]
Beta-Adrenergic Blocker
carvedilol
Coreg® [US/Can]
Calcium Channel Blocker
bepridil
Vascor® [US/Can]
Cardiac Glycoside
Digitek® [US]
digoxin
Lanoxicaps® [US/Can]
Lanoxin® Pediatric [US]
Lanoxin® [US/Can]
Cardiovascular Agent, Other
milrinone
Primacor® [US/Can]
Diuretic, Loop
Apo®-Furosemide [Can]
bumetanide

Bumex® [US/Can]
Burinex® [Can]
Demadex® [US]
Furocot® [US]
furosemide
Lasix® Special [Can]
Lasix® [US/Can]
torsemide
Diuretic, Potassium Sparing
amiloride
Dyrenium® [US/Can]
Midamor® [US/Can]
triamterene
Vasodilator
Apo®-Hydralazine [Can]
Apresoline® [US/Can]
hydralazine
Minitran™ [US/Can]
Nitrek® [US]
Nitro-Bid® Ointment [US]
Nitro-Dur® [US/Can]
Nitrogard® [US]
nitroglycerin
Nitrolingual® [US]
Nitrol® [US/Can]
Nitrong® SR [Can]
Nitropress® [US]
nitroprusside
NitroQuick® [US]
Nitrostat® [US/Can]
Nitro-Tab® [US]
NitroTime® [US]
Novo-Hylazin [Can]
Nu-Hydral [Can]
Transderm-Nitro® [Can]

CONJUNCTIVITIS (ALLERGIC)

Adrenal Corticosteroid
HMS Liquifilm® [US]
medrysone
Antihistamine
Acot-Tussin® Allergy [US-OTC]

Alercap® [US-OTC]
Aler-Dryl® [US-OTC]
Alertab® [US-OTC]
Aller-Chlor® [US-OTC]
Allerdryl® [Can]
Allermax® [US-OTC]
Allernix [Can]
Altaryl® [US-OTC]
Anti-Hist® [US-OTC]
ANX® [US]
Apo®-Dimenhydrinate [Can]
Apo®-Hydroxyzine [Can]
Atarax® [US/Can]
azatadine
Banaril® [US-OTC]
Banophen® [US-OTC]
Benadryl® [US/Can]
brompheniramine
chlorpheniramine
Chlor-Trimeton® [US-OTC]
Chlor-Tripolon® [Can]
Claritin® RediTabs® [US]
Claritin® [US/Can]
clemastine
Colhist® Solution [US-OTC]
cyproheptadine
Dermamycin® [US-OTC]
Derma-Pax® [US-OTC]
dexchlorpheniramine
dimenhydrinate
Dimetane® Extentabs® [US-OTC]
Dimetapp® Allergy Children's [US-OTC]
Dimetapp® Allergy [US-OTC]
Diphendryl® [US-OTC]
Diphenhist® [US-OTC]
diphenhydramine
Diphen® [US-OTC]
Diphenyl® [US-OTC]
Dramamine® Oral [US-OTC]
Dytuss® [US-OTC]
Genahist® [US-OTC]
Geridryl® [US-OTC]

Gravol® [Can]
Hydramine® [US-OTC]
Hydrate® [US]
hydroxyzine
Hyrexin® [US-OTC]
Hyzine-50® [US]
levocabastine
Livostin® [US/Can]
Lodrane® 12 Hour [US-OTC]
loratadine
Mediphedryl® [US-OTC]
Miles® Nervine [US-OTC]
ND-Stat® Solution [US-OTC]
Nolahist® [US/Can]
Novo-Hydroxyzin [Can]
olopatadine
Optimine® [US/Can]
Patanol® [US/Can]
Periactin® [US/Can]
phenindamine
PMS-Diphenhydramine [Can]
PMS-Hydroxyzine [Can]
Polaramine® [US]
Polydryl® [US-OTC]
Polytapp® Allergy Dye-Free Medication [US-OTC]
Q-Dryl® [US-OTC]
Quenalin® [US-OTC]
Restall® [US]
Siladryl® Allerfy® [US-OTC]
Silphen® [US-OTC]
Tavist®-1 [US-OTC]
Tavist® [US]
Vistacot® [US]
Vistaril® [US/Can]
Antihistamine/Decongestant
   Combination
Andehist NR Drops [US]
Carbaxefed RF [US]
carbinoxamine and pseudo-
   ephedrine
Hydro-Tussin™-CBX [US]
Palgic®-DS [US]

Palgic®-D [US]
Rondec® Drops [US]
Rondec® Tablets [US]
Rondec-TR® [US]
Antihistamine, H1 Blocker,
    Ophthalmic
Apo®-Ketotifen [Can]
Emadine® [US]
emedastine
ketotifen
Antihistamine, Ophthalmic
Astelin® [US/Can]
azelastine
Optivar™ [US]
Corticosteroid, Ophthalmic
Alrex™ [US/Can]
Lotemax™ [US/Can]
loteprednol
Mast Cell Stabilizer
Alamast™ [US/Can]
Alocril™ [US/Can]
nedocromil (ophthalmic)
pemirolast
Nonsteroidal Antiinflammatory Drug
    (NSAID)
Acular® PF [US]
Acular® [US/Can]
Apo®-Ketorolac [Can]
ketorolac
Novo-Ketorolac [Can]
Ophthalmic Agent, Miscellaneous
Alamast™ [US/Can]
pemirolast
Phenothiazine Derivative
Anergan® [US]
Phenergan® [US/Can]
promethazine

CONJUNCTIVITIS (BACTERIAL)

Antibiotic, Ophthalmic
levofloxacin
Quixin™ Ophthalmic [US]

CONJUNCTIVITIS (VERNAL)

Adrenal Corticosteroid
HMS Liquifilm® [US]
medrysone
Mast Cell Stabilizer
Alomide® [US/Can]
lodoxamide tromethamine

CONSTIPATION

Laxative
Acilac [Can]
Alophen® [US-OTC]
Apo®-Bisacodyl [Can]
Arlex® [US]
Bausch & Lomb® Computer Eye
    Drops [US-OTC]
Bisac-Evac™ [US-OTC]
bisacodyl
Black Draught® [US-OTC]
calcium polycarbophil
castor oil
Cholac® [US]
Cholan-HMB® [US-OTC]
Citrucel® [US-OTC]
Constilac® [US]
Constulose® [US]
dehydrocholic acid
Dulcolax® [US/Can]
Emulsoil® [US-OTC]
Enulose® [US]
Equalactin® Chewable Tablet [US-
    OTC]
Ex-Lax® Maximum Relief [US]
Ex-Lax® [US]
Feen-A-Mint® [US-OTC]
Femilax™ [US-OTC]
Fiberall® Chewable Tablet [US-
    OTC]
Fiberall® Powder [US-OTC]
Fiberall® Wafer [US-OTC]
FiberCon® Tablet [US-OTC]
Fiber-Lax® Tablet [US-OTC]

Fleet® Babylax® [US-OTC]
Fleet® Bisacodyl Enema [US-OTC]
Fleet® Enema [US/Can]
Fleet® Glycerin Suppositories Maximum Strength [US-OTC]
Fleet® Glycerin Suppositories [US-OTC]
Fleet® Liquid Glycerin Suppositories [US-OTC]
Fleet® Phospho®-Soda [US/Can]
Fleet® Stimulant Laxative [US-OTC]
Generlac® [US]
glycerin
Haley's M-O® [US-OTC]
Hydrocil® [US-OTC]
Konsyl-D® [US-OTC]
Konsyl® [US-OTC]
Kristalose™ [US]
lactulose
Laxilose [Can]
Mag-Gel® 600 [US]
magnesium hydroxide
magnesium hydroxide and mineral oil emulsion
magnesium oxide
magnesium sulfate
Mag-Ox® 400 [US-OTC]
malt soup extract
Maltsupex® [US-OTC]
Metamucil® Smooth Texture [US-OTC]
Metamucil® [US/Can]
methylcellulose
Mitrolan® Chewable Tablet [US-OTC]
Modane® Bulk [US-OTC]
Modane Tablets® [US-OTC]
Neoloid® [US-OTC]
Novo-Mucilax [Can]
Osmoglyn® [US]
Perdiem® Plain [US-OTC]
Phillips'® Milk of Magnesia [US-OTC]

PMS-Lactulose [Can]
psyllium
Purge® [US-OTC]
Reguloid® [US-OTC]
Sani-Supp® [US-OTC]
Senexon® [US-OTC]
senna
Senna-Gen® [US-OTC]
Senokot® [US-OTC]
Serutan® [US-OTC]
sodium phosphates
sorbitol
Syllact® [US-OTC]
Uro-Mag® [US-OTC]
Visicol™ [US]
X-Prep® [US-OTC]
Laxative/Stool Softener
Diocto C® [US-OTC]
docusate and casanthranol
Doxidan® [US-OTC]
Genasoft® Plus [US-OTC]
Peri-Colace® [US/Can]
Silace-C® [US-OTC]
Stool Softener
Colace® [US/Can]
Colax-C® [Can]
Diocto® [US-OTC]
docusate
DOS® Softgel® [US-OTC]
D-S-S® [US-OTC]
Ex-Lax® Stool Softener [US-OTC]
PMS-Docusate Calcium [Can]
PMS-Docusate Sodium [Can]
Regulex® [Can]
Selax® [Can]
Soflax™ [Can]
Surfak® [US-OTC]

CROHN DISEASE
5-Aminosalicylic Acid Derivative
Alti-Sulfasalazine® [Can]
Asacol® [US/Can]
Azulfidine® EN-tabs® [US]

Azulfidine® Tablet [US]
Canasa™ [US]
Dipentum® [US/Can]
mesalamine
Mesasal® [Can]
Novo-ASA [Can]
olsalazine
Pentasa® [US/Can]
Quintasa® [Can]
Rowasa® [US/Can]
Salazopyrin® [Can]
Salazopyrin En-Tabs® [Can]
Salofalk® [Can]
S.A.S.™ [Can]
sulfasalazine

CROUP
Adrenergic Agonist Agent
Adrenalin® Chloride [US/Can]
epinephrine
Primatene® Mist [US-OTC]
Vaponefrin® [Can]

CRYPTOCOCCOSIS
Antifungal Agent
Abelcet® [US/Can]
Amphocin® [US]
Amphotec® [US]
amphotericin B cholesteryl sulfate complex
amphotericin B (conventional)
amphotericin B lipid complex
Ancobon® [US/Can]
Apo®-Fluconazole [Can]
Diflucan® [US/Can]
fluconazole
flucytosine
Fungizone® [US/Can]
itraconazole
Sporanox® [US/Can]
Antifungal Agent, Systemic
AmBisome® [US/Can]
amphotericin B liposomal

CRYPTORCHIDISM
Gonadotropin
Chorex® [US]
chorionic gonadotropin (human)
Novarel™ [US]
Pregnyl® [US/Can]
Profasi® HP [Can]
Profasi® [US]

CURARE POISONING
Cholinergic Agent
edrophonium
Enlon® [US/Can]
Reversol® [US]
Tensilon® [US]

CUSHING SYNDROME
Antineoplastic Agent
aminoglutethimide
Cytadren® [US]

CYANIDE POISONING
Antidote
cyanide antidote kit
methylene blue
sodium thiosulfate
Urolene Blue® [US]
Vasodilator
amyl nitrite

CYCLOPLEGIA
Anticholinergic Agent
AK-Pentolate® [US]
atropine
Atropine-Care® [US]
Atropisol® [US/Can]
Cyclogyl® [US/Can]
cyclopentolate
Diopentolate® [Can]
Diotrope® [Can]
homatropine
Isopto® Atropine [US/Can]
Isopto® Homatropine [US]
Isopto® Hyoscine [US]

Mydriacyl® [US/Can]
Sal-Tropine™ [US]
scopolamine
tropicamide

CYCLOSERINE POISONING
Vitamin, Water Soluble
Aminoxin® [US-OTC]
pyridoxine

CYSTINURIA
Chelating Agent
Cuprimine® [US/Can]
Depen® [US/Can]
penicillamine

CYSTITIS (HEMORRHAGIC)
Antidote
mesna
Mesnex™ [US/Can]
Uromitexan™ [Can]

CYTOMEGALOVIRUS
Antiviral Agent
cidofovir
Cytovene® [US/Can]
foscarnet
Foscavir® [US/Can]
ganciclovir
Vistide® [US]
Vitrasert® [US/Can]
Antiviral Agent, Ophthalmic
fomivirsen
Vitravene™ [US/Can]
Immune Globulin
Carimune™ [US]
CytoGam® [US]
cytomegalovirus immune globulin
(intravenous-human)
Gamimune® N [US/Can]
Gammagard® S/D [US/Can]
Gammar®-P I.V. [US]
immune globulin (intravenous)

Iveegam EN [US]
Iveegam Immuno® [Can]
Panglobulin® [US]
Polygam® S/D [US]
Venoglobulin®-S [US]

DEBRIDEMENT OF CALLOUS TISSUE
Keratolytic Agent
trichloroacetic acid
Tri-Chlor® [US]

DEBRIDEMENT OF ESCHAR
Protectant, Topical
Granulex [US]
trypsin, balsam Peru, and castor oil

DECUBITUS ULCER
Enzyme
collagenase
Elase® [US]
fibrinolysin and desoxyribonuclease
Plaquase® [US]
Santyl® [US/Can]
Enzyme, Topical Debridement
Accuzyme™ [US]
papain and urea
Protectant, Topical
Granulex [US]
trypsin, balsam Peru, and castor oil
Topical Skin Product
Accuzyme™ [US]
Debrisan® [US-OTC]
dextranomer
papain and urea

DEEP VEIN THROMBOSIS (DVT)
Anticoagulant (Other)
Coumadin® [US/Can]
dalteparin
danaparoid

enoxaparin
Fragmin® [US/Can]
Hepalean® [Can]
Hepalean® Leo [Can]
Hepalean®-LOK [Can]
heparin
Hep-Lock® [US]
Innohep® [US/Can]
Lovenox® [US/Can]
Orgaran® [US/Can]
Taro-Warfarin [Can]
tinzaparin
warfarin
Factor Xa Inhibitor
Arixtra® [US]
fondaparinux
Low Molecular Weight Heparin
Fraxiparine™ [Can]
nadroparin (Canada only)

DEMENTIA

Acetylcholinesterase Inhibitor
Aricept® [US/Can]
donepezil
Antidepressant, Tricyclic (Tertiary
Amine)
Alti-Doxepin [Can]
Apo®-Doxepin [Can]
doxepin
Novo-Doxepin [Can]
Sinequan® [US/Can]
Benzodiazepine
Apo®-Diazepam [Can]
Diastat® [US/Can]
Diazemuls® [Can]
diazepam
Diazepam Intensol® [US]
Valium® [US/Can]
Ergot Alkaloid and Derivative
ergoloid mesylates
Germinal® [US]
Hydergine® LC [US]
Hydergine® [US/Can]

Phenothiazine Derivative
Apo®-Thioridazine [Can]
Mellaril® [US/Can]
thioridazine

DEPRESSION

Antidepressant
Celexa™ [US/Can]
citalopram
Antidepressant, Alpha-2 Antagonist
mirtazapine
Remeron® SolTab™ [US]
Remeron® [US]
Antidepressant, Aminoketone
bupropion
Wellbutrin® SR [US]
Wellbutrin® [US/Can]
Zyban® [US/Can]
Antidepressant, Miscellaneous
nefazodone
Serzone® [US/Can]
Antidepressant, Monoamine Oxidase
Inhibitor
Alti-Moclobemide [Can]
Apo®-Moclobemide [Can]
isocarboxazid
Manerix® [Can]
Marplan® [US]
moclobemide (Canada only)
Nardil® [US/Can]
Novo-Moclobemide [Can]
Nu-Moclobemide [Can]
Parnate® [US/Can]
phenelzine
tranylcypromine
Antidepressant, Phenethylamine
Effexor® [US/Can]
Effexor® XR [US/Can]
venlafaxine
Antidepressant/Phenothiazine
amitriptyline and perphenazine
Etrafon® [US/Can]
Triavil™ [US/Can]

Antidepressant, Selective Serotonin Reuptake Inhibitor
Alti-Fluoxetine [Can]
Alti-Fluvoxamine [Can]
Apo®-Fluoxetine [Can]
Apo®-Fluvoxamine [Can]
Apo®-Sertraline [Can]
escitalopram
fluoxetine
fluvoxamine
Gen-Fluoxetine [Can]
Gen-Fluvoxamine [Can]
Lexapro™ [US]
Luvox® [Can]
Novo-Fluoxetine [Can]
Novo-Fluvoxamine [Can]
Novo-Sertraline [Can]
Nu-Fluoxetine [Can]
Nu-Fluvoxamine [Can]
paroxetine
Paxil® CR™ [US/Can]
Paxil® [US/Can]
PMS-Fluoxetine [Can]
PMS-Fluvoxamine [Can]
Prozac® [US/Can]
Prozac® Weekly™ [US]
Rhoxal-fluoxetine [Can]
Sarafem™ [US]
sertraline
Zoloft® [US/Can]
Antidepressant, Tetracyclic
Ludiomil® [US/Can]
maprotiline
Antidepressant, Triazolopyridine
Alti-Trazodone [Can]
Apo®-Trazodone [Can]
Apo®-Trazodone D
Desyrel® [US/Can]
Gen-Trazodone [Can]
Novo-Trazodone [Can]
Nu-Trazodone [Can]
PMS-Trazodone [Can]
trazodone
Trazorel [Can]

Antidepressant, Tricyclic (Secondary Amine)
Alti-Desipramine [Can]
Alti-Nortriptyline [Can]
amoxapine
Apo®-Desipramine [Can]
Apo®-Nortriptyline [Can]
Aventyl® HCl [US/Can]
desipramine
Gen-Nortriptyline [Can]
Norpramin® [US/Can]
nortriptyline
Norventyl [Can]
Novo-Desipramine [Can]
Novo-Nortriptyline [Can]
Nu-Desipramine [Can]
Nu-Nortriptyline [Can]
Pamelor® [US/Can]
PMS-Desipramine
PMS-Nortriptyline [Can]
protriptyline
Vivactil® [US]
Antidepressant, Tricyclic (Tertiary Amine)
Alti-Doxepin [Can]
amitriptyline
amitriptyline and chlordiazepoxide
Apo®-Amitriptyline [Can]
Apo®-Doxepin [Can]
Apo®-Imipramine [Can]
Apo®-Trimip [Can]
doxepin
Elavil® [US/Can]
imipramine
Limbitrol® DS [US]
Limbitrol® [US/Can]
Novo-Doxepin [Can]
Novo-Tripramine [Can]
Nu-Trimipramine [Can]
Rhotrimine® [Can]
Sinequan® [US/Can]
Surmontil® [US/Can]
Tofranil-PM® [US]
Tofranil® [US/Can]

trimipramine
Vanatrip® [US]
Zonalon® Cream [US/Can]
Benzodiazepine
alprazolam
Alprazolam Intensol® [US]
Alti-Alprazolam [Can]
Apo®-Alpraz [Can]
Gen-Alprazolam [Can]
Novo-Alprazol [Can]
Nu-Alprax [Can]
Xana TS™ [Can]
Xanax® [US/Can]

DERMATOLOGIC DISORDER

Adrenal Corticosteroid
Acthar® [US]
Aeroseb-Dex® [US]
A-HydroCort® [US/Can]
Alti-Dexamethasone [Can]
A-methaPred® [US]
Apo®-Prednisone [Can]
Aristocort® Forte Injection [US]
Aristocort® Intralesional Injection [US]
Aristocort® Tablet [US/Can]
Aristospan® Intra-articular Injection [US/Can]
Aristospan® Intralesional Injection [US/Can]
Betaject™ [Can]
betamethasone (systemic)
Betnesol® [Can]
Celestone® Phosphate [US]
Celestone® Soluspan® [US/Can]
Celestone® [US]
Cel-U-Jec® [US]
Cortef® [US/Can]
corticotropin
cortisone acetate
Cortone® [Can]
Decadron®-LA [US]

Decadron® [US/Can]
Decaject-LA® [US]
Decaject® [US]
Delta-Cortef® [US]
Deltasone® [US]
Depo-Medrol® [US/Can]
Depopred® [US]
dexamethasone (systemic)
dexamethasone (topical)
Dexasone® L.A. [US]
Dexasone® [US/Can]
Dexone® LA [US]
Dexone® [US]
Emo-Cort® [Can]
Hexadrol® [US/Can]
H.P. Acthar® Gel [US]
Hycort® [US]
hydrocortisone (rectal)
hydrocortisone (systemic)
Hydrocortone® Acetate [US]
Kenalog® Injection [US/Can]
Key-Pred-SP® [US]
Key-Pred® [US]
Medrol® Tablet [US/Can]
methylprednisolone
Meticorten® [US]
Orapred™ [US]
Pediapred® [US/Can]
PMS-Dexamethasone [Can]
Prednicot® [US]
prednisolone (systemic)
Prednisol® TBA [US]
prednisone
Prelone® [US]
Solu-Cortef® [US/Can]
Solu-Medrol® [US/Can]
Solurex L.A.® [US]
Sterapred® DS [US]
Sterapred® [US]
Tac™-3 Injection [US]
Triam-A® Injection [US]
triamcinolone (systemic)
Triam Forte® Injection [US]
Winpred™ [Can]

DERMATOMYCOSIS
Antifungal Agent
Aloe Vesta® 2-n-1 Antifungal [US-OTC]
Apo®-Ketoconazole [Can]
Baza® Antifungal [US-OTC]
Carrington Antifungal [US-OTC]
Fulvicin® P/G [US]
Fulvicin-U/F® [US/Can]
Fungoid® Tincture [US-OTC]
Grifulvin® V [US]
griseofulvin
Gris-PEG® [US]
ketoconazole
Lotrimin® AF Powder/Spray [US-OTC]
Micatin® [US/Can]
miconazole
Micozole [Can]
Micro-Guard® [US-OTC]
Mitrazol® [US-OTC]
Monistat® 1 Combination Pack [US-OTC]
Monistat® 3 [US-OTC]
Monistat® 7 [US-OTC]
Monistat® [Can]
Monistat-Derm® [US]
naftifine
Naftin® [US]
Nizoral® A-D [US-OTC]
Nizoral® [US/Can]
Novo-Ketoconazole [Can]
oxiconazole
Oxistat® [US/Can]
Oxizole® [Can]
Zeasorb®-AF [US-OTC]

DERMATOSIS
Anesthetic/Corticosteroid
Lida-Mantle HC® [US]
lidocaine and hydrocortisone
Corticosteroid, Topical
Aclovate® [US]
Acticort® [US]
Aeroseb-HC® [US]
Ala-Cort® [US]
Ala-Scalp® [US]
alclometasone
Alphatrex® [US]
amcinonide
Anusol® HC-1 [US-OTC]
Anusol® HC-2.5% [US-OTC]
Aquacort® [Can]
Aristocort® A Topical [US]
Aristocort® Topical [US/Can]
Bactine® Hydrocortisone [US-OTC]
Betaderm® [Can]
Betamethacot® [US]
betamethasone (topical)
Betatrex® [US]
Beta-Val® [US]
Betnovate® [Can]
CaldeCORT® Anti-Itch Spray [US]
CaldeCORT® [US-OTC]
Capex™ [US/Can]
Carmol-HC® [US]
Celestoderm®-EV/2 [Can]
Celestoderm®-V [Can]
Cetacort®
clobetasol
Clocort® Maximum Strength [US-OTC]
clocortolone
Cloderm® [US/Can]
Cordran® SP [US]
Cordran® [US/Can]
Cormax® [US]
CortaGel® [US-OTC]
Cortaid® Maximum Strength [US-OTC]
Cortaid® with Aloe [US-OTC]
Cort-Dome® [US]
Cortizone®-5 [US-OTC]
Cortizone®-10 [US-OTC]
Cortoderm [Can]
Cutivate™ [US]

Cyclocort® [US/Can]
Del-Beta® [US]
Delcort® [US]
Dermacort® [US]
Dermarest Dricort® [US]
Derma-Smoothe/FS® [US/Can]
Dermatop® [US]
Dermolate® [US-OTC]
Dermovate® [Can]
Dermtex® HC with Aloe [US-OTC]
Desocort® [Can]
desonide
DesOwen® [US]
desoximetasone
diflorasone
Diprolene® AF [US]
Diprolene® [US/Can]
Diprosone® [US/Can]
Ectosone [Can]
Eldecort® [US]
Elocon® [US/Can]
fluocinolone
fluocinonide
Fluoderm [Can]
flurandrenolide
fluticasone (topical)
Gen-Clobetasol [Can]
Gynecort® [US-OTC]
halcinonide
halobetasol
Halog®-E [US]
Halog® [US/Can]
Hi-Cor-1.0® [US]
Hi-Cor-2.5® [US]
Hyderm [Can]
hydrocortisone (topical)
Hydrocort® [US]
Hydro-Tex® [US-OTC]
Hytone® [US]
Kenalog® in Orabase® [US/Can]
Kenalog® Topical [US/Can]
LactiCare-HC® [US]
Lanacort® [US-OTC]

Lidemol® [Can]
Lidex-E® [US]
Lidex® [US/Can]
Locoid® [US/Can]
Luxiq™ [US]
Lyderm® [Can]
Lydonide [Can]
Maxiflor® [US]
Maxivate® [US]
mometasone furoate
Nasonex® [US/Can]
Novo-Clobetasol [Can]
Nutracort® [US]
Olux™ [US]
Orabase® HCA [US]
Penecort® [US]
prednicarbate
Prevex® [Can]
Prevex® HC [Can]
Psorcon™ E [US]
Psorcon™ [US/Can]
Qualisone® [US]
Sarna® HC [Can]
Scalpicin® [US]
S-T Cort® [US]
Synacort® [US]
Synalar® [US/Can]
Taro-Desoximetasone [Can]
Taro-Sone® [Can]
Tegrin®-HC [US-OTC]
Temovate® [US]
Texacort® [US]
Tiamol® [Can]
Ti-U-Lac® H [Can]
Topicort®-LP [US]
Topicort® [US/Can]
Topilene® [Can]
Topisone®
Topsyn® [Can]
Triacet™ Topical [US] Oracort [Can]
Triaderm [Can]
triamcinolone (topical)
Tridesilon® [US]

U-Cort™ [US]
Ultravate™ [US/Can]
urea and hydrocortisone
Uremol® HC [Can]
Valisone® Scalp Lotion [Can]
Westcort® [US/Can]

DIABETES INSIPIDUS

Hormone, Posterior Pituitary
Pitressin® [US]
Pressyn® [Can]
vasopressin
Vasopressin Analog, Synthetic
DDAVP® [US/Can]
desmopressin acetate
Octostim® [Can]
Stimate™ [US]

DIABETES MELLITUS, INSULIN-DEPENDENT (IDDM)

Antidiabetic Agent, Parenteral
Humalog® Mix 75/25™ [US]
Humalog® [US/Can]
Humulin® 50/50 [US]
Humulin® 70/30 [US/Can]
Humulin® 80/20 [Can]
Humulin® L [US/Can]
Humulin® N [US/Can]
Humulin® R (Concentrated) U-500 [US]
Humulin® R [US/Can]
Humulin® U [US/Can]
insulin preparations
Lantus® [US]
Lente® Iletin® II [US]
Novolin® 70/30 [US]
Novolin®ge [Can]
Novolin® L [US]
Novolin® N [US]
Novolin® R [US]
NovoLog® [US]
NPH Iletin® II [US]

Regular Iletin® II [US]
Velosulin® BR (Buffered) [US]

DIABETES MELLITUS, NON-INSULIN-DEPENDENT (NIDDM)

Antidiabetic Agent
Actos® [US/Can]
Diamicron® [Can]
Gen-Gliclazide [Can]
gliclazide (Canada only)
nateglinide
Novo-Gliclazide [Can]
pioglitazone
Starlix® [US]
Antidiabetic Agent, Oral
acarbose
acetohexamide
Albert® Glyburide [Can]
Amaryl® [US/Can]
Apo®-Chlorpropamide [Can]
Apo®-Glyburide [Can]
Apo®-Metformin [Can]
Apo®-Tolbutamide [Can]
chlorpropamide
DiaBeta® [US/Can]
Diabinese® [US]
Euglucon® [Can]
Gen-Glybe [Can]
Gen-Metformin [Can]
glimepiride
glipizide
Glucophage® [US/Can]
Glucophage® XR [US]
Glucotrol® [US]
Glucotrol® XL [US]
Glucovance™ [US]
glyburide
glyburide and metformin
Glycon [Can]
Glynase™ PresTab™ [US]
Glyset™ [US/Can]
metformin

Micronase® [US]
miglitol
Novo-Glyburide [Can]
Novo-Metformin [Can]
Nu-Glyburide [Can]
Nu-Metformin [Can]
Orinase® Diagnostic [US]
PMS-Glyburide [Can]
Precose® [US/Can]
Rho®-Metformin [Can]
tolazamide
tolbutamide
Tolinase® [US/Can]
Tol-Tab® [US]
Antidiabetic Agent (Sulfonylurea)
Glucovance™ [US]
glyburide and metformin
Hypoglycemic Agent, Oral
Avandia® [US/Can]
Diamicron® [Can]
Gen-Gliclazide [Can]
gliclazide (Canada only)
GlucoNorm® [Can]
Novo-Gliclazide [Can]
Prandin™ [US/Can]
repaglinide
rosiglitazone
Sulfonylurea Agent
Diamicron® [Can]
Gen-Gliclazide [Can]
gliclazide (Canada only)
Novo-Gliclazide [Can]
Thiazolidinedione Derivative
Actos® [US/Can]
Avandia® [US/Can]
pioglitazone
rosiglitazone

DIABETIC GASTRIC STASIS

Gastrointestinal Agent, Prokinetic
Apo®-Metoclop [Can]
metoclopramide

Nu-Metoclopramide [Can]
Reglan® [US]

DIAPER RASH

Antifungal Agent
undecylenic acid and derivatives
Dietary Supplement
ME-500® [US]
methionine
Pedameth® [US]
Protectant, Topical
A and D™ Ointment [US-OTC]
Desitin® [US-OTC]
vitamin A and vitamin D
zinc oxide, cod liver oil, and talc
Topical Skin Product
Ammens® Medicated Deodorant
[US-OTC]
Balmex® [US-OTC]
Boudreaux's® Butt Paste [US-OTC]
Critic-Aid Skin Care® [US-OTC]
Desitin® Creamy [US-OTC]
methylbenzethonium chloride
Puri-Clens™ [US-OTC]
Sween Cream® [US-OTC]
Zincofax® [Can]
zinc oxide

DIARRHEA

Analgesic, Narcotic
opium tincture
paregoric
Anticholinergic Agent
Donnapectolin-PG® [US]
hyoscyamine, atropine, scopolamine,
kaolin, and pectin
hyoscyamine, atropine, scopolamine,
kaolin, pectin, and opium
Kapectolin PG® [US]
Antidiarrheal
Apo®-Loperamide [Can]
attapulgite
Children's Kaopectate® [US-OTC]
Diamode® [US-OTC]

Diarr-Eze [Can]
Diasorb® [US-OTC]
difenoxin and atropine
Diphenatol® [US]
diphenoxylate and atropine
Imodium® A-D [US-OTC]
Imodium® [US/Can]
Imogen® [US]
Imotil® [US]
Imperim® [US-OTC]
Kaodene® A-D [US-OTC]
Kaodene® NN [US-OTC]
kaolin and pectin
Kaolinpec® [US-OTC]
Kao-Paverin® [US-OTC]
Kaopectate® Advanced Formula
    [US-OTC]
Kaopectate® Maximum Strength
    Caplets [US-OTC]
Kaopectate® [US/Can]
Kao-Spen® [US-OTC]
Kapectolin® [US-OTC]
K-Pec® II [US-OTC]
K-Pek® [US-OTC]
Lomocot® [US]
Lomotil® [US/Can]
Lonox® [US]
loperamide
Lopercap [Can]
Motofen® [US]
Novo-Loperamide [Can]
PMS-Loperamine [Can]
Rhoxal-loperamine [Can]
Riva-Loperamine [Can]
Gastrointestinal Agent,
    Miscellaneous
Bacid® [US/Can]
Bismatrol® [US-OTC]
bismuth subgallate
bismuth subsalicylate
calcium polycarbophil
Devrom® [US-OTC]
Diotame® [US-OTC]

Equalactin® Chewable Tablet [US-
    OTC]
Fermalac [Can]
Fiberall® Chewable Tablet [US-
    OTC]
FiberCon® Tablet [US-OTC]
Fiber-Lax® Tablet [US-OTC]
Kala® [US-OTC]
Lactinex® [US-OTC]
Lactobacillus
Mitrolan® Chewable Tablet [US-
    OTC]
MoreDophilus® [US-OTC]
Pepto-Bismol® [US-OTC]
Pro-Bionate® [US-OTC]
Probiotica® [US-OTC]
Superdophilus® [US-OTC]
Somatostatin Analog
    octreotide
    Sandostatin LAR® [US/Can]
    Sandostatin® [US/Can]

DIARRHEA (BACTERIAL)
Aminoglycoside (Antibiotic)
    neomycin
    Neo-Rx [US]

DIGITALIS GLYCOSIDE POISONING
Antidote
    Digibind® [US/Can]
    DigiFab™ [US]
    digoxin immune Fab
Chelating Agent
    Chealamide® [US]
    Disotate® [US]
    edetate disodium
    Endrate® [US]

DIPHTHERIA
Antitoxin
    diphtheria antitoxin
Toxoid
    Adacel® [Can]

Daptacel™ [US]
diphtheria and tetanus toxoid
diphtheria, tetanus toxoids, and acellular pertussis vaccine
diphtheria, tetanus toxoids, and acellular pertussis vaccine and
  Haemophilus B conjugate vaccine
diphtheria, tetanus toxoids, and
  whole-cell pertussis vaccine
diphtheria, tetanus toxoids, whole-
  cell pertussis, and *Haemophilus* B
  conjugate vaccine
Infanrix® [US]
Pentacel™ [Can]
TriHIBit® [US]
Tripedia® [US]
Vaccine, Inactivated Bacteria
diphtheria, tetanus toxoids, and
  acellular pertussis vaccine and
  Haemophilus B conjugate vaccine
TriHIBit® [US]

DISCOID LUPUS ERYTHEMATOSUS (DLE)

Aminoquinoline (Antimalarial)
  Aralen® Phosphate [US/Can]
  chloroquine phosphate
  hydroxychloroquine
  Plaquenil® [US/Can]
Corticosteroid, Topical
  Aclovate® [US]
  Acticort® [US]
  Aeroseb-HC® [US]
  Ala-Cort® [US]
  Ala-Scalp® [US]
  alclometasone
  Alphatrex® [US]
  amcinonide
  Anusol® HC-1 [US-OTC]
  Anusol® HC-2.5% [US-OTC]
  Aquacort® [Can]
  Aristocort® A Topical [US]
  Aristocort® Topical [US/Can]

Bactine® Hydrocortisone [US-OTC]
Betaderm® [Can]
Betamethacot® [US]
betamethasone (topical)
Betatrex® [US]
Beta-Val® [US]
Betnovate® [Can]
CaldeCORT® Anti-Itch Spray [US]
CaldeCORT® [US-OTC]
Capex™ [US/Can]
Carmol-HC® [US]
Celestoderm®-EV/2 [Can]
Celestoderm®-V [Can]
Cetacort®
clobetasol
Clocort® Maximum Strength [US-
  OTC]
clocortolone
Cloderm® [US/Can]
Cordran® SP [US]
Cordran® [US/Can]
Cormax® [US]
CortaGel® [US-OTC]
Cortaid® Maximum Strength [US-
  OTC]
Cortaid® with Aloe [US-OTC]
Cort-Dome® [US]
Cortizone®-5 [US-OTC]
Cortizone®-10 [US-OTC]
Cortoderm [Can]
Cutivate™ [US]
Cyclocort® [US/Can]
Del-Beta® [US]
Delcort® [US]
Dermacort® [US]
Dermarest Dricort® [US]
Derma-Smoothe/FS® [US/Can]
Dermatop® [US]
Dermolate® [US-OTC]
Dermovate® [Can]
Dermtex® HC with Aloe [US-OTC]
Desocort® [Can]
desonide

DesOwen® [US]
desoximetasone
diflorasone
Diprolene® AF [US]
Diprolene® [US/Can]
Diprosone® [US/Can]
Ectosone [Can]
Eldecort® [US]
Elocon® [US/Can]
fluocinolone
fluocinonide
Fluoderm [Can]
flurandrenolide
fluticasone (topical)
Gen-Clobetasol [Can]
Gynecort® [US-OTC]
halcinonide
halobetasol
Halog®-E [US]
Halog® [US/Can]
Hi-Cor-1.0® [US]
Hi-Cor-2.5® [US]
Hyderm [Can]
hydrocortisone (topical)
Hydrocort® [US]
Hydro-Tex® [US-OTC]
Hytone® [US]
Kenalog® in Orabase® [US/Can]
Kenalog® Topical [US/Can]
LactiCare-HC® [US]
Lanacort® [US-OTC]
Lidemol® [Can]
Lidex-E® [US]
Lidex® [US/Can]
Locoid® [US/Can]
Luxiq™ [US]
Lyderm® [Can]
Lydonide [Can]
Maxiflor® [US]
Maxivate® [US]
mometasone furoate
Nasonex® [US/Can]
Novo-Clobetasol [Can]

Nutracort® [US]
Olux™ [US]
Orabase® HCA [US]
Penecort® [US]
prednicarbate
Prevex® [Can]
Prevex® HC [Can]
Psorcon™ E [US]
Psorcon™ [US/Can]
Qualisone® [US]
Sarna® HC [Can]
Scalpicin® [US]
S-T Cort® [US]
Synacort® [US]
Synalar® [US/Can]
Taro-Desoximetasone [Can]
Taro-Sone® [Can]
Tegrin®-HC [US-OTC]
Temovate® [US]
Texacort® [US]
Tiamol® [Can]
Ti-U-Lac® H [Can]
Topicort®-LP [US]
Topicort® [US/Can]
Topilene® [Can]
Topisone®
Topsyn® [Can]
Triacet™ Topical [US] Oracort [Can]
Triaderm [Can]
triamcinolone (topical)
Tridesilon® [US]
U-Cort™ [US]
Ultravate™ [US/Can]
urea and hydrocortisone
Uremol® HC [Can]
Valisone® Scalp Lotion [Can]
Westcort® [US/Can]

DIVERTICULITIS
Aminoglycoside (Antibiotic)
AKTob® [US]
Alcomicin® [Can]
Diogent® [Can]

Garamycin® [US/Can]
Garatec [Can]
Gentacidin® [US]
Gentak® [US]
gentamicin
Nebcin® [US/Can]
PMS-Tobramycin [Can]
tobramycin
Tobrex® [US/Can]
Tomycine™ [Can]
Antibiotic, Miscellaneous
Alti-Clindamycin [Can]
Apo®-Metronidazole [Can]
Azactam® [US/Can]
aztreonam
Cleocin HCl® [US]
Cleocin Pediatric® [US]
Cleocin Phosphate® [US]
Cleocin® [US]
Clindagel™ [US]
clindamycin
Dalacin® C [Can]
Flagyl ER® [US]
Flagyl® [US/Can]
metronidazole
Nidagel™ [Can]
Noritate™ [US/Can]
Novo-Nidazol [Can]
Carbapenem (Antibiotic)
imipenem and cilastatin
Primaxin® [US/Can]
Cephalosporin (Second Generation)
Cefotan® [US/Can]
cefotetan
cefoxitin
Mefoxin® [US/Can]
Penicillin
ampicillin
ampicillin and sulbactam
Apo®-Ampi [Can]
Marcillin® [US]
Novo-Ampicillin [Can]
Nu-Ampi [Can]

piperacillin and tazobactam sodium
Principen® [US]
Tazocin® [Can]
ticarcillin and clavulanate potassium
Timentin® [US/Can]
Unasyn® [US/Can]
Zosyn® [US]

DRUG DEPENDENCE (OPIOID)

Analgesic, Narcotic
Dolophine® [US/Can]
levomethadyl acetate hydrochloride
Metadol™ [Can]
methadone
Methadose® [US/Can]
ORLAAM® [US]

DUODENAL ULCER

Antacid
calcium carbonate and simethicone
Iosopan® Plus [US]
Lowsium® Plus [US]
magaldrate
magaldrate and simethicone
Mag-Gel® 600 [US]
magnesium hydroxide
magnesium oxide
Mag-Ox® 400 [US-OTC]
Phillips'® Milk of Magnesia [US-OTC]
Riopan Plus® Double Strength [US-OTC]
Riopan Plus® [US-OTC]
Riopan® [US-OTC]
Titralac® Plus Liquid [US-OTC]
Uro-Mag® [US-OTC]
Gastric Acid Secretion Inhibitor
Aciphex™ [US/Can]
lansoprazole
omeprazole
Prevacid® [US/Can]
Prilosec® [US/Can]
rabeprazole

Gastrointestinal Agent, Gastric or
    Duodenal Ulcer Treatment
    Apo®-Sucralate [Can]
    Carafate® [US]
    Novo-Sucralate [Can]
    Nu-Sucralate [Can]
    PMS-Sucralate [Can]
    ranitidine bismuth citrate
    sucralfate
    Sulcrate® [Can]
    Sulcrate® Suspension Plus [Can]
    Tritec® [US]
Histamine H2 Antagonist
    Acid Reducer 200® [US-OTC]
    Alti-Famotidine [Can]
    Alti-Ranitidine [Can]
    Apo®-Cimetidine [Can]
    Apo®-Famotidine [Can]
    Apo®-Nizatidine [Can]
    Apo®-Ranitidine [Can]
    Axid® AR [US-OTC]
    Axid® [US/Can]
    cimetidine
    famotidine
    Gen-Cimetidine [Can]
    Gen-Famotidine [Can]
    Gen-Ranitidine [Can]
    Heartburn 200® [US-OTC]
    Heartburn Relief 200® [US-OTC]
    nizatidine
    Novo-Cimetidine [Can]
    Novo-Famotidine [Can]
    Novo-Nizatidine [Can]
    Novo-Ranidine [Can]
    Nu-Cimet® [Can]
    Nu-Famotidine [Can]
    Nu-Ranit [Can]
    Pepcid® AC [US/Can]
    Pepcid® [US/Can]
    PMS-Cimetidine [Can]
    ranitidine hydrochloride
    Rhoxal-famotidine [Can]
    Tagamet® HB [US/Can]
    Tagamet® [US/Can]
    Ulcidine® [Can]
    Zantac® 75 [US-OTC]
    Zanta [Can]
    Zantac® [US/Can]

DYSMENORRHEA
Nonsteroidal Antiinflammatory Drug
    (NSAID)
    Advil® [US/Can]
    Aleve® [US-OTC]
    Alti-Flurbiprofen [Can]
    Alti-Piroxicam [Can]
    Anaprox® DS [US/Can]
    Anaprox® [US/Can]
    Ansaid® Oral [US/Can]
    Apo®-Diclo [Can]
    Apo®-Diclo SR [Can]
    Apo®-Diflunisal [Can]
    Apo®-Flurbiprofen [Can]
    Apo®-Ibuprofen [Can]
    Apo®-Keto [Can]
    Apo®-Keto-E [Can]
    Apo®-Keto SR [Can]
    Apo®-Mefenamic [Can]
    Apo®-Napro-Na [Can]
    Apo®-Napro-Na DS [Can]
    Apo®-Naproxen [Can]
    Apo®-Naproxen SR [Can]
    Apo®-Piroxicam [Can]
    Cataflam® [US/Can]
    diclofenac
    Diclotec [Can]
    diflunisal
    Dolobid® [US]
    EC-Naprosyn® [US]
    Feldene® [US/Can]
    flurbiprofen
    Froben® [Can]
    Froben-SR® [Can]
    Gen-Naproxen EC [Can]
    Gen-Piroxicam [Can]
    Genpril® [US-OTC]

Haltran® [US-OTC]
ibuprofen
Ibu-Tab® [US]
I-Prin [US-OTC]
ketoprofen
mefenamic acid
Menadol® [US-OTC]
Midol® Maximum Strength Cramp
    Formula [US-OTC]
Motrin® IB [US/Can]
Motrin® [US/Can]
Naprelan® [US]
Naprosyn® [US/Can]
naproxen
Naxen® [Can]
Novo-Difenac® [Can]
Novo-Difenac-K [Can]
Novo-Difenac® SR [Can]
Novo-Diflunisal [Can]
Novo-Flurprofen [Can]
Novo-Keto [Can]
Novo-Keto-EC [Can]
Novo-Naprox [Can]
Novo-Naprox Sodium [Can]
Novo-Naprox Sodium DS [Can]
Novo-Naprox SR [Can]
Novo-Pirocam® [Can]
Novo-Profen® [Can]
Nu-Diclo [Can]
Nu-Diclo-SR [Can]
Nu-Diflunisal [Can]
Nu-Flurprofen [Can]
Nu-Ibuprofen [Can]
Nu-Ketoprofen [Can]
Nu-Ketoprofen-E [Can]
Nu-Mefenamic [Can]
Nu-Naprox [Can]
Nu-Pirox [Can]
Orafen [Can]
Orudis® KT [US-OTC]
Orudis® SR [Can]
Oruvail® [US/Can]
Pexicam® [Can]

piroxicam
PMS-Diclofenac [Can]
PMS-Diclofenac SR [Can]
PMS-Mefenamic Acid [Can]
Ponstan® [Can]
Ponstel® [US/Can]
Rhodis™ [Can]
Rhodis-EC™ [Can]
Rhodis SR™ [Can]
Riva-Diclofenac [Can]
Riva-Diclofenac-K [Can]
Riva-Naproxen [Can]
Solaraze™ [US]
Synflex® [Can]
Synflex® DS [Can]
Voltaren Rapide® [Can]
Voltaren® [US/Can]
Voltaren®-XR [US]
Nonsteroidal Antiinflammatory Drug
    (NSAID), COX-2 Selective
    rofecoxib
    Vioxx® [US/Can]

DYSTONIA
Neuromuscular Blocker Agent,
    Toxin
    botulinum toxin type B
    Myobloc® [US]

DYSURIA
Analgesic, Urinary
    Azo-Dine® [US-OTC]
    Azo-Gesic® [US-OTC]
    Azo-Standard® [US]
    Baridium® [US]
    Phenazo™ [Can]
    phenazopyridine
    Prodium™ [US-OTC]
    Pyridiate® [US]
    Pyridium® [US/Can]
    Uristat® [US-OTC]
    Urodol® [US-OTC]
    Urofemme® [US-OTC]
    Urogesic® [US]

Antispasmodic Agent, Urinary
  flavoxate
  Urispas® [US/Can]
Sulfonamide
  sulfisoxazole and phenazopyridine

EAR WAX

Otic Agent, Ceruminolytic
  A/B® Otic [US]
  Allergan® Ear Drops [US]
  antipyrine and benzocaine
  Auralgan® [US/Can]
  Aurodex® [US]
  Auro® Ear Drops [US-OTC]
  Auroto® [US]
  Benzotic® [US]
  carbamide peroxide
  Cerumenex® [US/Can]
  Debrox® Otic [US-OTC]
  Dec-Agesic® A.B. [US]
  Dolotic® [US]
  E*R*O Ear [US-OTC]
  Mollifene® Ear Wax Removing Formula [US-OTC]
  Murine® Ear Drops [US-OTC]
  Rx-Otic® Drops [US]
  triethanolamine polypeptide oleate-condensate

ECLAMPSIA

Barbiturate
  Luminal® Sodium [US]
  phenobarbital
Benzodiazepine
  Apo®-Diazepam [Can]
  Diastat® [US/Can]
  Diazemuls® [Can]
  diazepam
  Diazepam Intensol® [US]
  Valium® [US/Can]

ECZEMA

Antibiotic/Corticosteroid, Topical
  Neo-Cortef® [Can]
  neomycin and hydrocortisone

Antifungal/Corticosteroid
  Ala-Quin® [US]
  clioquinol and hydrocortisone
  Dek-Quin® [US]
  Dermazene® [US]
  iodoquinol and hydrocortisone
  Vytone® [US]
Corticosteroid, Topical
  Aclovate® [US]
  Acticort® [US]
  Aeroseb-HC® [US]
  Ala-Cort® [US]
  Ala-Scalp® [US]
  alclometasone
  Alphatrex® [US]
  amcinonide
  Anusol® HC-1 [US-OTC]
  Anusol® HC-2.5% [US-OTC]
  Aquacort® [Can]
  Aristocort® A Topical [US]
  Aristocort® Topical [US/Can]
  Bactine® Hydrocortisone [US-OTC]
  Betaderm® [Can]
  Betamethacot® [US]
  betamethasone (topical)
  Betatrex® [US]
  Beta-Val® [US]
  Betnovate® [Can]
  CaldeCORT® Anti-Itch Spray [US]
  CaldeCORT® [US-OTC]
  Capex™ [US/Can]
  Carmol-HC® [US]
  Celestoderm®-EV/2 [Can]
  Celestoderm®-V [Can]
  Cetacort®
  clobetasol
  Clocort® Maximum Strength [US-OTC]
  clocortolone
  Cloderm® [US/Can]
  Cordran® SP [US]
  Cordran® [US/Can]
  Cormax® [US]

CortaGel® [US-OTC]
Cortaid® Maximum Strength [US-OTC]
Cortaid® with Aloe [US-OTC]
Cort-Dome® [US]
Cortizone®-5 [US-OTC]
Cortizone®-10 [US-OTC]
Cortoderm [Can]
Cutivate™ [US]
Cyclocort® [US/Can]
Del-Beta® [US]
Delcort® [US]
Dermacort® [US]
Dermarest Dricort® [US]
Derma-Smoothe/FS® [US/Can]
Dermatop® [US]
Dermolate® [US-OTC]
Dermovate® [Can]
Dermtex® HC with Aloe [US-OTC]
Desocort® [Can]
desonide
DesOwen® [US]
desoximetasone
diflorasone
Diprolene® AF [US]
Diprolene® [US/Can]
Diprosone® [US/Can]
Ectosone [Can]
Eldecort® [US]
Elocon® [US/Can]
fluocinolone
fluocinonide
Fluoderm [Can]
flurandrenolide
fluticasone (topical)
Gen-Clobetasol [Can]
Gynecort® [US-OTC]
halcinonide
halobetasol
Halog®-E [US]
Halog® [US/Can]
Hi-Cor-1.0® [US]
Hi-Cor-2.5® [US]

Hyderm [Can]
hydrocortisone (topical)
Hydrocort® [US]
Hydro-Tex® [US-OTC]
Hytone® [US]
Kenalog® in Orabase® [US/Can]
Kenalog® Topical [US/Can]
LactiCare-HC® [US]
Lanacort® [US-OTC]
Lidemol® [Can]
Lidex-E® [US]
Lidex® [US/Can]
Locoid® [US/Can]
Luxiq™ [US]
Lyderm® [Can]
Lydonide [Can]
Maxiflor® [US]
Maxivate® [US]
mometasone furoate
Nasonex® [US/Can]
Novo-Clobetasol [Can]
Nutracort® [US]
Olux™ [US]
Orabase® HCA [US]
Penecort® [US]
prednicarbate
Prevex® [Can]
Prevex® HC [Can]
Psorcon™ E [US]
Psorcon™ [US/Can]
Qualisone® [US]
Sarna® HC [Can]
Scalpicin® [US]
S-T Cort® [US]
Synacort® [US]
Synalar® [US/Can]
Taro-Desoximetasone [Can]
Taro-Sone® [Can]
Tegrin®-HC [US-OTC]
Temovate® [US]
Texacort® [US]
Tiamol® [Can]
Ti-U-Lac® H [Can]

Topicort®-LP [US]
Topicort® [US/Can]
Topilene® [Can]
Topisone®
Topsyn® [Can]
Triacet™ Topical [US] Oracort [Can]
Triaderm [Can]
triamcinolone (topical)
Tridesilon® [US]
U-Cort™ [US]
Ultravate™ [US/Can]
urea and hydrocortisone
Uremol® HC [Can]
Valisone® Scalp Lotion [Can]
Westcort® [US/Can]

EDEMA
Antihypertensive Agent, Combination
Aldactazide® [US/Can]
Aldoril® [US]
Apo®-Methazide [Can]
Apo®-Triazide [Can]
atenolol and chlorthalidone
benazepril and hydrochlorothiazide
Capozide® [US/Can]
captopril and hydrochlorothiazide
clonidine and chlorthalidone
Combipres® [US]
Dyazide® [US]
enalapril and hydrochlorothiazide
Enduronyl® Forte [US/Can]
Enduronyl® [US/Can]
hydralazine and hydrochlorothiazide
hydralazine, hydrochlorothiazide, and
    reserpine
Hydra-Zide® [US]
hydrochlorothiazide and spironolac-
    tone
hydrochlorothiazide and triamterene
Hyserp® [US]
Hyzaar® [US/Can]
Inderide® LA [US]
Inderide® [US]

lisinopril and hydrochlorothiazide
losartan and hydrochlorothiazide
Lotensin® HCT [US]
Maxzide® [US]
methyclothiazide and deserpidine
methyldopa and hydrochlorothiazide
Minizide® [US]
Novo-Spirozine [Can]
Novo-Triamzide [Can]
Nu-Triazide [Can]
prazosin and polythiazide
Prinzide® [US/Can]
propranolol and hydrochlorothiazide
Tenoretic® [US/Can]
Vaseretic® [US/Can]
Zestoretic® [US/Can]
Diuretic, Combination
amiloride and hydrochlorothiazide
Apo®-Amilzide [Can]
Moduret® [Can]
Moduretic® [US/Can]
Novamilor [Can]
Nu-Amilzide [Can]
Diuretic, Loop
Apo®-Furosemide [Can]
bumetanide
Bumex® [US/Can]
Burinex® [Can]
Demadex® [US]
Edecrin® [US/Can]
ethacrynic acid
Furocot® [US]
furosemide
Lasix® Special [Can]
Lasix® [US/Can]
torsemide
Diuretic, Miscellaneous
Apo®-Chlorthalidone [Can]
Apo®-Indapamide [Can]
caffeine and sodium benzoate
chlorthalidone
Gen-Indapamide [Can]
indapamide

Lozide® [Can]
Lozol® [US/Can]
metolazone
Mykrox® [US/Can]
Novo-Indapamide [Can]
Nu-Indapamide [Can]
PMS-Indapamide [Can]
Thalitone® [US]
Zaroxolyn® [US/Can]
Diuretic, Osmotic
mannitol
Osmitrol® [US/Can]
Resectisol® Irrigation Solution [US]
Diuretic, Potassium Sparing
Aldactone® [US/Can]
amiloride
Dyrenium® [US/Can]
Midamor® [US/Can]
Novo-Spiroton [Can]
spironolactone
triamterene
Diuretic, Thiazide
Apo®-Hydro [Can]
Aquacot® [US]
Aquatensen® [US/Can]
Aquazide H® [US]
bendroflumethiazide
chlorothiazide
Diuril® [US/Can]
Enduron® [US/Can]
Ezide® [US]
hydrochlorothiazide
Hydrocot® [US]
HydroDIURIL® [US/Can]
Metatensin® [Can]
methyclothiazide
Microzide™ [US]
Naqua® [US/Can]
Naturetin® [US]
Oretic® [US]
polythiazide
Renese® [US]
Trichlorex® [Can]

trichlormethiazide
Zide® [US]

EMBOLISM
Anticoagulant (Other)
Coumadin® [US/Can]
dicumarol
enoxaparin
Hepalean® [Can]
Hepalean® Leo [Can]
Hepalean®-LOK [Can]
heparin
Hep-Lock® [US]
Innohep® [US/Can]
Lovenox® [US/Can]
Taro-Warfarin [Can]
tinzaparin
warfarin
Antiplatelet Agent
Apo®-ASA [Can]
Apo®-Dipyridamole FC [Can]
Asaphen [Can]
Asaphen E.C. [Can]
aspirin
Bayer® Aspirin Regimen Adult Low
Strength [US-OTC]
Bayer® Aspirin Regimen Adult Low
Strength with Calcium
[US-OTC]
dipyridamole
Ecotrin® Low Adult Strength [US-
OTC]
Halfprin® [US-OTC]
Novo-Dipiradol [Can]
Persantine® [US/Can]
Fibrinolytic Agent
Abbokinase® [US]
Activase® rt-PA [Can]
Activase® [US]
alteplase
Retavase® [US/Can]
reteplase
Streptase® [US/Can]

streptokinase
urokinase

EMPHYSEMA
Adrenergic Agonist Agent
AccuNeb™ [US]
Adrenalin® Chloride [US/Can]
albuterol
Alti-Salbutamol [Can]
Alupent® [US]
Apo®-Salvent [Can]
bitolterol
Brethine® [US]
Bricanyl® [Can]
Bronchial Mist® [US]
ephedrine
epinephrine
isoproterenol
Isuprel® [US]
metaproterenol
Novo-Salmol [Can]
Primatene® Mist [US-OTC]
Proventil® HFA [US]
Proventil® Repetabs® [US]
Proventil® [US]
terbutaline
Tornalate® [US/Can]
Vaponefrin® [Can]
Ventolin® HFA [US]
Ventolin® [US]
Volmax® [US]
Anticholinergic Agent
Alti-Ipratropium [Can]
Apo®-Ipravent [Can]
Atrovent® [US/Can]
Gen-Ipratropium [Can]
ipratropium
Novo-Ipramide [Can]
Nu-Ipratropium [Can]
PMS-Ipratropium [Can]
Expectorant
potassium iodide
SSKI® [US]

Mucolytic Agent
acetylcysteine
Acys-5® [US]
Mucomyst® [US/Can]
Parvolex® [Can]
Theophylline Derivative
Aerolate III® [US]
Aerolate JR® [US]
Aerolate SR® [US]
aminophylline
Apo®-Theo LA [Can]
Choledyl SA® [US]
Dilor® [US/Can]
dyphylline
Elixophyllin® GG [US]
Elixophyllin® [US]
Lufyllin® [US/Can]
Neoasma® [US]
Novo-Theophyl SR [Can]
oxtriphylline
Phyllocontin®-350 [Can]
Phyllocontin® [Can]
Quibron®-T/SR [US/Can]
Quibron®-T [US]
Quibron® [US]
Slo-Phyllin® [US]
Theo-24® [US]
Theochron® [US]
Theocon® [US]
Theo-Dur® [US/Can]
Theolair™ [US/Can]
Theolate® [US]
Theomar® GG [US]
theophylline
theophylline and guaifenesin
T-Phyl® [US]
Uniphyl® [US/Can]

ENCEPHALITIS (HERPESVIRUS)
Antiviral Agent
acyclovir
Apo®-Acyclovir [Can]

Avirax™ [Can]
Gen-Acyclovir [Can]
Nu-Acyclovir [Can]
Zovirax® [US/Can]

ENDOCARDITIS TREATMENT

Aminoglycoside (Antibiotic)
  Alcomicin® [Can]
  amikacin
  Amikin® [US/Can]
  Diogent® [Can]
  Garamycin® [US/Can]
  Garatec [Can]
  gentamicin
  Nebcin® [US/Can]
  PMS-Tobramycin [Can]
  tobramycin
  Tobrex® [US/Can]
  Tomycine™ [Can]
Antibiotic, Miscellaneous
  Vancocin® [US/Can]
  Vancoled® [US]
  vancomycin
Antibiotic, Penicillin
  pivampicillin (Canada only)
  Pondocillin® [Can]
Antifungal Agent
  Amphocin® [US]
  amphotericin B (conventional)
  Fungizone® [US/Can]
Cephalosporin (First Generation)
  Ancef® [US/Can]
  Cefadyl® [US/Can]
  cefazolin
  cephalothin
  cephapirin
  Ceporacin® [Can]
  Kefzol® [US/Can]
Penicillin
  ampicillin
  Apo®-Ampi [Can]
  Marcillin® [US]

nafcillin
Novo-Ampicillin [Can]
Nu-Ampi [Can]
oxacillin
penicillin G (parenteral/aqueous)
Pfizerpen® [US/Can]
Principen® [US]
Quinolone
  ciprofloxacin
  Cipro® [US/Can]

ENDOMETRIOSIS

Androgen
  Cyclomen® [Can]
  danazol
  Danocrine® [US/Can]
Contraceptive, Oral
  Alesse® [US/Can]
  Apri® [US]
  Aviane™ [US]
  Brevicon® [US]
  Cryselle™ [US]
  Cyclessa® [US]
  Demulen® 30 [Can]
  Demulen® [US]
  Desogen® [US]
  Enpresse™ [US]
  Estrostep® Fe [US]
  ethinyl estradiol and desogestrel
  ethinyl estradiol and ethynodiol
    diacetate
  ethinyl estradiol and levonorgestrel
  ethinyl estradiol and norethindrone
  ethinyl estradiol and norgestimate
  ethinyl estradiol and norgestrel
  femhrt® [US/Can]
  Jenest™-28 [US]
  Kariva™ [US]
  Lessina™ [US]
  Levlen® [US]
  Levlite™ [US]
  Levora® [US]
  Loestrin® Fe [US]

Loestrin® [US/Can]
Lo/Ovral® [US]
Low-Ogestrel® [US]
Marvelon® [Can]
mestranol and norethindrone
Microgestin™ Fe [US]
Minestrin™ 1/20 [Can]
Min-Ovral® [Can]
Mircette® [US]
Modicon® [US]
Necon® 0.5/35 [US]
Necon® 1/35 [US]
Necon® 1/50 [US]
Necon® 10/11 [US]
Nordette® [US]
Norinyl® 1+35 [US]
Norinyl® 1+50 [US]
Nortrel™ [US]
Ogestrel®
Ortho-Cept® [US/Can]
Ortho-Cyclen® [US/Can]
Ortho-Novum® 1/50 [US/Can]
Ortho-Novum® [US]
Ortho-Tri-Cyclen® Lo [US]
Ortho Tri-Cyclen® [US/Can]
Ovcon® [US]
Ovral® [US/Can]
Portia™ [US]
PREVEN™ [US]
Select™ 1/35 [Can]
Synphasic® [Can]
Tri-Levlen® [US]
Tri-Norinyl® [US]
Triphasil® [US/Can]
Triquilar® [Can]
Trivora® [US]
Zovia™ [US]
Contraceptive, Progestin Only
Aygestin® [US]
Micronor® [US/Can]
norethindrone
norgestrel
Norlutate® [Can]

Nor-QD® [US]
Ovrette® [US/Can]
Gonadotropin-Releasing Hormone
    Analog
histrelin
Supprelin™ [US]
Hormone, Posterior Pituitary
nafarelin
Synarel® [US/Can]
Progestin
hydroxyprogesterone caproate
Hylutin® [US]
Prodrox® [US]

ENURESIS
Anticholinergic Agent
belladonna
Antidepressant, Tricyclic (Tertiary
    Amine)
Apo®-Imipramine [Can]
imipramine
Tofranil-PM® [US]
Tofranil® [US/Can]
Antispasmodic Agent, Urinary
Ditropan® [US/Can]
Ditropan® XL [US]
Gen-Oxybutynin [Can]
Novo-Oxybutynin [Can]
Nu-Oxybutyn [Can]
oxybutynin
PMS-Oxybutynin [Can]
Vasopressin Analog, Synthetic
DDAVP® [US/Can]
desmopressin acetate
Octostim® [Can]
Stimate™ [US]

EPICONDYLITIS
Nonsteroidal Antiinflammatory Drug
    (NSAID)
Advil® Children's [US-OTC]
Advil® Infants' Concentrated Drops
    [US-OTC]
Advil® Junior [US-OTC]

Advil® [US/Can]
Aleve® [US-OTC]
Anaprox® DS [US/Can]
Anaprox® [US/Can]
Apo®-Ibuprofen [Can]
Apo®-Indomethacin [Can]
Apo®-Napro-Na [Can]
Apo®-Napro-Na DS [Can]
Apo®-Naproxen [Can]
Apo®-Naproxen SR [Can]
EC-Naprosyn® [US]
Gen-Naproxen EC [Can]
Genpril® [US-OTC]
Haltran® [US-OTC]
ibuprofen
Ibu-Tab® [US]
Indocid® [Can]
Indocid® P.D.A. [Can]
Indocin® SR [US]
Indocin® [US]
Indo-Lemmon [Can]
indomethacin
Indotec [Can]
I-Prin [US-OTC]
Menadol® [US-OTC]
Motrin® Children's [US/Can]
Motrin® IB [US/Can]
Motrin® Infants' [US-OTC]
Motrin® Junior Strength [US-OTC]
Motrin® [US/Can]
Naprelan® [US]
Naprosyn® [US/Can]
naproxen
Naxen® [Can]
Novo-Methacin [Can]
Novo-Naprox [Can]
Novo-Naprox Sodium [Can]
Novo-Naprox Sodium DS [Can]
Novo-Naprox SR [Can]
Novo-Profen® [Can]
Nu-Ibuprofen [Can]
Nu-Indo [Can]
Nu-Naprox [Can]

Rhodacine® [Can]
Riva-Naproxen [Can]
Synflex® [Can]
Synflex® DS [Can]

EPILEPSY
Anticonvulsant
acetazolamide
Alti-Clobazam [Can]
Alti-Divalproex [Can]
Apo®-Acetazolamide [Can]
Apo®-Carbamazepine [Can]
Apo®-Divalproex [Can]
carbamazepine
Carbatrol® [US]
Celontin® [US/Can]
clobazam (Canada only)
Depacon® [US]
Depakene® [US/Can]
Depakote® Delayed Release [US]
Depakote® ER [US]
Depakote® Sprinkle® [US]
Diamox Sequels® [US]
Diamox® [US/Can]
Epitol® [US]
Epival® I.V. [Can]
ethosuximide
felbamate
Felbatol® [US]
Frisium® [Can]
gabapentin
Gabitril® [US/Can]
Gen-Carbamazepine CR [Can]
Gen-Divalproex [Can]
Lamictal® [US/Can]
lamotrigine
magnesium sulfate
methsuximide
Neurontin® [US/Can]
Novo-Carbamaz [Can]
Novo-Clobazam [Can]
Novo-Divalproex [Can]
Nu-Carbamazepine® [Can]

Nu-Divalproex [Can]
PMS-Carbamazepine [Can]
PMS-Valproic Acid [Can]
PMS-Valproic Acid E.C.
  [Can]
Rhoxal-valproic [Can]
Sabril® [US/Can]
Taro-Carbamazepin [Can]
Tegretol® [US/Can]
Tegretol®-XR [US]
tiagabine
Topamax® [US/Can]
topiramate
valproic acid and derivatives
vigabatrin (Canada only)
Zarontin® [US/Can]
Anticonvulsant, Miscellaneous
Keppra® [US/Can]
levetiracetam
oxcarbazepine
Trileptal® [US/Can]
Anticonvulsant, Sulfonamide
Zonegran™ [US/Can]
zonisamide
Antidepressant
Alti-Clobazam [Can]
clobazam (Canada only)
Frisium® [Can]
Novo-Clobazam [Can]
Barbiturate
amobarbital
Amytal® [US/Can]
Apo®-Primidone [Can]
Luminal® Sodium [US]
Mebaral® [US/Can]
mephobarbital
Mysoline® [US/Can]
phenobarbital
primidone
Benzodiazepine
Alti-Clonazepam [Can]
Apo®-Clonazepam [Can]
Apo®-Clorazepate [Can]

Apo®-Oxazepam [Can]
Clonapam [Can]
clonazepam
clorazepate
Gen-Clonazepam [Can]
Klonopin™ [US/Can]
Novo-Clonazepam [Can]
Novo-Clopate [Can]
Nu-Clonazepam [Can]
oxazepam
PMS-Clonazepam [Can]
Rho-Clonazepam [Can]
Rivotril® [Can]
Serax® [US]
Tranxene® [US/Can]
Hydantoin
Cerebyx® [US/Can]
Dilantin® [US/Can]
ethotoin
fosphenytoin
Peganone® [US/Can]
Phenytek™ [US]
phenytoin

EROSIVE ESOPHAGITIS
Proton Pump Inhibitor
  esomeprazole
  Nexium™ [US]

ESOPHAGEAL VARICES
Hormone, Posterior Pituitary
  Pitressin® [US]
  Pressyn® [Can]
  vasopressin
Sclerosing Agent
  Ethamolin® [US]
  ethanolamine oleate
  sodium tetradecyl
  Sotradecol® [US]
  Trombovar® [Can]
Variceal Bleeding (Acute) Agent
  somatostatin (Canada only)
  Stilamin® [Can]

ESOPHAGITIS
Gastric Acid Secretion Inhibitor
lansoprazole
omeprazole
Prevacid® [US/Can]
Prilosec® [US/Can]

ESSENTIAL THROMBOCYTHEMIA (ET)
Platelet Reducing Agent
Agrylin® [US/Can]
anagrelide

ETHYLENE GLYCOL POISONING
Pharmaceutical Aid
alcohol (ethyl)

EXTRAPYRAMIDAL SYMPTOM
Anticholinergic Agent
Akineton® [US/Can]
Apo®-Benztropine [Can]
Apo®-Trihex [Can]
Artane® [US]
benztropine
biperiden
Cogentin® [US/Can]
Kemadrin® [US/Can]
Procyclid™ [Can]
procyclidine
trihexyphenidyl

EYE INFECTION
Antibiotic/Corticosteroid, Ophthalmic
AK-Cide® [US]
AK-Trol® [US]
bacitracin, neomycin, polymyxin B, and hydrocortisone
Blephamide® [US/Can]
Cortimyxin® [Can]
Cortisporin® Ophthalmic [US/Can]
Dexacidin® [US]
Dexacine™ [US]
Dioptimyd® [Can]
Dioptrol® [Can]
FML-S® [US]
Maxitrol® [US/Can]
Metimyd® [US]
Neo-Cortef® [Can]
NeoDecadron® Ocumeter® [US]
neomycin and dexamethasone
neomycin and hydrocortisone
neomycin, polymyxin B, and dexamethasone
neomycin, polymyxin B, and hydrocortisone
neomycin, polymyxin B, and prednisolone
Poly-Pred® [US]
Pred-G® [US]
prednisolone and gentamicin
sulfacetamide and prednisolone
sulfacetamide sodium and fluorometholone
TobraDex® [US/Can]
tobramycin and dexamethasone
Vasocidin® [US/Can]
Antibiotic, Ophthalmic
Akne-Mycin® [US]
AK-Poly-Bac® [US]
AK-Spore® Ophthalmic Solution [US]
AK-Sulf® [US]
AKTob® [US]
AK-Tracin® [US]
Alcomicin® [Can]
Apo®-Oflox [Can]
Apo®-Tetra [Can]
A/T/S® [US]
Baciguent® [US/Can]
bacitracin
bacitracin and polymyxin B
bacitracin, neomycin, and polymyxin B
Bleph®-10 [US]
Brodspec® [US]

Carmol® Scalp [US]
Cetamide® [US/Can]
chloramphenicol
Chloromycetin® Parenteral [US/Can]
Chloroptic® Ophthalmic [US]
Ciloxan™ [US/Can]
ciprofloxacin
Cipro® [US/Can]
Diochloram® [Can]
Diogent® [Can]
Diosulf™ [Can]
Emgel® [US]
EmTet® [US]
Erycette® [US]
EryDerm® [US]
Erygel® [US]
Erythra-Derm™ [US]
erythromycin (ophthalmic/topical)
Floxin® [US/Can]
Garamycin® [US/Can]
Garatec [Can]
Genoptic® [US]
Gentacidin® [US]
Gentak® [US]
gentamicin
Klaron® [US]
Levaquin® [US/Can]
levofloxacin
LID-Pack® [Can]
Mycitracin® [US-OTC]
Nebcin® [US/Can]
neomycin, polymyxin B, and grami-
  cidin
Neosporin® Ophthalmic Ointment
  [US/Can]
Neosporin® Ophthalmic Solution
  [US/Can]
Neosporin® Topical [US/Can]
Neotopic® [Can]
Novo-Tetra [Can]
Nu-Tetra [Can]
Ocu-Chlor® Ophthalmic [US]
Ocuflox® [US/Can]
Ocu-Sul® [US]

ofloxacin
Optimyxin® Ophthalmic [Can]
Optimyxin Plus® [Can]
oxytetracycline and polymyxin B
Pentamycetin® [Can]
PMS-Polytrimethoprim [Can]
PMS-Tobramycin [Can]
Polycidin® Ophthalmic
Polysporin® Ophthalmic [US]
Polysporin® Topical [US-OTC]
Polytrim® [US/Can]
Quixin™ Ophthalmic [US]
Romycin® [US]
Sebizon® [US]
Sodium Sulamyd® [US/Can]
Staticin® [US]
Sulf-10® [US]
sulfacetamide
Sumycin® [US]
Terramycin® w/Polymyxin B
  Ophthalmic [US]
tetracycline
Theramycin Z® [US]
TOBI™ [US/Can]
tobramycin
Tobrex® [US/Can]
Tomycine™ [Can]
trimethoprim and polymyxin B
Triple Antibiotic® [US]
T-Stat® [US]
Wesmycin® [US]

EYE IRRITATION
Adrenergic Agonist Agent
  AK-Con™ [US]
  Albalon® [US]
  Allersol® [US]
  Clear Eyes® ACR [US-OTC]
  Clear Eyes® [US-OTC]
  naphazoline
  Naphcon Forte® [Can]
  Naphcon® [US-OTC]
  phenylephrine and zinc sulfate
  Privine® [US-OTC]

VasoClear® [US-OTC]
Vasocon® [Can]
Zincfrin® [US/Can]
Ophthalmic Agent, Miscellaneous
Akwa Tears® [US-OTC]
AquaSite® [US-OTC]
artificial tears
Bion® Tears [US-OTC]
HypoTears PF [US-OTC]
HypoTears [US-OTC]
Isopto® Tears [US/Can]
Liquifilm® Tears [US-OTC]
Moisture® Eyes PM [US-OTC]
Moisture® Eyes [US-OTC]
Murine® Tears [US-OTC]
Murocel® [US-OTC]
Nature's Tears® [US-OTC]
Nu-Tears® II [US-OTC]
Nu-Tears® [US-OTC]
OcuCoat® PF [US-OTC]
OcuCoat® [US/Can]
Puralube® Tears [US-OTC]
Refresh® Plus [US/Can]
Refresh® Tears [US/Can]
Refresh® [US-OTC]
Teardrops® [Can]
Teargen® II [US-OTC]
Teargen® [US-OTC]
Tearisol® [US-OTC]
Tears Again® [US-OTC]
Tears Naturale® Free [US-OTC]
Tears Naturale® II [US-OTC]
Tears Naturale® [US-OTC]
Tears Plus® [US-OTC]
Tears Renewed® [US-OTC]
Ultra Tears® [US-OTC]
Viva-Drops® [US-OTC]

EYELID INFECTION

Antibiotic, Ophthalmic
mercuric oxide
Ocu-Merox® [US]
Pharmaceutical Aid
boric acid

FACTOR IX DEFICIENCY

Antihemophilic Agent
AlphaNine® SD [US]
BeneFix™ [US]
factor IX complex (human)
Hemonyne® [US]
Konyne® 80 [US]
Profilnine® SD [US]
Proplex® T [US]

FACTOR VIII DEFICIENCY

Blood Product Derivative
Alphanate® [US]
antihemophilic factor (human)
Hemofil® M [US/Can]
Humate-P® [US/Can]
Kōate®-DVI [US]
Monarc® M [US]
Monoclate-P® [US]
Hemophilic Agent
antiinhibitor coagulant complex
Autoplex® T [US]
Feiba VH Immuno® [US/Can]

FEBRILE NEUTROPENIA

Quinolone
ciprofloxacin
Cipro® [US/Can]

FIBROMYOSITIS

Antidepressant, Tricyclic (Tertiary Amine)
amitriptyline
Apo®-Amitriptyline [Can]
Elavil® [US/Can]
Vanatrip® [US]

GAG REFLEX SUPPRESSION

Analgesic, Topical
Anestacon® [US]
Dermaflex® Gel [US]
lidocaine
Lidodan™ [Can]
Xylocaine® [US/Can]

Local Anesthetic
Americaine® [US-OTC]
benzocaine
benzocaine, butyl aminobenzoate, tetracaine, and benzalkonium chloride
Cetacaine® [US]
Dyclone® [US]
dyclonine
Hurricaine® [US]
Pontocaine® [US/Can]
tetracaine
Trocaine® [US-OTC]

GALACTORRHEA
Ergot Alkaloid and Derivative
Apo® Bromocriptine [Can]
bromocriptine
Parlodel® [US/Can]
PMS-Bromocriptine [Can]

GALLBLADDER DISEASE (DIAGNOSTIC)
Diagnostic Agent
Kinevac® [US]
sincalide

GAS PAIN
Antiflatulent
aluminum hydroxide, magnesium hydroxide, and simethicone
calcium carbonate and simethicone
Diovol Plus® [Can]
Flatulex® [US-OTC]
Gas-X® [US-OTC]
Iosopan® Plus [US]
Lowsium® Plus [US]
Maalox® Anti-Gas [US-OTC]
Maalox® Fast Release Liquid [US-OTC]
Maalox® Max [US-OTC]
magaldrate and simethicone
Mylanta® [Can]
Mylanta™ Double Strength

Mylanta™ Extra Strength [Can]
Mylanta® Extra Strength Liquid [US-OTC]
Mylanta® Gas [US-OTC]
Mylanta® Liquid [US-OTC]
Mylanta™ Regular Strength [Can]
Mylicon® [US-OTC]
Ovol® [Can]
Phazyme® [Can]
Riopan Plus® Double Strength [US-OTC]
Riopan Plus® [US-OTC]
simethicone
Titralac® Plus Liquid [US-OTC]

GASTRIC ULCER
Antacid
calcium carbonate and simethicone
Iosopan® Plus [US]
Lowsium® Plus [US]
magaldrate
magaldrate and simethicone
Mag-Gel® 600 [US]
magnesium hydroxide
magnesium oxide
Mag-Ox® 400 [US-OTC]
Phillips'® Milk of Magnesia [US-OTC]
Riopan Plus® Double Strength [US-OTC]
Riopan Plus® [US-OTC]
Riopan® [US-OTC]
Titralac® Plus Liquid [US-OTC]
Uro-Mag® [US-OTC]
Histamine H2 Antagonist
Acid Reducer 200® [US-OTC]
Alti-Famotidine [Can]
Alti-Ranitidine [Can]
Apo®-Cimetidine [Can]
Apo®-Famotidine [Can]
Apo®-Nizatidine [Can]
Apo®-Ranitidine [Can]
Axid® AR [US-OTC]

Axid® [US/Can]
cimetidine
famotidine
Gen-Cimetidine [Can]
Gen-Famotidine [Can]
Gen-Ranitidine [Can]
Heartburn 200® [US-OTC]
Heartburn Relief 200® [US-OTC]
nizatidine
Novo-Cimetidine [Can]
Novo-Famotidine [Can]
Novo-Nizatidine [Can]
Novo-Ranidine [Can]
Nu-Cimet® [Can]
Nu-Famotidine [Can]
Nu-Ranit [Can]
Pepcid® AC [US/Can]
Pepcid® [US/Can]
PMS-Cimetidine [Can]
ranitidine hydrochloride
Rhoxal-famotidine [Can]
Tagamet® HB [US/Can]
Tagamet® [US/Can]
Ulcidine® [Can]
Zantac® 75 [US-OTC]
Zanta [Can]
Zantac® [US/Can]
Prostaglandin
Cytotec® [US/Can]
misoprostol

GASTRITIS
Antacid
aluminum hydroxide and magnesium hydroxide
Diovol® [Can]
Diovol® Ex [Can]
Gelusil® [Can]
Gelusil® Extra Strength [Can]
Maalox® TC (Therapeutic Concentrate) [US-OTC]
Maalox® [US-OTC]
Univol® [Can]

Histamine H2 Antagonist
Acid Reducer 200® [US-OTC]
Alti-Ranitidine [Can]
Apo®-Cimetidine [Can]
Apo®-Ranitidine [Can]
cimetidine
Gen-Cimetidine [Can]
Gen-Ranitidine [Can]
Heartburn 200® [US-OTC]
Heartburn Relief 200® [US-OTC]
Novo-Cimetidine [Can]
Novo-Ranidine [Can]
Nu-Cimet® [Can]
Nu-Ranit [Can]
PMS-Cimetidine [Can]
ranitidine hydrochloride
Tagamet® HB [US/Can]
Tagamet® [US/Can]
Zantac® 75 [US-OTC]
Zanta [Can]
Zantac® [US/Can]

GASTROESOPHAGEAL REFLUX DISEASE (GERD)
Cholinergic Agent
bethanechol
Duvoid® [Can]
Myotonachol™ [Can]
Urecholine® [US]
Gastric Acid Secretion Inhibitor
Aciphex™ [US/Can]
lansoprazole
omeprazole
Prevacid® [US/Can]
Prilosec® [US/Can]
rabeprazole
Gastrointestinal Agent, Prokinetic
Apo®-Metoclop [Can]
cisapride
metoclopramide
Nu-Metoclopramide [Can]
Propulsid® [US]
Reglan® [US]

Histamine H2 Antagonist
Acid Reducer 200®
[US-OTC]
Alti-Famotidine [Can]
Alti-Ranitidine [Can]
Apo®-Cimetidine [Can]
Apo®-Famotidine [Can]
Apo®-Nizatidine [Can]
Apo®-Ranitidine [Can]
Axid® AR [US-OTC]
Axid® [US/Can]
cimetidine
famotidine
Gen-Cimetidine [Can]
Gen-Famotidine [Can]
Gen-Ranitidine [Can]
Heartburn 200® [US-OTC]
Heartburn Relief 200®
[US-OTC]
nizatidine
Novo-Cimetidine [Can]
Novo-Famotidine [Can]
Novo-Nizatidine [Can]
Novo-Ranidine [Can]
Nu-Cimet® [Can]
Nu-Famotidine [Can]
Nu-Ranit [Can]
Pepcid® AC [US/Can]
Pepcid® [US/Can]
PMS-Cimetidine [Can]
ranitidine hydrochloride
Rhoxal-famotidine [Can]
Tagamet® HB [US/Can]
Tagamet® [US/Can]
Ulcidine® [Can]
Zantac® 75 [US-OTC]
Zanta [Can]
Zantac® [US/Can]
Proton Pump Inhibitor
Panto™ IV [Can]
Pantoloc™ [Can]
pantoprazole
Protonix® [US/Can]

GENITAL HERPES
Antiviral Agent
famciclovir
Famvir™ [US/Can]
valacyclovir
Valtrex® [US/Can]

GENITAL WART
Immune Response Modifier
Aldara™ [US/Can]
imiquimod

GIANT PAPILLARY CONJUNCTIVITIS
Mast Cell Stabilizer
Crolom® [US]
cromolyn sodium

GIARDIASIS
Amebicide
Apo®-Metronidazole [Can]
Flagyl ER® [US]
Flagyl® [US/Can]
Humatin® [US/Can]
metronidazole
Nidagel™ [Can]
Noritate™ [US/Can]
Novo-Nidazol [Can]
paromomycin
Anthelmintic
albendazole
Albenza® [US]
Antiprotozoal
furazolidone
Furoxone® [US/Can]

GLAUCOMA
Adrenergic Agonist Agent
AK-Dilate® Ophthalmic [US]
AK-Nefrin® Ophthalmic [US]
Dionephrine® [Can]
dipivefrin
Epifrin® [US]
Epinal® [US]

epinephrine
epinephryl borate
Mydfrin® Ophthalmic [US/Can]
Neo-Synephrine® Ophthalmic [US]
Ophtho-Dipivefrin™ [Can]
phenylephrine
PMS-Dipivefrin [Can]
Prefrin™ Ophthalmic [US]
Primatene® Mist [US-OTC]
Propine® [US/Can]
Alpha2-Adrenergic Agonist Agent,
  Ophthalmic
Alphagan® P [US/Can]
apraclonidine
brimonidine
Iopidine® [US/Can]
Beta-Adrenergic Blocker
Apo®-Timol [Can]
Apo®-Timop [Can]
Betagan® [US/Can]
betaxolol
Betimol® [US]
Betoptic® S [US/Can]
carteolol
Cartrol® Oral [US/Can]
Cosopt® [US/Can]
dorzolamide and timolol
Gen-Timolol [Can]
Kerlone® [US]
levobunolol
metipranolol
Novo-Levobunolol [Can]
Nu-Timolol [Can]
Ocupress® Ophthalmic
  [US/Can]
Optho-Bunolol® [Can]
OptiPranolol® [US/Can]
Phoxal-timolol [Can]
PMS-Levobunolol [Can]
PMS-Timolol [Can]
Tim-AK [Can]
timolol
Timoptic® OcuDose® [US]

Timoptic® [US/Can]
Timoptic-XE® [US/Can]
Beta-Adrenergic Blocker, Ophthalmic
Betaxon® [US/Can]
levobetaxolol
Carbonic Anhydrase Inhibitor
acetazolamide
Apo®-Acetazolamide [Can]
Azopt® [US/Can]
brinzolamide
Cosopt® [US/Can]
Daranide® [US/Can]
Diamox Sequels® [US]
Diamox® [US/Can]
dichlorphenamide
dorzolamide
dorzolamide and timolol
methazolamide
Neptazane® [US/Can]
Trusopt® [US/Can]
Cholinergic Agent
carbachol
Carbastat® [US/Can]
Carboptic® [US]
Diocarpine [Can]
Isopto® Carbachol [US/Can]
Isopto® Carpine [US/Can]
Miocarpine® [Can]
Miostat® Intraocular
  [US/Can]
P6E1® [US]
pilocarpine
pilocarpine and epinephrine
Pilocar® [US]
Pilopine HS® [US/Can]
Piloptic® [US]
Salagen® [US/Can]
Cholinesterase Inhibitor
echothiophate iodide
Phospholine Iodide® [US]
physostigmine
Diuretic, Osmotic
mannitol

Osmitrol® [US/Can]
urea
Ophthalmic Agent, Miscellaneous
 Bausch & Lomb® Computer Eye
  Drops [US-OTC]
 bimatoprost
 glycerin
 Lumigan™ [US]
 Osmoglyn® [US]
 unoprostone
Prostaglandin
 latanoprost
 Xalatan® [US/Can]
Prostaglandin, Ophthalmic
 Travatan™ [US]
 travoprost

GLIOMA

Antineoplastic Agent
 CeeNU® [US/Can]
 lomustine
Antiviral Agent
 interferon alfa-2b and ribavirin combination pack
 Rebetron™ [US/Can]
Biological Response Modulator
 interferon alfa-2b
 interferon alfa-2b and ribavirin combination pack
 Intron® A [US/Can]
 Rebetron™ [US/Can]

GOITER

Thyroid Product
 Armour® Thyroid [US]
 Cytomel® [US/Can]
 Eltroxin® [Can]
 Levothroid® [US]
 levothyroxine
 Levo-T™ [US]
 Levoxyl® [US]
 liothyronine
 liotrix
 Nature-Throid® NT [US]

Novothyrox [US]
Synthroid® [US/Can]
thyroid
Thyrolar® [US/Can]
Triostat™ [US]
Unithroid™ [US]
Westhroid® [US]

GOLD POISONING

Chelating Agent
 BAL in Oil® [US]
 dimercaprol

GONORRHEA

Antibiotic, Macrolide
 Rovamycine® [Can]
 spiramycin (Canada only)
Antibiotic, Miscellaneous
 spectinomycin
 Trobicin® [US]
Antibiotic, Quinolone
 gatifloxacin
 Tequin® [US/Can]
Cephalosporin (Second Generation)
 cefoxitin
 Ceftin® [US/Can]
 cefuroxime
 Kefurox® [US/Can]
 Mefoxin® [US/Can]
 Zinacef® [US/Can]
Cephalosporin (Third Generation)
 cefixime
 ceftriaxone
 Rocephin® [US/Can]
 Suprax® [US/Can]
Quinolone
 Apo®-Oflox [Can]
 ciprofloxacin
 Cipro® [US/Can]
 Floxin® [US/Can]
 ofloxacin
Tetracycline Derivative
 Adoxa™ [US]
 Apo®-Doxy [Can]

Apo®-Doxy Tabs [Can]
Apo®-Tetra [Can]
Brodspec® [US]
Doryx® [US]
Doxy-100™ [US]
Doxycin [Can]
doxycycline
Doxytec [Can]
EmTet® [US]
Monodox® [US]
Novo-Doxylin [Can]
Novo-Tetra [Can]
Nu-Doxycycline [Can]
Nu-Tetra [Can]
Sumycin® [US]
tetracycline
Vibramycin® [US]
Vibra-Tabs® [US/Can]
Wesmycin® [US]

GOUT

Antigout Agent
  colchicine
  colchicine and probenecid
Nonsteroidal Antiinflammatory Drug
    (NSAID)
  Advil® Children's [US-OTC]
  Advil® Infants' Concentrated Drops
    [US-OTC]
  Advil® Junior [US-OTC]
  Advil® [US/Can]
  Aleve® [US-OTC]
  Anaprox® DS [US/Can]
  Anaprox® [US/Can]
  Apo®-Diclo [Can]
  Apo®-Diclo SR [Can]
  Apo®-Ibuprofen [Can]
  Apo®-Indomethacin [Can]
  Apo®-Napro-Na [Can]
  Apo®-Napro-Na DS [Can]
  Apo®-Naproxen [Can]
  Apo®-Naproxen SR [Can]
  Apo®-Sulin [Can]

Cataflam® [US/Can]
Clinoril® [US]
diclofenac
Diclotec [Can]
EC-Naprosyn® [US]
Gen-Naproxen EC [Can]
Genpril® [US-OTC]
Haltran® [US-OTC]
ibuprofen
Ibu-Tab® [US]
Indocid® [Can]
Indocid® P.D.A. [Can]
Indocin® SR [US]
Indocin® [US]
Indo-Lemmon [Can]
indomethacin
Indotec [Can]
I-Prin [US-OTC]
Menadol® [US-OTC]
Motrin® IB [US/Can]
Motrin® [US/Can]
Naprelan® [US]
Naprosyn® [US/Can]
naproxen
Naxen® [Can]
Novo-Difenac® [Can]
Novo-Difenac-K [Can]
Novo-Difenac® SR [Can]
Novo-Methacin [Can]
Novo-Naprox [Can]
Novo-Naprox Sodium [Can]
Novo-Naprox Sodium DS [Can]
Novo-Naprox SR [Can]
Novo-Profen® [Can]
Novo-Sundac [Can]
Nu-Diclo [Can]
Nu-Diclo-SR [Can]
Nu-Ibuprofen [Can]
Nu-Indo [Can]
Nu-Naprox [Can]
Nu-Sundac [Can]
PMS-Diclofenac [Can]
PMS-Diclofenac SR [Can]

Rhodacine® [Can]
Riva-Diclofenac [Can]
Riva-Diclofenac-K [Can]
Riva-Naproxen [Can]
Solaraze™ [US]
sulindac
Synflex® [Can]
Synflex® DS [Can]
Voltaren Rapide® [Can]
Voltaren® [US/Can]
Voltaren®-XR [US]
Uricosuric Agent
Anturane® [US]
Apo®-Sulfinpyrazone [Can]
Benuryl™ [Can]
Nu-Sulfinpyrazone [Can]
probenecid
sulfinpyrazone
Xanthine Oxidase Inhibitor
allopurinol
Aloprim™ [US]
Apo®-Allopurinol [Can]
Zyloprim® [US/Can]

GRAFT VS. HOST DISEASE

Immunosuppressant Agent
Atgam® [US/Can]
CellCept® [US/Can]
cyclosporine
Gengraf™ [US]
lymphocyte immune globulin
muromonab-CD3
mycophenolate
Neoral® [US/Can]
Orthoclone OKT® 3 [US/Can]
Prograf® [US/Can]
Protopic® [US]
Sandimmune® [US/Can]
tacrolimus

GRAM-NEGATIVE INFECTION

Aminoglycoside (Antibiotic)
AKTob® [US]

Alcomicin® [Can]
amikacin
Amikin® [US/Can]
Diogent® [Can]
Garamycin® [US/Can]
Garatec [Can]
Genoptic® [US]
Gentacidin® [US]
Gentak® [US]
gentamicin
kanamycin
Kantrex® [US/Can]
Nebcin® [US/Can]
PMS-Tobramycin [Can]
TOBI™ [US/Can]
tobramycin
Tobrex® [US/Can]
Tomycine™ [Can]
Antibiotic, Carbapenem
ertapenem
Invanz™ [US]
Antibiotic, Miscellaneous
Apo®-Nitrofurantoin [Can]
Azactam® [US/Can]
aztreonam
colistimethate
Coly-Mycin® M [US/Can]
Furadantin® [US]
Macrobid® [US/Can]
Macrodantin® [US/Can]
nitrofurantoin
Novo-Furantoin [Can]
Antibiotic, Penicillin
pivampicillin (Canada only)
Pondocillin® [Can]
Antibiotic, Quinolone
gatifloxacin
Levaquin® [US/Can]
levofloxacin
Tequin® [US/Can]
Carbapenem (Antibiotic)
imipenem and cilastatin
meropenem

Merrem® I.V. [US/Can]
Primaxin® [US/Can]
Cephalosporin (First Generation)
Ancef® [US/Can]
Apo®-Cefadroxil [Can]
Apo®-Cephalex [Can]
Biocef® [US]
cefadroxil
Cefadyl® [US/Can]
cefazolin
cephalexin
cephalothin
cephapirin
cephradine
Ceporacin® [Can]
Duricef® [US/Can]
Keflex® [US]
Keftab® [US/Can]
Kefzol® [US/Can]
Novo-Cefadroxil [Can]
Novo-Lexin® [Can]
Nu-Cephalex® [Can]
Velosef® [US]
Cephalosporin (Second Generation)
Apo®-Cefaclor [Can]
Ceclor® CD [US]
Ceclor® [US/Can]
cefaclor
cefamandole
Cefotan® [US/Can]
cefotetan
cefoxitin
cefpodoxime
cefprozil
Ceftin® [US/Can]
cefuroxime
Cefzil® [US/Can]
Kefurox® [US/Can]
Mandol® [US]
Mefoxin® [US/Can]
Novo-Cefaclor [Can]
Nu-Cefaclor [Can]
PMS-Cefaclor [Can]

Vantin® [US/Can]
Zinacef® [US/Can]
Cephalosporin (Third Generation)
Cedax® [US]
cefixime
Cefizox® [US/Can]
Cefobid® [US/Can]
cefoperazone
cefotaxime
ceftazidime
ceftibuten
ceftizoxime
ceftriaxone
Ceptaz® [US/Can]
Claforan® [US/Can]
Fortaz® [US/Can]
Rocephin® [US/Can]
Suprax® [US/Can]
Tazicef® [US]
Tazidime® [US/Can]
Cephalosporin (Fourth Generation)
cefepime
Maxipime® [US/Can]
Genitourinary Irrigant
neomycin and polymyxin B
Neosporin® G.U. Irrigant [US/Can]
Macrolide (Antibiotic)
Apo®-Erythro Base [Can]
Apo®-Erythro E-C [Can]
Apo®-Erythro-ES [Can]
Apo®-Erythro-S [Can]
azithromycin
Biaxin® [US/Can]
Biaxin® XL [US]
clarithromycin
Diomycin® [Can]
dirithromycin
Dynabac® [US]
E.E.S.® [US/Can]
Erybid™ [Can]
Eryc® [US/Can]
EryPed® [US]
Ery-Tab® [US]

Erythrocin® [US/Can]
erythromycin and sulfisoxazole
erythromycin (systemic)
Eryzole® [US]
Lincocin® [US/Can]
lincomycin
Lincorex® [US]
Nu-Erythromycin-S [Can]
PCE® [US/Can]
Pediazole® [US/Can]
PMS-Erythromycin [Can]
Tao® [US]
troleandomycin
Zithromax® [US/Can]
Z-PAK® [US/Can]
Penicillin
  amoxicillin
  amoxicillin and clavulanate potassium
  Amoxicot® [US]
  Amoxil® [US/Can]
  ampicillin
  ampicillin and sulbactam
  Apo®-Amoxi [Can]
  Apo®-Ampi [Can]
  Apo®-Pen VK [Can]
  Augmentin ES-600™ [US]
  Augmentin® [US/Can]
  Bicillin® C-R 900/300 [US]
  Bicillin® C-R [US]
  Bicillin® L-A [US]
  carbenicillin
  Clavulin® [Can]
  Gen-Amoxicillin [Can]
  Geocillin® [US]
  Lin-Amox [Can]
  Marcillin® [US]
  Moxilin® [US]
  Nadopen-V® [Can]
  Novamoxin® [Can]
  Novo-Ampicillin [Can]
  Novo-Pen-VK® [Can]
  Nu-Amoxi [Can]
  Nu-Ampi [Can]

Nu-Pen-VK® [Can]
penicillin G benzathine
penicillin G benzathine and procaine
  combined
penicillin G procaine
penicillin V potassium
Permapen® [US]
piperacillin
piperacillin and tazobactam sodium
Pipracil® [US/Can]
Principen® [US]
PVF® K [Can]
Suspen® [US]
Tazocin® [Can]
ticarcillin
ticarcillin and clavulanate potassium
Ticar® [US]
Timentin® [US/Can]
Trimox® [US]
Truxcillin® [US]
Unasyn® [US/Can]
Veetids® [US]
Wycillin® [US/Can]
Wymox® [US]
Zosyn® [US]
Quinolone
  Apo®-Norflox [Can]
  Apo®-Oflox [Can]
  Cinobac® [US/Can]
  cinoxacin
  ciprofloxacin
  Cipro® [US/Can]
  Floxin® [US/Can]
  lomefloxacin
  Maxaquin® [US]
  nalidixic acid
  NegGram® [US/Can]
  norfloxacin
  Noroxin® [US/Can]
  Novo-Norfloxacin [Can]
  Ocuflox® [US/Can]
  ofloxacin
  Riva-Norfloxacin [Can]

sparfloxacin
Zagam® [US]
Sulfonamide
  Apo®-Sulfatrim [Can]
  Bactrim™ DS [US]
  Bactrim™ [US]
  erythromycin and sulfisoxazole
  Eryzole® [US]
  Gantrisin® Pediatric Suspension [US]
  Novo-Trimel [Can]
  Novo-Trimel D.S. [Can]
  Nu-Cotrimox® [Can]
  Pediazole® [US/Can]
  Septra® DS [US/Can]
  Septra® [US/Can]
  sulfadiazine
  sulfamethoxazole and trimethoprim
  Sulfatrim® DS [US]
  Sulfatrim® [US]
  sulfisoxazole
  sulfisoxazole and phenazopyridine
  Sulfizole® [Can]
  Truxazole® [US]
Tetracycline Derivative
  Adoxa™ [US]
  Alti-Minocycline [Can]
  Apo®-Doxy [Can]
  Apo®-Doxy Tabs [Can]
  Apo®-Minocycline [Can]
  Apo®-Tetra [Can]
  Brodspec® [US]
  Doryx® [US]
  Doxy-100™ [US]
  Doxycin [Can]
  doxycycline
  Doxytec [Can]
  Dynacin® [US]
  EmTet® [US]
  Gen-Minocycline [Can]
  Minocin® [US/Can]
  minocycline
  Monodox® [US]
  Novo-Doxylin [Can]
  Novo-Minocycline [Can]
  Novo-Tetra [Can]
  Nu-Doxycycline [Can]
  Nu-Tetra [Can]
  oxytetracycline
  Periostat® [US]
  Rhoxal-Minocycline [Can]
  Sumycin® [US]
  Terramycin® I.M. [US/Can]
  tetracycline
  Vibramycin® [US]
  Vibra-Tabs® [US/Can]
  Wesmycin® [US]

GRANULOMATOUS DISEASE, CHRONIC
Biological Response Modulator
  Actimmune® [US/Can]
  interferon gamma-1b

GROWTH HORMONE (DIAGNOSTIC)
Diagnostic Agent
  Geref® Diagnostic [US]
  Geref® [US]
  sermorelin acetate

GUILLAIN-BARRÉ SYNDROME
Immune Globulin
  Carimune™ [US]
  Gamimune® N [US/Can]
  Gammagard® S/D [US/Can]
  Gammar®-P I.V. [US]
  immune globulin (intravenous)
  Iveegam EN [US]
  Iveegam Immuno® [Can]
  Panglobulin® [US]
  Polygam® S/D [US]
  Venoglobulin®-S [US]

HAY FEVER
Adrenergic Agonist Agent
  Afrin® Extra Moisturizing [US-OTC]

Afrin® Original [US-OTC]
Afrin® Severe Congestion [US-OTC]
Afrin® Sinus [US-OTC]
Afrin® [US-OTC]
Dristan® Long Lasting Nasal [Can]
Drixoral® Nasal [Can]
Duramist® Plus [US-OTC]
Duration® [US-OTC]
Genasal [US-OTC]
Neo-Synephrine® 12 Hour Extra
   Moisturizing [US-OTC]
Neo-Synephrine® 12 Hour [US-OTC]
Nōstrilla® [US-OTC]
oxymetazoline
Twice-A-Day® [US-OTC]
Vicks Sinex® 12 Hour Ultrafine Mist
   [US-OTC]
Visine® L.R. [US-OTC]
4-Way® Long Acting [US-OTC]
Antihistamine
   Allegra® [US/Can]
   fexofenadine
Antihistamine/Decongestant
   Combination
acrivastine and pseudoephedrine
Actanol® [US-OTC]
Actedril® [US-OTC]
Actifed® [US/Can]
Allerest® Maximum Strength [US-
   OTC]
Allerfed® [US-OTC]
Allerfrim® [US-OTC]
Allerphed® [US-OTC]
Altafed® [US-OTC]
Aphedrid™ [US-OTC]
Aprodine® [US-OTC]
Biofed-PE® [US-OTC]
Cenafed® Plus Tablet [US-OTC]
chlorpheniramine and pseu-
   doephedrine
Chlor-Trimeton® Allergy/Deconges-
   tant [US-OTC]
Codimal-LA® Half [US-OTC]

Codimal-LA® [US-OTC]
Deconamine® SR [US-OTC]
Deconamine® [US-OTC]
Genac® Tablet [US-OTC]
Hayfebrol® [US-OTC]
Histafed® [US-OTC]
Histalet® [US-OTC]
Hista-Tabs® [US-OTC]
Pseudocot-T® [US-OTC]
Rhinosyn-PD® [US-OTC]
Rhinosyn® [US-OTC]
Ridifed® [US-OTC]
Ritifed® [US-OTC]
Ryna® [US-OTC]
Semprex®-D [US]
Silafed® [US-OTC]
Sudafed® Cold & Allergy [US-OTC]
Triacin® [US-OTC]
Tri-Fed® [US-OTC]
Triphed® [US-OTC]
Triposed® Tablet [US-OTC]
triprolidine and pseudoephedrine
Tri-Pseudafed® [US-OTC]
Tri-Sofed® [US-OTC]
Tri-Sudo® [US-OTC]
Uni-Fed® [US-OTC]
Vi-Sudo® [US-OTC]

HEADACHE (SINUS)

Analgesic, Nonnarcotic
   acetaminophen and diphenhydramine
   acetaminophen and phenyltoloxam-
      ine
   Anacin® PM Aspirin Free [US-OTC]
   Excedrin® P.M. [US-OTC]
   Genesec® [US-OTC]
   Goody's PM® Powder [US-OTC]
   Legatrin PM® [US-OTC]
   Percogesic® [US-OTC]
   Phenylgesic® [US-OTC]
   Tylenol® PM Extra Strength [US-
      OTC]
   Tylenol® Severe Allergy [US-OTC]

Antihistamine/Analgesic
chlorpheniramine and acetaminophen
Coricidin® [US-OTC]
Antihistamine/Decongestant/Analgesic
acetaminophen, chlorpheniramine,
and pseudoephedrine
Alka-Seltzer® Plus Cold Liqui-Gels®
[US-OTC]
Children's Tylenol® Cold
[US-OTC]
Comtrex® Allergy-Sinus [US-OTC]
Sinutab® Sinus & Allergy [Can]
Sinutab® Sinus Allergy Maximum
Strength [US-OTC]
Thera-Flu® Flu and Cold [US]
Tylenol® Allergy Sinus [US/Can]
Cold Preparation
acetaminophen, dextromethorphan,
and pseudoephedrine
Alka-Seltzer® Plus Flu Liqui-Gels®
[US-OTC]
Comtrex® Non-Drowsy Cough and
Cold [US-OTC]
Contac® Cough, Cold and Flu Day &
Night™ [Can]
Contac® Severe Cold and Flu/Non-
Drowsy [US-OTC]
Infants' Tylenol® Cold Plus Cough
Concentrated Drops [US-OTC]
Sudafed® Cold & Cough Extra
Strength [Can]
Sudafed® Severe Cold [US-OTC]
Thera-Flu® Non-Drowsy Flu, Cold
and Cough [US-OTC]
Triaminic® Sore Throat Formula
[US-OTC]
Tylenol® Cold [Can]
Tylenol® Cold Non-Drowsy [US-
OTC]
Tylenol® Flu Non-Drowsy Maximum
Strength [US-OTC]
Vicks® DayQuil® Cold and Flu Non-
Drowsy [US-OTC]

Decongestant/Analgesic
acetaminophen and pseudoephedrine
Advil® Cold & Sinus Caplets [US-
OTC]
Advil® Cold & Sinus Tablet [Can]
Alka-Seltzer Plus® Cold and Sinus
[US-OTC]
Children's Tylenol® Sinus [US-OTC]
Dristan® N.D. [Can]
Dristan® N.D., Extra Strength [Can]
Dristan® Sinus Caplets [US]
Dristan® Sinus Tablet [Can]
Infants Tylenol® Cold [US-OTC]
Medi-Synal [US-OTC]
Ornex® Maximum Strength [US-
OTC]
Ornex® [US-OTC]
pseudoephedrine and ibuprofen
Sinus-Relief® [US-OTC]
Sinutab® Non Drowsy [Can]
Sinutab® Sinus Maximum Strength
Without Drowsiness [US-OTC]
Sudafed® Cold and Sinus [US-OTC]
Sudafed® Head Cold and Sinus Extra
Strength [Can]
Sudafed® Sinus Headache [US-OTC]
Tylenol® Decongestant [Can]
Tylenol® Sinus [Can]
Tylenol® Sinus Non-Drowsy [US-
OTC]

HEADACHE (SPINAL PUNCTURE)

Diuretic, Miscellaneous
caffeine and sodium benzoate

HEADACHE (TENSION)

Analgesic, Narcotic
butalbital compound and codeine
Fiorinal®-C 1/2 [Can]
Fiorinal®-C 1/4 [Can]
Fiorinal® With Codeine [US]
Tecnal C 1/2 [Can]
Tecnal C 1/4 [Can]

Analgesic, Nonnarcotic
  acetaminophen, isometheptene, and
    dichloralphenazone
  Advil® Migraine [US-OTC]
  Advil® [US/Can]
  Apo®-Ibuprofen [Can]
  Genpril® [US-OTC]
  Haltran® [US-OTC]
  ibuprofen
  Ibu-Tab® [US]
  I-Prin [US-OTC]
  Menadol® [US-OTC]
  Midrin® [US]
  Migratine® [US]
  Motrin® IB [US/Can]
  Motrin® Migraine Pain [US-OTC]
  Motrin® [US/Can]
  Novo-Profen® [Can]
  Nu-Ibuprofen [Can]
Barbiturate/Analgesic
  Anolor 300® [US]
  Arcet® [US]
  Axocet® [US]
  Bucet™ [US]
  Bupap® [US]
  butalbital, acetaminophen, and
    caffeine
  butalbital, aspirin, and caffeine
  Butalbital Compound® [US]
  Butex Forte® [US]
  Cephadyn® [US]
  Dolgic® [US]
  Esgic-Plus™ [US]
  Esgic® [US]
  Ezol® [US]
  Farbital® [US]
  Fioricet® [US]
  Fiorinal® [US/Can]
  Fortabs® [US]
  Geone® [US]
  Laniroif® [US]
  Margesic® [US]
  Marten-Tab® [US]

  Medigesic® [US]
  Nonbac® [US]
  Pacaps® [US]
  Phrenilin Forte® [US]
  Phrenilin® [US]
  Promacet® [US]
  Repan CF® [US]
  Repan® [US]
  Sedapap® [US]
  Tecnal® [Can]
  Tenake® [US]
  Tencon® [US]
  Triad® [US]
  Trianal® [Can]
  Zebutal® [US]
Benzodiazepine
  Apo®-Diazepam [Can]
  Diastat® [US/Can]
  Diazemuls® [Can]
  diazepam
  Diazepam Intensol® [US]
  Valium® [US/Can]
Skeletal Muscle Relaxant
  aspirin and meprobamate
  Equagesic® [US]
  292 MEP® [Can]

HEADACHE (VASCULAR)

Analgesic, Nonnarcotic
  Advil® Migraine [US-OTC]
  Advil® [US/Can]
  Aleve® [US-OTC]
  Anaprox® DS [US/Can]
  Anaprox® [US/Can]
  Apo®-Diflunisal [Can]
  Apo®-Ibuprofen [Can]
  Apo®-Keto [Can]
  Apo®-Keto-E [Can]
  Apo®-Keto SR [Can]
  Apo®-Mefenamic [Can]
  Apo®-Napro-Na [Can]
  Apo®-Napro-Na DS [Can]
  Apo®-Naproxen [Can]

Apo®-Naproxen SR [Can]
diflunisal
Dolobid® [US]
EC-Naprosyn® [US]
Gen-Naproxen EC [Can]
Genpril® [US-OTC]
Haltran® [US-OTC]
ibuprofen
Ibu-Tab® [US]
I-Prin [US-OTC]
ketoprofen
meclofenamate
mefenamic acid
Menadol® [US-OTC]
Motrin® Migraine Pain [US-OTC]
Motrin® [US/Can]
Naprelan® [US]
Naprosyn® [US/Can]
naproxen
Naxen® [Can]
Novo-Diflunisal [Can]
Novo-Keto [Can]
Novo-Keto-EC [Can]
Novo-Naprox [Can]
Novo-Naprox Sodium [Can]
Novo-Naprox Sodium DS [Can]
Novo-Naprox SR [Can]
Novo-Profen® [Can]
Nu-Diflunisal [Can]
Nu-Ibuprofen [Can]
Nu-Ketoprofen [Can]
Nu-Ketoprofen-E [Can]
Nu-Mefenamic [Can]
Nu-Naprox [Can]
Orafen [Can]
Orudis® KT [US-OTC]
Orudis® SR [Can]
Oruvail® [US/Can]
PMS-Mefenamic Acid [Can]
Ponstan® [Can]
Ponstel® [US/Can]
Rhodis™ [Can]
Rhodis-EC™ [Can]

Rhodis SR™ [Can]
Riva-Naproxen [Can]
Synflex® [Can]
Synflex® DS [Can]
Beta-Adrenergic Blocker
Apo®-Propranolol [Can]
Inderal® LA [US/Can]
Inderal® [US/Can]
Nu-Propranolol [Can]
propranolol
Decongestant/Analgesic
Advil® Cold & Sinus Caplets [US-OTC]
Advil® Cold & Sinus Tablet [Can]
Dristan® Sinus Caplets [US]
Dristan® Sinus Tablet [Can]
pseudoephedrine and ibuprofen
Ergot Alkaloid and Derivative
Cafergot® [US/Can]
D.H.E. 45® [US]
dihydroergotamine
ergotamine
methysergide
Migranal® [US/Can]
Sansert® [US/Can]
Wigraine® [US]

HEART BLOCK
Adrenergic Agonist Agent
Adrenalin® Chloride [US/Can]
epinephrine
isoproterenol
Isuprel® [US]

HEARTBURN
Antacid
Alka-Mints® [US-OTC]
Amitone® [US-OTC]
Apo®-Cal [Can]
Cal Carb-HD® [US-OTC]
Calci-Chew™ [US-OTC]
Calci-Mix™ [US-OTC]
calcium carbonate
calcium carbonate and simethicone

Caltrate® 600 [US/Can]
Chooz® [US-OTC]
famotidine, calcium carbonate, and
    magnesium hydroxide
Florical® [US-OTC]
Mallamint® [US-OTC]
Nephro-Calci® [US-OTC]
Os-Cal® 500 [US/Can]
Oyst-Cal 500 [US-OTC]
Oystercal® 500 [US]
Pepcid® Complete [US-OTC]
Rolaids® Calcium Rich [US-OTC]
Titralac® Plus Liquid [US-OTC]
Tums® E-X Extra Strength Tablet
    [US-OTC]
Tums® Ultra [US-OTC]
Tums® [US-OTC]
Histamine H2 Antagonist
Acid Reducer 200® [US-OTC]
Apo®-Cimetidine [Can]
cimetidine
famotidine, calcium carbonate, and
    magnesium hydroxide
Gen-Cimetidine [Can]
Heartburn 200® [US-OTC]
Heartburn Relief 200® [US-OTC]
Novo-Cimetidine [Can]
Nu-Cimet® [Can]
Pepcid® Complete [US-OTC]
PMS-Cimetidine [Can]
Tagamet® HB [US/Can]
Tagamet® [US/Can]
Proton Pump Inhibitor
Panto™ IV [Can]
Pantoloc™ [Can]
pantoprazole
Protonix® [US/Can]

HEAVY METAL POISONING
Antidote
deferoxamine
Desferal® [US/Can]

HELICOBACTER PYLORI
Antibiotic, Miscellaneous
Apo®-Metronidazole [Can]
Flagyl ER® [US]
Flagyl® [US/Can]
metronidazole
Nidagel™ [Can]
Noritate™ [US/Can]
Novo-Nidazol [Can]
Antidiarrheal
bismuth subsalicylate, metronidazole,
    and tetracycline
Helidac™ [US]
Gastrointestinal Agent, Gastric or
    Duodenal Ulcer Treatment
ranitidine bismuth citrate
Tritec® [US]
Gastrointestinal Agent, Miscellaneous
Bismatrol® [US-OTC]
bismuth subsalicylate
Diotame® [US-OTC]
Pepto-Bismol® [US-OTC]
Macrolide (Antibiotic)
Biaxin® [US/Can]
Biaxin® XL [US]
clarithromycin
Penicillin
amoxicillin
Amoxicot® [US]
Amoxil® [US/Can]
Apo®-Amoxi [Can]
Gen-Amoxicillin [Can]
Lin-Amox [Can]
Moxilin® [US]
Novamoxin® [Can]
Nu-Amoxi [Can]
Trimox® [US]
Wymox® [US]
Tetracycline Derivative
Apo®-Tetra [Can]
Brodspec® [US]
EmTet® [US]
Novo-Tetra [Can]

Nu-Tetra [Can]
Sumycin® [US]
tetracycline
Wesmycin® [US]

HEMATOLOGIC DISORDER
Adrenal Corticosteroid
Acthar® [US]
A-HydroCort® [US/Can]
Alti-Dexamethasone [Can]
A-methaPred® [US]
Apo®-Prednisone [Can]
Aristocort® Forte Injection [US]
Aristocort® Intralesional Injection [US]
Aristocort® Tablet [US/Can]
Aristospan® Intra-articular Injection [US/Can]
Aristospan® Intralesional Injection [US/Can]
Betaject™ [Can]
betamethasone (systemic)
Betnesol® [Can]
Celestone® Phosphate [US]
Celestone® Soluspan® [US/Can]
Celestone® [US]
Cel-U-Jec® [US]
Cortef® [US/Can]
corticotropin
cortisone acetate
Cortone® [Can]
Decadron®-LA [US]
Decadron® [US/Can]
Decaject-LA® [US]
Decaject® [US]
Delta-Cortef® [US]
Deltasone® [US]
Depo-Medrol® [US/Can]
Depopred® [US]
dexamethasone (systemic)
Dexasone® L.A. [US]
Dexasone® [US/Can]
Dexone® LA [US]

Dexone® [US]
Hexadrol® [US/Can]
H.P. Acthar® Gel [US]
hydrocortisone (systemic)
Hydrocortone® Acetate [US]
Kenalog® Injection [US/Can]
Key-Pred-SP® [US]
Key-Pred® [US]
Medrol® Tablet [US/Can]
methylprednisolone
Meticorten® [US]
Orapred™ [US]
Pediapred® [US/Can]
PMS-Dexamethasone [Can]
Prednicot® [US]
prednisolone (systemic)
Prednisol® TBA [US]
prednisone
Prelone® [US]
Solu-Cortef® [US/Can]
Solu-Medrol® [US/Can]
Solurex L.A.® [US]
Sterapred® DS [US]
Sterapred® [US]
Tac™-3 Injection [US]
Triam-A® Injection [US]
triamcinolone (systemic)
Triam Forte® Injection [US]
Winpred™ [Can]

HEMOLYTIC DISEASE OF THE NEWBORN
Immune Globulin
BayRho-D® Full-Dose [US]
BayRho-D® Mini-Dose [US]
Rho(D) immune globulin
RhoGAM® [US]
WinRho SDF® [US]

HEMOPHILIA
Antihemophilic Agent
antihemophilic factor (porcine)
Hyate®:C [US]

Coagulation Factor
  eptacog alfa (activated) (Canada
    only)
  NiaStase® [Can]
Vasopressin Analog, Synthetic
  DDAVP® [US/Can]
  desmopressin acetate
  Octostim® [Can]
  Stimate™ [US]

HEMOPHILIA A

Antihemophilic Agent
  factor VIIa (recombinant)
  Novo-Seven® [US]
Blood Product Derivative
  Alphanate® [US]
  antihemophilic factor (human)
  antihemophilic factor (recombinant)
  factor VIIa (recombinant)
  Helixate® FS [US]
  Hemofil® M [US/Can]
  Humate-P® [US/Can]
  Kōate®-DVI [US]
  Kogenate® FS [US/Can]
  Monarc® M [US]
  Monoclate-P® [US]
  Novo-Seven® [US]
  Recombinate™ [US/Can]

HEMOPHILIA B

Antihemophilic Agent
  factor IX (purified/human)
  factor VIIa (recombinant)
  Immunine® VH [Can]
  Mononine® [US]
  Novo-Seven® [US]
Blood Product Derivative
  factor VIIa (recombinant)
  Novo-Seven® [US]

HEMORRHAGE

Adrenergic Agonist Agent
  Adrenalin® Chloride [US/Can]
  epinephrine

Antihemophilic Agent
  AlphaNine® SD [US]
  BeneFix™ [US]
  factor IX complex (human)
  Hemonyne® [US]
  Kōnyne® 80 [US]
  Profilnine® SD [US]
  Proplex® T [US]
Ergot Alkaloid and Derivative
  ergonovine
  Ergotrate® Maleate Injection [US]
Hemostatic Agent
  Amicar® [US/Can]
  aminocaproic acid
  aprotinin
  Avitene® [US]
  cellulose, oxidized
  gelatin (absorbable)
  Gelfilm® [US]
  Gelfoam® [US]
  Helistat® [US]
  Hemotene® [US]
  microfibrillar collagen hemostat
  Oxycel® [US]
  Surgicel® [US]
  thrombin (topical)
  Thrombogen® [US]
  Thrombostat® [Can]
  Trasylol® [US/Can]
Progestin
  Alti-MPA [Can]
  Aygestin® [US]
  Crinone® [US/Can]
  Depo-Provera® [US/Can]
  Gen-Medroxy [Can]
  hydroxyprogesterone caproate
  Hylutin® [US]
  medroxyprogesterone acetate
  Micronor® [US/Can]
  norethindrone
  Norlutate® [Can]
  Nor-QD® [US]
  Novo-Medrone [Can]

Prodrox® [US]
Progestasert® [US]
progesterone
Prometrium® [US/Can]
Provera® [US/Can]
Sclerosing Agent
sodium tetradecyl
Sotradecol® [US]
Trombovar® [Can]
Vitamin, Fat Soluble
AquaMEPHYTON® [US/Can]
Mephyton® [US/Can]
phytonadione

HEMORRHOID
Adrenal Corticosteroid
Anusol-HC® Suppository [US]
Colocort™ [US]
Cortifoam® [US/Can]
Emo-Cort® [Can]
Hycort® [US]
hydrocortisone (rectal)
Proctocort™ Rectal [US]
ProctoCream ® HC Cream [US]
Anesthetic/Corticosteroid
Analpram-HC® [US]
Corticaine® [US]
dibucaine and hydrocortisone
Enzone® [US]
Epifoam® [US]
Pramosone® [US]
Pramox® HC [Can]
pramoxine and hydrocortisone
ProctoFoam®-HC [US/Can]
Zone-A Forte® [US]
Astringent
Preparation H® Cleansing Pads [Can]
Tucks® [US-OTC]
witch hazel
Local Anesthetic
Americaine® Anesthetic Lubricant [US]
benzocaine

Benzodent® [US-OTC]
dibucaine
Fleet® Pain Relief [US-OTC]
Foille® Medicated First Aid [US-OTC]
Foille® Plus [US-OTC]
Foille® [US-OTC]
Orabase®-B [US-OTC]
PrameGel® [US-OTC]
pramoxine
Prax® [US-OTC]
ProctoFoam® NS [US-OTC]
tetracaine
Tronolane® [US-OTC]
Tronothane® [US-OTC]

HEMOSIDEROSIS
Antidote
deferoxamine
Desferal® [US/Can]

HEMOSTASIS
Hemostatic Agent
fibrin sealant kit
Tisseel® VH Fibrin Sealant Kit [US/Can]

HEPARIN POISONING
Antidote
protamine sulfate

HEPATIC CIRRHOSIS
Diuretic, Potassium Sparing
amiloride
Midamor® [US/Can]

HEPATIC COMA (ENCEPHALOPATHY)
Amebicide
Humatin® [US/Can]
paromomycin
Aminoglycoside (Antibiotic)
Myciguent [US-OTC]
Neo-Rx [US]

Ammonium Detoxicant
  Acilac [Can]
  Cholac® [US]
  Constilac® [US]
  Constulose® [US]
  Enulose® [US]
  Generlac® [US]
  Kristalose™ [US]
  lactulose
  Laxilose [Can]
  PMS-Lactulose [Can]

HEPATITIS A

Immune Globulin
  BayGam® [US/Can]
  immune globulin (intramuscular)
Vaccine
  hepatitis A inactivated and hepatitis
    B (recombinant) vaccine
  Twinrix® [US/Can]
Vaccine, Inactivated Virus
  Avaxim® [Can]
  Epaxal Berna® [Can]
  Havrix® [US/Can]
  hepatitis A vaccine
  VAQTA® [US/Can]

HEPATITIS B

Antiretroviral Agent, Non-nucleoside
    Reverse Transcriptase Inhibitor
    (NNRTI)
  adefovir
  Hepsera™ [US]
Antiviral Agent
  Epivir®-HBV™ [US]
  Epivir® [US]
  Heptovir® [Can]
  interferon alfa-2b and ribavirin com-
    bination pack
  lamivudine
  Rebetron™ [US/Can]
  3TC® [Can]
Biological Response Modulator
  interferon alfa-2b

interferon alfa-2b and ribavirin com-
    bination pack
  Intron® A [US/Can]
  Rebetron™ [US/Can]
Immune Globulin
  BayHep B™ [US/Can]
  hepatitis B immune globulin
  Nabi-HB® [US]
Vaccine
  hepatitis A inactivated and hepatitis
    B (recombinant) vaccine
  Twinrix® [US/Can]
Vaccine, Inactivated Virus
  Comvax® [US]
  Engerix-B® [US/Can]
  Haemophilus B conjugate and hepati-
    tis B vaccine
  hepatitis B vaccine
  Recombivax HB® [US/Can]

HEPATITIS C

Antiviral Agent
  interferon alfa-2b and ribavirin com-
    bination pack
  Rebetron™ [US/Can]
Biological Response Modulator
  interferon alfa-2b
  interferon alfa-2b and ribavirin com-
    bination pack
  Intron® A [US/Can]
  Rebetron™ [US/Can]
Interferon
  Infergen® [US/Can]
  interferon alfacon-1
  peginterferon alfa-2b
  PEG-Intron™ [US]

HERPES SIMPLEX

Antiviral Agent
  acyclovir
  Apo®-Acyclovir [Can]
  Avirax™ [Can]
  Cytovene® [US/Can]

famciclovir
Famvir™ [US/Can]
foscarnet
Foscavir® [US/Can]
ganciclovir
Gen-Acyclovir [Can]
Nu-Acyclovir [Can]
trifluridine
vidarabine
Vira-A® [US]
Viroptic® [US/Can]
Vitrasert® [US/Can]
Zovirax® [US/Can]
Antiviral Agent, Topical
Abreva™ [US-OTC]
docosanol

HERPES ZOSTER
Analgesic, Topical
Antiphogistine Rub A-535 Capsaicin [Can]
Arth Dr® [US]
Arthricare Hand & Body® [US]
Born Again Super Pain Relieving® [US]
Caprex Plus® [US]
Caprex® [US]
Capsagel Extra Strength® [US]
Capsagel Maximum Strength® [US]
Capsagel® [US]
Capsagesic-HP Arthritis Relief® [US]
capsaicin
Capsin® [US-OTC]
D-Care Circulation Stimulator® [US]
Double Cap® [US]
Icy Hot Arthritis Therapy® [US]
Pain Enz® [US]
Pharmacist's Capsaicin® [US]
Rid-A-Pain-HP® [US]
Rid-A-Pain® [US]
Sloan's Liniment® [US]
Sportsmed® [US]
Theragen HP® [US]

Theragen® [US]
Therapatch Warm® [US]
Trixaicin HP® [US]
Trixaicin® [US]
Zostrix High Potency® [US]
Zostrix®-HP [US/Can]
Zostrix Sports® [US]
Zostrix® [US/Can]
Antiviral Agent
acyclovir
Apo®-Acyclovir [Can]
Avirax™ [Can]
famciclovir
Famvir™ [US/Can]
Gen-Acyclovir [Can]
Nu-Acyclovir [Can]
valacyclovir
Valtrex® [US/Can]
vidarabine
Vira-A® [US]
Zovirax® [US/Can]

HIATAL HERNIA
Antacid
calcium carbonate and simethicone
Iosopan® Plus [US]
Lowsium® Plus [US]
magaldrate
magaldrate and simethicone
Riopan Plus® Double Strength [US-OTC]
Riopan Plus® [US-OTC]
Riopan® [US-OTC]
Titralac® Plus Liquid [US-OTC]

HICCUPS
Phenothiazine Derivative
Chlorpromanyl® [Can]
chlorpromazine
Largactil® [Can]
Thorazine® [US]
triflupromazine
Vesprin® [US/Can]

HAEMOPHILUS INFLUENZAE

Toxoid
  diphtheria, tetanus toxoids, and acel-
  lular pertussis vaccine and
  Haemophilus B conjugate vaccine
  TriHIBit® [US]
Vaccine, Inactivated Bacteria
  ActHIB® [US/Can]
  diphtheria, tetanus toxoids, and acel-
  lular pertussis vaccine and
  Haemophilus B conjugate vaccine
  Haemophilus B conjugate vaccine
  HibTITER® [US]
  PedvaxHIB® [US/Can]
  TriHIBit® [US]
Vaccine, Inactivated Virus
  Comvax® [US]
  Haemophilus B conjugate and hepati-
  tis B vaccine

HISTOPLASMOSIS

Antifungal Agent
  Amphocin® [US]
  amphotericin B (conventional)
  Apo®-Ketoconazole [Can]
  Fungizone® [US/Can]
  itraconazole
  ketoconazole
  Nizoral® A-D [US-OTC]
  Nizoral® [US/Can]
  Novo-Ketoconazole [Can]
  Sporanox® [US/Can]

HODGKIN DISEASE

Antineoplastic Agent
  Adriamycin® [Can]
  Adriamycin PFS® [US]
  Adriamycin RDF® [US]
  BiCNU® [US/Can]
  Blenoxane® [US/Can]
  bleomycin
  Caelyx® [Can]
  carmustine
  CeeNU® [US/Can]
  chlorambucil
  cisplatin
  cyclophosphamide
  Cytoxan® [US/Can]
  dacarbazine
  doxorubicin
  DTIC® [Can]
  DTIC-Dome® [US]
  Gliadel® [US]
  Idamycin® [Can]
  Idamycin PFS® [US]
  idarubicin
  Leukeran® [US/Can]
  lomustine
  Matulane® [US/Can]
  mechlorethamine
  Mustargen® [US/Can]
  Natulan® [Can]
  Neosar® [US]
  Oncovin® [US/Can]
  Platinol®-AQ [US]
  Platinol® [US]
  procarbazine
  Procytox® [Can]
  Rubex® [US]
  streptozocin
  Thioplex® [US]
  thiotepa
  Velban® [US/Can]
  vinblastine
  Vincasar® PFS® [US/Can]
  vincristine
  Zanosar® [US/Can]

HOMOCYSTINURIA

Urinary Tract Product
  betaine anhydrous
  Cystadane® [US/Can]

HOOKWORMS

Anthelmintic
  albendazole

Albenza® [US]
Ascarel® [US-OTC]
Combantrin™ [Can]
mebendazole
Pamix® [US-OTC]
Pin-X® [US-OTC]
pyrantel pamoate
Reese's® Pinworm Medicine [US-OTC]
Vermox® [US/Can]

HORMONAL IMBALANCE (FEMALE)
Progestin
Alti-MPA [Can]
Aygestin® [US]
Crinone® [US/Can]
Depo-Provera® [US/Can]
Gen-Medroxy [Can]
hydroxyprogesterone caproate
Hylutin® [US]
medroxyprogesterone acetate
Micronor® [US/Can]
norethindrone
Norlutate® [Can]
Nor-QD® [US]
Novo-Medrone [Can]
Prodrox® [US]
Progestasert® [US]
progesterone
Prometrium® [US/Can]
Provera® [US/Can]

HUNTINGTON CHOREA
Monoamine Depleting Agent
Nitoman® [Can]
tetrabenazine (Canada only)

HYDATIDIFORM MOLE (BENIGN)
Prostaglandin
Cervidil® Vaginal Insert [US/Can]
dinoprostone
Prepidil® Vaginal Gel [US/Can]
Prostin E2® Vaginal Suppository [US/Can]

HYPERAMMONEMIA
Ammonium Detoxicant
Acilac [Can]
Cholac® [US]
Constilac® [US]
Constulose® [US]
Enulose® [US]
Generlac® [US]
Kristalose™ [US]
lactulose
Laxilose [Can]
PMS-Lactulose [Can]
sodium phenylacetate and sodium benzoate
Ucephan® [US]

HYPERCALCEMIA
Antidote
gallium nitrate
Ganite™ [US]
Mithracin® [US/Can]
plicamycin
Bisphosphonate Derivative
Actonel™ [US/Can]
alendronate
Aredia® [US/Can]
Bonefos® [US/Can]
clodronate disodium (Canada only)
Didronel® [US/Can]
etidronate disodium
Fosamax® [US/Can]
Ostac® [US/Can]
pamidronate
risedronate
zoledronic acid
Zometa® [US/Can]
Chelating Agent
Chealamide® [US]
Disotate® [US]
edetate disodium
Endrate® [US]

Polypeptide Hormone
  Calcimar® [Can]
  calcitonin
  Caltine® [Can]
  Miacalcin® [US/Can]
Urinary Tract Product
  Calcibind® [US/Can]
  cellulose sodium phosphate

HYPERCHOLES-TEROLEMIA

Antihyperlipidemic Agent,
    Miscellaneous
  colesevelam
  Colestid® [US/Can]
  colestipol
  WelChol™ [US/Can]
Bile Acid Sequestrant
  cholestyramine resin
  colesevelam
  LoCHOLEST® Light [US]
  LoCHOLEST® [US]
  Novo-Cholamine [Can]
  Novo-Cholamine Light [Can]
  PMS-Cholestyramine [Can]
  Prevalite® [US]
  Questran® Light [US/Can]
  Questran® Powder [US/Can]
  WelChol™ [US/Can]
HMG-CoA Reductase Inhibitor
  Advicor™ [US]
  Altocor™ [US]
  Apo®-Lovastatin [Can]
  atorvastatin
  fluvastatin
  Lescol® [US/Can]
  Lescol® XL [US]
  Lin-Pravastatin [Can]
  Lipitor® [US/Can]
  lovastatin
  Mevacor® [US/Can]
  niacin and lovastatin
  Pravachol® [US/Can]

  pravastatin
  simvastatin
  Zocor® [US/Can]
Vitamin, Water Soluble
  Advicor™ [US]
  niacin and lovastatin

HYPERHIDROSIS
Topical Skin Product
  aluminum chloride hexahydrate
  Drysol™ [US]

HYPERKALEMIA
Antidote
  Kayexalate® [US/Can]
  Kionex™ [US]
  PMS-Sodium Polystyrene Sulfonate
    [Can]
  sodium polystyrene sulfonate
  SPS® [US]
Electrolyte Supplement, Oral
  Alka-Mints® [US-OTC]
  Amitone® [US-OTC]
  Apo®-Cal [Can]
  Calbon® [US]
  Cal Carb-HD® [US-OTC]
  Calci-Chew™ [US-OTC]
  Calci-Mix™ [US-OTC]
  Calcionate® [US-OTC]
  Calciquid® [US-OTC]
  Cal-Citrate® 250 [US-OTC]
  calcium carbonate
  calcium citrate
  calcium glubionate
  calcium gluceptate
  calcium lactate
  calcium phosphate (dibasic)
  Cal-Lac® [US]
  Caltrate® 600 [US/Can]
  Chooz® [US-OTC]
  Citracal® [US-OTC]
  Florical® [US-OTC]
  Mallamint® [US-OTC]
  Nephro-Calci® [US-OTC]

Neut® [US]
Os-Cal® 500 [US/Can]
Oyst-Cal 500 [US-OTC]
Oystercal® 500 [US]
Posture® [US-OTC]
Ridactate® [US]
Rolaids® Calcium Rich [US-OTC]
sodium bicarbonate
Tums® E-X Extra Strength Tablet
[US-OTC]
Tums® Ultra [US-OTC]
Tums® [US-OTC]

HYPERKERATOSIS (FOLLICULARIS)
Keratolytic Agent
Compound W® [US-OTC]
Dr Scholl's® Disk [US-OTC]
Dr Scholl's® Wart Remover [US-OTC]
DuoFilm® [US-OTC]
Duoforte® 27 [Can]
DuoPlant® [US-OTC]
Freezone® [US-OTC]
Gordofilm® [US-OTC]
Mediplast® Plaster [US-OTC]
Mosco® [US-OTC]
Occlusal™ [Can]
Occlusal®-HP [US/Can]
Off-Ezy® Wart Remover [US-OTC]
Psor-a-set® Soap [US-OTC]
Sal-Acid® Plaster [US-OTC]
Salactic® Film [US-OTC]
salicylic acid
Sal-Plant® [US-OTC]
Sebcur® [Can]
Soluver® [Can]
Soluver® Plus [Can]
Trans-Ver-Sal® AdultPatch [US-OTC]
Trans-Ver-Sal® [Can]
Trans-Ver-Sal® PediaPatch [US-OTC]
Trans-Ver-Sal® PlantarPatch [US-OTC]
Wart-Off® [US-OTC]

HYPERLIPIDEMIA
Antihyperlipidemic Agent, Miscellaneous
Apo®-Fenofibrate [Can]
Apo®-Feno-Micro [Can]
Apo®-Gemfibrozil [Can]
bezafibrate (Canada only)
Bezalip® [Can]
Colestid® [US/Can]
colestipol
fenofibrate
gemfibrozil
Gen-Fenofibrat Micro [Can]
Gen-Gemfibrozil [Can]
Lipidil Micro® [Can]
Lipidil Supra® [Can]
Lopid® [US/Can]
Novo-Gemfibrozil [Can]
Nu-Fenofibrate [Can]
Nu-Gemfibrozil [Can]
PMS-Bezafibrate [Can]
PMS-Fenofibrate Micro [Can]
PMS-Gemfibrozil [Can]
TriCor® [US/Can]
Bile Acid Sequestrant
cholestyramine resin
LoCHOLEST® Light [US]
LoCHOLEST® [US]
Novo-Cholamine [Can]
Novo-Cholamine Light [Can]
PMS-Cholestyramine [Can]
Prevalite® [US]
Questran® Light [US/Can]
Questran® Powder [US/Can]
HMG-CoA Reductase Inhibitor
Advicor™ [US]
niacin and lovastatin
Vitamin, Water Soluble
Advicor™ [US]

niacin
niacin and lovastatin
Niacor® [US]
Niaspan® [US/Can]
Nicotinex [US-OTC]
Slo-Niacin® [US-OTC]

HYPERMAGNESEMIA

Diuretic, Loop
  Apo®-Furosemide [Can]
  bumetanide
  Bumex® [US/Can]
  Burinex® [Can]
  Demadex® [US]
  Edecrin® [US/Can]
  ethacrynic acid
  Furocot® [US]
  furosemide
  Lasix® Special [Can]
  Lasix® [US/Can]
  torsemide
Electrolyte Supplement, Oral
  calcium chloride
  calcium gluceptate
  calcium gluconate
  Calfort® [US]
  Cal-G® [US]

HYPERMENORRHEA (TREATMENT)

Contraceptive, Oral
  Alesse® [US/Can]
  Apri® [US]
  Aviane™ [US]
  Brevicon® [US]
  Cryselle™ [US]
  Cyclessa® [US]
  Demulen® 30 [Can]
  Demulen® [US]
  Desogen® [US]
  Enpresse™ [US]
  Estrostep® Fe [US]
  ethinyl estradiol and desogestrel
  ethinyl estradiol and ethynodiol
    diacetate
  ethinyl estradiol and levonorgestrel
  ethinyl estradiol and norethindrone
  ethinyl estradiol and norgestimate
  ethinyl estradiol and norgestrel
  femhrt® [US/Can]
  Jenest™-28 [US]
  Kariva™ [US]
  Lessina™ [US]
  Levlen® [US]
  Levlite™ [US]
  Levora® [US]
  Loestrin® Fe [US]
  Loestrin® [US/Can]
  Lo/Ovral® [US]
  Low-Ogestrel® [US]
  Marvelon® [Can]
  mestranol and norethindrone
  Microgestin™ Fe [US]
  Minestrin™ 1/20 [Can]
  Min-Ovral® [Can]
  Mircette® [US]
  Modicon® [US]
  Necon® 0.5/35 [US]
  Necon® 1/35 [US]
  Necon® 1/50 [US]
  Necon® 10/11 [US]
  Nordette® [US]
  Norinyl® 1+35 [US]
  Norinyl® 1+50 [US]
  Nortrel™ [US]
  Ogestrel®
  Ortho-Cept® [US/Can]
  Ortho-Cyclen® [US/Can]
  Ortho-Novum® 1/50 [US/Can]
  Ortho-Novum® [US]
  Ortho-Tri-Cyclen® Lo [US]
  Ortho Tri-Cyclen® [US/Can]
  Ovcon® [US]
  Ovral® [US/Can]
  Portia™ [US]
  PREVEN™ [US]

Select™ 1/35 [Can]
Synphasic® [Can]
Tri-Levlen® [US]
Tri-Norinyl® [US]
Triphasil® [US/Can]
Triquilar® [Can]
Trivora® [US]
Zovia™ [US]
Contraceptive, Progestin Only
norgestrel
Ovrette® [US/Can]

HYPERPARATHYROIDISM
Vitamin D Analog
doxercalciferol
Hectorol® [US/Can]
paricalcitol
Zemplar™ [US/Can]

HYPERPHOSPHATEMIA
Antacid
ALternaGel® [US-OTC]
Alu-Cap® [US-OTC]
aluminum hydroxide
Amphojel® [Can]
Basaljel® [Can]
Electrolyte Supplement, Oral
Alka-Mints® [US-OTC]
Amitone® [US-OTC]
Apo®-Cal [Can]
Cal Carb-HD® [US-OTC]
Calci-Chew™ [US-OTC]
Calci-Mix™ [US-OTC]
calcium acetate
calcium carbonate
Caltrate® 600 [US/Can]
Chooz® [US-OTC]
Florical® [US-OTC]
Mallamint® [US-OTC]
Nephro-Calci® [US-OTC]
Os-Cal® 500 [US/Can]
Oyst-Cal 500 [US-OTC]
Oystercal® 500 [US]
PhosLo® [US]

Rolaids® Calcium Rich
[US-OTC]
Tums® E-X Extra Strength Tablet
[US-OTC]
Tums® Ultra [US-OTC]
Tums® [US-OTC]
Phosphate Binder
Renagel® [US/Can]
sevelamer

HYPERPLASIA, VULVAR SQUAMOUS
Estrogen Derivative
Alora® [US]
Cenestin™ [US/Can]
Climara® [US/Can]
Congest [Can]
Delestrogen® [US/Can]
Depo®-Estradiol [US/Can]
Esclim® [US]
Estrace® [US/Can]
Estraderm® [US/Can]
estradiol
Estratab® [US]
Estring® [US/Can]
Estrogel® [Can]
estrogens (conjugated A/synthetic)
estrogens (conjugated/equine)
estrogens (esterified)
estrone
estropipate
Gynodiol™ [US]
Kestrone® [US/Can]
Menest® [US]
Oesclim® [Can]
Oestrilin [Can]
Ogen® [US/Can]
Ortho-Est® [US]
PMS-Conjugated Estrogens [Can]
Premarin® [US/Can]
Vagifem® [US/Can]
Vivelle-Dot® [US]
Vivelle® [US/Can]

HYPERPROLACTINEMIA
Ergot Alkaloid and Derivative
  Apo® Bromocriptine [Can]
  bromocriptine
  Parlodel® [US/Can]
  PMS-Bromocriptine [Can]
Ergot-like Derivative
  cabergoline
  Dostinex® [US]

HYPERTENSION (ARTERIAL)
Beta-Adrenergic Blocker
  Levatol® [US/Can]
  penbutolol

HYPERTENSION (CEREBRAL)
Barbiturate
  Pentothal® Sodium [US/Can]
  thiopental
Diuretic, Osmotic
  mannitol
  urea

HYPERTENSION (CORONARY)
Vasodilator
  nitroglycerin
  Nitrol® [US/Can]

HYPERTENSION (OCULAR)
Alpha2-Adrenergic Agonist Agent,
    Ophthalmic
  Alphagan® P [US/Can]
  brimonidine
Beta-Adrenergic Blocker
  Betagan® [US/Can]
  levobunolol
  Novo-Levobunolol [Can]
  Optho-Bunolol® [Can]
  PMS-Levobunolol [Can]

HYPERTHERMIA (MALIGNANT)
Skeletal Muscle Relaxant
  Dantrium® [US/Can]
  dantrolene

HYPERTHYROIDISM
Antithyroid Agent
  methimazole
  Pima® [US]
  potassium iodide
  propylthiouracil
  Propyl-Thyracil® [Can]
  Tapazole® [US/Can]
  Thyro-Block® [Can]
Beta-Adrenergic Blocker
  Apo®-Propranolol [Can]
  Inderal® LA [US/Can]
  Inderal® [US/Can]
  Nu-Propranolol [Can]
  propranolol

HYPERTRIGLY-CERIDEMIA
Antihyperlipidemic Agent,
    Miscellaneous
  Apo®-Gemfibrozil [Can]
  gemfibrozil
  Gen-Gemfibrozil [Can]
  Lopid® [US/Can]
  Novo-Gemfibrozil [Can]
  Nu-Gemfibrozil [Can]
  PMS-Gemfibrozil [Can]
HMG-CoA Reductase
    Inhibitor
  simvastatin
  Zocor® [US/Can]
Vitamin, Water Soluble
  niacin
  Niacor® [US]
  Niaspan® [US/Can]
  Nicotinex [US-OTC]
  Slo-Niacin® [US-OTC]

HYPERTROPHIC CARDIOMYOPATHY
Calcium Channel Blocker
  Adalat® CC [US]
  Adalat® XL® [Can]
  Apo®-Nifed [Can]
  Apo®-Nifed PA [Can]
  Nifedical™ XL [US]
  nifedipine
  Novo-Nifedin [Can]
  Nu-Nifed [Can]
  Procardia® [US/Can]
  Procardia XL® [US]

HYPERURICEMIA
Enzyme
  Elitek™ [US]
  rasburicase
Uricosuric Agent
  Anturane® [US]
  Apo®-Sulfinpyrazone [Can]
  Benuryl™ [Can]
  Nu-Sulfinpyrazone [Can]
  probenecid
  sulfinpyrazone
Xanthine Oxidase Inhibitor
  allopurinol
  Aloprim™ [US]
  Apo®-Allopurinol [Can]
  Zyloprim® [US/Can]

HYPOALDOSTERONISM
Diuretic, Potassium Sparing
  amiloride
  Midamor® [US/Can]

HYPOCALCEMIA
Electrolyte Supplement, Oral
  Alka-Mints® [US-OTC]
  Amitone® [US-OTC]
  Apo®-Cal [Can]
  Calbon® [US]
  Cal Carb-HD® [US-OTC]
  Calci-Chew™ [US-OTC]
  Calci-Mix™ [US-OTC]
  Calcionate® [US-OTC]
  Calciquid® [US-OTC]
  Cal-Citrate® 250 [US-OTC]
  calcium carbonate
  calcium chloride
  calcium citrate
  calcium glubionate
  calcium gluceptate
  calcium gluconate
  calcium lactate
  calcium phosphate (dibasic)
  Calfort® [US]
  Cal-G® [US]
  Cal-Lac® [US]
  Caltrate® 600 [US/Can]
  Chooz® [US-OTC]
  Citracal® [US-OTC]
  Florical® [US-OTC]
  Mallamint® [US-OTC]
  Nephro-Calci® [US-OTC]
  Os-Cal® 500 [US/Can]
  Oyst-Cal 500 [US-OTC]
  Oystercal® 500 [US]
  Posture® [US-OTC]
  Ridactate® [US]
  Rolaids® Calcium Rich
    [US-OTC]
  Tums® E-X Extra Strength Tablet
    [US-OTC]
  Tums® Ultra [US-OTC]
  Tums® [US-OTC]
Vitamin D Analog
  calcifediol
  Calciferol™ [US]
  Calcijex™ [US]
  calcitriol
  Calderol® [US/Can]
  DHT™ [US]
  dihydrotachysterol
  Drisdol® [US/Can]
  ergocalciferol
  Hytakerol® [US/Can]

Ostoforte® [Can]
Rocaltrol® [US/Can]

HYPOCHLOREMIA
Electrolyte Supplement, Oral
  ammonium chloride

HYPOCHLORHYDRIA
Gastrointestinal Agent, Miscellaneous
  Feracid® [US]
  glutamic acid

HYPOGLYCEMIA
Antihypoglycemic Agent
  B-D™ Glucose [US-OTC]
  Dex4 Glucose [US-OTC]
  diazoxide
  GlucaGen® Diagnostic Kit [US]
  GlucaGen® [US]
  glucagon
  Glucagon Diagnostic Kit [US]
  Glucagon Emergency Kit [US]
  glucose (instant)
  Glutol™ [US-OTC]
  Glutose™ [US-OTC]
  Hyperstat® I.V. [US/Can]
  Insta-Glucose® [US-OTC]
  Proglycem® [US/Can]

HYPOKALEMIA
Diuretic, Potassium Sparing
  Aldactone® [US/Can]
  amiloride
  Dyrenium® [US/Can]
  Midamor® [US/Can]
  Novo-Spiroton [Can]
  spironolactone
  triamterene
Electrolyte Supplement, Oral
  Apo®-K [Can]
  Cena-K® [US]
  Effer-K™ [US]
  Glu-K® [US-OTC]
  K+ 10® [US]

Kaochlor® [US]
Kaon-Cl-10® [US]
Kaon-Cl® [US]
Kaon® [US/Can]
Kay Ciel® [US]
K+ Care® ET [US]
K+ Care® [US]
K-Dur® 10 [US/Can]
K-Dur® 20 [US/Can]
Klor-Con® 8 [US]
Klor-Con® 10 [US]
Klor-Con®/25 [US]
Klor-Con®/EF [US]
Klor-Con® [US]
K-Lor™ [US/Can]
Klorvess® [US]
Klotrix® [US]
K-Lyte/Cl® [US/Can]
K-Lyte® [US/Can]
K-Phos® MF [US]
K-Phos® Neutral [US]
K-Phos® No. 2 [US]
K-Tab® [US]
Micro-K® 10 Extencaps® [US]
Micro-K® Extencaps [US/Can]
Neutra-Phos®-K [US]
Neutra-Phos® Powder [US]
potassium acetate
potassium acetate, potassium bicar-
  bonate, and potassium citrate
potassium bicarbonate
potassium bicarbonate and potassium
  chloride, effervescent
potassium bicarbonate and potassium
  citrate, effervescent
potassium chloride
potassium citrate and potassium gluconate
potassium gluconate
potassium phosphate
potassium phosphate and sodium
  phosphate
Roychlor® [Can]

Rum-K® [US]
Slow-K® [Can]
Tri-K® [US]
Twin-K® [US]
Uro-KP-Neutral® [US]

HYPOMAGNESEMIA
Electrolyte Supplement, Oral
Chloromag® [US]
Mag Delay® [US]
Mag-Gel® 600 [US]
magnesium chloride
magnesium gluconate
magnesium hydroxide
magnesium oxide
magnesium sulfate
Magonate® [US-OTC]
Mag-Ox® 400 [US-OTC]
Mag-SR® [US]
Phillips'® Milk of Magnesia [US-OTC]
Slow-Mag® [US/Can]
Uro-Mag® [US-OTC]

HYPONATREMIA
Electrolyte Supplement, Oral
sodium acetate
sodium bicarbonate
sodium chloride
sodium phosphates

HYPOPARATHYROIDISM
Diagnostic Agent
Parathar™ [US]
teriparatide
Vitamin D Analog
Calciferol™ [US]
Calcijex™ [US]
calcitriol
DHT™ [US]
dihydrotachysterol
Drisdol® [US/Can]
ergocalciferol
Hytakerol® [US/Can]

Ostoforte® [Can]
Rocaltrol® [US/Can]

HYPOPHOSPHATEMIA
Electrolyte Supplement, Oral
K-Phos® MF [US]
K-Phos® Neutral [US]
K-Phos® No. 2 [US]
Neutra-Phos®-K [US]
Neutra-Phos® Powder [US]
potassium phosphate
potassium phosphate and sodium phosphate
Uro-KP-Neutral® [US]
Vitamin D Analog
calcifediol
Calciferol™ [US]
Calcijex™ [US]
calcitriol
Calderol® [US/Can]
DHT™ [US]
dihydrotachysterol
Drisdol® [US/Can]
ergocalciferol
Hytakerol® [US/Can]
Ostoforte® [Can]
Rocaltrol® [US/Can]

HYPOPROTHROMBINEMIA
Vitamin, Fat Soluble
AquaMEPHYTON® [US/Can]
Mephyton® [US/Can]
phytonadione

HYPOTENSION (ORTHOSTATIC)
Adrenergic Agonist Agent
ephedrine
phenylephrine
Alpha-Adrenergic Agonist
Amatine® [Can]
midodrine
ProAmatine [US]

Central Nervous System Stimulant,
 Nonamphetamine
 Concerta™ [US]
 Metadate® CD [US]
 Metadate™ ER [US]
 Methylin™ ER [US]
 Methylin™ [US]
 methylphenidate
 PMS-Methylphenidate [Can]
 Riphenidate [Can]
 Ritalin® LA [US]
 Ritalin-SR® [US/Can]
 Ritalin® [US/Can]

HYPOTHYROIDISM
Thyroid Product
 Armour® Thyroid [US]
 Cytomel® [US/Can]
 Eltroxin® [Can]
 Levothroid® [US]
 levothyroxine
 Levo-T™ [US]
 Levoxyl® [US]
 liothyronine
 liotrix
 Nature-Throid® NT [US]
 Novothyrox [US]
 Synthroid® [US/Can]
 thyroid
 Thyrolar® [US/Can]
 Triostat™ [US]
 Unithroid™ [US]
 Westhroid® [US]

HYPOXIC RESPIRATORY FAILURE
Vasodilator, Pulmonary
 INOmax® [US/Can]
 nitric oxide

ICHTHYOSIS
Keratolytic Agent
 Duofilm® Solution [US]
 Keralyt® Gel [US-OTC]
 salicylic acid and lactic acid
 salicylic acid and propylene glycol

IDIOPATHIC THROMBOCYTOPENIA PURPURA (ITP)
Immune Globulin
 BayGam® [US/Can]
 Carimune™ [US]
 Gamimune® N [US/Can]
 Gammagard® S/D [US/Can]
 Gammar®-P I.V. [US]
 immune globulin
  (intramuscular)
 immune globulin (intravenous)
 Iveegam EN [US]
 Iveegam Immuno® [Can]
 Panglobulin® [US]
 Polygam® S/D [US]
 Venoglobulin®-S [US]

IMPETIGO
Antibiotic, Topical
 bacitracin, neomycin, and
  polymyxin B
 Bactroban® [US/Can]
 mupirocin
 Mycitracin® [US-OTC]
 Neosporin® Topical [US/Can]
 Neotopic® [Can]
 Triple Antibiotic® [US]
Penicillin
 Apo®-Pen VK [Can]
 Nadopen-V® [Can]
 Novo-Pen-VK® [Can]
 Nu-Pen-VK® [Can]
 penicillin G procaine
 penicillin V potassium
 PVF® K [Can]
 Suspen® [US]
 Truxcillin® [US]
 Veetids® [US]
 Wycillin® [US/Can]

INFLAMMATION (NONRHEUMATIC)

Adrenal Corticosteroid
  Acthar® [US]
  A-HydroCort® [US/Can]
  Alti-Dexamethasone [Can]
  A-methaPred® [US]
  Apo®-Prednisone [Can]
  Aristocort® Forte Injection [US]
  Aristocort® Intralesional Injection [US]
  Aristocort® Tablet [US/Can]
  Aristospan® Intra-articular Injection [US/Can]
  Aristospan® Intralesional Injection [US/Can]
  Betaject™ [Can]
  betamethasone (systemic)
  Betnesol® [Can]
  Celestone® Phosphate [US]
  Celestone® Soluspan® [US/Can]
  Celestone® [US]
  Cel-U-Jec® [US]
  Cortef® [US/Can]
  corticotropin
  cortisone acetate
  Cortone® [Can]
  Decadron®-LA [US]
  Decadron® [US/Can]
  Decaject-LA® [US]
  Decaject® [US]
  Delta-Cortef® [US]
  Deltasone® [US]
  Depo-Medrol® [US/Can]
  Depopred® [US]
  dexamethasone (systemic)
  Dexasone® L.A. [US]
  Dexasone® [US/Can]
  Dexone® LA [US]
  Dexone® [US]
  Hexadrol® [US/Can]
  H.P. Acthar® Gel [US]
  hydrocortisone (systemic)
  Hydrocortone® Acetate [US]
  Kenalog® Injection [US/Can]
  Key-Pred-SP® [US]
  Key-Pred® [US]
  Medrol® Tablet [US/Can]
  methylprednisolone
  Meticorten® [US]
  Orapred™ [US]
  Pediapred® [US/Can]
  PMS-Dexamethasone [Can]
  Prednicot® [US]
  prednisolone (systemic)
  Prednisol® TBA [US]
  prednisone
  Prelone® [US]
  Solu-Cortef® [US/Can]
  Solu-Medrol® [US/Can]
  Solurex L.A.® [US]
  Sterapred® DS [US]
  Sterapred® [US]
  Tac™-3 Injection [US]
  Triam-A® Injection [US]
  triamcinolone (systemic)
  Triam Forte® Injection [US]
  Winpred™ [Can]

INFLAMMATORY BOWEL DISEASE

5-Aminosalicylic Acid Derivative
  Alti-Sulfasalazine® [Can]
  Asacol® [US/Can]
  Azulfidine® EN-tabs® [US]
  Azulfidine® Tablet [US]
  Canasa™ [US]
  Dipentum® [US/Can]
  mesalamine
  Mesasal® [Can]
  Novo-ASA [Can]
  olsalazine
  Pentasa® [US/Can]
  Quintasa® [Can]
  Rowasa® [US/Can]
  Salazopyrin® [Can]

Salazopyrin En-Tabs® [Can]
Salofalk® [Can]
S.A.S.™ [Can]
sulfasalazine

INFLUENZA
Antiviral Agent
amantadine
Endantadine® [Can]
Flumadine® [US/Can]
PMS-Amantadine [Can]
rimantadine
Symmetrel® [US/Can]
Antiviral Agent, Inhalation Therapy
Relenza® [US/Can]
zanamivir
Antiviral Agent, Oral
oseltamivir
Tamiflu™ [US/Can]
Vaccine, Inactivated Virus
FluShield® [US]
Fluviral S/F® [Can]
Fluvirin® [US]
Fluzone® [US/Can]
influenza virus vaccine
Vaxigrip® [Can]

INFLUENZA A
Antiviral Agent
amantadine
Endantadine® [Can]
Flumadine® [US/Can]
PMS-Amantadine [Can]
rimantadine
Symmetrel® [US/Can]

INSOMNIA
Antihistamine
ANX® [US]
Apo®-Hydroxyzine [Can]
Atarax® [US/Can]
Benadryl® [US/Can]
Compoz® Nighttime Sleep Aid [US-OTC]

Diphendryl® [US-OTC]
Diphenhist® [US-OTC]
diphenhydramine
Diphen® [US-OTC]
Diphenyl® [US-OTC]
Dormin® Sleep Aid [US-OTC]
doxylamine
Genahist® [US-OTC]
Geridryl® [US-OTC]
Hydramine® [US-OTC]
hydroxyzine
Hyrexin® [US-OTC]
Hyzine-50® [US]
Mediphedryl® [US-OTC]
Medi-Sleep® [US-OTC]
Miles® Nervine [US-OTC]
Night-Time Sleep Aid US-OTC]
Novo-Hydroxyzin [Can]
Nytol™ [Can]
Nytol™ Extra Strength [Can]
Nytol® Quickcaps® [US-OTC]
PMS-Diphenhydramine [Can]
PMS-Hydroxyzine [Can]
Polydryl® [US-OTC]
Q-Dryl® [US-OTC]
Quenalin® [US-OTC]
Restall® [US]
Siladryl® Allerfy® [US-OTC]
Silphen® [US-OTC]
Simply Sleep® [US-OTC]
Sleep-Aid® [US-OTC]
Sleepinal® [US-OTC]
Sleep® Tabs [US-OTC]
Sominex® [US-OTC]
Truxadryl® [US-OTC]
Twilite® [US-OTC]
Unisom® [US-OTC]
Unison® Sleepgels® Maximum Strength [US-OTC]
Vistacot® [US]
Vistaril® [US/Can]

Barbiturate
  amobarbital
  amobarbital and secobarbital
  Amytal® [US/Can]
  butabarbital sodium
  Butisol Sodium® [US]
  Nembutal® [US/Can]
  pentobarbital
  phenobarbital
  secobarbital
  Seconal™ [US]
  Tuinal® [US]
Benzodiazepine
  Apo®-Diazepam [Can]
  Apo®-Flurazepam [Can]
  Apo®-Lorazepam [Can]
  Apo®-Temazepam [Can]
  Apo®-Triazo [Can]
  Ativan® [US/Can]
  Dalmane® [US/Can]
  Diastat® [US/Can]
  Diazemuls® [Can]
  diazepam
  Diazepam Intensol® [US]
  Doral® [US/Can]
  estazolam
  flurazepam
  Gen-Temazepam [Can]
  Gen-Triazolam [Can]
  Halcion® [US/Can]
  lorazepam
  Novo-Lorazem® [Can]
  Novo-Temazepam [Can]
  Nu-Loraz [Can]
  Nu-Temazepam [Can]
  PMS-Temazepam [Can]
  ProSom™ [US]
  quazepam
  Restoril® [US/Can]
  Riva-Lorazepam [Can]
  temazepam
  triazolam
  Valium® [US/Can]

Hypnotic
  Apo®-Zopiclone [Can]
  Gen-Zopiclone [Can]
  Imovane® [Can]
  Nu-Zopiclone [Can]
  Rhovane® [Can]
  zopiclone (Canada only)
Hypnotic, Nonbarbiturate
  Ambien® [US/Can]
  Aquachloral® Supprettes® [US]
  chloral hydrate
  ethchlorvynol
  Placidyl® [US]
  PMS-Chloral Hydrate [Can]
  Somnote® [US]
  zolpidem
Hypnotic, Nonbenzodiazepine
    (Pyrazolopyrimidine)
  Sonata® [US/Can]
  Starnoc® [Can]
  zaleplon

INTERMITTENT CLAUDICATION
Platelet Aggregation Inhibitor
  cilostazol
  Pletal® [US/Can]

INTERSTITIAL CYSTITIS
Analgesic, Urinary
  Elmiron® [US/Can]
  pentosan polysulfate sodium
Urinary Tract Product
  dimethyl sulfoxide
  Kemsol® [Can]
  Rimso®-50 [US/Can]

INTRACRANIAL PRESSURE
Barbiturate
  Pentothal® Sodium [US/Can]
  thiopental
Diuretic, Osmotic
  mannitol
  Osmitrol® [US/Can]

INTRAOCULAR PRESSURE
Ophthalmic Agent, Miscellaneous
glycerin
Osmoglyn® [US]

IRON DEFICIENCY ANEMIA
Iron Salt
ferric gluconate
Ferrlecit® [US]

IRON POISONING
Antidote
deferoxamine
Desferal® [US/Can]

IRRITABLE BOWEL SYNDROME (IBS)
Anticholinergic Agent
Antispas® Tablet [US]
Apo®-Chlorax [Can]
atropine
Atropine-Care® [US]
Atropisol® [US/Can]
Bentylol® [Can]
Bentyl® [US]
clidinium and chlordiazepoxide
Dicyclocot® [US]
dicyclomine
Donnapine® [US]
Donnatal® [US]
Formulex® [Can]
Haponal® [US]
Hyonatol® [US]
hyoscyamine, atropine, scopolamine, and phenobarbital
Hypersed® [US]
Isopto® Atropine [US/Can]
Librax® [US/Can]
Lomine [Can]
Propanthel™ [Can]
propantheline
Sal-Tropine™ [US]

Antispasmodic Agent, Gastrointestinal
Modulon® [Can]
trimebutine (Canada only)
Calcium Antagonist
Dicetel® [Can]
pinaverium (Canada only)
Gastrointestinal Agent, Miscellaneous
Dicetel® [Can]
pinaverium (Canada only)
Laxative
Fiberall® Powder [US-OTC]
Fiberall® Wafer [US-OTC]
Hydrocil® [US-OTC]
Konsyl-D® [US-OTC]
Konsyl® [US-OTC]
Metamucil® Smooth Texture [US-OTC]
Metamucil® [US/Can]
Modane® Bulk [US-OTC]
Novo-Mucilax [Can]
Perdiem® Plain [US-OTC]
psyllium
Reguloid® [US-OTC]
Serutan® [US-OTC]
Syllact® [US-OTC]
Serotonin 5-HT4 Receptor Agonist
tegaserod
Zelnorm™ [US]

ISCHEMIA
Blood Viscosity Reducer Agent
Albert® Pentoxifylline [Can]
Apo®-Pentoxifylline SR [Can]
Nu-Pentoxifylline SR [Can]
pentoxifylline
Trental® [US/Can]
Platelet Aggregation Inhibitor
abciximab
ReoPro® [US/Can]
Vasodilator
ethaverine
Ethavex-100® [US]
Papacon® [US]

papaverine
Para-Time S.R.® [US]
Pavacot® [US]

ISONIAZID POISONING
Vitamin, Water Soluble
Aminoxin® [US-OTC]
pyridoxine

JAPANESE ENCEPHALITIS
Vaccine, Inactivated Virus
Japanese encephalitis virus vaccine
(inactivated)
JE-VAX® [US/Can]

KAPOSI SARCOMA
Antineoplastic Agent
daunorubicin citrate (liposomal)
DaunoXome® [US]
Doxil® [US/Can]
doxorubicin (liposomal)
Onxol™ [US]
paclitaxel
Taxol® [US/Can]
Velban® [US/Can]
vinblastine
Antineoplastic Agent, Miscellaneous
alitretinoin
Panretin™ [US]
Biological Response Modulator
interferon alfa-2a
interferon alfa-2b
Intron® A [US/Can]
Roferon-A® [US/Can]
Retinoic Acid Derivative
alitretinoin
Panretin™ [US]

KAWASAKI DISEASE
Immune Globulin
BayGam® [US/Can]
Carimune™ [US]
Gamimune® N [US/Can]
Gammagard® S/D [US/Can]

Gammar®-P I.V. [US]
immune globulin (intramuscular)
immune globulin (intravenous)
Iveegam EN [US]
Iveegam Immuno® [Can]
Panglobulin® [US]
Polygam® S/D [US]
Venoglobulin®-S [US]

KERATITIS (FUNGAL)
Antifungal Agent
Natacyn® [US/Can]
natamycin

KERATITIS (HERPES SIMPLEX)
Antiviral Agent
trifluridine
vidarabine
Vira-A® [US]
Viroptic® [US/Can]

KERATITIS (VERNAL)
Antiviral Agent
trifluridine
Viroptic® [US/Can]
Mast Cell Stabilizer
Alomide® [US/Can]
lodoxamide tromethamine

KERATOCONJUNCTIVITIS (VERNAL)
Mast Cell Stabilizer
Alomide® [US/Can]
lodoxamide tromethamine

KERATOSIS (ACTINIC)
Porphyrin Agent, Topical
aminolevulinic acid
Levulan® Kerastick™ [US/Can]

KIDNEY STONE
Alkalinizing Agent
Polycitra® [US]
potassium citrate

sodium citrate and potassium citrate
mixture
Urocit®-K [US]
Chelating Agent
Cuprimine® [US/Can]
Depen® [US/Can]
penicillamine
Electrolyte Supplement, Oral
K-Phos® MF [US]
K-Phos® Neutral [US]
K-Phos® No. 2 [US]
Neutra-Phos®-K [US]
Neutra-Phos® Powder [US]
potassium phosphate
potassium phosphate and sodium
phosphate
Uro-KP-Neutral® [US]
Irrigating Solution
citric acid bladder mixture
Renacidin® [US]
Urinary Tract Product
Calcibind® [US/Can]
cellulose sodium phosphate
Thiola™ [US/Can]
tiopronin
Xanthine Oxidase Inhibitor
allopurinol
Aloprim™ [US]
Apo®-Allopurinol [Can]
Zyloprim® [US/Can]

LABOR (PREMATURE)
Adrenergic Agonist Agent
Brethine® [US]
Bricanyl® [Can]
terbutaline

LACTATION (SUPPRESSION)
Ergot Alkaloid and Derivative
Apo® Bromocriptine [Can]
bromocriptine
Parlodel® [US/Can]
PMS-Bromocriptine [Can]

LACTOSE INTOLERANCE
Nutritional Supplement
Dairyaid® [Can]
Dairy Ease® [US-OTC]
Lactaid® [US-OTC]
lactase
Lactrase® [US-OTC]

LEAD POISONING
Chelating Agent
BAL in Oil® [US]
Calcium Disodium Versenate® [US]
Chemet® [US/Can]
Cuprimine® [US/Can]
Depen® [US/Can]
dimercaprol
edetate calcium disodium
penicillamine
succimer

LEUKEMIA
Antineoplastic Agent
Adriamycin® [Can]
Adriamycin PFS® [US]
Adriamycin RDF® [US]
asparaginase
busulfan
Busulfex® [US/Can]
Caelyx® [Can]
Cerubidine® [US/Can]
chlorambucil
cladribine
cyclophosphamide
cytarabine
Cytosar® [Can]
Cytosar-U® [US]
Cytoxan® [US/Can]
daunorubicin hydrochloride
doxorubicin
Droxia™ [US]
Elspar® [US/Can]
etoposide
fludarabine
Fludara® [US/Can]

Hydrea® [US/Can]
hydroxyurea
Ifex® [US/Can]
ifosfamide
Kidrolase® [Can]
Lanvis® [Can]
Leukeran® [US/Can]
Leustatin™ [US/Can]
mechlorethamine
mercaptopurine
methotrexate
Mithracin® [US/Can]
mitoxantrone
Mustargen® [US/Can]
Myleran® [US/Can]
Mylocel™ [US]
Neosar® [US]
Nipent™ [US/Can]
Novantrone® [US/Can]
Oncaspar® [US/Can]
Oncovin® [US/Can]
pegaspargase
pentostatin
plicamycin
Procytox® [Can]
Purinethol® [US/Can]
Rheumatrex® [US]
Rubex® [US]
teniposide
thioguanine
Toposar® [US]
tretinoin (oral)
Trexall™ [US]
VePesid® [US/Can]
Vesanoid® [US/Can]
Vincasar® PFS® [US/Can]
vincristine
Vumon® [US/Can]
Antineoplastic Agent, Miscellaneous
   arsenic trioxide
   Trisenox™ [US]
Antineoplastic Agent, Monoclonal
   Antibody

   alemtuzumab
   Campath® [US]
Antineoplastic Agent, Natural Source
   (Plant) Derivative
   gemtuzumab ozogamicin
   Mylotarg™ [US/Can]
Antineoplastic, Tyrosine Kinase
   Inhibitor
   Gleevec™ [US]
   imatinib
Antiviral Agent
   interferon alfa-2b and ribavirin com-
      bination pack
   Rebetron™ [US/Can]
Biological Response Modulator
   interferon alfa-2a
   interferon alfa-2b
   interferon alfa-2b and ribavirin com-
      bination pack
   Intron® A [US/Can]
   Rebetron™ [US/Can]
   Roferon-A® [US/Can]
Immune Globulin
   Carimune™ [US]
   Gamimune® N [US/Can]
   Gammagard® S/D [US/Can]
   Gammar®-P I.V. [US]
   immune globulin (intravenous)
   Iveegam EN [US]
   Iveegam Immuno® [Can]
   Panglobulin® [US]
   Polygam® S/D [US]
   Venoglobulin®-S [US]
Immune Modulator
   Ergamisol® [US/Can]
   levamisole

LICE

Scabicides/Pediculicides
   A-200™ Lice [US-OTC]
   A-200™ [US-OTC]
   Acticin® [US]
   Elimite® [US]

End Lice® [US-OTC]
Hexit™ [Can]
Kwellada-P™ [Can]
lindane
malathion
Nix® Dermal Cream [Can]
Nix® [US/Can]
Ovide™ [US]
permethrin
PMS-Lindane [Can]
Pronto® [US-OTC]
pyrethrins
Pyrinex® Pediculicide
   [US-OTC]
Pyrinyl Plus® [US-OTC]
Pyrinyl® [US-OTC]
R & C™ II [Can]
R & C® Lice [US]
R & C™ Shampoo/Conditioner
   [Can]
R & C® [US-OTC]
RID® Mousse [Can]
RID® Spray [US-OTC]
RID® [US-OTC]
Tisit® Blue Gel [US-OTC]
Tisit® [US-OTC]

LYME DISEASE

Antibiotic, Penicillin
   pivampicillin (Canada only)
   Pondocillin® [Can]
Cephalosporin (Third Generation)
   ceftriaxone
   Rocephin® [US/Can]
Macrolide (Antibiotic)
   Apo®-Erythro Base [Can]
   Apo®-Erythro E-C [Can]
   Apo®-Erythro-ES [Can]
   Apo®-Erythro-S [Can]
   Diomycin® [Can]
   E.E.S.® [US/Can]
   Erybid™ [Can]
   Eryc® [US/Can]

EryPed® [US]
Ery-Tab® [US]
Erythrocin® [US/Can]
erythromycin (systemic)
Nu-Erythromycin-S [Can]
PCE® [US/Can]
PMS-Erythromycin [Can]
Penicillin
   amoxicillin
   Amoxicot® [US]
   Amoxil® [US/Can]
   ampicillin
   Apo®-Amoxi [Can]
   Apo®-Ampi [Can]
   Apo®-Pen VK [Can]
   Gen-Amoxicillin [Can]
   Lin-Amox [Can]
   Marcillin® [US]
   Moxilin® [US]
   Nadopen-V® [Can]
   Novamoxin® [Can]
   Novo-Ampicillin [Can]
   Novo-Pen-VK® [Can]
   Nu-Amoxi [Can]
   Nu-Ampi [Can]
   Nu-Pen-VK® [Can]
   penicillin V potassium
   Principen® [US]
   PVF® K [Can]
   Suspen® [US]
   Trimox® [US]
   Truxcillin® [US]
   Veetids® [US]
   Wymox® [US]
Tetracycline Derivative
   Adoxa™ [US]
   Apo®-Doxy [Can]
   Apo®-Doxy Tabs [Can]
   Apo®-Tetra [Can]
   Brodspec® [US]
   Doryx® [US]
   Doxy-100™ [US]
   Doxycin [Can]

doxycycline
Doxytec [Can]
EmTet® [US]
Monodox® [US]
Novo-Doxylin [Can]
Novo-Tetra [Can]
Nu-Doxycycline [Can]
Nu-Tetra [Can]
Sumycin® [US]
tetracycline
Vibramycin® [US]
Vibra-Tabs® [US/Can]
Wesmycin® [US]

LYMPHOMA

Antineoplastic Agent
Adriamycin® [Can]
Adriamycin PFS® [US]
Adriamycin RDF® [US]
asparaginase
BiCNU® [US/Can]
Blenoxane® [US/Can]
bleomycin
Caelyx® [Can]
carmustine
CeeNU® [US/Can]
chlorambucil
cisplatin
cyclophosphamide
cytarabine
Cytosar® [Can]
Cytosar-U® [US]
Cytoxan® [US/Can]
doxorubicin
Elspar® [US/Can]
etoposide
Gliadel® [US]
Idamycin® [Can]
Idamycin PFS® [US]
idarubicin
Ifex® [US/Can]
ifosfamide
Kidrolase® [Can]

Leukeran® [US/Can]
lomustine
Matulane® [US/Can]
mechlorethamine
methotrexate
mitoxantrone
Mustargen® [US/Can]
Natulan® [Can]
Neosar® [US]
Novantrone® [US/Can]
Oncaspar® [US/Can]
Oncovin® [US/Can]
pegaspargase
Platinol®-AQ [US]
Platinol® [US]
procarbazine
Procytox® [Can]
Rheumatrex® [US]
Rituxan® [US/Can]
rituximab
Rubex® [US]
teniposide
Thioplex® [US]
thiotepa
Toposar® [US]
Trexall™ [US]
Velban® [US/Can]
VePesid® [US/Can]
vinblastine
Vincasar® PFS® [US/Can]
vincristine
Vumon® [US/Can]
Antineoplastic Agent, Monoclonal
    Antibody
ibritumomab
Zevalin™ [US]
Antiviral Agent
interferon alfa-2b and ribavirin com-
    bination pack
Rebetron™ [US/Can]
Biological Response Modulator
interferon alfa-2a
interferon alfa-2b

A191

interferon alfa-2b and ribavirin combination pack
Intron® A [US/Can]
Rebetron™ [US/Can]
Roferon-A® [US/Can]
Colony-Stimulating Factor
Leukine™ [US/Can]
sargramostim
Radiopharmaceutical
ibritumomab
Zevalin™ [US]

LYMPHOMATOUS MENINGITIS

Antineoplastic Agent, Antimetabolite (Purine)
cytarabine (liposomal)
DepoCyt™ [US/Can]

MACULAR DEGENERATION

Ophthalmic Agent
verteporfin
Visudyne™ [US/Can]

MALIGNANT EFFUSION

Antineoplastic Agent
Thioplex® [US]
thiotepa

MANIA

Anticonvulsant
Alti-Divalproex [Can]
Apo®-Divalproex [Can]
Depacon® [US]
Depakene® [US/Can]
Depakote® Delayed Release [US]
Depakote® ER [US]
Depakote® Sprinkle® [US]
Epival® I.V. [Can]
Gen-Divalproex [Can]
Novo-Divalproex [Can]
Nu-Divalproex [Can]
PMS-Valproic Acid [Can]

PMS-Valproic Acid E.C. [Can]
Rhoxal-valproic [Can]
valproic acid and derivatives
Antimanic Agent
Carbolith™ [Can]
Duralith® [Can]
Eskalith CR® [US]
Eskalith® [US]
Lithane™ [Can]
lithium
Lithobid® [US]
PMS-Lithium Carbonate [Can]
PMS-Lithium Citrate [Can]
Phenothiazine Derivative
Chlorpromanyl® [Can]
chlorpromazine
Largactil® [Can]
Thorazine® [US]

MARFAN SYNDROME

Rauwolfia Alkaloid
reserpine

MEASLES (RUBELLA)

Vaccine, Live Virus
measles and rubella vaccines, combined
M-R-VAX® II [US]

MEASLES (RUBEOLA)

Immune Globulin
BayGam® [US/Can]
immune globulin (intramuscular)
Vaccine, Live Virus
measles and rubella vaccines, combined
M-R-VAX® II [US]

MELANOMA

Antineoplastic Agent
Blenoxane® [US/Can]
bleomycin
CeeNU® [US/Can]

cisplatin
Cosmegen® [US/Can]
dacarbazine
dactinomycin
Droxia™ [US]
DTIC® [Can]
DTIC-Dome® [US]
Hydrea® [US/Can]
hydroxyurea
lomustine
Mylocel™ [US]
Platinol®-AQ [US]
Platinol® [US]
teniposide
Vumon® [US/Can]
Antiviral Agent
interferon alfa-2b and ribavirin combination pack
Rebetron™ [US/Can]
Biological Response Modulator
interferon alfa-2a
interferon alfa-2b
interferon alfa-2b and ribavirin combination pack
Intron® A [US/Can]
Rebetron™ [US/Can]
Roferon-A® [US/Can]

MÉNIERE DISEASE
Antihistamine
Antivert® [US/Can]
betahistine (Canada only)
Bonamine™ [Can]
Bonine® [US/Can]
Dramamine® II [US-OTC]
meclizine
Meni-D® [US]
Serc® [Can]

MENINGITIS (TUBERCULOUS)
Antitubercular Agent
streptomycin

MENORRHAGIA
Androgen
Cyclomen® [Can]
danazol
Danocrine® [US/Can]

MERCURY POISONING
Chelating Agent
BAL in Oil® [US]
dimercaprol

METHANOL POISONING
Pharmaceutical Aid
alcohol (ethyl)
Biobase™ [Can]
Dilusol® [Can]
Duonalc® [Can]
Duonalc-E® Mild [Can]
Lavacol® [US-OTC]

METHOTREXATE POISONING
Folic Acid Derivative
leucovorin
Wellcovorin® [US]

MIGRAINE
Analgesic, Nonnarcotic
acetaminophen, isometheptene, and dichloralphenazone
Advil® Migraine [US-OTC]
Advil® [US/Can]
Aleve® [US-OTC]
Anaprox® DS [US/Can]
Anaprox® [US/Can]
Apo®-Diflunisal [Can]
Apo®-Ibuprofen [Can]
Apo®-Keto [Can]
Apo®-Keto-E [Can]
Apo®-Keto SR [Can]
Apo®-Mefenamic [Can]
Apo®-Napro-Na [Can]
Apo®-Napro-Na DS [Can]
Apo®-Naproxen [Can]

Apo®-Naproxen SR [Can]
diflunisal
Dolobid® [US]
EC-Naprosyn® [US]
Gen-Naproxen EC [Can]
Genpril® [US-OTC]
Haltran® [US-OTC]
ibuprofen
Ibu-Tab® [US]
I-Prin [US-OTC]
ketoprofen
meclofenamate
mefenamic acid
Menadol® [US-OTC]
Migratine® [US]
Motrin® Migraine Pain [US-OTC]
Motrin® [US/Can]
Naprelan® [US]
Naprosyn® [US/Can]
naproxen
Naxen® [Can]
Novo-Diflunisal [Can]
Novo-Keto [Can]
Novo-Keto-EC [Can]
Novo-Naprox [Can]
Novo-Naprox Sodium [Can]
Novo-Naprox Sodium DS [Can]
Novo-Naprox SR [Can]
Novo-Profen® [Can]
Nu-Diflunisal [Can]
Nu-Ibuprofen [Can]
Nu-Ketoprofen [Can]
Nu-Ketoprofen-E [Can]
Nu-Mefenamic [Can]
Nu-Naprox [Can]
Orafen [Can]
Orudis® KT [US-OTC]
Orudis® SR [Can]
Oruvail® [US/Can]
PMS-Mefenamic Acid [Can]
Ponstan® [Can]
Ponstel® [US/Can]
Rhodis™ [Can]

Rhodis-EC™ [Can]
Rhodis SR™ [Can]
Riva-Naproxen [Can]
Synflex® [Can]
Synflex® DS [Can]

Antidepressant, Tricyclic (Tertiary Amine)
amitriptyline
Apo®-Amitriptyline [Can]
Elavil® [US/Can]
Vanatrip® [US]

Antimigraine Agent
Amerge® [US/Can]
frovatriptan
Frova™ [US]
Imitrex® [US/Can]
Maxalt-MLT™ [US]
Maxalt RPD™ [Can]
Maxalt® [US/Can]
naratriptan
rizatriptan
sumatriptan succinate
zolmitriptan
Zomig® [US/Can]
Zomig-ZMT™ [US]

Beta-Adrenergic Blocker
Alti-Nadolol [Can]
Apo®-Nadol [Can]
Apo®-Propranolol [Can]
Apo®-Timol [Can]
Apo®-Timop [Can]
Betimol® [US]
Blocadren® [US]
Corgard® [US/Can]
Gen-Timolol [Can]
Inderal® LA [US/Can]
Inderal® [US/Can]
nadolol
Novo-Nadolol [Can]
Nu-Propranolol [Can]
Nu-Timolol [Can]
Phoxal-timolol [Can]
PMS-Timolol [Can]

propranolol
Tim-AK [Can]
timolol
Timoptic® OcuDose® [US]
Timoptic® [US/Can]
Timoptic-XE® [US/Can]
Calcium-Entry Blocker (Selective)
flunarizine (Canada only)
Sibelium® [Can]
Decongestant/Analgesic
Advil® Cold & Sinus Caplets [US-OTC]
Advil® Cold & Sinus Tablet [Can]
Dristan® Sinus Caplets [US]
Dristan® Sinus Tablet [Can]
pseudoephedrine and ibuprofen
Ergot Alkaloid and Derivative
belladonna, phenobarbital, and ergot-amine tartrate
Bellamine S [US]
Bellergal® Spacetabs® [Can]
Bel-Phen-Ergot S® [US]
Bel-Tabs [US]
Cafergot® [US/Can]
D.H.E. 45® [US]
dihydroergotamine
ergotamine
methysergide
Migranal® [US/Can]
Sansert® [US/Can]
Wigraine® [US]
Serotonin 5-HT1B, 1D Receptor Agonist
frovatriptan
Frova™ [US]
Serotonin 5-HT1D Receptor Agonist
almotriptan
Axert™ [US]
Serotonin Agonist
Amerge® [US/Can]
Maxalt-MLT™ [US]
Maxalt RPD™ [Can]
Maxalt® [US/Can]

naratriptan
rizatriptan
zolmitriptan
Zomig® [US/Can]
Zomig-ZMT™ [US]

MIGRAINE (PROPHYLAXIS)
Antimigraine Agent
pizotifen (Canada only)
Sandomigran® [Can]
Sandomigran DS® [Can]

MITRAL VALVE PROLAPSE
Beta-Adrenergic Blocker
Apo®-Propranolol [Can]
Inderal® LA [US/Can]
Inderal® [US/Can]
Nu-Propranolol [Can]
propranolol

MOTION SICKNESS
Anticholinergic Agent
scopolamine
Transderm Scōp® [US]
Transderm-V® [Can]
Antihistamine
Antivert® [US/Can]
Benadryl® [US/Can]
Bonamine™ [Can]
Bonine® [US/Can]
dimenhydrinate
diphenhydramine
Dramamine® II [US-OTC]
Dramamine® Oral [US-OTC]
meclizine
Mediphedryl® [US-OTC]
Meni-D® [US]
Miles® Nervine [US-OTC]
Nytol™ [Can]
Nytol™ Extra Strength [Can]
Nytol® Quickcaps® [US-OTC]
PMS-Diphenhydramine [Can]
Polydryl® [US-OTC]

Q-Dryl® [US-OTC]
Quenalin® [US-OTC]
Siladryl® Allerfy® [US-OTC]
Silphen® [US-OTC]
Simply Sleep® [US-OTC]
Sleepinal® [US-OTC]
Sleep® Tabs [US-OTC]
Sominex® [US-OTC]
TripTone® Caplets® [US-OTC]
Truxadryl® [US-OTC]
Tusstat® [US-OTC]
Twilite® [US-OTC]
Unison® Sleepgels® Maximum
    Strength [US-OTC]
Phenothiazine Derivative
    Anergan® [US]
    Phenergan® [US/Can]
    promethazine

MOUTH PAIN
Pharmaceutical Aid
    Cēpastat® [US-OTC]
    Chloraseptic® [US-OTC]
    phenol
    Ulcerease® [US-OTC]

MULTIPLE SCLEROSIS
Antigout Agent
    colchicine
Biological, Miscellaneous
    Copaxone® [US/Can]
    glatiramer acetate
Biological Response Modulator
    Avonex® [US/Can]
    Betaseron® [US/Can]
    interferon beta-1a
    interferon beta-1b
    Rebif® [US/Can]
Skeletal Muscle Relaxant
    Apo®-Baclofen [Can]
    baclofen
    Dantrium® [US/Can]
    dantrolene
    Gen-Baclofen [Can]

Lioresal® [US/Can]
Liotec [Can]
Nu-Baclo [Can]
PMS-Baclofen [Can]

MUSCARINE POISONING
Anticholinergic Agent
    atropine

MUSCLE SPASM
Skeletal Muscle Relaxant
    Apo®-Cyclobenzaprine [Can]
    Aspirin® Backache [Can]
    carisoprodol
    carisoprodol and aspirin
    carisoprodol, aspirin, and codeine
    chlorzoxazone
    cyclobenzaprine
    Flexeril® [US/Can]
    Flexitec [Can]
    Gen-Cyclobenzaprine [Can]
    metaxalone
    methocarbamol
    methocarbamol and aspirin
    Methoxisal [Can]
    Methoxisal-C [Can]
    Mivacron® [US/Can]
    mivacurium
    Norflex™ [US/Can]
    Norgesic™ Forte [US/Can]
    Norgesic™ [US/Can]
    Novo-Cycloprine [Can]
    Nu-Cyclobenzaprine [Can]
    orphenadrine
    orphenadrine, aspirin, and caffeine
    Orphengesic Forte [US]
    Orphengesic [US]
    Parafon Forte® [Can]
    Parafon Forte™ DSC [US]
    Rhoxal-orphendrine [Can]
    Robaxin® [US/Can]
    Robaxisal® Extra Strength [Can]
    Robaxisal® [US/Can]
    Skelaxin® [US/Can]

Soma® Compound [US]
Soma® Compound w/Codeine [US]
Soma® [US/Can]
Strifon Forte® [Can]

MYASTHENIA GRAVIS
Cholinergic Agent
  ambenonium
  edrophonium
  Enlon® [US/Can]
  Mestinon®-SR [Can]
  Mestinon® Timespan® [US]
  Mestinon® [US/Can]
  Mytelase® [US/Can]
  neostigmine
  Prostigmin® [US/Can]
  pyridostigmine
  Regonol® [US]
  Reversol® [US]
  Tensilon® [US]
Skeletal Muscle Relaxant
  tubocurarine

MYCOBACTERIUM AVIUM-INTRACELLULARE
Antibiotic, Aminoglycoside
  streptomycin
Antibiotic, Miscellaneous
  Mycobutin® [US/Can]
  rifabutin
  Rifadin® [US/Can]
  rifampin
  Rimactane® [US]
  Rofact™ [Can]
Antimycobacterial Agent
  ethambutol
  Etibi® [Can]
  Myambutol® [US]
Antitubercular Agent
  streptomycin
Carbapenem (Antibiotic)
  imipenem and cilastatin
  meropenem

Merrem® I.V. [US/Can]
Primaxin® [US/Can]
Leprostatic Agent
  clofazimine
  Lamprene® [US/Can]
Macrolide (Antibiotic)
  azithromycin
  Biaxin® [US/Can]
  Biaxin® XL [US]
  clarithromycin
  Zithromax® [US/Can]
  Z-PAK® [US/Can]
Quinolone
  ciprofloxacin
  Cipro® [US/Can]

MYELOMA
Antineoplastic Agent
  Adriamycin® [Can]
  Adriamycin PFS® [US]
  Adriamycin RDF® [US]
  Alkeran® [US/Can]
  BiCNU® [US/Can]
  Caelyx® [Can]
  carmustine
  cisplatin
  cyclophosphamide
  Cytoxan® [US/Can]
  doxorubicin
  Gliadel® [US]
  melphalan
  Neosar® [US]
  Platinol®-AQ [US]
  Platinol® [US]
  Procytox® [Can]
  Rubex® [US]
  teniposide
  Vumon® [US/Can]

MYOCARDIAL INFARCTION
Anticoagulant (Other)
  Coumadin® [US/Can]
  enoxaparin

Hepalean® [Can]
Hepalean® Leo [Can]
Hepalean®-LOK [Can]
heparin
Hep-Lock® [US]
Lovenox® [US/Can]
Taro-Warfarin [Can]
warfarin
Antiplatelet Agent
Apo®-ASA [Can]
Apo®-Dipyridamole FC [Can]
aspirin
Bayer® Aspirin Regimen Adult Low
Strength [US-OTC]
Bayer® Aspirin Regimen Adult Low
Strength with Calcium
[US-OTC]
clopidogrel
dipyridamole
Ecotrin® Low Adult Strength [US-OTC]
Halfprin® [US-OTC]
Persantine® [US/Can]
Plavix® [US/Can]
Beta-Adrenergic Blocker
Alti-Nadolol [Can]
Apo®-Atenol [Can]
Apo®-Metoprolol [Can]
Apo®-Nadol [Can]
Apo®-Propranolol [Can]
Apo®-Timol [Can]
Apo®-Timop [Can]
atenolol
Betaloc® [Can]
Betaloc® Durules®
Betimol® [US]
Blocadren® [US]
Corgard® [US/Can]
Gen-Atenolol [Can]
Gen-Metoprolol [Can]
Gen-Timolol [Can]
Inderal® LA [US/Can]
Inderal® [US/Can]

Lopressor® [US/Can]
metoprolol
nadolol
Novo-Atenol [Can]
Novo-Metoprolol [Can]
Novo-Nadolol [Can]
Nu-Atenol
Nu-Metop [Can]
Nu-Propranolol [Can]
Nu-Timolol [Can]
Phoxal-timolol [Can]
PMS-Atenolol [Can]
PMS-Metoprolol [Can]
PMS-Timolol [Can]
propranolol
Rhoxal-atenolol [Can]
Tenolin [Can]
Tenormin® [US/Can]
Tim-AK [Can]
timolol
Timoptic® OcuDose® [US]
Timoptic® [US/Can]
Timoptic-XE® [US/Can]
Toprol-XL® [US/Can]
Fibrinolytic Agent
Activase® rt-PA [Can]
Activase® [US]
alteplase
Retavase® [US/Can]
reteplase
Streptase® [US/Can]
streptokinase
Thrombolytic Agent
tenecteplase
TNKase™ [US]

NARCOTIC DETOXIFICATION
Analgesic, Narcotic
Dolophine® [US/Can]
Metadol™ [Can]
methadone
Methadose® [US/Can]

NAUSEA
Anticholinergic Agent
  scopolamine
    Transderm Scōp® [US]
    Transderm-V® [Can]
Antiemetic
  Benzacot® [US]
  dronabinol
  droperidol
  Emetrol® [US-OTC]
  Inapsine® [US]
  Marinol® [US/Can]
  Nausetrol® [US-OTC]
  phosphorated carbohydrate solution
  Tigan® [US/Can]
  trimethobenzamide
Antihistamine
  Apo®-Dimenhydrinate [Can]
  Calm-X® Oral [US-OTC]
  dimenhydrinate
  Dramamine® Oral [US-OTC]
  Gravol® [Can]
  Hydrate® [US]
  TripTone® Caplets® [US-OTC]
Gastrointestinal Agent, Prokinetic
  Apo®-Metoclop [Can]
  metoclopramide
  Nu-Metoclopramide [Can]
  Reglan® [US]
Phenothiazine Derivative
  Anergan® [US]
  Apo®-Perphenazine [Can]
  Chlorpromanyl® [Can]
  chlorpromazine
  Compazine® [US/Can]
  Compro™ [US]
  Largactil® [Can]
  Nu-Prochlor [Can]
  perphenazine
  Phenergan® [US/Can]
  prochlorperazine
  promethazine
  Stemetil® [Can]
  thiethylperazine
  Thorazine® [US]
  Torecan® [US]
  triflupromazine
  Trilafon® [US/Can]
  Vesprin® [US/Can]
Selective 5-HT3 Receptor Antagonist
  granisetron
  Kytril™ [US/Can]
  ondansetron
  Zofran® ODT [US/Can]
  Zofran® [US/Can]

NEISSERIA MENINGITIDIS
Vaccine, Live Bacteria
  meningococcal polysaccharide vaccine (groups A, C, Y and W-135)
  Menomune®-A/C/Y/W-135 [US]

NEOPLASTIC DISEASE (TREATMENT ADJUNCT)
Adrenal Corticosteroid
  Acthar® [US]
  A-HydroCort® [US/Can]
  Alti-Dexamethasone [Can]
  A-methaPred® [US]
  Apo®-Prednisone [Can]
  Aristocort® Forte Injection [US]
  Aristocort® Intralesional Injection [US]
  Aristocort® Tablet [US/Can]
  Aristospan® Intra-articular Injection [US/Can]
  Aristospan® Intralesional Injection [US/Can]
  Betaject™ [Can]
  betamethasone (systemic)
  Betnesol® [Can]
  Celestone® Phosphate [US]
  Celestone® Soluspan® [US/Can]
  Celestone® [US]
  Cel-U-Jec® [US]
  Cortef® [US/Can]
  corticotropin

cortisone acetate
Cortone® [Can]
Decadron®-LA [US]
Decadron® [US/Can]
Decaject-LA® [US]
Decaject® [US]
Delta-Cortef® [US]
Deltasone® [US]
Depo-Medrol® [US/Can]
Depopred® [US]
dexamethasone (systemic)
Dexasone® L.A. [US]
Dexasone® [US/Can]
Dexone® LA [US]
Dexone® [US]
Hexadrol® [US/Can]
H.P. Acthar® Gel [US]
hydrocortisone (systemic)
Hydrocortone® Acetate [US]
Kenalog® Injection [US/Can]
Key-Pred-SP® [US]
Key-Pred® [US]
Medrol® Tablet [US/Can]
methylprednisolone
Meticorten® [US]
Orapred™ [US]
Pediapred® [US/Can]
PMS-Dexamethasone [Can]
Prednicot® [US]
prednisolone (systemic)
Prednisol® TBA [US]
prednisone
Prelone® [US]
Solu-Cortef® [US/Can]
Solu-Medrol® [US/Can]
Solurex L.A.® [US]
Sterapred® DS [US]
Sterapred® [US]
Tac™-3 Injection [US]
Triam-A® Injection [US]
triamcinolone (systemic)
Triam Forte® Injection [US]
Winpred™ [Can]

NEPHROLITHIASIS
Alkalinizing Agent
  potassium citrate
  Urocit®-K [US]

NEPHROTIC SYNDROME
Adrenal Corticosteroid
  Acthar® [US]
  A-HydroCort® [US/Can]
  Alti-Dexamethasone [Can]
  A-methaPred® [US]
  Apo®-Prednisone [Can]
  Aristocort® Forte Injection [US]
  Aristocort® Intralesional Injection
    [US]
  Aristocort® Tablet [US/Can]
  Aristospan® Intra-articular Injection
    [US/Can]
  Aristospan® Intralesional Injection
    [US/Can]
  Betaject™ [Can]
  betamethasone (systemic)
  Betnesol® [Can]
  Celestone® Phosphate [US]
  Celestone® Soluspan® [US/Can]
  Celestone® [US]
  Cel-U-Jec® [US]
  Cortef® [US/Can]
  corticotropin
  cortisone acetate
  Cortone® [Can]
  Decadron®-LA [US]
  Decadron® [US/Can]
  Decaject-LA® [US]
  Decaject® [US]
  Delta-Cortef® [US]
  Deltasone® [US]
  Depo-Medrol® [US/Can]
  Depopred® [US]
  dexamethasone (systemic)
  Dexasone® L.A. [US]
  Dexasone® [US/Can]
  Dexone® LA [US]

Dexone® [US]
Hexadrol® [US/Can]
H.P. Acthar® Gel [US]
hydrocortisone (systemic)
Hydrocortone® Acetate [US]
Kenalog® Injection [US/Can]
Key-Pred-SP® [US]
Key-Pred® [US]
Medrol® Tablet [US/Can]
methylprednisolone
Meticorten® [US]
Orapred™ [US]
Pediapred® [US/Can]
PMS-Dexamethasone [Can]
Prednicot® [US]
prednisolone (systemic)
Prednisol® TBA [US]
prednisone
Prelone® [US]
Solu-Cortef® [US/Can]
Solu-Medrol® [US/Can]
Solurex L.A.® [US]
Sterapred® DS [US]
Sterapred® [US]
Tac™-3 Injection [US]
Triam-A® Injection [US]
triamcinolone (systemic)
Triam Forte® Injection [US]
Winpred™ [Can]
Antihypertensive Agent, Combination
Aldactazide® [US/Can]
Apo®-Triazide [Can]
Dyazide® [US]
hydrochlorothiazide and spironolactone
hydrochlorothiazide and triamterene
Maxzide® [US]
Novo-Spirozine [Can]
Novo-Triamzide [Can]
Nu-Triazide [Can]
Antineoplastic Agent
chlorambucil
cyclophosphamide

Cytoxan® [US/Can]
Leukeran® [US/Can]
Neosar® [US]
Procytox® [Can]
Diuretic, Loop
Apo®-Furosemide [Can]
bumetanide
Bumex® [US/Can]
Burinex® [Can]
Demadex® [US]
Furocot® [US]
furosemide
Lasix® Special [Can]
Lasix® [US/Can]
torsemide
Diuretic, Miscellaneous
Apo®-Chlorthalidone [Can]
Apo®-Indapamide [Can]
chlorthalidone
Gen-Indapamide [Can]
indapamide
Lozide® [Can]
Lozol® [US/Can]
metolazone
Mykrox® [US/Can]
Novo-Indapamide [Can]
Nu-Indapamide [Can]
PMS-Indapamide [Can]
Thalitone® [US]
Zaroxolyn® [US/Can]
Diuretic, Thiazide
Apo®-Hydro [Can]
Aquacot® [US]
Aquatensen® [US/Can]
Aquazide H® [US]
bendroflumethiazide
chlorothiazide
Diuril® [US/Can]
Enduron® [US/Can]
Ezide® [US]
hydrochlorothiazide
Hydrocot® [US]
HydroDIURIL® [US/Can]

Metatensin® [Can]
methyclothiazide
Microzide™ [US]
Naqua® [US/Can]
Naturetin® [US]
Oretic® [US]
Trichlorex® [Can]
trichlormethiazide
Zide® [US]
Immunosuppressant Agent
    Alti-Azathioprine [Can]
    azathioprine
    cyclosporine
    Gen-Azathioprine [Can]
    Gengraf™ [US]
    Imuran® [US/Can]
    Neoral® [US/Can]
    Sandimmune® [US/Can]

NEPHROTOXICITY (CISPLATIN-INDUCED)

Antidote
    amifostine
    Ethyol® [US/Can]

NEURALGIA

Analgesic, Nonnarcotic
    Arthropan® [US-OTC]
    choline salicylate
    Teejel® [Can]
Analgesic, Topical
    Antiphlogistine Rub A-535 No
        Odour [Can]
    Antiphogistine Rub A-535 Capsaicin
        [Can]
    Arth Dr® [US]
    Arthricare Hand & Body® [US]
    Born Again Super Pain Relieving®
        [US]
    Caprex Plus® [US]
    Caprex® [US]
    Capsagel Extra Strength® [US]
    Capsagel Maximum Strength®
        [US]

Capsagel® [US]
Capsagesic-HP Arthritis Relief® [US]
capsaicin
Capsin® [US-OTC]
D-Care Circulation Stimulator® [US]
Double Cap® [US]
Icy Hot Arthritis Therapy® [US]
Myoflex® [US/Can]
Pain Enz® [US]
Pharmacist's Capsaicin® [US]
Rid-A-Pain-HP® [US]
Rid-A-Pain® [US]
Sloan's Liniment® [US]
Sportscreme® [US-OTC]
Sportsmed® [US]
Theragen HP® [US]
Theragen® [US]
Therapatch Warm® [US]
triethanolamine salicylate
Trixaicin HP® [US]
Trixaicin® [US]
Zostrix High Potency® [US]
Zostrix®-HP [US/Can]
Zostrix Sports® [US]
Zostrix® [US/Can]
Nonsteroidal Antiinflammatory Drug
    (NSAID)
    Apo®-ASA [Can]
    Asaphen [Can]
    Asaphen E.C. [Can]
    Ascriptin® Arthritis Pain [US-OTC]
    Ascriptin® Enteric [US-OTC]
    Ascriptin® Extra Strength [US-OTC]
    Ascriptin® [US-OTC]
    Aspercin Extra [US-OTC]
    Aspercin [US-OTC]
    Aspergum® [US-OTC]
    aspirin
    Bayer® Aspirin Extra Strength [US-
        OTC]
    Bayer® Aspirin Regimen Regular
        Strength [US-OTC]
    Bayer® Aspirin [US-OTC]

Bayer® Plus Extra Strength [US-OTC]
Bufferin® Arthritis Strength [US-OTC]
Bufferin® Extra Strength [US-OTC]
Bufferin® [US-OTC]
Easprin® [US]
Ecotrin® Maximum Strength [US-OTC]
Ecotrin® [US-OTC]
Entrophen® [Can]
Novasen [Can]
St. Joseph® Pain Reliever [US-OTC]
ZORprin® [US]

NEURITIS (OPTIC)
Adrenal Corticosteroid
A-HydroCort® [US/Can]
Alti-Dexamethasone [Can]
A-methaPred® [US]
Apo®-Prednisone [Can]
Aristocort® Forte Injection [US]
Aristocort® Intralesional Injection [US]
Aristocort® Tablet [US/Can]
Aristospan® Intra-articular Injection [US/Can]
Aristospan® Intralesional Injection [US/Can]
Betaject™ [Can]
betamethasone (systemic)
Betnesol® [Can]
Celestone® Phosphate [US]
Celestone® Soluspan® [US/Can]
Celestone® [US]
Cel-U-Jec® [US]
Cortef® [US/Can]
cortisone acetate
Cortone® [Can]
Decadron®-LA [US]
Decadron® [US/Can]
Decaject-LA® [US]
Decaject® [US]

Delta-Cortef® [US]
Deltasone® [US]
Depo-Medrol® [US/Can]
Depopred® [US]
dexamethasone (systemic)
Dexasone® L.A. [US]
Dexasone® [US/Can]
Dexone® LA [US]
Dexone® [US]
Hexadrol® [US/Can]
hydrocortisone (systemic)
Hydrocortone® Acetate [US]
Kenalog® Injection [US/Can]
Key-Pred-SP® [US]
Key-Pred® [US]
Medrol® Tablet [US/Can]
methylprednisolone
Meticorten® [US]
Orapred™ [US]
Pediapred® [US/Can]
PMS-Dexamethasone [Can]
Prednicot® [US]
prednisolone (systemic)
Prednisol® TBA [US]
prednisone
Prelone® [US]
Solu-Cortef® [US/Can]
Solu-Medrol® [US/Can]
Solurex L.A.® [US]
Sterapred® DS [US]
Sterapred® [US]
Tac™-3 Injection [US]
Triam-A® Injection [US]
triamcinolone (systemic)
Triam Forte® Injection [US]
Winpred™ [Can]

NEUROBLASTOMA
Antineoplastic Agent
Adriamycin® [Can]
Adriamycin PFS® [US]
Adriamycin RDF® [US]
Alkeran® [US/Can]

Caelyx® [Can]
Cosmegen® [US/Can]
cyclophosphamide
Cytoxan® [US/Can]
dacarbazine
dactinomycin
doxorubicin
DTIC® [Can]
DTIC-Dome® [US]
melphalan
Neosar® [US]
Oncovin® [US/Can]
Procytox® [Can]
Rubex® [US]
teniposide
Vincasar® PFS® [US/Can]
vincristine
Vumon® [US/Can]

NEUROGENIC BLADDER

Antispasmodic Agent, Urinary
Ditropan® [US/Can]
Ditropan® XL [US]
Gen-Oxybutynin [Can]
Novo-Oxybutynin [Can]
Nu-Oxybutyn [Can]
oxybutynin
PMS-Oxybutynin [Can]

NEUROLOGIC DISEASE

Adrenal Corticosteroid
Acthar® [US]
A-HydroCort® [US/Can]
Alti-Dexamethasone [Can]
A-methaPred® [US]
Apo®-Prednisone [Can]
Aristocort® Forte Injection [US]
Aristocort® Intralesional Injection
[US]
Aristocort® Tablet [US/Can]
Aristospan® Intra-articular Injection
[US/Can]
Aristospan® Intralesional Injection
[US/Can]

Betaject™ [Can]
betamethasone (systemic)
Betnesol® [Can]
Celestone® Phosphate [US]
Celestone® Soluspan® [US/Can]
Celestone® [US]
Cel-U-Jec® [US]
Cortef® [US/Can]
corticotropin
cortisone acetate
Cortone® [Can]
Decadron®-LA [US]
Decadron® [US/Can]
Decaject-LA® [US]
Decaject® [US]
Delta-Cortef® [US]
Deltasone® [US]
Depo-Medrol® [US/Can]
Depopred® [US]
dexamethasone (systemic)
Dexasone® L.A. [US]
Dexasone® [US/Can]
Dexone® LA [US]
Dexone® [US]
Hexadrol® [US/Can]
H.P. Acthar® Gel [US]
hydrocortisone (systemic)
Hydrocortone® Acetate [US]
Kenalog® Injection [US/Can]
Key-Pred-SP® [US]
Key-Pred® [US]
Medrol® Tablet [US/Can]
methylprednisolone
Meticorten® [US]
Orapred™ [US]
Pediapred® [US/Can]
PMS-Dexamethasone [Can]
Prednicot® [US]
prednisolone (systemic)
Prednisol® TBA [US]
prednisone
Prelone® [US]
Solu-Cortef® [US/Can]

Solu-Medrol® [US/Can]
Solurex L.A.® [US]
Sterapred® DS [US]
Sterapred® [US]
Tac™-3 Injection [US]
Triam-A® Injection [US]
triamcinolone (systemic)
Triam Forte® Injection [US]
Winpred™ [Can]

NEUTROPENIA
Colony-Stimulating Factor
filgrastim
Neupogen® [US/Can]

NOCTURIA
Antispasmodic Agent, Urinary
flavoxate
Urispas® [US/Can]

OBSESSIVE-COMPULSIVE DISORDER (OCD)
Antidepressant, Selective Serotonin
Reuptake Inhibitor
Alti-Fluoxetine [Can]
Alti-Fluvoxamine [Can]
Apo®-Fluoxetine [Can]
Apo®-Fluvoxamine [Can]
Apo®-Sertraline [Can]
fluoxetine
fluvoxamine
Gen-Fluoxetine [Can]
Gen-Fluvoxamine [Can]
Luvox® [Can]
Novo-Fluoxetine [Can]
Novo-Fluvoxamine [Can]
Novo-Sertraline [Can]
Nu-Fluoxetine [Can]
Nu-Fluvoxamine [Can]
paroxetine
Paxil® CR™ [US/Can]
Paxil® [US/Can]
PMS-Fluoxetine [Can]
PMS-Fluvoxamine [Can]

Prozac® [US/Can]
Prozac® Weekly™ [US]
Rhoxal-fluoxetine [Can]
Sarafem™ [US]
sertraline
Zoloft® [US/Can]
Antidepressant, Tricyclic (Tertiary
Amine)
Anafranil® [US/Can]
Apo®-Clomipramine [Can]
clomipramine
Gen-Clomipramine [Can]
Novo-Clopramine [Can]

ONYCHOMYCOSIS
Antifungal Agent
Fulvicin® P/G [US]
Fulvicin-U/F® [US/Can]
Grifulvin® V [US]
griseofulvin
Gris-PEG® [US]
Lamisil® Oral [US/Can]
terbinafine (oral)

OPIOID POISONING
Antidote
nalmefene
naloxone
naltrexone
Narcan® [US/Can]
Revex® [US]
ReVia® [US/Can]

ORAL LESIONS
Local Anesthetic
benzocaine, gelatin, pectin, and
sodium carboxymethylcellulose
Orabase® With Benzocaine [US-
OTC]

ORGAN REJECTION
Immunosuppressant Agent
daclizumab
Zenapax® [US/Can]

ORGAN TRANSPLANT
Immunosuppressant Agent
  basiliximab
  CellCept® [US/Can]
  cyclosporine
  Gengraf™ [US]
  muromonab-CD3
  mycophenolate
  Neoral® [US/Can]
  Orthoclone OKT® 3 [US/Can]
  Prograf® [US/Can]
  Protopic® [US]
  Rapamune® [US/Can]
  Sandimmune® [US/Can]
  Simulect® [US/Can]
  sirolimus
  tacrolimus

OSTEODYSTROPHY
Vitamin D Analog
  calcifediol
  Calciferol™ [US]
  Calcijex™ [US]
  calcitriol
  Calderol® [US/Can]
  DHT™ [US]
  dihydrotachysterol
  Drisdol® [US/Can]
  ergocalciferol
  Hytakerol® [US/Can]
  Ostoforte® [Can]
  Rocaltrol® [US/Can]

OSTEOMALACIA
Vitamin D Analog
  Calciferol™ [US]
  Drisdol® [US/Can]
  ergocalciferol
  Ostoforte® [Can]

OSTEOMYELITIS
Antibiotic, Miscellaneous
  Alti-Clindamycin [Can]
  Cleocin HCl® [US]

Cleocin Pediatric® [US]
Cleocin Phosphate® [US]
Cleocin® [US]
clindamycin
Dalacin® C [Can]
Vancocin® [US/Can]
Vancoled® [US]
vancomycin
Antifungal Agent, Systemic
  Fucidin® [Can]
  fusidic acid (Canada only)
Carbapenem (Antibiotic)
  imipenem and cilastatin
  meropenem
  Merrem® I.V. [US/Can]
  Primaxin® [US/Can]
Cephalosporin (First Generation)
  Ancef® [US/Can]
  Cefadyl® [US/Can]
  cefazolin
  cephalothin
  cephapirin
  Ceporacin® [Can]
  Kefzol® [US/Can]
Cephalosporin (Second Generation)
  Cefotan® [US/Can]
  cefotetan
  cefoxitin
  Ceftin® [US/Can]
  cefuroxime
  Kefurox® [US/Can]
  Mefoxin® [US/Can]
  Zinacef® [US/Can]
Cephalosporin (Third Generation)
  Cefizox® [US/Can]
  Cefobid® [US/Can]
  cefoperazone
  cefotaxime
  ceftazidime
  ceftizoxime
  ceftriaxone
  Ceptaz® [US/Can]
  Claforan® [US/Can]

Fortaz® [US/Can]
Rocephin® [US/Can]
Tazicef® [US]
Tazidime® [US/Can]
Penicillin
  ampicillin and sulbactam
  dicloxacillin
  Dynapen® [US]
  nafcillin
  oxacillin
  ticarcillin and clavulanate potassium
  Timentin® [US/Can]
  Unasyn® [US/Can]
Quinolone
  ciprofloxacin
  Cipro® [US/Can]

OSTEOPOROSIS
Bisphosphonate Derivative
  alendronate
  Aredia® [US/Can]
  Didronel® [US/Can]
  etidronate disodium
  Fosamax® [US/Can]
  pamidronate
Electrolyte Supplement, Oral
  Calbon® [US]
  Calcionate® [US-OTC]
  Calciquid® [US-OTC]
  calcium glubionate
  calcium lactate
  calcium phosphate (dibasic)
  Cal-Lac® [US]
  Posture® [US-OTC]
  Ridactate® [US]
Estrogen and Progestin Combination
  estrogens and medroxyprogesterone
  Premphase® [US/Can]
  Prempro™ [US/Can]
Estrogen Derivative
  Alora® [US]
  Cenestin™ [US/Can]
  Climara® [US/Can]

Congest [Can]
Delestrogen® [US/Can]
Depo®-Estradiol [US/Can]
diethylstilbestrol
Esclim® [US]
Estinyl® [US]
Estrace® [US/Can]
Estraderm® [US/Can]
estradiol
Estratab® [US]
Estring® [US/Can]
Estrogel® [Can]
estrogens (conjugated A/synthetic)
estrogens (conjugated/equine)
estrogens (esterified)
ethinyl estradiol
Gynodiol™ [US]
Honvol® [Can]
Menest® [US]
Oesclim® [Can]
PMS-Conjugated Estrogens [Can]
Premarin® [US/Can]
Stilphostrol® [US]
Vagifem® [US/Can]
Vivelle-Dot® [US]
Vivelle® [US/Can]
Mineral, Oral
  fluoride
Polypeptide Hormone
  Calcimar® [Can]
  calcitonin
  Caltine® [Can]
  Miacalcin® [US/Can]
Selective Estrogen Receptor Modulator
  (SERM)
  Evista® [US/Can]
  raloxifene

OSTEOSARCOMA
Antineoplastic Agent
  Adriamycin® [Can]
  Adriamycin PFS® [US]
  Adriamycin RDF® [US]

Caelyx® [Can]
cisplatin
doxorubicin
methotrexate
Platinol®-AQ [US]
Platinol® [US]
Rheumatrex® [US]
Rubex® [US]
Trexall™ [US]

OTITIS EXTERNA
Aminoglycoside (Antibiotic)
  AKTob® [US]
  Alcomicin® [Can]
  amikacin
  Amikin® [US/Can]
  Diogent® [Can]
  Garamycin® [US/Can]
  Genoptic® [US]
  Gentacidin® [US]
  Gentak® [US]
  gentamicin
  kanamycin
  Kantrex® [US/Can]
  Myciguent [US-OTC]
  Nebcin® [US/Can]
  Neo-Fradin™ [US]
  neomycin
  Neo-Rx [US]
  PMS-Tobramycin [Can]
  TOBI™ [US/Can]
  tobramycin
  Tobrex® [US/Can]
  Tomycine™ [Can]
Antibacterial, Otic
  acetic acid
  VōSol® [US]
Antibiotic/Corticosteroid, Otic
  Acetasol® HC [US]
  acetic acid, propylene glycol diacetate, and hydrocortisone
  AntibiOtic® Ear [US]
  ciprofloxacin and hydrocortisone

Cipro® HC Otic [US/Can]
Coly-Mycin® S Otic [US]
Cortimyxin® [Can]
Cortisporin® Otic [US/Can]
Cortisporin®-TC Otic [US]
neomycin, colistin, hydrocortisone, and thonzonium
neomycin, polymyxin B, and hydrocortisone
PediOtic® [US]
VōSol® HC [US/Can]
Antibiotic, Otic
  chloramphenicol
  Diochloram® [Can]
  Floxin® [US/Can]
  ofloxacin
Antifungal/Corticosteroid
  Dermazene® [US]
  iodoquinol and hydrocortisone
  Vytone® [US]
Cephalosporin (Third Generation)
  ceftazidime
  Ceptaz® [US/Can]
  Fortaz® [US/Can]
  Tazicef® [US]
  Tazidime® [US/Can]
Corticosteroid, Topical
  Aclovate® [US]
  Acticort® [US]
  Aeroseb-HC® [US]
  alclometasone
  Alphatrex® [US]
  amcinonide
  Aquacort® [Can]
  Aristocort® A Topical [US]
  Aristocort® Topical [US/Can]
  Betaderm® [Can]
  Betamethacot® [US]
  betamethasone (topical)
  Betatrex® [US]
  Beta-Val® [US]
  Betnovate® [Can]
  CaldeCORT® Anti-Itch Spray [US]

CaldeCORT® [US-OTC]
Capex™ [US/Can]
Carmol-HC® [US]
Celestoderm®-EV/2 [Can]
Celestoderm®-V [Can]
Cetacort®
clobetasol
Clocort® Maximum Strength [US-OTC]
clocortolone
Cloderm® [US/Can]
Cordran® SP [US]
Cordran® [US/Can]
Cormax® [US]
CortaGel® [US-OTC]
Cortaid® Maximum Strength [US-OTC]
Cortaid® with Aloe [US-OTC]
Cort-Dome® [US]
Cortizone®-5 [US-OTC]
Cortizone®-10 [US-OTC]
Cortoderm [Can]
Cutivate™ [US]
Cyclocort® [US/Can]
Del-Beta® [US]
Delcort® [US]
Dermacort® [US]
Dermarest Dricort® [US]
Derma-Smoothe/FS® [US/Can]
Dermatop® [US]
Dermolate® [US-OTC]
Dermovate® [Can]
Dermtex® HC with Aloe [US-OTC]
Desocort® [Can]
desonide
DesOwen® [US]
desoximetasone
diflorasone
Diprolene® AF [US]
Diprolene® [US/Can]
Diprosone® [US/Can]
Ectosone [Can]
Eldecort® [US]

Elocon® [US/Can]
fluocinolone
fluocinonide
Fluoderm [Can]
flurandrenolide
fluticasone (topical)
Gen-Clobetasol [Can]
halcinonide
halobetasol
Halog®-E [US]
Halog® [US/Can]
Hi-Cor-1.0® [US]
Hi-Cor-2.5® [US]
Hyderm [Can]
hydrocortisone (topical)
Hydrocort® [US]
Hydro-Tex® [US-OTC]
Hytone® [US]
LactiCare-HC® [US]
Lanacort® [US-OTC]
Lidemol® [Can]
Lidex-E® [US]
Lidex® [US/Can]
Locoid® [US/Can]
Luxiq™ [US]
Lyderm® [Can]
Lydonide [Can]
Maxiflor® [US]
Maxivate® [US]
mometasone furoate
Novo-Clobetasol [Can]
Nutracort® [US]
Olux™ [US]
Orabase® HCA [US]
Penecort® [US]
prednicarbate
Prevex® [Can]
Prevex® HC [Can]
Psorcon™ E [US]
Psorcon™ [US/Can]
Qualisone® [US]
Sarna® HC [Can]
S-T Cort® [US]

Synacort® [US]
Synalar® [US/Can]
Taro-Desoximetasone [Can]
Taro-Sone® [Can]
Tegrin®-HC [US-OTC]
Temovate® [US]
Texacort® [US]
Tiamol® [Can]
Ti-U-Lac® H [Can]
Topicort®-LP [US]
Topicort® [US/Can]
Topilene® [Can]
Topisone®
Topsyn® [Can]
Triacet™ Topical [US] Oracort [Can]
Triaderm [Can]
triamcinolone (topical)
Tridesilon® [US]
U-Cort™ [US]
Ultravate™ [US/Can]
urea and hydrocortisone
Uremol® HC [Can]
Valisone® Scalp Lotion [Can]
Westcort® [US/Can]
Local Anesthetic
Americaine® [US-OTC]
benzocaine
Otic Agent, Analgesic
A/B® Otic [US]
Allergan® Ear Drops [US]
antipyrine and benzocaine
Auralgan® [US/Can]
Aurodex® [US]
Auroto® [US]
Benzotic® [US]
Dec-Agesic® A.B. [US]
Dolotic® [US]
Rx-Otic® Drops [US]
Otic Agent, Antiinfective
aluminum acetate and acetic acid
Cresylate® [US]
m-cresyl acetate
Otic Domeboro® [US]

Quinolone
ciprofloxacin
Cipro® [US/Can]
lomefloxacin
Maxaquin® [US]
nalidixic acid
NegGram® [US/Can]

OTITIS MEDIA
Antibiotic, Carbacephem
Lorabid™ [US/Can]
loracarbef
Antibiotic, Miscellaneous
Primsol® [US]
Proloprim® [US/Can]
trimethoprim
Antibiotic, Otic
Apo®-Oflox [Can]
Floxin® [US/Can]
ofloxacin
Antibiotic, Penicillin
pivampicillin (Canada only)
Pondocillin® [Can]
Cephalosporin (First Generation)
Apo®-Cefadroxil [Can]
Apo®-Cephalex [Can]
Biocef® [US]
cefadroxil
cephalexin
Duricef® [US/Can]
Keflex® [US]
Keftab® [US/Can]
Novo-Cefadroxil [Can]
Novo-Lexin® [Can]
Nu-Cephalex® [Can]
Cephalosporin (Second
    Generation)
Apo®-Cefaclor [Can]
Ceclor® CD [US]
Ceclor® [US/Can]
cefaclor
cefpodoxime
cefprozil

Ceftin® [US/Can]
cefuroxime
Cefzil® [US/Can]
Kefurox® [US/Can]
Novo-Cefaclor [Can]
Nu-Cefaclor [Can]
PMS-Cefaclor [Can]
Vantin® [US/Can]
Zinacef® [US/Can]
Cephalosporin (Third Generation)
Cedax® [US]
cefdinir
cefixime
ceftibuten
Omnicef® [US/Can]
Suprax® [US/Can]
Macrolide (Antibiotic)
Apo®-Erythro Base [Can]
Apo®-Erythro E-C [Can]
Apo®-Erythro-ES [Can]
Apo®-Erythro-S [Can]
Diomycin® [Can]
E.E.S.® [US/Can]
Erybid™ [Can]
Eryc® [US/Can]
EryPed® [US]
Ery-Tab® [US]
Erythrocin® [US/Can]
erythromycin and sulfisoxazole
erythromycin (systemic)
Eryzole® [US]
Nu-Erythromycin-S [Can]
PCE® [US/Can]
Pediazole® [US/Can]
PMS-Erythromycin [Can]
Otic Agent, Analgesic
A/B® Otic [US]
Allergan® Ear Drops [US]
antipyrine and benzocaine
Auralgan® [US/Can]
Aurodex® [US]
Auroto® [US]
Benzotic® [US]

Dec-Agesic® A.B. [US]
Dolotic® [US]
Rx-Otic® Drops [US]
Penicillin
amoxicillin
amoxicillin and clavulanate
potassium
Amoxicot® [US]
Amoxil® [US/Can]
ampicillin
Apo®-Amoxi [Can]
Apo®-Ampi [Can]
Augmentin ES-600™ [US]
Augmentin® [US/Can]
Clavulin® [Can]
Gen-Amoxicillin [Can]
Lin-Amox [Can]
Marcillin® [US]
Moxilin® [US]
Novamoxin® [Can]
Novo-Ampicillin [Can]
Nu-Amoxi [Can]
Nu-Ampi [Can]
Principen® [US]
Trimox® [US]
Wymox® [US]
Sulfonamide
Apo®-Sulfatrim [Can]
Bactrim™ DS [US]
Bactrim™ [US]
erythromycin and sulfisoxazole
Eryzole® [US]
Gantrisin® Pediatric Suspension
[US]
Novo-Trimel [Can]
Novo-Trimel D.S. [Can]
Nu-Cotrimox® [Can]
Pediazole® [US/Can]
Septra® DS [US/Can]
Septra® [US/Can]
sulfamethoxazole and tri-
methoprim
Sulfatrim® DS [US]

Sulfatrim® [US]
sulfisoxazole
Sulfizole® [Can]
Truxazole® [US]
Tetracycline Derivative
Adoxa™ [US]
Alti-Minocycline [Can]
Apo®-Doxy [Can]
Apo®-Doxy Tabs [Can]
Apo®-Minocycline [Can]
Apo®-Tetra [Can]
Brodspec® [US]
Doryx® [US]
Doxy-100™ [US]
Doxycin [Can]
doxycycline
Doxytec [Can]
Dynacin® [US]
EmTet® [US]
Gen-Minocycline [Can]
Minocin® [US/Can]
minocycline
Monodox® [US]
Novo-Doxylin [Can]
Novo-Minocycline [Can]
Novo-Tetra [Can]
Nu-Doxycycline [Can]
Nu-Tetra [Can]
oxytetracycline
Periostat® [US]
Rhoxal-Minocycline [Can]
Sumycin® [US]
Terramycin® I.M. [US/Can]
tetracycline
Vibramycin® [US]
Vibra-Tabs® [US/Can]
Wesmycin® [US]

OVERACTIVE BLADDER
Anticholinergic Agent
Detrol® LA [US]
Detrol® [US/Can]
tolterodine

OVULATION INDUCTION
Gonadotropin
Chorex® [US]
chorionic gonadotropin (human)
chorionic gonadotropin (recombinant)
Humegon™ [US]
menotropins
Novarel™ [US]
Ovidrel® [US]
Pergonal® [US/Can]
Pregnyl® [US/Can]
Profasi® HP [Can]
Profasi® [US]
Repronex® [US]
Ovulation Stimulator
chorionic gonadotropin (recombinant)
Clomid® [US/Can]
clomiphene
Fertinex® [US]
Fertinorm® H.P. [Can]
Metrodin® [US]
Ovidrel® [US]
Serophene® [US/Can]
urofollitropin

PAGET DISEASE OF BONE
Antidote
Mithracin® [US/Can]
plicamycin
Bisphosphonate Derivative
alendronate
Aredia® [US/Can]
Didronel® [US/Can]
etidronate disodium
Fosamax® [US/Can]
pamidronate
Skelid® [US]
tiludronate
Polypeptide Hormone
Calcimar® [Can]
calcitonin

Caltine® [Can]
Miacalcin® [US/Can]

PAIN (ANOGENITAL)
Anesthetic/Corticosteroid
Analpram-HC® [US]
Enzone® [US]
Epifoam® [US]
Pramosone® [US]
Pramox® HC [Can]
pramoxine and hydrocortisone
ProctoFoam®-HC [US/Can]
Zone-A Forte® [US]
Local Anesthetic
Americaine® Anesthetic Lubricant
[US]
Americaine® [US-OTC]
Ametop™ [Can]
Anbesol® Baby [US/Can]
Anbesol® Maximum Strength [US-
OTC]
Anbesol® [US-OTC]
Anusol® [US-OTC]
Babee® Teething® [US-OTC]
benzocaine
Benzodent® [US-OTC]
Chiggerex® [US-OTC]
Chiggertox® [US-OTC]
Cylex® [US-OTC]
Detane® [US-OTC]
dibucaine
Dyclone® [US]
dyclonine
Fleet® Pain Relief [US-OTC]
Foille® Medicated First Aid [US-
OTC]
Foille® Plus [US-OTC]
Foille® [US-OTC]
HDA® Toothache [US-OTC]
Hurricaine® [US]
Itch-X® [US-OTC]
Mycinettes® [US-OTC]
Nupercainal® [US-OTC]

Orabase®-B [US-OTC]
Orajel® Baby Nighttime [US-OTC]
Orajel® Baby [US-OTC]
Orajel® Maximum Strength [US-
OTC]
Orajel® [US-OTC]
Orasol® [US-OTC]
Phicon® [US-OTC]
Pontocaine® [US/Can]
PrameGel® [US-OTC]
pramoxine
Prax® [US-OTC]
ProctoFoam® NS [US-OTC]
Solarcaine® [US-OTC]
Sucrets® [US-OTC]
tetracaine
Trocaine® [US-OTC]
Tronolane® [US-OTC]
Tronothane® [US-OTC]
Zilactin® Baby [US/Can]
Zilactin®-B [US/Can]

PAIN (BONE)
Radiopharmaceutical
Metastron® [US/Can]
strontium-89

PAIN (DIABETIC NEUROPATHY NEURALGIA)
Analgesic, Topical
Antiphogistine Rub A-535 Capsaicin
[Can]
Arth Dr® [US]
Arthricare Hand & Body® [US]
Born Again Super Pain Relieving®
[US]
Caprex Plus® [US]
Caprex® [US]
Capsagel Extra Strength® [US]
Capsagel Maximum Strength® [US]
Capsagel® [US]
Capsagesic-HP Arthritis Relief® [US]

capsaicin
Capsin® [US-OTC]
D-Care Circulation Stimulator® [US]
Double Cap® [US]
Icy Hot Arthritis Therapy® [US]
Pain Enz® [US]
Pharmacist's Capsaicin® [US]
Rid-A-Pain-HP® [US]
Rid-A-Pain® [US]
Sloan's Liniment® [US]
Sportsmed® [US]
Theragen HP® [US]
Theragen® [US]
Therapatch Warm® [US]
Trixaicin HP® [US]
Trixaicin® [US]
Zostrix High Potency® [US]
Zostrix®-HP [US/Can]
Zostrix Sports® [US]
Zostrix® [US/Can]

PAIN (LUMBAR PUNCTURE)
Analgesic, Topical
EMLA® [US/Can]
lidocaine and prilocaine

PAIN (MUSCLE)
Analgesic, Topical
dichlorodifluoromethane and
trichloromonofluoromethane
Fluori-Methane® [US]

PAIN (SKIN GRAFT HARVESTING)
Analgesic, Topical
EMLA® [US/Can]
lidocaine and prilocaine

PANCREATIC EXOCRINE INSUFFICIENCY
Enzyme
Cotazym-S® [US]
Cotazym® [US/Can]

Creon® 5 [US/Can]
Creon® 10 [US/Can]
Creon® 20 [US/Can]
Creon® 25 [Can]
Kutrase® [US]
Ku-Zyme® HP [US]
Ku-Zyme® [US]
Lipram® [US]
Pancrease® MT 4 [US/Can]
Pancrease® MT 10 [US/Can]
Pancrease® MT 16 [US/Can]
Pancrease® MT 20 [US/Can]
Pancrease® [US]
Pancrecarb MS-4® [US]
Pancrecarb MS-8® [US]
pancrelipase
Ultrase® MT12 [US/Can]
Ultrase® MT18 [US/Can]
Ultrase® MT20 [US/Can]
Ultrase® [US/Can]
Viokase® [US/Can]

PANCREATIC EXOCRINE INSUFFICIENCY (DIAGNOSTIC)
Diagnostic Agent
SecreFlo™ [US]
secretin

PANCREATITIS
Anticholinergic Agent
Propanthel™ [Can]
propantheline

PANIC ATTACK
Benzodiazepine
alprazolam
Alprazolam Intensol® [US]
Alti-Alprazolam [Can]
Apo®-Alpraz [Can]
Apo®-Temazepam [Can]
Gen-Alprazolam [Can]
Gen-Temazepam [Can]
Novo-Alprazol [Can]

Novo-Temazepam [Can]
Nu-Alprax [Can]
Nu-Temazepam [Can]
PMS-Temazepam [Can]
Restoril® [US/Can]
temazepam
Xana TS™ [Can]
Xanax® [US/Can]

PANIC DISORDER (PD)

Antidepressant, Selective Serotonin
    Reuptake Inhibitor
paroxetine
Paxil® CR™ [US/Can]
Paxil® [US/Can]

PARALYTIC ILEUS (PROPHYLAXIS)

Gastrointestinal Agent, Stimulant
dexpanthenol
D-Pan® Plus [US-OTC]
D-Pan® [US]

PARKINSONISM

Anti-Parkinson Agent
Akineton® [US/Can]
amantadine
Apo®-Benztropine [Can]
Apo® Bromocriptine [Can]
Apo®-Trihex [Can]
Artane® [US]
benserazide and levodopa (Canada
    only)
benztropine
biperiden
bromocriptine
Cogentin® [US/Can]
Comtan® [US/Can]
Endantadine® [Can]
entacapone
Kemadrin® [US/Can]
Parlodel® [US/Can]
PMS-Amantadine [Can]
PMS-Bromocriptine [Can]

Procyclid™ [Can]
procyclidine
Prolapa® [Can]
ReQuip® [US/Can]
ropinirole
Symmetrel® [US/Can]
Tasmar® [US]
tolcapone
trihexyphenidyl
Dopaminergic Agent (Anti-Parkinson)
Apo®-Levocarb [Can]
Apo®-Selegiline [Can]
Atapryl® [US]
carbidopa
Eldepryl® [US/Can]
Endo®-Levodopa/Carbidopa [Can]
Gen-Selegiline [Can]
levodopa
levodopa and carbidopa
Lodosyn® [US]
Mirapex® [US/Can]
Novo-Selegiline [Can]
Nu-Levocarb [Can]
Nu-Selegiline [Can]
pergolide
Permax® [US/Can]
pramipexole
selegiline
Selpak® [US]
Sinemet® CR [US/Can]
Sinemet® [US/Can]
Reverse COMT Inhibitor
Comtan® [US/Can]
entacapone

PARKINSON DISEASE

Anti-Parkinson Agent
ethopropazine (Canada only)
Parsitan® [Can]

PELVIC INFLAMMATORY DISEASE (PID)

Aminoglycoside (Antibiotic)
AKTob® [US]

Alcomicin® [Can]
amikacin
Amikin® [US/Can]
Diogent® [Can]
Garamycin® [US/Can]
Garatec [Can]
Gentacidin® [US]
Gentak® [US]
gentamicin
Nebcin® [US/Can]
PMS-Tobramycin [Can]
TOBI™ [US/Can]
tobramycin
Tobrex® [US/Can]
Tomycine™ [Can]
Cephalosporin (Second Generation)
Cefotan® [US/Can]
cefotetan
cefoxitin
Mefoxin® [US/Can]
Cephalosporin (Third Generation)
Cefizox® [US/Can]
Cefobid® [US/Can]
cefoperazone
cefotaxime
ceftizoxime
ceftriaxone
Claforan® [US/Can]
Rocephin® [US/Can]
Macrolide (Antibiotic)
Apo®-Erythro Base [Can]
Apo®-Erythro E-C [Can]
Apo®-Erythro-ES [Can]
Apo®-Erythro-S [Can]
azithromycin
Diomycin® [Can]
E.E.S.® [US/Can]
Erybid™ [Can]
Eryc® [US/Can]
EryPed® [US]
Ery-Tab® [US]
Erythrocin® [US/Can]
erythromycin (systemic)

Nu-Erythromycin-S [Can]
PCE® [US/Can]
PMS-Erythromycin [Can]
Zithromax® [US/Can]
Z-PAK® [US/Can]
Penicillin
ampicillin and sulbactam
piperacillin
piperacillin and tazobactam sodium
Pipracil® [US/Can]
Tazocin® [Can]
ticarcillin
ticarcillin and clavulanate
  potassium
Ticar® [US]
Timentin® [US/Can]
Unasyn® [US/Can]
Zosyn® [US]
Quinolone
Apo®-Oflox [Can]
ciprofloxacin
Cipro® [US/Can]
Floxin® [US/Can]
ofloxacin
Tetracycline Derivative
Adoxa™ [US]
Apo®-Doxy [Can]
Apo®-Doxy Tabs [Can]
Apo®-Tetra [Can]
Brodspec® [US]
Doryx® [US]
Doxy-100™ [US]
Doxycin [Can]
doxycycline
Doxytec [Can]
EmTet® [US]
Monodox® [US]
Novo-Doxylin [Can]
Novo-Tetra [Can]
Nu-Doxycycline [Can]
Nu-Tetra [Can]
Periostat® [US]
Sumycin® [US]

tetracycline
Vibramycin® [US]
Vibra-Tabs® [US/Can]
Wesmycin® [US]

PEPTIC ULCER
Antibiotic, Miscellaneous
   Apo®-Metronidazole [Can]
   Flagyl ER® [US]
   Flagyl® [US/Can]
   metronidazole
   Nidagel™ [Can]
   Noritate™ [US/Can]
   Novo-Nidazol [Can]
Anticholinergic Agent
   Anaspaz® [US]
   Antispas® Tablet [US]
   Apo®-Chlorax [Can]
   A-Spas® S/L [US]
   atropine
   belladonna
   Cantil® [US/Can]
   clidinium and chlordiazepoxide
   Cystospaz-M® [US]
   Cystospaz® [US/Can]
   Donnapine® [US]
   Donnatal® [US]
   glycopyrrolate
   Haponal® [US]
   Hyonatol® [US]
   hyoscyamine
   hyoscyamine, atropine, scopolamine,
     and phenobarbital
   Hyosine [US]
   Hypersed® [US]
   Levbid® [US]
   Levsinex® [US]
   Levsin/SL® [US]
   Levsin® [US/Can]
   Librax® [US/Can]
   mepenzolate
   methscopolamine
   NuLev™ [US]

Pamine® [US/Can]
Propanthel™ [Can]
propantheline
Robinul® Forte [US]
Robinul® [US]
Spacol T/S [US]
Spacol [US]
Symax SL [US]
Symax SR [US]
Antidiarrheal
   bismuth subsalicylate, metronidazole,
     and tetracycline
   Helidac™ [US]
Gastric Acid Secretion Inhibitor
   lansoprazole
   omeprazole
   Prevacid® [US/Can]
   Prilosec® [US/Can]
Gastrointestinal Agent, Gastric or
    Duodenal Ulcer Treatment
   Apo®-Sucralate [Can]
   Carafate® [US]
   Novo-Sucralate [Can]
   Nu-Sucralate [Can]
   PMS-Sucralate [Can]
   sucralfate
   Sulcrate® [Can]
   Sulcrate® Suspension Plus [Can]
Gastrointestinal Agent, Miscellaneous
   Bismatrol® [US-OTC]
   bismuth subsalicylate
   Diotame® [US-OTC]
   Pepto-Bismol® [US-OTC]
Histamine H2 Antagonist
   Acid Reducer 200® [US-OTC]
   Alti-Famotidine [Can]
   Alti-Ranitidine [Can]
   Apo®-Cimetidine [Can]
   Apo®-Famotidine [Can]
   Apo®-Nizatidine [Can]
   Apo®-Ranitidine [Can]
   Axid® AR [US-OTC]
   Axid® [US/Can]

cimetidine
famotidine
Gen-Cimetidine [Can]
Gen-Famotidine [Can]
Gen-Ranitidine [Can]
Heartburn 200® [US-OTC]
Heartburn Relief 200®
   [US-OTC]
nizatidine
Novo-Cimetidine [Can]
Novo-Famotidine [Can]
Novo-Nizatidine [Can]
Novo-Ranidine [Can]
Nu-Cimet® [Can]
Nu-Famotidine [Can]
Nu-Ranit [Can]
Pepcid® AC [US/Can]
Pepcid® [US/Can]
PMS-Cimetidine [Can]
ranitidine hydrochloride
Rhoxal-famotidine [Can]
Tagamet® HB [US/Can]
Tagamet® [US/Can]
Ulcidine® [Can]
Zantac® 75 [US-OTC]
Zanta [Can]
Zantac® [US/Can]
Macrolide (Antibiotic)
Biaxin® [US/Can]
Biaxin® XL [US]
clarithromycin
Penicillin
amoxicillin
Amoxicot® [US]
Amoxil® [US/Can]
Apo®-Amoxi [Can]
Gen-Amoxicillin [Can]
Lin-Amox [Can]
Moxilin® [US]
Novamoxin® [Can]
Nu-Amoxi [Can]
Trimox® [US]
Wymox® [US]

PERIANAL WART
Immune Response Modifier
Aldara™ [US/Can]
imiquimod

PERIPHERAL VASCULAR DISEASE
Vasodilator, Peripheral
cyclandelate

PERIPHERAL VASOSPASTIC DISORDER
Alpha-Adrenergic Blocking Agent
Priscoline® [US]
tolazoline

PERSISTENT PULMONARY HYPERTENSION OF THE NEWBORN (PPHN)
Alpha-Adrenergic Blocking Agent
Priscoline® [US]
tolazoline

PERSISTENT PULMONARY VASOCONSTRICTION
Alpha-Adrenergic Blocking Agent
Priscoline® [US]
tolazoline

PERTUSSIS
Toxoid
Adacel® [Can]
Daptacel™ [US]
diphtheria, tetanus toxoids, and acellular pertussis vaccine
diphtheria, tetanus toxoids, and acellular pertussis vaccine and
   Haemophilus B conjugate
   vaccine
diphtheria, tetanus toxoids, and
   whole-cell pertussis vaccine
diphtheria, tetanus toxoids, whole-
   cell pertussis, and *Haemophilus* B
   conjugate vaccine

Infanrix® [US]
Pentacel™ [Can]
TriHIBit® [US]
Tripedia® [US]
Vaccine, Inactivated Bacteria
diphtheria, tetanus toxoids, and acel-
lular pertussis vaccine and
Haemophilus B conjugate vaccine
TriHIBit® [US]

PHARYNGITIS
Antibiotic, Penicillin
pivampicillin (Canada only)
Pondocillin® [Can]
Cephalosporin (First Generation)
Apo®-Cefadroxil [Can]
Apo®-Cephalex [Can]
Biocef® [US]
cefadroxil
cephalexin
Duricef® [US/Can]
Keflex® [US]
Keftab® [US/Can]
Novo-Cefadroxil [Can]
Novo-Lexin® [Can]
Nu-Cephalex® [Can]
Cephalosporin (Second Generation)
cefpodoxime
cefprozil
Ceftin® [US/Can]
cefuroxime
Cefzil® [US/Can]
Kefurox® [US/Can]
Vantin® [US/Can]
Zinacef® [US/Can]
Cephalosporin (Third Generation)
Cedax® [US]
ceftibuten
Macrolide (Antibiotic)
Apo®-Erythro Base [Can]
Apo®-Erythro E-C [Can]
Apo®-Erythro-ES [Can]
Apo®-Erythro-S [Can]

azithromycin
Diomycin® [Can]
E.E.S.® [US/Can]
Erybid™ [Can]
Eryc® [US/Can]
EryPed® [US]
Ery-Tab® [US]
Erythrocin® [US/Can]
erythromycin (systemic)
Nu-Erythromycin-S [Can]
PCE® [US/Can]
PMS-Erythromycin [Can]
Zithromax® [US/Can]
Z-PAK® [US/Can]
Penicillin
amoxicillin
Amoxicot® [US]
Amoxil® [US/Can]
ampicillin
Apo®-Amoxi [Can]
Apo®-Ampi [Can]
Apo®-Pen VK [Can]
Bicillin® C-R 900/300 [US]
Bicillin® C-R [US]
Bicillin® L-A [US]
Gen-Amoxicillin [Can]
Lin-Amox [Can]
Marcillin® [US]
Moxilin® [US]
Nadopen-V® [Can]
Novamoxin® [Can]
Novo-Ampicillin [Can]
Novo-Pen-VK® [Can]
Nu-Amoxi [Can]
Nu-Ampi [Can]
Nu-Pen-VK® [Can]
penicillin G benzathine
penicillin G benzathine and procaine
combined
penicillin G procaine
penicillin V potassium
Permapen® [US]
Principen® [US]

PVF® K [Can]
Suspen® [US]
Trimox® [US]
Truxcillin® [US]
Veetids® [US]
Wycillin® [US/Can]
Wymox® [US]
Tetracycline Derivative
Adoxa™ [US]
Alti-Minocycline [Can]
Apo®-Doxy [Can]
Apo®-Doxy Tabs [Can]
Apo®-Minocycline [Can]
Apo®-Tetra [Can]
Brodspec® [US]
Doryx® [US]
Doxy-100™ [US]
Doxycin [Can]
doxycycline
Doxytec [Can]
Dynacin® [US]
EmTet® [US]
Gen-Minocycline [Can]
Minocin® [US/Can]
minocycline
Monodox® [US]
Novo-Doxylin [Can]
Novo-Minocycline [Can]
Novo-Tetra [Can]
Nu-Doxycycline [Can]
Nu-Tetra [Can]
oxytetracycline
Periostat® [US]
Rhoxal-Minocycline [Can]
Sumycin® [US]
Terramycin® I.M. [US/Can]
tetracycline
Vibramycin® [US]
Vibra-Tabs® [US/Can]
Wesmycin® [US]

PINWORMS
Anthelmintic
Ascarel® [US-OTC]
Combantrin™ [Can]
mebendazole
Pamix® [US-OTC]
Pin-X® [US-OTC]
pyrantel pamoate
Reese's® Pinworm Medicine [US-OTC]
Vermox® [US/Can]

PLANTAR WART
Keratolytic Agent
Duofilm® Solution [US]
salicylic acid and lactic acid
Topical Skin Product
silver nitrate

PNEUMOCYSTIS CARINII
Antibiotic, Miscellaneous
Neutrexin® [US]
Primsol® [US]
Proloprim® [US/Can]
trimethoprim
trimetrexate glucuronate
Antiprotozoal
atovaquone
Mepron™ [US/Can]
NebuPent™ [US]
Pentacarinat® [Can]
Pentam-300® [US]
pentamidine
Sulfonamide
Apo®-Sulfatrim [Can]
Bactrim™ DS [US]
Bactrim™ [US]
Novo-Trimel [Can]
Novo-Trimel D.S. [Can]
Nu-Cotrimox® [Can]
Septra® DS [US/Can]
Septra® [US/Can]
sulfamethoxazole and trimethoprim
Sulfatrim® DS [US]
Sulfatrim® [US]
Sulfone
dapsone

PNEUMONIA

Aminoglycoside (Antibiotic)
  AKTob® [US]
  Alcomicin® [Can]
  amikacin
  Amikin® [US/Can]
  Diogent® [Can]
  Garamycin® [US/Can]
  Garatec [Can]
  Gentacidin® [US]
  Gentak® [US]
  gentamicin
  Nebcin® [US/Can]
  PMS-Tobramycin [Can]
  tobramycin
  Tobrex® [US/Can]
  Tomycine™ [Can]
Antibiotic, Carbapenem
  ertapenem
  Invanz™ [US]
Antibiotic, Miscellaneous
  Alti-Clindamycin [Can]
  Azactam® [US/Can]
  aztreonam
  Cleocin HCl® [US]
  Cleocin Pediatric® [US]
  Cleocin Phosphate® [US]
  Cleocin® [US]
  clindamycin
  Dalacin® C [Can]
  Vancocin® [US/Can]
  Vancoled® [US]
  vancomycin
Antibiotic, Penicillin
  pivampicillin (Canada only)
  Pondocillin® [Can]
Antibiotic, Quinolone
  gatifloxacin
  Levaquin® [US/Can]
  levofloxacin
  Tequin® [US/Can]
Carbapenem (Antibiotic)
  imipenem and cilastatin

  meropenem
  Merrem® I.V. [US/Can]
  Primaxin® [US/Can]
Cephalosporin (First Generation)
  Ancef® [US/Can]
  Apo®-Cefadroxil [Can]
  Apo®-Cephalex [Can]
  Biocef® [US]
  cefadroxil
  Cefadyl® [US/Can]
  cefazolin
  cephalexin
  cephalothin
  cephapirin
  cephradine
  Ceporacin® [Can]
  Duricef® [US/Can]
  Keflex® [US]
  Keftab® [US/Can]
  Kefzol® [US/Can]
  Novo-Cefadroxil [Can]
  Novo-Lexin® [Can]
  Nu-Cephalex® [Can]
  Velosef® [US]
Cephalosporin (Second Generation)
  Cefotan® [US/Can]
  cefotetan
  cefoxitin
  cefpodoxime
  cefprozil
  Ceftin® [US/Can]
  cefuroxime
  Cefzil® [US/Can]
  Kefurox® [US/Can]
  Mefoxin® [US/Can]
  Vantin® [US/Can]
  Zinacef® [US/Can]
Cephalosporin (Third Generation)
  cefdinir
  cefixime
  Cefizox® [US/Can]
  Cefobid® [US/Can]
  cefoperazone

cefotaxime
ceftazidime
ceftizoxime
ceftriaxone
Ceptaz® [US/Can]
Claforan® [US/Can]
Fortaz® [US/Can]
Omnicef® [US/Can]
Rocephin® [US/Can]
Suprax® [US/Can]
Tazicef® [US]
Tazidime® [US/Can]
Cephalosporin (Fourth Generation)
cefepime
Maxipime® [US/Can]
Macrolide (Antibiotic)
Apo®-Erythro Base [Can]
Apo®-Erythro E-C [Can]
Apo®-Erythro-ES [Can]
Apo®-Erythro-S [Can]
azithromycin
Biaxin® [US/Can]
Biaxin® XL [US]
clarithromycin
Diomycin® [Can]
dirithromycin
Dynabac® [US]
E.E.S.® [US/Can]
Erybid™ [Can]
Eryc® [US/Can]
EryPed® [US]
Ery-Tab® [US]
Erythrocin® [US/Can]
erythromycin (systemic)
Nu-Erythromycin-S [Can]
PCE® [US/Can]
PMS-Erythromycin [Can]
Zithromax® [US/Can]
Z-PAK® [US/Can]
Penicillin
amoxicillin
amoxicillin and clavulanate
  potassium

Amoxicot® [US]
Amoxil® [US/Can]
ampicillin
ampicillin and sulbactam
Apo®-Amoxi [Can]
Apo®-Ampi [Can]
Apo®-Cloxi [Can]
Apo®-Pen VK [Can]
Augmentin ES-600™ [US]
Augmentin® [US/Can]
Bicillin® C-R 900/300 [US]
Bicillin® C-R [US]
Bicillin® L-A [US]
carbenicillin
Clavulin® [Can]
cloxacillin
dicloxacillin
Dynapen® [US]
Gen-Amoxicillin [Can]
Geocillin® [US]
Lin-Amox [Can]
Marcillin® [US]
Moxilin® [US]
Nadopen-V® [Can]
nafcillin
Novamoxin® [Can]
Novo-Ampicillin [Can]
Novo-Cloxin [Can]
Novo-Pen-VK® [Can]
Nu-Amoxi [Can]
Nu-Ampi [Can]
Nu-Cloxi® [Can]
Nu-Pen-VK® [Can]
oxacillin
penicillin G benzathine
penicillin G benzathine and procaine
  combined
penicillin G (parenteral/aqueous)
penicillin G procaine
penicillin V potassium
Permapen® [US]
Pfizerpen® [US/Can]
piperacillin

piperacillin and tazobactam sodium
Pipracil® [US/Can]
Principen® [US]
PVF® K [Can]
Suspen® [US]
Tazocin® [Can]
ticarcillin
ticarcillin and clavulanate potassium
Ticar® [US]
Timentin® [US/Can]
Trimox® [US]
Truxcillin® [US]
Unasyn® [US/Can]
Veetids® [US]
Wycillin® [US/Can]
Wymox® [US]
Zosyn® [US]
Quinolone
Apo®-Oflox [Can]
ciprofloxacin
Cipro® [US/Can]
Floxin® [US/Can]
lomefloxacin
Maxaquin® [US]
ofloxacin
sparfloxacin
Zagam® [US]
Sulfonamide
Apo®-Sulfatrim [Can]
Bactrim™ DS [US]
Bactrim™ [US]
Novo-Trimel [Can]
Novo-Trimel D.S. [Can]
Nu-Cotrimox® [Can]
Septra® DS [US/Can]
Septra® [US/Can]
sulfamethoxazole and trimethoprim
Sulfatrim® DS [US]
Sulfatrim® [US]
Vaccine
pneumococcal conjugate vaccine (7-valent)
Prevnar™ [US]

Vaccine, Inactivated Bacteria
Pneumo 23™ [Can]
pneumococcal vaccine
Pneumovax® 23 [US/Can]
Pnu-Imune® 23 [US]

PNEUMONIA, COMMUNITY-ACQUIRED
Antibiotic, Quinolone
ABC Pack™ (Avelox®) [US]
Avelox® [US/Can]
moxifloxacin

POISON IVY
Protectant, Topical
bentoquatam
IvyBlock® [US-OTC]

POISON OAK
Protectant, Topical
bentoquatam
IvyBlock® [US-OTC]

POISON SUMAC
Protectant, Topical
bentoquatam
IvyBlock® [US-OTC]

POLIOMYELITIS
Vaccine, Live Virus
Orimune® [US]
poliovirus vaccine, live, trivalent, oral
Vaccine, Live Virus and Inactivated Virus
IPOL™ [US/Can]
poliovirus vaccine (inactivated)

POLYCYTHEMIA VERA
Antineoplastic Agent
busulfan
Busulfex® [US/Can]
mechlorethamine
Mustargen® [US/Can]
Myleran® [US/Can]

POLYMYOSITIS

Antineoplastic
    Agent
  chlorambucil
  cyclophosphamide
  Cytoxan® [US/Can]
  Leukeran® [US/Can]
  methotrexate
  Neosar® [US]
  Procytox® [Can]
  Rheumatrex® [US]
  Trexall™ [US]
Immunosuppressant
    Agent
  Alti-Azathioprine [Can]
  azathioprine
  Gen-Azathioprine [Can]
  Imuran® [US/Can]

PORPHYRIA

Blood Modifiers
  hemin
  Panhematin® [US]
Phenothiazine Derivative
  Chlorpromanyl® [Can]
  chlorpromazine
  Largactil® [Can]
  Thorazine® [US]

PORTAL-SYSTEMIC ENCEPHALOPATHY (PSE)

Ammonium Detoxicant
  Acilac [Can]
  Cholac® [US]
  Constilac® [US]
  Constulose® [US]
  Enulose® [US]
  Generlac® [US]
  Kristalose™ [US]
  lactulose
  Laxilose [Can]
  PMS-Lactulose [Can]

POSTPARTUM HEMORRHAGE

Uteronic Agent
  carbetocin (Canada only)
  Duratocin™ [Can]

PREECLAMPSIA

Electrolyte Supplement, Oral
  magnesium sulfate

PREMENSTRUAL DYSPHORIC DISORDER (PMDD)

Antidepressant, Selective Serotonin
    Reuptake Inhibitor
  Alti-Fluoxetine [Can]
  Apo®-Fluoxetine [Can]
  fluoxetine
  Gen-Fluoxetine [Can]
  Novo-Fluoxetine [Can]
  Nu-Fluoxetine [Can]
  PMS-Fluoxetine [Can]
  Prozac® [US/Can]
  Prozac® Weekly™ [US]
  Rhoxal-fluoxetine [Can]
  Sarafem™ [US]

PRIMARY PULMONARY HYPERTENSION (PPH)

Platelet Inhibitor
  epoprostenol
  Flolan® [US/Can]

PROCTITIS

5-Aminosalicylic Acid Derivative
  Asacol® [US/Can]
  Canasa™ [US]
  mesalamine
  Mesasal® [Can]
  Novo-ASA [Can]
  Pentasa® [US/Can]
  Quintasa® [Can]
  Rowasa® [US/Can]
  Salofalk® [Can]

PROCTOSIGMOIDITIS
5-Aminosalicylic Acid Derivative
  Asacol® [US/Can]
  Canasa™ [US]
  mesalamine
  Mesasal® [Can]
  Novo-ASA [Can]
  Pentasa® [US/Can]
  Quintasa® [Can]
  Rowasa® [US/Can]
  Salofalk® [Can]

PROSTATITIS
Quinolone
  Apo®-Oflox [Can]
  Floxin® [US/Can]
  ofloxacin
Sulfonamide
  Apo®-Sulfatrim [Can]
  Bactrim™ DS [US]
  Bactrim™ [US]
  Novo-Trimel [Can]
  Novo-Trimel D.S. [Can]
  Nu-Cotrimox® [Can]
  Septra® DS [US/Can]
  Septra® [US/Can]
  sulfamethoxazole and trimethoprim
  Sulfatrim® DS [US]
  Sulfatrim® [US]

PROTOZOAL INFECTION
Antiprotozoal
  Apo®-Metronidazole [Can]
  Flagyl ER® [US]
  Flagyl® [US/Can]
  furazolidone
  Furoxone® [US/Can]
  metronidazole
  NebuPent™ [US]
  Nidagel™ [Can]
  Noritate™ [US/Can]
  Novo-Nidazol [Can]
  Pentacarinat® [Can]

Pentam-300® [US]
pentamidine

PRURITUS
Antihistamine
  Acot-Tussin® Allergy [US-OTC]
  Alercap® [US-OTC]
  Aler-Dryl® [US-OTC]
  Alertab® [US-OTC]
  Aller-Chlor® [US-OTC]
  Allerdryl® [Can]
  Allermax® [US-OTC]
  Allernix [Can]
  Altaryl® [US-OTC]
  Anti-Hist® [US-OTC]
  ANX® [US]
  Apo®-Hydroxyzine [Can]
  Atarax® [US/Can]
  azatadine
  Banaril® [US-OTC]
  Banophen® [US-OTC]
  Benadryl® [US/Can]
  brompheniramine
  chlorpheniramine
  Chlor-Trimeton® [US-OTC]
  Chlor-Tripolon® [Can]
  Claritin® RediTabs® [US]
  Claritin® [US/Can]
  clemastine
  Colhist® Solution [US-OTC]
  Compoz® Nighttime Sleep Aid [US-OTC]
  cyproheptadine
  Dermamycin® [US-OTC]
  Derma-Pax® [US-OTC]
  dexchlorpheniramine
  Dimetane® Extentabs® [US-OTC]
  Dimetapp® Allergy Children's [US-OTC]
  Dimetapp® Allergy [US-OTC]
  Diphendryl® [US-OTC]
  Diphenhist® [US-OTC]
  diphenhydramine

Diphen® [US-OTC]
Diphenyl® [US-OTC]
Dormin® Sleep Aid [US-OTC]
Dytuss® [US-OTC]
Genahist® [US-OTC]
Geridryl® [US-OTC]
Hydramine® [US-OTC]
hydroxyzine
Hyrexin® [US-OTC]
Hyzine-50® [US]
Lodrane® 12 Hour [US-OTC]
loratadine
Mediphedryl® [US-OTC]
Miles® Nervine [US-OTC]
ND-Stat® Solution [US-OTC]
Nolahist® [US/Can]
Novo-Hydroxyzin [Can]
Nytol™ [Can]
Nytol™ Extra Strength [Can]
Nytol® Quickcaps® [US-OTC]
Optimine® [US/Can]
Panectyl® [Can]
Periactin® [US/Can]
phenindamine
PMS-Diphenhydramine [Can]
PMS-Hydroxyzine [Can]
Polaramine® [US]
Polydryl® [US-OTC]
Polytapp® Allergy Dye-Free Medication [US-OTC]
Q-Dryl® [US-OTC]
Quenalin® [US-OTC]
Restall® [US]
Siladryl® Allerfy® [US-OTC]
Silphen® [US-OTC]
Simply Sleep® [US-OTC]
Sleepinal® [US-OTC]
Sleep® Tabs [US-OTC]
Sominex® [US-OTC]
Tavist®-1 [US-OTC]
Tavist® [US]
trimeprazine (Canada only)
Truxadryl® [US-OTC]

Tusstat® [US-OTC]
Twilite® [US-OTC]
Unison® Sleepgels® Maximum Strength [US-OTC]
Vistacot® [US]
Vistaril® [US/Can]
Phenothiazine Derivative
Anergan® [US]
Phenergan® [US/Can]
promethazine

PSEUDOHYPOPARATHY-ROIDISM

Vitamin D Analog
Calciferol™ [US]
Calcijex™ [US]
calcitriol
DHT™ [US]
dihydrotachysterol
Drisdol® [US/Can]
ergocalciferol
Hytakerol® [US/Can]
Ostoforte® [Can]
Rocaltrol® [US/Can]

PSORIASIS

Antibiotic/Corticosteroid, Topical
Neo-Cortef® [Can]
neomycin and hydrocortisone
Antineoplastic Agent
methotrexate
Rheumatrex® [US]
Trexall™ [US]
Antipsoriatic Agent
Balnetar® [US/Can]
calcipotriene
coal tar
coal tar and salicylic acid
coal tar, lanolin, and mineral oil
Denorex® [US-OTC]
DHS® Tar [US-OTC]
Dovonex® [US]
Duplex® T [US-OTC]
Estar® [US/Can]

etretinate
Fototar® [US-OTC]
Neutrogena® T/Derm [US]
Neutrogena® T/Sal [US-OTC]
Oxipor® VHC [US-OTC]
Pentrax® [US-OTC]
Polytar® [US-OTC]
psoriGel® [US-OTC]
P & S Plus® [US-OTC]
Sebcur/T® [Can]
Targel® [Can]
Tegison® [US]
Tegrin® Dandruff Shampoo [US-OTC]
T/Gel® [US-OTC]
X-Seb™ T [US-OTC]
Zetar® [US/Can]
Corticosteroid, Topical
Aclovate® [US]
Acticort® [US]
Aeroseb-HC® [US]
Ala-Cort® [US]
Ala-Scalp® [US]
alclometasone
Alphatrex® [US]
amcinonide
Aquacort® [Can]
Aristocort® A Topical [US]
Aristocort® Topical [US/Can]
Bactine® Hydrocortisone [US-OTC]
Betaderm® [Can]
Betamethacot® [US]
betamethasone (topical)
Betatrex® [US]
Beta-Val® [US]
Betnovate® [Can]
CaldeCORT® Anti-Itch Spray [US]
CaldeCORT® [US-OTC]
Capex™ [US/Can]
Carmol-HC® [US]
Celestoderm®-EV/2 [Can]
Celestoderm®-V [Can]
Cetacort®

clobetasol
Clocort® Maximum Strength [US-OTC]
clocortolone
Cloderm® [US/Can]
Cordran® SP [US]
Cordran® [US/Can]
Cormax® [US]
CortaGel® [US-OTC]
Cortaid® Maximum Strength [US-OTC]
Cortaid® with Aloe [US-OTC]
Cort-Dome® [US]
Cortizone®-5 [US-OTC]
Cortizone®-10 [US-OTC]
Cortoderm [Can]
Cutivate™ [US]
Cyclocort® [US/Can]
Del-Beta® [US]
Delcort® [US]
Dermacort® [US]
Dermarest Dricort® [US]
Derma-Smoothe/FS® [US/Can]
Dermatop® [US]
Dermolate® [US-OTC]
Dermovate® [Can]
Dermtex® HC with Aloe [US-OTC]
Desocort® [Can]
desonide
DesOwen® [US]
desoximetasone
diflorasone
Diprolene® AF [US]
Diprolene® [US/Can]
Diprosone® [US/Can]
Ectosone [Can]
Eldecort® [US]
Elocon® [US/Can]
fluocinolone
fluocinonide
Fluoderm [Can]
flurandrenolide
fluticasone (topical)

Gen-Clobetasol [Can]
Gynecort® [US-OTC]
halcinonide
halobetasol
Halog®-E [US]
Halog® [US/Can]
Hi-Cor-1.0® [US]
Hi-Cor-2.5® [US]
Hyderm [Can]
hydrocortisone (topical)
Hydrocort® [US]
Hydro-Tex® [US-OTC]
Hytone® [US]
Kenalog® in Orabase® [US/Can]
Kenalog® Topical [US/Can]
LactiCare-HC® [US]
Lanacort® [US-OTC]
Lidemol® [Can]
Lidex-E® [US]
Lidex® [US/Can]
Locoid® [US/Can]
Luxiq™ [US]
Lyderm® [Can]
Lydonide [Can]
Maxiflor® [US]
Maxivate® [US]
mometasone furoate
Nasonex® [US/Can]
Novo-Clobetasol [Can]
Nutracort® [US]
Olux™ [US]
Penecort® [US]
prednicarbate
Prevex® [Can]
Prevex® HC [Can]
Psorcon™ E [US]
Psorcon™ [US/Can]
Qualisone® [US]
Sarna® HC [Can]
Scalpicin® [US]
S-T Cort® [US]
Synacort® [US]
Synalar® [US/Can]

Taro-Desoximetasone [Can]
Taro-Sone® [Can]
Tegrin®-HC [US-OTC]
Temovate® [US]
Texacort® [US]
Tiamol® [Can]
Ti-U-Lac® H [Can]
Topicort®-LP [US]
Topicort® [US/Can]
Topilene® [Can]
Topisone®
Topsyn® [Can]
Triacet™ Topical [US] Oracort
[Can]
Triaderm [Can]
triamcinolone (topical)
Tridesilon® [US]
U-Cort™ [US]
Ultravate™ [US/Can]
urea and hydrocortisone
Uremol® HC [Can]
Valisone® Scalp Lotion [Can]
Westcort® [US/Can]
Keratolytic Agent
Anthraforte® [Can]
anthralin
Anthranol® [Can]
Anthrascalp® [Can]
Drithocreme® [US]
Psor-a-set® Soap [US-OTC]
Sal-Acid® Plaster [US-OTC]
Salactic® Film [US-OTC]
salicylic acid
salicylic acid and propylene glycol
Sal-Plant® [US-OTC]
Sebcur® [Can]
Soluver® [Can]
Soluver® Plus [Can]
tazarotene
Tazorac® [US/Can]
Psoralen
methoxsalen
8-MOP® [US/Can]

Oxsoralen® Lotion [US/Can]
Oxsoralen-Ultra® [US/Can]
Ultramop™ [Can]
Uvadex® [US/Can]
Retinoid-like Compound
acitretin
Soriatane® [US/Can]

PSYCHOSIS

Antipsychotic Agent
Clopixol-Acuphase® [Can]
Clopixol® [Can]
Clopixol® Depot [Can]
olanzapine
quetiapine
Seroquel® [US/Can]
zuclopenthixol (Canada only)
Zyprexa® [US/Can]
Zyprexa® Zydis® [US]
Antipsychotic Agent, Benzisoxazole
Risperdal Consta™ [Investigational]
[US]
Risperdal® [US/Can]
risperidone
Antipsychotic Agent, Butyrophenone
Apo®-Haloperidol [Can]
droperidol
Haldol® Decanoate [US]
Haldol® [US/Can]
haloperidol
Inapsine® [US]
Novo-Peridol [Can]
Peridol [Can]
PMS-Haloperidol LA [Can]
Rho®-Haloperidol Decanoate [Can]
Antipsychotic Agent, Dibenzoxazepine
Apo®-Loxapine [Can]
loxapine
Loxitane® C [US]
Loxitane® I.M. [US]
Loxitane® [US]
Nu-Loxapine [Can]
PMS-Loxapine [Can]

Antipsychotic Agent, Dihydroindoline
Moban® [US/Can]
molindone
Phenothiazine Derivative
Apo®-Fluphenazine [Can]
Apo®-Perphenazine [Can]
Apo®-Thioridazine [Can]
Apo®-Trifluoperazine [Can]
Chlorpromanyl® [Can]
chlorpromazine
Compazine® [US/Can]
Compro™ [US]
fluphenazine
Largactil® [Can]
Mellaril® [US/Can]
mesoridazine
Modecate® [Can]
Moditen® Enanthate [Can]
Moditen® HCl [Can]
Neuleptil® [Can]
Nu-Prochlor [Can]
pericyazine (Canada only)
perphenazine
PMS-Fluphenazine Decanoate
[Can]
prochlorperazine
Prolixin Decanoate® [US]
Prolixin Enanthate® [US]
Prolixin® [US]
promazine
Rho®-Fluphenazin Decanoate [Can]
Serentil® [US/Can]
Stelazine® [US]
Stemetil® [Can]
thioridazine
Thorazine® [US]
trifluoperazine
triflupromazine
Trilafon® [US/Can]
Vesprin® [US/Can]
Thioxanthene Derivative
Navane® [US/Can]
thiothixene

PULMONARY ARTERY HYPERTENSION (PAH)
Endothelin Antagonist
  bosentan
  Tracleer™ [US]
Vasodilator
  Remodulin™ [US]
  treprostinil

PULMONARY EMBOLISM
Anticoagulant (Other)
  Coumadin® [US/Can]
  dicumarol
  enoxaparin
  Hepalean® [Can]
  Hepalean® Leo [Can]
  Hepalean®-LOK [Can]
  heparin
  Hep-Lock® [US]
  Lovenox® [US/Can]
  Taro-Warfarin [Can]
  warfarin
Fibrinolytic Agent
  Abbokinase® [US]
  Activase® rt-PA [Can]
  Activase® [US]
  alteplase
  Streptase® [US/Can]
  streptokinase
  urokinase
Low Molecular Weight Heparin
  Fraxiparine™ [Can]
  nadroparin (Canada only)

PULMONARY TUBERCULOSIS
Antitubercular Agent
  Priftin® [US/Can]
  rifapentine

PURPURA
Immune Globulin
  Carimune™ [US]

  Gamimune® N [US/Can]
  Gammagard® S/D [US/Can]
  Gammar®-P I.V. [US]
  immune globulin (intravenous)
  Iveegam EN [US]
  Iveegam Immuno® [Can]
  Panglobulin® [US]
  Polygam® S/D [US]
  Venoglobulin®-S [US]
Immunosuppressant Agent
  Alti-Azathioprine [Can]
  azathioprine
  Gen-Azathioprine [Can]
  Imuran® [US/Can]

PURPURA (THROMBOCYTOPENIC)
Antineoplastic Agent
  Oncovin® [US/Can]
  Vincasar® PFS® [US/Can]
  vincristine

PYELONEPHRITIS
Antibiotic, Carbapenem
  ertapenem
  Invanz™ [US]
Antibiotic, Quinolone
  gatifloxacin
  Tequin® [US/Can]

PYRIMETHAMINE POISONING
Folic Acid Derivative
  leucovorin
  Wellcovorin® [US]

RABIES
Immune Globulin
  BayRab® [US/Can]
  Imogam® Rabies Pasteurized [Can]
  Imogam® [US]
  rabies immune globulin (human)
Vaccine, Inactivated Virus
  Imovax® Rabies [US/Can]
  rabies virus vaccine

RAT-BITE FEVER
Antibiotic, Aminoglycoside
  streptomycin

RATTLESNAKE BITE
Antivenin
  antivenin *(Crotalidae)* polyvalent
  Antivenin Polyvalent [Equine] [US]
  CroFab™ [Ovine] [US]

RAYNAUD DISEASE
Vasodilator
  isoxsuprine
  Vasodilan® [US]

RENAL ALLOGRAFT REJECTION
Immunosuppressant Agent
  antithymocyte globulin (rabbit)
  Thymoglobulin® [US]

RENAL COLIC
Analgesic, Nonnarcotic
  Apo®-Ketorolac [Can]
  ketorolac
  Novo-Ketorolac [Can]
  Toradol® [US/Can]
Anticholinergic Agent
  Antispas® Tablet [US]
  Donnapine® [US]
  Donnatal® [US]
  Haponal® [US]
  Hyonatol® [US]
  hyoscyamine, atropine, scopolamine, and phenobarbital
  Hypersed® [US]

RESPIRATORY DISTRESS SYNDROME (RDS)
Lung Surfactant
  beractant
  calfactant
  colfosceril palmitate
  Curosurf® [US/Can]

Exosurf® Neonatal™ [US/Can]
  Infasurf® [US]
  poractant alfa
  Survanta® [US/Can]

RESPIRATORY SYNCYTIAL VIRUS (RSV)
Antiviral Agent
  Rebetol® [US]
  ribavirin
  Virazole® [US/Can]
Immune Globulin
  RespiGam™ [US]
  respiratory syncytial virus immune globulin (intravenous)
Monoclonal Antibody
  palivizumab
  Synagis® [US]

RESPIRATORY TRACT INFECTION
Aminoglycoside (Antibiotic)
  AKTob® [US]
  Alcomicin® [Can]
  Diogent® [Can]
  Garamycin® [US/Can]
  Garatec [Can]
  Gentacidin® [US]
  Gentak® [US]
  gentamicin
  Nebcin® [US/Can]
  PMS-Tobramycin [Can]
  tobramycin
  Tobrex® [US/Can]
  Tomycine™ [Can]
Antibiotic, Carbacephem
  Lorabid™ [US/Can]
  loracarbef
Antibiotic, Macrolide
  Rovamycine® [Can]
  spiramycin (Canada only)
Antibiotic, Miscellaneous
  Alti-Clindamycin [Can]

Azactam® [US/Can]
aztreonam
Cleocin HCl® [US]
Cleocin Pediatric® [US]
Cleocin Phosphate® [US]
Cleocin® [US]
clindamycin
Dalacin® C [Can]
Antibiotic, Penicillin
  pivampicillin (Canada only)
  Pondocillin® [Can]
Antibiotic, Quinolone
  gatifloxacin
  Levaquin® [US/Can]
  levofloxacin
  Quixin™ Ophthalmic [US]
  Tequin® [US/Can]
Cephalosporin (First Generation)
  Ancef® [US/Can]
  Apo®-Cefadroxil [Can]
  Apo®-Cephalex [Can]
  Biocef® [US]
  cefadroxil
  Cefadyl® [US/Can]
  cefazolin
  cephalexin
  cephalothin
  cephapirin
  cephradine
  Ceporacin® [Can]
  Duricef® [US/Can]
  Keflex® [US]
  Keftab® [US/Can]
  Kefzol® [US/Can]
  Novo-Cefadroxil [Can]
  Novo-Lexin® [Can]
  Nu-Cephalex® [Can]
  Velosef® [US]
Cephalosporin (Second Generation)
  Apo®-Cefaclor [Can]
  Ceclor® CD [US]
  Ceclor® [US/Can]
  cefaclor

cefamandole
Cefotan® [US/Can]
cefotetan
cefoxitin
cefpodoxime
cefprozil
Ceftin® [US/Can]
cefuroxime
Cefzil® [US/Can]
Kefurox® [US/Can]
Mandol® [US]
Mefoxin® [US/Can]
Novo-Cefaclor [Can]
Nu-Cefaclor [Can]
PMS-Cefaclor [Can]
Vantin® [US/Can]
Zinacef® [US/Can]
Cephalosporin (Third Generation)
  Cedax® [US]
  cefixime
  Cefizox® [US/Can]
  Cefobid® [US/Can]
  cefoperazone
  cefotaxime
  ceftazidime
  ceftibuten
  ceftizoxime
  ceftriaxone
  Ceptaz® [US/Can]
  Claforan® [US/Can]
  Fortaz® [US/Can]
  Rocephin® [US/Can]
  Suprax® [US/Can]
  Tazicef® [US]
  Tazidime® [US/Can]
Cephalosporin (Fourth Generation)
  cefepime
  Maxipime® [US/Can]
Macrolide (Antibiotic)
  Apo®-Erythro Base [Can]
  Apo®-Erythro E-C [Can]
  Apo®-Erythro-ES [Can]
  Apo®-Erythro-S [Can]

azithromycin
Biaxin® [US/Can]
Biaxin® XL [US]
clarithromycin
Diomycin® [Can]
dirithromycin
Dynabac® [US]
E.E.S.® [US/Can]
Erybid™ [Can]
Eryc® [US/Can]
EryPed® [US]
Ery-Tab® [US]
Erythrocin® [US/Can]
erythromycin and sulfisoxazole
erythromycin (systemic)
Eryzole® [US]
Nu-Erythromycin-S [Can]
PCE® [US/Can]
Pediazole® [US/Can]
PMS-Erythromycin [Can]
Zithromax® [US/Can]
Z-PAK® [US/Can]
Penicillin
amoxicillin
amoxicillin and clavulanate
  potassium
Amoxicot® [US]
Amoxil® [US/Can]
ampicillin
ampicillin and sulbactam
Apo®-Amoxi [Can]
Apo®-Ampi [Can]
Apo®-Cloxi [Can]
Apo®-Pen VK [Can]
Augmentin ES-600™ [US]
Augmentin® [US/Can]
Bicillin® C-R 900/300 [US]
Bicillin® C-R [US]
Bicillin® L-A [US]
carbenicillin
Clavulin® [Can]
cloxacillin
dicloxacillin

Dynapen® [US]
Gen-Amoxicillin [Can]
Geocillin® [US]
Lin-Amox [Can]
Marcillin® [US]
Moxilin® [US]
Nadopen-V® [Can]
nafcillin
Novamoxin® [Can]
Novo-Ampicillin [Can]
Novo-Cloxin [Can]
Novo-Pen-VK® [Can]
Nu-Amoxi [Can]
Nu-Ampi [Can]
Nu-Cloxi® [Can]
Nu-Pen-VK® [Can]
oxacillin
penicillin G benzathine
penicillin G benzathine and procaine
  combined
penicillin G (parenteral/aqueous)
penicillin G procaine
penicillin V potassium
Permapen® [US]
Pfizerpen® [US/Can]
piperacillin
piperacillin and tazobactam sodium
Pipracil® [US/Can]
Principen® [US]
PVF® K [Can]
Suspen® [US]
Tazocin® [Can]
ticarcillin
ticarcillin and clavulanate potassium
Ticar® [US]
Timentin® [US/Can]
Trimox® [US]
Truxcillin® [US]
Unasyn® [US/Can]
Veetids® [US]
Wycillin® [US/Can]
Wymox® [US]
Zosyn® [US]

Quinolone
  Apo®-Oflox [Can]
  ciprofloxacin
  Cipro® [US/Can]
  Floxin® [US/Can]
  lomefloxacin
  Maxaquin® [US]
  ofloxacin
  sparfloxacin
  Zagam® [US]
Sulfonamide
  erythromycin and sulfisoxazole
  Eryzole® [US]
  Pediazole® [US/Can]

RETINOBLASTOMA

Antineoplastic Agent
  Cosmegen® [US/Can]
  cyclophosphamide
  Cytoxan® [US/Can]
  dactinomycin
  Neosar® [US]
  Procytox® [Can]

REYE SYNDROME

Diuretic, Osmotic
  mannitol
  Osmitrol® [US/Can]
Ophthalmic Agent, Miscellaneous
  glycerin
  Osmoglyn® [US]
Vitamin, Fat Soluble
  AquaMEPHYTON® [US/Can]
  Mephyton® [US/Can]
  phytonadione

RHABDOMYOSARCOMA

Antineoplastic Agent
  Alkeran® [US/Can]
  Cosmegen® [US/Can]
  cyclophosphamide
  Cytoxan® [US/Can]
  dactinomycin
  etoposide
  melphalan
  Neosar® [US]
  Oncovin® [US/Can]
  Procytox® [Can]
  Toposar® [US]
  VePesid® [US/Can]
  Vincasar® PFS® [US/Can]
  vincristine

RHEUMATIC DISORDER

Adrenal Corticosteroid
  Acthar® [US]
  A-HydroCort® [US/Can]
  Alti-Dexamethasone [Can]
  A-methaPred® [US]
  Apo®-Prednisone [Can]
  Aristocort® Forte Injection [US]
  Aristocort® Intralesional Injection
    [US]
  Aristocort® Tablet [US/Can]
  Aristospan® Intra-articular Injection
    [US/Can]
  Aristospan® Intralesional Injection
    [US/Can]
  Betaject™ [Can]
  betamethasone (systemic)
  Betnesol® [Can]
  Celestone® Phosphate [US]
  Celestone® Soluspan® [US/Can]
  Celestone® [US]
  Cel-U-Jec® [US]
  Cortef® [US/Can]
  corticotropin
  cortisone acetate
  Cortone® [Can]
  Decadron®-LA [US]
  Decadron® [US/Can]
  Decaject-LA® [US]
  Decaject® [US]
  Delta-Cortef® [US]
  Deltasone® [US]
  Depo-Medrol® [US/Can]
  Depopred® [US]

dexamethasone (systemic)
Dexasone® L.A. [US]
Dexasone® [US/Can]
Dexone® LA [US]
Dexone® [US]
Hexadrol® [US/Can]
H.P. Acthar® Gel [US]
hydrocortisone (systemic)
Hydrocortone® Acetate [US]
Kenalog® Injection [US/Can]
Key-Pred-SP® [US]
Key-Pred® [US]
Medrol® Tablet [US/Can]
methylprednisolone
Meticorten® [US]
Orapred™ [US]
Pediapred® [US/Can]
PMS-Dexamethasone [Can]
Prednicot® [US]
prednisolone (systemic)
Prednisol® TBA [US]
prednisone
Prelone® [US]
Solu-Cortef® [US/Can]
Solu-Medrol® [US/Can]
Solurex L.A.® [US]
Sterapred® DS [US]
Sterapred® [US]
Tac™-3 Injection [US]
Triam-A® Injection [US]
triamcinolone (systemic)
Triam Forte® Injection [US]
Winpred™ [Can]

RHEUMATIC FEVER
Nonsteroidal Antiinflammatory Drug
(NSAID)
Amigesic® [US/Can]
Argesic®-SA [US]
Arthropan® [US-OTC]
Backache Pain Relief Extra Strength
[US]
choline magnesium trisalicylate

choline salicylate
Disalcid® [US]
Doan's®, Original [US-OTC]
Extra Strength Doan's® [US-OTC]
Keygesic-10® [US]
magnesium salicylate
Mobidin® [US]
Momentum® [US-OTC]
Mono-Gesic® [US]
Salflex® [US/Can]
salsalate
Teejel® [Can]
Tricosal® [US]
Trilisate® [US/Can]
Penicillin
Bicillin® C-R 900/300 [US]
Bicillin® C-R [US]
penicillin G benzathine and procaine
combined

RHEUMATOID ARTHRITIS
Analgesic, Nonnarcotic
Arthrotec® [US/Can]
diclofenac and misoprostol
Nonsteroidal Antiinflammatory Drug
(NSAID), COX-2 Selective
Bextra™ [US]
valdecoxib
Prostaglandin
Arthrotec® [US/Can]
diclofenac and misoprostol

RHINITIS
Adrenal Corticosteroid
beclomethasone
Beconase® AQ [US]
Beconase® [US]
budesonide
Dexacort® Phosphate Turbinaire®
[US]
dexamethasone (nasal)
dexamethasone (systemic)
Dexasone® L.A. [US]
Dexasone® [US/Can]

Dexone® LA [US]
Dexone® [US]
Flonase® [US]
flunisolide
fluticasone (nasal)
Gen-Budesonide AQ [Can]
Nasalide® [US/Can]
Nasarel® [US]
Pulmicort Turbuhaler® [US/Can]
Rhinalar® [Can]
Rhinocort® Aqua™ [US/Can]
Rhinocort® [US/Can]
Rivanase AQ [Can]
Vancenase® AQ 84 mcg [US]
Vancenase® Pockethaler® [US]
Adrenergic Agonist Agent
Afrin® Extra Moisturizing [US-OTC]
Afrin® Original [US-OTC]
Afrin® Severe Congestion [US-OTC]
Afrin® Sinus [US-OTC]
Afrin® [US-OTC]
Balminil® Decongestant [Can]
Cenafed® [US-OTC]
Children's Silfedrine® [US-OTC]
Children's Sudafed® Nasal Decon-
gestant [US-OTC]
Decofed® [US-OTC]
Decongest [Can]
Dimetapp® Decongestant Liqui-
Gels® [US-OTC]
Dristan® Long Lasting Nasal [Can]
Drixoral® Nasal [Can]
Duramist® Plus [US-OTC]
Duration® [US-OTC]
Efidac/24® [US-OTC]
Eltor® [Can]
ephedrine
Genaphed® [US-OTC]
Genasal [US-OTC]
Geneye® [US-OTC]
Neo-Synephrine® 12 Hour Extra
Moisturizing [US-OTC]
Neo-Synephrine® 12 Hour [US-OTC]

Nōstrilla® [US-OTC]
oxymetazoline
PediaCare® Decongestant Infants
[US-OTC]
PMS-Pseudoephedrine [Can]
Pretz-D® [US-OTC]
pseudoephedrine
Pseudofrin [Can]
Robidrine® [Can]
Sudafed® 12 Hour [US-OTC]
Sudafed® Children's [US-OTC]
Sudafed® Decongestant [Can]
Sudafed® [US-OTC]
tetrahydrozoline
Triaminic® AM Decongestant For-
mula [US-OTC]
Triaminic® Infant Decongestant
[US/Can]
Twice-A-Day® [US-OTC]
Tyzine® [US]
Vicks Sinex® 12 Hour Ultrafine Mist
[US-OTC]
4-Way® Long Acting [US-OTC]
xylometazoline
Antihistamine
Allegra® [US/Can]
Aller-Chlor® [US-OTC]
Apo®-Cetirizine [Can]
azatadine
brompheniramine
cetirizine
chlorpheniramine
Chlor-Trimeton® [US-OTC]
Chlor-Tripolon® [Can]
Claritin® RediTabs® [US]
Claritin® [US/Can]
clemastine
Colhist® Solution [US-OTC]
cyproheptadine
dexchlorpheniramine
Dimetane® Extentabs® [US-OTC]
Dimetapp® Allergy Children's [US-
OTC]

Dimetapp® Allergy [US-OTC]
fexofenadine
Lodrane® 12 Hour [US-OTC]
loratadine
ND-Stat® Solution [US-OTC]
Nolahist® [US/Can]
Optimine® [US/Can]
Periactin® [US/Can]
phenindamine
Polaramine® [US]
Polytapp® Allergy Dye-Free Medication [US-OTC]
Reactine™ [Can]
Tavist®-1 [US-OTC]
Tavist® [US]
Zyrtec® [US]
Antihistamine/Decongestant/
   Antitussive
   Cerose-DM® [US-OTC]
   chlorpheniramine, phenylephrine,
     and codeine
   chlorpheniramine, phenylephrine,
     and dextromethorphan
   Pediacof® [US]
   Pedituss® [US]
Antihistamine/Decongestant
   Combination
   Allegra-D® [US/Can]
   Andehist NR Syrup [US]
   Benadryl® Decongestant Allergy
     [US-OTC]
   Brofed® [US]
   Bromanate® [US-OTC]
   Bromfed-PD® [US-OTC]
   Bromfed® [US-OTC]
   Bromfenex® PD [US]
   Bromfenex® [US]
   brompheniramine and pseu-
     doephedrine
   Children's Dimetapp® Elixir Cold &
     Allergy [US-OTC]
   chlorpheniramine, phenylephrine,
     and phenyltoloxamine

Chlor-Tripolon ND® [Can]
Claritin-D® 12-Hour [US]
Claritin-D® 24-Hour [US]
Claritin® Extra [Can]
Comhist® LA [US]
Comhist® [US]
diphenhydramine and pseu-
   doephedrine
fexofenadine and pseudoephedrine
loratadine and pseudoephedrine
Rondec® Syrup [US]
Touro™ Allergy [US]
Antihistamine, Nonsedating
   Clarinex® [US]
   desloratadine
Corticosteroid, Intranasal
   Elocon® [US/Can]
   mometasone furoate
   Nasonex® [US/Can]
Corticosteroid, Topical
   Nasacort® AQ [US/Can]
   Nasacort® [US/Can]
   triamcinolone (inhalation, nasal)
   Trinasal® [Can]
Decongestant/Analgesic
   Advil® Cold & Sinus Caplets [US-
     OTC]
   Advil® Cold & Sinus Tablet [Can]
   Dristan® Sinus Caplets [US]
   Dristan® Sinus Tablet [Can]
   pseudoephedrine and ibuprofen
Mast Cell Stabilizer
   Apo®-Cromolyn [Can]
   Crolom® [US]
   cromolyn sodium
   Gastrocrom® [US]
   Intal® [US/Can]
   Nalcrom® [Can]
   Nasalcrom® [US-OTC]
   Nu-Cromolyn [Can]
   Opticrom® [US/Can]
Phenothiazine Derivative
   Anergan® [US]

Phenergan® [US/Can]
promethazine

RHINITIS (ALLERGIC)
Antihistamine/Decongestant
    Combination
cetirizine and pseudoephedrine
Zyrtec-D 12 Hour™ [US]
Corticosteroid, Intranasal
    Elocon® [US/Can]
    mometasone furoate
    Nasonex® [US/Can]

RHINORRHEA
Anticholinergic Agent
    Alti-Ipratropium [Can]
    Apo®-Ipravent [Can]
    Atrovent® [US/Can]
    Gen-Ipratropium [Can]
    ipratropium
    Novo-Ipramide [Can]
    Nu-Ipratropium [Can]
    PMS-Ipratropium [Can]

ROUNDWORMS
Anthelmintic
    Ascarel® [US-OTC]
    Combantrin™ [Can]
    mebendazole
    Pamix® [US-OTC]
    Pin-X® [US-OTC]
    pyrantel pamoate
    Reese's® Pinworm Medicine [US-OTC]
    Vermox® [US/Can]

RUBELLA
Vaccine, Live Virus
    Biavax® II [US]
    measles, mumps, and rubella vaccines, combined
    Meruvax® II [US]
    M-M-R® II [US/Can]
    Priorix™ [Can]

rubella and mumps vaccines, combined
rubella virus vaccine (live)

SARCOIDOSIS
Corticosteroid, Topical
    Aclovate® [US]
    Acticort® [US]
    Aeroseb-HC® [US]
    Ala-Cort® [US]
    Ala-Scalp® [US]
    alclometasone
    Alphatrex® [US]
    amcinonide
    Aquacort® [Can]
    Aristocort® A Topical [US]
    Aristocort® Topical [US/Can]
    Bactine® Hydrocortisone [US-OTC]
    Betaderm® [Can]
    Betamethacot® [US]
    betamethasone (topical)
    Betatrex® [US]
    Beta-Val® [US]
    Betnovate® [Can]
    CaldeCORT® Anti-Itch Spray [US]
    CaldeCORT® [US-OTC]
    Capex™ [US/Can]
    Carmol-HC® [US]
    Celestoderm®-EV/2 [Can]
    Celestoderm®-V [Can]
    Cetacort®
    clobetasol
    Clocort® Maximum Strength [US-OTC]
    clocortolone
    Cloderm® [US/Can]
    Cordran® SP [US]
    Cordran® [US/Can]
    Cormax® [US]
    CortaGel® [US-OTC]
    Cortaid® Maximum Strength [US-OTC]
    Cortaid® with Aloe [US-OTC]

Cort-Dome® [US]
Cortizone®-5 [US-OTC]
Cortizone®-10 [US-OTC]
Cortoderm [Can]
Cutivate™ [US]
Cyclocort® [US/Can]
Del-Beta® [US]
Delcort® [US]
Dermacort® [US]
Dermarest Dricort® [US]
Derma-Smoothe/FS® [US/Can]
Dermatop® [US]
Dermolate® [US-OTC]
Dermovate® [Can]
Dermtex® HC with Aloe [US-OTC]
Desocort® [Can]
desonide
DesOwen® [US]
desoximetasone
diflorasone
Diprolene® AF [US]
Diprolene® [US/Can]
Diprosone® [US/Can]
Ectosone [Can]
Eldecort® [US]
Elocon® [US/Can]
fluocinolone
fluocinonide
Fluoderm [Can]
flurandrenolide
fluticasone (topical)
Gen-Clobetasol [Can]
Gynecort® [US-OTC]
halcinonide
halobetasol
Halog®-E [US]
Halog® [US/Can]
Hi-Cor-1.0® [US]
Hi-Cor-2.5® [US]
Hyderm [Can]
hydrocortisone (topical)
Hydrocort® [US]
Hydro-Tex® [US-OTC]

Hytone® [US]
Kenalog® in Orabase® [US/Can]
Kenalog® Topical [US/Can]
LactiCare-HC® [US]
Lanacort® [US-OTC]
Lidemol® [Can]
Lidex-E® [US]
Lidex® [US/Can]
Locoid® [US/Can]
Luxiq™ [US]
Lyderm® [Can]
Lydonide [Can]
Maxiflor® [US]
Maxivate® [US]
mometasone furoate
Nasonex® [US/Can]
Novo-Clobetasol [Can]
Nutracort® [US]
Olux™ [US]
Orabase® HCA [US]
Penecort® [US]
prednicarbate
Prevex® [Can]
Prevex® HC [Can]
Psorcon™ E [US]
Psorcon™ [US/Can]
Qualisone® [US]
Sarna® HC [Can]
Scalpicin® [US]
S-T Cort® [US]
Synacort® [US]
Synalar® [US/Can]
Taro-Desoximetasone [Can]
Taro-Sone® [Can]
Tegrin®-HC [US-OTC]
Temovate® [US]
Texacort® [US]
Tiamol® [Can]
Ti-U-Lac® H [Can]
Topicort®-LP [US]
Topicort® [US/Can]
Topilene® [Can]
Topisone®

Topsyn® [Can]
Triacet™ Topical [US] Oracort [Can]
Triaderm [Can]
triamcinolone (topical)
Tridesilon® [US]
U-Cort™ [US]
Ultravate™ [US/Can]
urea and hydrocortisone
Uremol® HC [Can]
Valisone® Scalp Lotion [Can]
Westcort® [US/Can]

SARCOMA
Antineoplastic Agent
Adriamycin® [Can]
Adriamycin PFS® [US]
Adriamycin RDF® [US]
Blenoxane® [US/Can]
bleomycin
Caelyx® [Can]
cisplatin
Cosmegen® [US/Can]
dacarbazine
dactinomycin
doxorubicin
DTIC® [Can]
DTIC-Dome® [US]
Ifex® [US/Can]
ifosfamide
methotrexate
Oncovin® [US/Can]
Platinol®-AQ [US]
Platinol® [US]
Rheumatrex® [US]
Rubex® [US]
Trexall™ [US]
Velban® [US/Can]
vinblastine
Vincasar® PFS® [US/Can]
vincristine

SCABIES
Scabicides/Pediculicides
A-200™ Lice [US-OTC]

A-200™ [US-OTC]
Acticin® [US]
crotamiton
Elimite® [US]
End Lice® [US-OTC]
Eurax® Topical [US]
Hexit™ [Can]
Kwellada-P™ [Can]
lindane
Nix® Dermal Cream [Can]
Nix® [US/Can]
permethrin
PMS-Lindane [Can]
Pronto® [US-OTC]
pyrethrins
Pyrinex® Pediculicide [US-OTC]
Pyrinyl Plus® [US-OTC]
Pyrinyl® [US-OTC]
R & C™ II [Can]
R & C® Lice [US]
R & C™ Shampoo/Conditioner [Can]
R & C® [US-OTC]
RID® Mousse [Can]
RID® Spray [US-OTC]
RID® [US-OTC]
Tisit® Blue Gel [US-OTC]
Tisit® [US-OTC]

SCHIZOPHRENIA
Antipsychotic Agent
Clopixol-Acuphase® [Can]
Clopixol® [Can]
Clopixol® Depot [Can]
Fluanxol® Depot [Can]
Fluanxol® Tablet [Can]
flupenthixol (Canada only)
olanzapine
quetiapine
Seroquel® [US/Can]
zuclopenthixol (Canada only)
Zyprexa® [US/Can]
Zyprexa® Zydis® [US]

Antipsychotic Agent, Benzisoxazole
  Risperdal Consta™ [Investigational] [US]
  Risperdal® [US/Can]
  risperidone
Antipsychotic Agent, Dibenzodiazepine
  clozapine
  Clozaril® [US/Can]
Neuroleptic Agent
  Apo®-Methoprazine [Can]
  Majeptil® [Can]
  methotrimeprazine (Canada only)
  Novo-Meprazine [Can]
  Nozinan® [Can]
  thioproperazine (Canada only)
Thioxanthene Derivative
  Fluanxol® Depot [Can]
  Fluanxol® Tablet [Can]
  flupenthixol (Canada only)

SCLERODERMA
Aminoquinoline (Antimalarial)
  Aralen® Phosphate [US/Can]
  chloroquine phosphate
Chelating Agent
  Cuprimine® [US/Can]
  Depen® [US/Can]
  penicillamine

SEBORRHEIC DERMATITIS
Antiseborrheic Agent, Topical
  Aveeno® Cleansing Bar [US-OTC]
  Balnetar® [US/Can]
  Capitrol® [US/Can]
  chloroxine
  coal tar
  coal tar and salicylic acid
  coal tar, lanolin, and mineral oil
  Denorex® [US-OTC]
  DHS® Tar [US-OTC]
  DHS Zinc® [US-OTC]
  Duplex® T [US-OTC]
  Estar® [US/Can]
  Exsel® [US]
  Fostex® [US-OTC]
  Fototar® [US-OTC]
  Head & Shoulders® Intensive Treatment [US-OTC]
  Head & Shoulders® [US-OTC]
  Neutrogena® T/Derm [US]
  Neutrogena® T/Sal [US-OTC]
  Novacet® [US]
  Oxipor® VHC [US-OTC]
  Pentrax® [US-OTC]
  Pernox® [US-OTC]
  Polytar® [US-OTC]
  psoriGel® [US-OTC]
  P & S Plus® [US-OTC]
  pyrithione zinc
  Sastid® Plain Therapeutic Shampoo and Acne Wash [US-OTC]
  Sebcur/T® [Can]
  selenium sulfide
  Selsun Blue® [US-OTC]
  Selsun Gold® for Women [US-OTC]
  Selsun® [US]
  Sulfacet-R® [US]
  sulfur and salicylic acid
  sulfur and sulfacetamide
  Targel® [Can]
  Tegrin® Dandruff Shampoo [US-OTC]
  T/Gel® [US-OTC]
  Theraplex Z® [US-OTC]
  Versel® [Can]
  X-Seb™ T [US-OTC]
  Zetar® [US/Can]
  Zincon® [US-OTC]
  ZNP® Bar [US-OTC]
Keratolytic Agent
  Compound W® [US-OTC]
  Dr Scholl's® Disk [US-OTC]
  Dr Scholl's® Wart Remover [US-OTC]
  DuoFilm® [US-OTC]
  Duoforte® 27 [Can]
  DuoPlant® [US-OTC]

Freezone® [US-OTC]
Gordofilm® [US-OTC]
Mediplast® Plaster [US-OTC]
Mosco® [US-OTC]
Occlusal™ [Can]
Occlusal®-HP [US/Can]
Off-Ezy® Wart Remover
  [US-OTC]
Psor-a-set® Soap [US-OTC]
Sal-Acid® Plaster [US-OTC]
Salactic® Film [US-OTC]
salicylic acid
Sal-Plant® [US-OTC]
Sebcur® [Can]
Soluver® [Can]
Soluver® Plus [Can]
Trans-Ver-Sal® AdultPatch [US-
  OTC]
Trans-Ver-Sal® [Can]
Trans-Ver-Sal® PediaPatch [US-
  OTC]
Trans-Ver-Sal® PlantarPatch [US-
  OTC]
Wart-Off® [US-OTC]

SEPSIS
Protein C (Activated)
  drotrecogin alfa
  Xigris™ [US]

SINUSITIS
Adrenergic Agonist Agent
  Balminil® Decongestant [Can]
  Cenafed® [US-OTC]
  Children's Silfedrine® [US-OTC]
  Children's Sudafed® Nasal Decon-
    gestant [US-OTC]
  Contac® Cold 12 Hour Relief Non
    Drowsy
  Decofed® [US-OTC]
  Dimetapp® Decongestant Liqui-
    Gels® [US-OTC]
  Efidac/24® [US-OTC]
  Eltor® [Can]

Genaphed® [US-OTC]
PediaCare® Decongestant Infants
  [US-OTC]
PMS-Pseudoephedrine [Can]
pseudoephedrine
Pseudofrin [Can]
Robidrine® [Can]
Sudafed® 12 Hour [US-OTC]
Sudafed® Children's [US-OTC]
Sudafed® Decongestant [Can]
Sudafed® [US-OTC]
Triaminic® AM Decongestant For-
  mula [US-OTC]
Triaminic® Infant Decongestant
  [US/Can]
Aminoglycoside (Antibiotic)
  Alcomicin® [Can]
  Diogent® [Can]
  Garamycin® [US/Can]
  Garatec [Can]
  Gentacidin® [US]
  Gentak® [US]
  gentamicin
Antibiotic, Miscellaneous
  Alti-Clindamycin [Can]
  Cleocin HCl® [US]
  Cleocin Pediatric® [US]
  Cleocin Phosphate® [US]
  Cleocin® [US]
  clindamycin
  Dalacin® C [Can]
Antibiotic, Penicillin
  pivampicillin (Canada only)
  Pondocillin® [Can]
Antibiotic, Quinolone
  ABC Pack™ (Avelox®) [US]
  Avelox® [US/Can]
  gatifloxacin
  Levaquin® [US/Can]
  levofloxacin
  moxifloxacin
  Quixin™ Ophthalmic [US]
  Tequin® [US/Can]

Antihistamine/Decongestant
    Combination
  Benadryl® Decongestant Allergy
    [US-OTC]
  diphenhydramine and pseu-
    doephedrine
Cephalosporin (First Generation)
  Apo®-Cefadroxil [Can]
  Apo®-Cephalex [Can]
  Biocef® [US]
  cefadroxil
  cephalexin
  cephradine
  Duricef® [US/Can]
  Keflex® [US]
  Keftab® [US/Can]
  Novo-Cefadroxil [Can]
  Novo-Lexin® [Can]
  Nu-Cephalex® [Can]
  Velosef® [US]
Cephalosporin (Second Generation)
  Apo®-Cefaclor [Can]
  Ceclor® CD [US]
  Ceclor® [US/Can]
  cefaclor
  cefpodoxime
  cefprozil
  Ceftin® [US/Can]
  cefuroxime
  Cefzil® [US/Can]
  Kefurox® [US/Can]
  Novo-Cefaclor [Can]
  Nu-Cefaclor [Can]
  PMS-Cefaclor [Can]
  Vantin® [US/Can]
  Zinacef® [US/Can]
Cephalosporin (Third Generation)
  Cedax® [US]
  cefdinir
  cefixime
  ceftibuten
  Omnicef® [US/Can]
  Suprax® [US/Can]

Cold Preparation
  Aquatab® C [US]
  Balminil DM + Decongestant +
    Expectorant [Can]
  Benylin® DM-D-E [Can]
  Endal® [US]
  Entex® LA [US]
  guaifenesin and phenylephrine
  guaifenesin, pseudoephedrine, and
    dextromethorphan
  Guiatuss™ CF [US]
  Koffex DM + Decongestant +
    Expectorant [Can]
  Liquibid-D [US]
  Maxifed® DM [US]
  Novahistex® DM Decongestant
    Expectorant [Can]
  Novahistine® DM Decongestant
    Expectorant [Can]
  PanMist®-DM [US]
  Prolex-D [US]
  Robitussin® Cold and Congestion
    [US-OTC]
  Robitussin® Cough and Cold Infant
    [US-OTC]
  Touro™ CC [US]
Decongestant/Analgesic
  Advil® Cold & Sinus Caplets [US-
    OTC]
  Advil® Cold & Sinus Tablet [Can]
  Dristan® Sinus Caplets [US]
  Dristan® Sinus Tablet [Can]
  pseudoephedrine and ibuprofen
Expectorant/Decongestant
  Ami-Tex PSE [US]
  Anatuss LA [US]
  Aquatab® D Dose Pack [US]
  Aquatab® [US]
  Congestac® [US]
  Deconsal® II [US]
  Defen-LA® [US]
  Duratuss™ GP [US]
  Duratuss™ [US]

Entex® PSE [US]
Eudal®-SR [US]
G-Phed-PD [US]
G-Phed [US]
Guaifed-PD® [US]
Guaifed® [US-OTC]
guaifenesin and pseudoephedrine
Guaifenex® GP [US]
Guaifenex® PSE [US]
Guaifen PSE [US]
Guai-Vent™/PSE [US]
Maxifed-G® [US]
Maxifed® [US]
Miraphen PSE [US]
Novahistex® Expectorant With De-
    congestant [Can]
PanMist® Jr. [US]
PanMist® LA [US]
PanMist® S [US]
Profen® II [US-OTC]
Pseudo GG TR [US]
Pseudovent™, Pseudovent™-Ped
    [US]
Respa-1st® [US]
Respaire®-60 SR [US]
Respaire®-120 SR [US]
Robitussin-PE® [US-OTC]
Robitussin® Severe Congestion [US-
    OTC]
Touro LA® [US]
V-Dec-M® [US]
Versacaps® [US]
Zephrex LA® [US]
Zephrex® [US]
Macrolide (Antibiotic)
Apo®-Erythro Base [Can]
Apo®-Erythro E-C [Can]
Apo®-Erythro-ES [Can]
Apo®-Erythro-S [Can]
Biaxin® [US/Can]
Biaxin® XL [US]
clarithromycin

Diomycin® [Can]
dirithromycin
Dynabac® [US]
E.E.S.® [US/Can]
Erybid™ [Can]
Eryc® [US/Can]
EryPed® [US]
Ery-Tab® [US]
Erythrocin® [US/Can]
erythromycin (systemic)
Nu-Erythromycin-S [Can]
PCE® [US/Can]
PMS-Erythromycin [Can]
Penicillin
amoxicillin
amoxicillin and clavulanate
    potassium
Amoxicot® [US]
Amoxil® [US/Can]
ampicillin
Apo®-Amoxi [Can]
Apo®-Ampi [Can]
Apo®-Cloxi [Can]
Augmentin ES-600™ [US]
Augmentin® [US/Can]
Clavulin® [Can]
cloxacillin
Gen-Amoxicillin [Can]
Lin-Amox [Can]
Marcillin® [US]
Moxilin® [US]
nafcillin
Novamoxin® [Can]
Novo-Ampicillin [Can]
Novo-Cloxin [Can]
Nu-Amoxi [Can]
Nu-Ampi [Can]
Nu-Cloxi® [Can]
oxacillin
Principen® [US]
Trimox® [US]
Wymox® [US]

Quinolone
   Apo®-Oflox [Can]
   ciprofloxacin
   Cipro® [US/Can]
   Floxin® [US/Can]
   lomefloxacin
   Maxaquin® [US]
   ofloxacin
   sparfloxacin
   Zagam® [US]
Sulfonamide
   Apo®-Sulfatrim [Can]
   Bactrim™ DS [US]
   Bactrim™ [US]
   Novo-Trimel [Can]
   Novo-Trimel D.S. [Can]
   Nu-Cotrimox® [Can]
   Septra® DS [US/Can]
   Septra® [US/Can]
   sulfamethoxazole and trimethoprim
   Sulfatrim® DS [US]
   Sulfatrim® [US]
Tetracycline Derivative
   Adoxa™ [US]
   Alti-Minocycline [Can]
   Apo®-Doxy [Can]
   Apo®-Doxy Tabs [Can]
   Apo®-Minocycline [Can]
   Apo®-Tetra [Can]
   Brodspec® [US]
   Doryx® [US]
   Doxy-100™ [US]
   Doxycin [Can]
   doxycycline
   Doxytec [Can]
   Dynacin® [US]
   EmTet® [US]
   Gen-Minocycline [Can]
   Minocin® [US/Can]
   minocycline
   Monodox® [US]
   Novo-Doxylin [Can]

Novo-Minocycline [Can]
Novo-Tetra [Can]
Nu-Doxycycline [Can]
Nu-Tetra [Can]
oxytetracycline
Periostat® [US]
Rhoxal-Minocycline [Can]
Sumycin® [US]
Terramycin® I.M. [US/Can]
tetracycline
Vibramycin® [US]
Vibra-Tabs® [US/Can]
Wesmycin® [US]

SJÖGREN SYNDROME
Cholinergic Agent
   cevimeline
   Evoxac™ [US/Can]

SKIN ULCER
Enzyme
   collagenase
   Elase® [US]
   fibrinolysin and desoxyribonuclease
   Plaquase® [US]
   Santyl® [US/Can]
Topical Skin Product
   Debrisan® [US-OTC]
   dextranomer

SPASTICITY
Alpha2-Adrenergic Agonist Agent
   tizanidine
   Zanaflex® [US/Can]
Benzodiazepine
   Apo®-Diazepam [Can]
   Diastat® [US/Can]
   Diazemuls® [Can]
   diazepam
   Diazepam Intensol® [US]
   Valium® [US/Can]
Skeletal Muscle Relaxant
   Apo®-Baclofen [Can]
   baclofen

Dantrium® [US/Can]
dantrolene
Gen-Baclofen [Can]
Lioresal® [US/Can]
Liotec [Can]
Nu-Baclo [Can]
PMS-Baclofen [Can]

SPONDYLITIS (ANKYLOSING)

Nonsteroidal Antiinflammatory Drug
  (NSAID)
  Alti-Piroxicam [Can]
  Apo®-Diclo [Can]
  Apo®-Diclo SR [Can]
  Apo®-Piroxicam [Can]
  Cataflam® [US/Can]
  diclofenac
  Diclotec [Can]
  Feldene® [US/Can]
  Gen-Piroxicam [Can]
  Novo-Difenac® [Can]
  Novo-Difenac-K [Can]
  Novo-Difenac® SR [Can]
  Novo-Pirocam® [Can]
  Nu-Diclo [Can]
  Nu-Diclo-SR [Can]
  Nu-Pirox [Can]
  Pexicam® [Can]
  piroxicam
  PMS-Diclofenac [Can]
  PMS-Diclofenac SR [Can]
  Riva-Diclofenac [Can]
  Riva-Diclofenac-K [Can]
  Solaraze™ [US]
  Voltaren Rapide® [Can]
  Voltaren® [US/Can]
  Voltaren®-XR [US]
  Voltare Ophtha® [Can]

STATUS EPILEPTICUS

Anticonvulsant
  paraldehyde
  Paral® [US]

Barbiturate
  amobarbital
  Amytal® [US/Can]
  Luminal® Sodium [US]
  Nembutal® [US/Can]
  pentobarbital
  phenobarbital
Benzodiazepine
  Apo®-Diazepam [Can]
  Apo®-Lorazepam [Can]
  Ativan® [US/Can]
  Diastat® [US/Can]
  Diazemuls® [Can]
  diazepam
  Diazepam Intensol® [US]
  lorazepam
  Novo-Lorazem® [Can]
  Nu-Loraz [Can]
  Riva-Lorazepam [Can]
  Valium® [US/Can]
Hydantoin
  Dilantin® [US/Can]
  Phenytek™ [US]
  phenytoin

STOMATITIS

Local Anesthetic
  Dyclone® [US]
  dyclonine
  Sucrets® [US-OTC]

STRABISMUS

Cholinesterase Inhibitor
  echothiophate iodide
  Phospholine Iodide® [US]
Ophthalmic Agent, Toxin
  Botox® [US/Can]
  botulinum toxin type A

STROKE

Antiplatelet Agent
  Alti-Ticlopidine [Can]
  Apo®-ASA [Can]
  Apo®-Ticlopidine [Can]

Asaphen [Can]
Asaphen E.C. [Can]
aspirin
Bayer® Aspirin Regimen Adult Low
  Strength [US-OTC]
Bayer® Aspirin Regimen Adult Low
  Strength with Calcium [US-OTC]
Ecotrin® Low Adult Strength [US-
  OTC]
Halfprin® [US-OTC]
Nu-Ticlopidine [Can]
Sureprin 81™ [US-OTC]
Ticlid® [US/Can]
ticlopidine
Fibrinolytic Agent
  Activase® rt-PA [Can]
  Activase® [US]
  alteplase
Skeletal Muscle Relaxant
  Dantrium® [US/Can]
  dantrolene

SUNBURN
Nonsteroidal Antiinflammatory Drug
    (NSAID)
  Alti-Piroxicam [Can]
  Apo®-Piroxicam [Can]
  Feldene® [US/Can]
  Gen-Piroxicam [Can]
  Novo-Pirocam® [Can]
  Nu-Pirox [Can]
  Pexicam® [Can]
  piroxicam

SYNCOPE
Adrenergic Agonist Agent
  Adrenalin® Chloride [US/Can]
  epinephrine
  isoproterenol
  Isuprel® [US]
Respiratory Stimulant
  ammonia spirit (aromatic)
  Aromatic Ammonia Aspirols®
    [US]

SYNDROME OF INAPPRO-PRIATE SECRETION OF ANTIDIURETIC HORMONE (SIADH)
Tetracycline Derivative
  Declomycin® [US/Can]
  demeclocycline

SYPHILIS
Antibiotic, Miscellaneous
  chloramphenicol
  Chloromycetin® Parenteral [US/Can]
Penicillin
  Bicillin® L-A [US]
  penicillin G benzathine
  penicillin G (parenteral/aqueous)
  penicillin G procaine
  Permapen® [US]
  Pfizerpen® [US/Can]
  Wycillin® [US/Can]
Tetracycline Derivative
  Adoxa™ [US]
  Apo®-Doxy [Can]
  Apo®-Doxy Tabs [Can]
  Apo®-Tetra [Can]
  Brodspec® [US]
  Doryx® [US]
  Doxy-100™ [US]
  Doxycin [Can]
  doxycycline
  Doxytec [Can]
  EmTet® [US]
  Monodox® [US]
  Novo-Doxylin [Can]
  Novo-Tetra [Can]
  Nu-Doxycycline [Can]
  Nu-Tetra [Can]
  Periostat® [US]
  Sumycin® [US]
  tetracycline
  Vibramycin® [US]
  Vibra-Tabs® [US/Can]
  Wesmycin® [US]

SYSTEMIC LUPUS ERYTHEMATOSUS (SLE)
Aminoquinoline (Antimalarial)
  hydroxychloroquine
  Plaquenil® [US/Can]
Antineoplastic Agent
  cyclophosphamide
  Cytoxan® [US/Can]
  Neosar® [US]
  Procytox® [Can]

TAPEWORM INFESTATION
Amebicide
  Humatin® [US/Can]
  paromomycin

TARDIVE DYSKINESIA
Anticonvulsant
  Sabril® [US/Can]
  vigabatrin (Canada only)
Monoamine Depleting Agent
  Nitoman® [Can]
  tetrabenazine (Canada only)
Skeletal Muscle Relaxant
  Apo®-Baclofen [Can]
  baclofen
  Gen-Baclofen [Can]
  Lioresal® [US/Can]
  Liotec [Can]
  Nu-Baclo [Can]
  PMS-Baclofen [Can]

TETANUS
Antibiotic, Miscellaneous
  Apo®-Metronidazole [Can]
  Flagyl ER® [US]
  Flagyl® [US/Can]
  metronidazole
  Nidagel™ [Can]
  Noritate™ [US/Can]
  Novo-Nidazol [Can]
Immune Globulin
  BayTet™ [US/Can]
  tetanus immune globulin (human)

Toxoid
  Adacel® [Can]
  Daptacel™ [US]
  diphtheria and tetanus toxoid
  diphtheria, tetanus toxoids, and acellular pertussis vaccine
  diphtheria, tetanus toxoids, and acellular pertussis vaccine and *Haemophilus* B conjugate vaccine
  diphtheria, tetanus toxoids, and whole-cell pertussis vaccine
  diphtheria, tetanus toxoids, whole-cell pertussis, and *Haemophilus* B conjugate vaccine
  Infanrix® [US]
  Pentacel™ [Can]
  tetanus toxoid (adsorbed)
  tetanus toxoid (fluid)
  TriHIBit® [US]
  Tripedia® [US]
Vaccine, Inactivated Bacteria
  diphtheria, tetanus toxoids, and acellular pertussis vaccine and *Haemophilus* B conjugate vaccine
  TriHIBit® [US]

THREADWORM (NONDISSEMINATED INTESTINAL)
Antibiotic, Miscellaneous
  ivermectin
  Stromectol® [US]

THROMBOCYTOPENIA
Anticoagulant, Thrombin Inhibitor
  argatroban
Enzyme
  alglucerase
  Ceredase® [US]
Platelet Growth Factor
  Neumega® [US]
  oprelvekin

THROMBOCYTOPENIA (HEPARIN-INDUCED)
Anticoagulant (Other)
  lepirudin
  Refludan® [US/Can]

THROMBOCYTOSIS
Antineoplastic Agent
  Droxia™ [US]
  Hydrea® [US/Can]
  hydroxyurea
  Mylocel™ [US]

THROMBOLYTIC THERAPY
Anticoagulant (Other)
  anisindione
  Coumadin® [US/Can]
  dalteparin
  dicumarol
  enoxaparin
  Fragmin® [US/Can]
  Hepalean® [Can]
  Hepalean® Leo [Can]
  Hepalean®-LOK [Can]
  heparin
  Hep-Lock® [US]
  Innohep® [US/Can]
  Lovenox® [US/Can]
  Miradon® [US]
  Taro-Warfarin [Can]
  tinzaparin
  warfarin
Fibrinolytic Agent
  Abbokinase® [US]
  Activase® rt-PA [Can]
  Activase® [US]
  alteplase
  Retavase® [US/Can]
  reteplase
  Streptase® [US/Can]
  streptokinase
  urokinase

THROMBOSIS (ARTERIAL)
Fibrinolytic Agent
  Streptase® [US/Can]
  streptokinase

THYROTOXIC CRISIS
Antithyroid Agent
  methimazole
  Pima® [US]
  potassium iodide
  propylthiouracil
  Propyl-Thyracil® [Can]
  SSKI® [US]
  Tapazole® [US/Can]
  Thyro-Block® [Can]

TOURETTE DISEASE
Antipsychotic Agent, Butyrophenone
  Apo®-Haloperidol [Can]
  Haldol® Decanoate [US]
  Haldol® [US/Can]
  haloperidol
  Novo-Peridol [Can]
  Peridol [Can]
  PMS-Haloperidol LA [Can]
  Rho®-Haloperidol Decanoate [Can]
Neuroleptic Agent
  Orap™ [US/Can]
  pimozide
Phenothiazine Derivative
  Chlorpromanyl® [Can]
  chlorpromazine
  Largactil® [Can]
  Thorazine® [US]

TOXOPLASMOSIS
Antibiotic, Miscellaneous
  Alti-Clindamycin [Can]
  Cleocin HCl® [US]
  Cleocin Pediatric® [US]
  Cleocin Phosphate® [US]
  Cleocin® [US]
  clindamycin
  Dalacin® C [Can]

Folic Acid Antagonist (Antimalarial)
  Daraprim® [US/Can]
  pyrimethamine
Sulfonamide
  sulfadiazine

TRANSFUSION REACTION

Antihistamine
  Alercap® [US-OTC]
  Aler-Dryl® [US-OTC]
  Alertab® [US-OTC]
  Aller-Chlor® [US-OTC]
  Allerdryl® [Can]
  Allermax® [US-OTC]
  Allernix [Can]
  Altaryl® [US-OTC]
  Anti-Hist® [US-OTC]
  ANX® [US]
  Apo®-Hydroxyzine [Can]
  Atarax® [US/Can]
  azatadine
  Banaril® [US-OTC]
  Banophen® [US-OTC]
  Benadryl® [US/Can]
  brompheniramine
  chlorpheniramine
  Chlor-Trimeton® [US-OTC]
  Chlor-Tripolon® [Can]
  Claritin® RediTabs® [US]
  Claritin® [US/Can]
  clemastine
  Colhist® Solution [US-OTC]
  cyproheptadine
  Dermamycin® [US-OTC]
  Derma-Pax® [US-OTC]
  dexchlorpheniramine
  Dimetane® Extentabs® [US-OTC]
  Dimetapp® Allergy Children's [US-OTC]
  Dimetapp® Allergy [US-OTC]
  Diphendryl® [US-OTC]
  Diphenhist® [US-OTC]
  diphenhydramine
  Diphen® [US-OTC]
  Diphenyl® [US-OTC]
  Dytuss® [US-OTC]
  Genahist® [US-OTC]
  Geridryl® [US-OTC]
  Hydramine® [US-OTC]
  hydroxyzine
  Hyrexin® [US-OTC]
  Hyzine-50® [US]
  Lodrane® 12 Hour [US-OTC]
  loratadine
  Mediphedryl® [US-OTC]
  Nolahist® [US/Can]
  Novo-Hydroxyzin [Can]
  Optimine® [US/Can]
  Periactin® [US/Can]
  phenindamine
  PMS-Diphenhydramine [Can]
  PMS-Hydroxyzine [Can]
  Polaramine® [US]
  Polydryl® [US-OTC]
  Polytapp® Allergy Dye-Free Medication [US-OTC]
  Q-Dryl® [US-OTC]
  Quenalin® [US-OTC]
  Siladryl® Allerfy® [US-OTC]
  Silphen® [US-OTC]
  Tavist®-1 [US-OTC]
  Tavist® [US]
  Vistacot® [US]
  Vistaril® [US/Can]
Phenothiazine Derivative
  Anergan® [US]
  Phenergan® [US/Can]
  promethazine

TRANSIENT ISCHEMIC ATTACK (TIA)

Anticoagulant (Other)
  enoxaparin
  Hepalean® [Can]
  Hepalean® Leo [Can]
  Hepalean®-LOK [Can]

heparin
Hep-Lock® [US]
Lovenox® [US/Can]
Antiplatelet Agent
aspirin
Bayer® Aspirin Regimen Adult Low
Strength [US-OTC]
Bayer® Aspirin Regimen Adult Low
Strength with Calcium [US-OTC]
Ecotrin® Low Adult Strength [US-
OTC]
Halfprin® [US-OTC]
Sureprin 81™ [US-OTC]

TUBERCULOSIS
Antibiotic, Aminoglycoside
streptomycin
Antibiotic, Miscellaneous
Capastat® Sulfate [US]
capreomycin
cycloserine
Rifadin® [US/Can]
Rifamate® [US/Can]
rifampin
rifampin and isoniazid
rifampin, isoniazid, and pyrazinamide
Rifater® [US/Can]
Rimactane® [US]
Rofact™ [Can]
Seromycin® Pulvules® [US]
Antimycobacterial Agent
ethambutol
ethionamide
Etibi® [Can]
Myambutol® [US]
Trecator®-SC [US/Can]
Antitubercular Agent
isoniazid
Isotamine® [Can]
Nydrazid® [US]
PMS-Isoniazid [Can]
pyrazinamide
streptomycin

Tebrazid™ [Can]
Biological Response Modulator
BCG vaccine
ImmuCyst® [Can]
Oncotice™ [Can]
Pacis™ [Can]
TheraCys® [US]
TICE® BCG [US]
Nonsteroidal Antiinflammatory Drug
(NSAID)
aminosalicylate sodium
Nemasol® Sodium [Can]

TUBERCULOSIS (DIAGNOSTIC)
Diagnostic Agent
Aplisol® [US]
Tine Test PPD [US]
tuberculin tests
Tubersol® [US]

TUMOR (BRAIN)
Antineoplastic Agent
BiCNU® [US/Can]
carboplatin
carmustine
CeeNU® [US/Can]
Gliadel® [US]
lomustine
Matulane® [US/Can]
mechlorethamine
Mustargen® [US/Can]
Natulan® [Can]
Paraplatin-AQ [Can]
Paraplatin® [US]
procarbazine
Biological Response Modulator
interferon alfa-2b
Intron® A [US/Can]

TURNER SYNDROME
Androgen
Oxandrin® [US]
oxandrolone

ULCER, DIABETIC FOOT OR LEG
Topical Skin Product
  becaplermin
  Regranex® [US/Can]

ULCER (DUODENAL)
Proton Pump Inhibitor
  Panto™ IV [Can]
  Pantoloc™ [Can]
  pantoprazole
  Protonix® [US/Can]

ULCER (GASTRIC)
Proton Pump Inhibitor
  Panto™ IV [Can]
  Pantoloc™ [Can]
  pantoprazole
  Protonix® [US/Can]

URINARY BLADDER SPASM
Anticholinergic Agent
  Propanthel™ [Can]
  propantheline

URINARY RETENTION
Antispasmodic Agent,
    Urinary
  Ditropan® [US/Can]
  Ditropan® XL [US]
  Gen-Oxybutynin [Can]
  Novo-Oxybutynin [Can]
  Nu-Oxybutyn [Can]
  oxybutynin
  PMS-Oxybutynin [Can]
Cholinergic Agent
  bethanechol
  Duvoid® [Can]
  Myotonachol™ [Can]
  neostigmine
  Prostigmin® [US/Can]
  Urecholine® [US]

URINARY TRACT INFECTION
Antibiotic, Carbacephem
  Lorabid™ [US/Can]
  loracarbef
Antibiotic, Miscellaneous
  Apo®-Nitrofurantoin
    [Can]
  Azactam® [US/Can]
  aztreonam
  Dehydral® [Can]
  fosfomycin
  Furadantin® [US]
  Hip-Rex™ [Can]
  Hiprex® [US/Can]
  Macrobid® [US/Can]
  Macrodantin® [US/Can]
  Mandelamine® [Can]
  methenamine
  Monurol™ [US/Can]
  nitrofurantoin
  Novo-Furantoin [Can]
  Primsol® [US]
  Proloprim® [US/Can]
  trimethoprim
  Urasal® [Can]
  Urex® [US/Can]
  Vancocin® [US/Can]
  Vancoled® [US]
  vancomycin
Antibiotic, Penicillin
  pivampicillin (Canada only)
  Pondocillin® [Can]
Antibiotic, Quinolone
  gatifloxacin
  Levaquin® [US/Can]
  levofloxacin
  Quixin™ Ophthalmic
    [US]
  Tequin® [US/Can]
Antibiotic, Urinary Antiinfective
  Atrosept® [US]
  Dolsed® [US]

methenamine, phenyl salicylate, atropine, hyoscyamine, benzoic acid, and methylene blue
UAA® [US]
Uridon Modified® [US]
Urised® [US]
Uritin® [US]
Cephalosporin (First Generation)
  Ancef® [US/Can]
  Apo®-Cefadroxil [Can]
  Apo®-Cephalex [Can]
  Biocef® [US]
  cefadroxil
  Cefadyl® [US/Can]
  cefazolin
  cephalexin
  cephalothin
  cephapirin
  cephradine
  Ceporacin® [Can]
  Duricef® [US/Can]
  Keflex® [US]
  Keftab® [US/Can]
  Kefzol® [US/Can]
  Novo-Cefadroxil [Can]
  Novo-Lexin® [Can]
  Nu-Cephalex® [Can]
  Velosef® [US]
Cephalosporin (Second Generation)
  Apo®-Cefaclor [Can]
  Ceclor® CD [US]
  Ceclor® [US/Can]
  cefaclor
  cefamandole
  Cefotan® [US/Can]
  cefotetan
  cefoxitin
  cefpodoxime
  cefprozil
  Ceftin® [US/Can]
  cefuroxime
  Cefzil® [US/Can]
  Kefurox® [US/Can]

Mandol® [US]
Mefoxin® [US/Can]
Novo-Cefaclor [Can]
Nu-Cefaclor [Can]
PMS-Cefaclor [Can]
Vantin® [US/Can]
Zinacef® [US/Can]
Cephalosporin (Third Generation)
  Cedax® [US]
  cefixime
  Cefizox® [US/Can]
  Cefobid® [US/Can]
  cefoperazone
  cefotaxime
  ceftazidime
  ceftibuten
  ceftizoxime
  ceftriaxone
  Ceptaz® [US/Can]
  Claforan® [US/Can]
  Fortaz® [US/Can]
  Rocephin® [US/Can]
  Suprax® [US/Can]
  Tazicef® [US]
  Tazidime® [US/Can]
Cephalosporin (Fourth Generation)
  cefepime
  Maxipime® [US/Can]
Genitourinary Irrigant
  neomycin and polymyxin B
  Neosporin® G.U. Irrigant [US/Can]
Irrigating Solution
  citric acid bladder mixture
  Renacidin® [US]
Penicillin
  amoxicillin
  amoxicillin and clavulanate potassium
  Amoxicot® [US]
  Amoxil® [US/Can]
  ampicillin
  ampicillin and sulbactam
  Apo®-Amoxi [Can]

Apo®-Ampi [Can]
Apo®-Cloxi [Can]
Apo®-Pen VK [Can]
Augmentin ES-600™ [US]
Augmentin® [US/Can]
Bicillin® C-R 900/300 [US]
Bicillin® C-R [US]
Bicillin® L-A [US]
carbenicillin
Clavulin® [Can]
cloxacillin
dicloxacillin
Dynapen® [US]
Gen-Amoxicillin [Can]
Geocillin® [US]
Lin-Amox [Can]
Marcillin® [US]
Moxilin® [US]
Nadopen-V® [Can]
nafcillin
Novamoxin® [Can]
Novo-Ampicillin [Can]
Novo-Cloxin [Can]
Novo-Pen-VK® [Can]
Nu-Amoxi [Can]
Nu-Ampi [Can]
Nu-Cloxi® [Can]
Nu-Pen-VK® [Can]
oxacillin
penicillin G benzathine
penicillin G benzathine and procaine
    combined
penicillin G (parenteral/aqueous)
penicillin G procaine
penicillin V potassium
Permapen® [US]
Pfizerpen® [US/Can]
piperacillin
piperacillin and tazobactam sodium
Pipracil® [US/Can]
Principen® [US]
PVF® K [Can]
Suspen® [US]

Tazocin® [Can]
ticarcillin and clavulanate
    potassium
Timentin® [US/Can]
Trimox® [US]
Truxcillin® [US]
Unasyn® [US/Can]
Veetids® [US]
Wycillin® [US/Can]
Wymox® [US]
Zosyn® [US]
Quinolone
    Apo®-Norflox [Can]
    Apo®-Oflox [Can]
    Cinobac® [US/Can]
    cinoxacin
    Floxin® [US/Can]
    lomefloxacin
    Maxaquin® [US]
    nalidixic acid
    NegGram® [US/Can]
    norfloxacin
    Noroxin® [US/Can]
    Novo-Norfloxacin [Can]
    Ocuflox® [US/Can]
    ofloxacin
    Riva-Norfloxacin [Can]
    sparfloxacin
    Zagam® [US]
Sulfonamide
    Apo®-Sulfatrim [Can]
    Bactrim™ DS [US]
    Bactrim™ [US]
    Gantrisin® Pediatric Suspension [US]
    Novo-Trimel [Can]
    Novo-Trimel D.S. [Can]
    Nu-Cotrimox® [Can]
    Septra® DS [US/Can]
    Septra® [US/Can]
    sulfadiazine
    sulfamethoxazole and trimethoprim
    Sulfatrim® DS [US]
    Sulfatrim® [US]

sulfisoxazole
sulfisoxazole and phenazopyridine
Sulfizole® [Can]
Truxazole® [US]
Urinary Tract Product
acetohydroxamic acid
Atrosept® [US]
Dolsed® [US]
Lithostat® [US]
methenamine, phenyl salicylate, atropine, hyoscyamine, benzoic acid, and methylene blue
UAA® [US]
Uridon Modified® [US]
Urised® [US]
Uritin® [US]

UVEITIS
Adrenal Corticosteroid
rimexolone
Vexol® [US/Can]
Adrenergic Agonist Agent
AK-Dilate® Ophthalmic [US]
AK-Nefrin® Ophthalmic [US]
Dionephrine® [Can]
Mydfrin® Ophthalmic [US/Can]
Neo-Synephrine® Ophthalmic [US]
phenylephrine
Prefrin™ Ophthalmic [US]
Anticholinergic Agent
atropine
Atropine-Care® [US]
Atropisol® [US/Can]
homatropine
Isopto® Atropine [US/Can]
Isopto® Homatropine [US]
Isopto® Hyoscine [US]
scopolamine

VAGINITIS
Antibiotic, Vaginal
sulfabenzamide, sulfacetamide, and sulfathiazole
V.V.S.® [US]

Estrogen and Progestin Combination
estrogens and medroxyprogesterone
Premphase® [US/Can]
Prempro™ [US/Can]
Estrogen Derivative
Alora® [US]
Cenestin™ [US/Can]
Climara® [US/Can]
Congest [Can]
Delestrogen® [US/Can]
Depo®-Estradiol [US/Can]
diethylstilbestrol
Esclim® [US]
Estinyl® [US]
Estrace® [US/Can]
Estraderm® [US/Can]
estradiol
Estring® [US/Can]
Estrogel® [Can]
estrogens (conjugated A/synthetic)
estrogens (conjugated/equine)
estrone
ethinyl estradiol
Gynodiol™ [US]
Honvol® [Can]
Kestrone® [US/Can]
Oesclim® [Can]
Oestrilin [Can]
PMS-Conjugated Estrogens [Can]
Premarin® [US/Can]
Stilphostrol® [US]
Vagifem® [US/Can]
Vivelle-Dot® [US]
Vivelle® [US/Can]

VALPROIC ACID POISONING
Dietary Supplement
Carnitor® [US/Can]
levocarnitine
Mito-Carn® [US]

VANCOMYCIN-RESISTANT *ENTEROCOCCUS FAECIUM* BACTEREMIA (VRE)
Antibiotic, Oxazolidinone
  linezolid
  Zyvox™ [US]
Antibiotic, Streptogramin
  quinupristin and dalfopristin
  Synercid® [US/Can]

VARICELLA
Antiviral Agent
  acyclovir
  Apo®-Acyclovir [Can]
  Avirax™ [Can]
  foscarnet
  Foscavir® [US/Can]
  Gen-Acyclovir [Can]
  Nu-Acyclovir [Can]
  Zovirax® [US/Can]
Immune Globulin
  BayGam® [US/Can]
  immune globulin (intramuscular)
  varicella-zoster immune globulin
    (human)

VARICELLA-ZOSTER
Vaccine, Live Virus
  varicella virus vaccine
  Varivax® [US/Can]

VARICOSE ULCER
Protectant, Topical
  Granulex [US]
  trypsin, balsam Peru, and castor oil

VASCULAR DISORDER
Vasodilator
  isoxsuprine
  Vasodilan® [US]

VENEREAL WART
Biological Response Modulator
  Alferon® N [US/Can]
  interferon alfa-n3

VERTIGO
Antihistamine
  Antivert® [US/Can]
  Apo®-Dimenhydrinate [Can]
  Bonamine™ [Can]
  Bonine® [US/Can]
  Calm-X® Oral [US-OTC]
  Compoz® Nighttime Sleep Aid [US-OTC]
  dimenhydrinate
  diphenhydramine
  Dramamine® II [US-OTC]
  Dramamine® Oral [US-OTC]
  meclizine
  TripTone® Caplets® [US-OTC]

VITAMIN B DEFICIENCY
Vitamin, Water Soluble
  Allbee® With C [US-OTC]
  Berocca® [US]
  Nephrocaps® [US]
  Penta/3B®+C [Can]
  Surbex-T® Filmtabs® [US-OTC]
  Surbex® With C Filmtabs® [US-OTC]
  Vicon-C® [US-OTC]
  Vita 3B+C [Can]
  vitamin B complex with vitamin C
  vitamin B complex with vitamin C
    and folic acid

VITAMIN B5 DEFICIENCY
Vitamin, Water Soluble
  pantothenic acid

VITAMIN B6 DEFICIENCY
Vitamin, Water Soluble
  Aminoxin® [US-OTC]
  pyridoxine

VITAMIN B12 DEFICIENCY
Vitamin, Water Soluble
  Bedoz [Can]

Cobal® [US]
Cobolin-M® [US]
cyanocobalamin
LA-12® [US]
Nascobal® [US]
Neuroforte-R® [US]
Twelve Resin-K® [US]
Vita® #12 [US]
Vitabee® 12 [US]

VITAMIN C DEFICIENCY
Vitamin, Water Soluble
Allbee® With C [US-OTC]
Apo®-C [Can]
ascorbic acid
Berocca® [US]
C-500-GR™ [US-OTC]
Cecon® [US-OTC]
Cenolate® [US]
Cevi-Bid® [US-OTC]
C-Gram [US-OTC]
Dull-C® [US-OTC]
Nephrocaps® [US]
Penta/3B®+C [Can]
Proflavanol C™ [Can]
Revitalose C-1000® [Can]
sodium ascorbate
Surbex-T® Filmtabs® [US-OTC]
Surbex® With C Filmtabs® [US-OTC]
Vicon-C® [US-OTC]
Vita 3B+C [Can]
Vita-C® [US-OTC]
vitamin B complex with vitamin C
vitamin B complex with vitamin C
and folic acid

VITAMIN D DEFICIENCY
Vitamin D Analog
Calciferol™ [US]
cholecalciferol
Delta-D® [US]
Drisdol® [US/Can]
D-Vi-Sol® [Can]
ergocalciferol
Ostoforte® [Can]

VITAMIN E DEFICIENCY
Vitamin, Fat Soluble
Liqui-E® [US]
tocophersolan

VITAMIN K DEFICIENCY
Vitamin, Fat Soluble
AquaMEPHYTON® [US/Can]
Mephyton® [US/Can]
phytonadione

VITILIGO
Psoralen
methoxsalen
8-MOP® [US/Can]
Oxsoralen® Lotion [US/Can]
Oxsoralen-Ultra® [US/Can]
trioxsalen
Trisoralen® [US]
Ultramop™ [Can]
Uvadex® [US/Can]
Topical Skin Product
Benoquin® [US]
monobenzone

VOMITING
Anticholinergic Agent
Isopto® Hyoscine [US]
Scopace® [US]
scopolamine
Transderm Scōp® [US]
Transderm-V® [Can]
Antiemetic
Anergan® [US]
ANX® [US]
Apo®-Hydroxyzine [Can]
Atarax® [US/Can]
Benzacot® [US]
dronabinol
droperidol
hydroxyzine

Hyzine-50® [US]
Inapsine® [US]
Marinol® [US/Can]
Novo-Hydroxyzin [Can]
Phenergan® [US/Can]
PMS-Hydroxyzine [Can]
promethazine
Restall® [US]
Tigan® [US/Can]
trimethobenzamide
Vistacot® [US]
Vistaril® [US/Can]
Antihistamine
Apo®-Dimenhydrinate [Can]
Calm-X® Oral [US-OTC]
dimenhydrinate
Dramamine® Oral [US-OTC]
Gravol® [Can]
Hydrate® [US]
TripTone® Caplets® [US-OTC]
Phenothiazine Derivative
Apo®-Perphenazine [Can]
Chlorpromanyl® [Can]
chlorpromazine
Compazine® [US/Can]
Compro™ [US]
Largactil® [Can]
Nu-Prochlor [Can]
perphenazine
prochlorperazine
Stemetil® [Can]
thiethylperazine
Thorazine® [US]
Torecan® [US]
triflupromazine
Trilafon® [US/Can]
Vesprin® [US/Can]

VOMITING, CHEMOTHERAPY-RELATED
Selective 5-HT3 Receptor Antagonist
Anzemet® [US/Can]

dolasetron
granisetron
Kytril™ [US/Can]
ondansetron
Zofran® ODT [US/Can]
Zofran® [US/Can]

WHIPWORMS
Anthelmintic
mebendazole
Vermox® [US/Can]

XEROSTOMIA
Cholinergic Agent
pilocarpine
Salagen® [US/Can]

ZOLLINGER-ELLISON SYNDROME
Antacid
calcium carbonate and simethicone
Iosopan® Plus [US]
Lowsium® Plus [US]
magaldrate
magaldrate and simethicone
Mag-Gel® 600 [US]
magnesium hydroxide
magnesium oxide
Mag-Ox® 400 [US-OTC]
Phillips'® Milk of Magnesia [US-OTC]
Riopan Plus® Double Strength [US-OTC]
Riopan Plus® [US-OTC]
Riopan® [US-OTC]
Titralac® Plus Liquid [US-OTC]
Uro-Mag® [US-OTC]
Antineoplastic Agent
streptozocin
Zanosar® [US/Can]
Gastric Acid Secretion Inhibitor
Aciphex™ [US/Can]
lansoprazole
omeprazole

Prevacid® [US/Can]
Prilosec® [US/Can]
rabeprazole
Histamine H2 Antagonist
  Acid Reducer 200®
    [US-OTC]
  Alti-Famotidine [Can]
  Alti-Ranitidine [Can]
  Apo®-Cimetidine [Can]
  Apo®-Famotidine [Can]
  Apo®-Ranitidine [Can]
  cimetidine
  famotidine
  Gen-Cimetidine [Can]
  Gen-Famotidine [Can]
  Gen-Ranitidine [Can]
  Heartburn 200® [US-OTC]
  Heartburn Relief 200® [US-OTC]
  Novo-Cimetidine [Can]

Novo-Famotidine [Can]
Novo-Ranidine [Can]
Nu-Cimet® [Can]
Nu-Famotidine [Can]
Nu-Ranit [Can]
Pepcid® AC [US/Can]
Pepcid® [US/Can]
PMS-Cimetidine [Can]
ranitidine hydrochloride
Rhoxal-famotidine [Can]
Tagamet® HB [US/Can]
Tagamet® [US/Can]
Ulcidine® [Can]
Zantac® 75 [US-OTC]
Zanta [Can]
Zantac® [US/Can]
Prostaglandin
  Cytotec® [US/Can]
  misoprostol

Appendix 4
Fractures

abduction fracture
abduction-external rotation fracture
accessory navicular fracture
accessory ossicle fracture
acetabular posterior wall fracture
acetabular rim fracture
acute avulsion fracture
acute fracture
acute on chronic fracture
adduction fracture
agenetic fracture
Aitken epiphysial fracture
Allen calcaneal fracture
alveolar bone fracture
alveolar process fracture
alveolar socket wall fracture
anatomic fracture
anatomic neck fracture
Anderson-Hutchins unstable tibial shaft
   fracture
angle fracture
angulated fracture
angulation fracture
ankle mortise fracture
anterior calcaneal process fracture
anterior column fracture
anterior fracture
anterior inferior iliac spine fracture
anterior rib fracture
anteroinferior corner fracture
anterolateral compression fracture
anular fracture
apex fracture
apophysial fracture
arch fracture
articular mass separation fracture
articular pillar fracture
artificial fracture
Ashhurst-Bromer ankle fracture
Atkin epiphysial fracture

atlantal fracture
atlas burst fracture
atlas-axis combination fracture
atrophic fracture
avulsion chip fracture
avulsion stress fracture
axial compression fracture
axial load 3-part, 2-plane fracture
axial load teardrop fracture
axial loading fracture
axis fracture
axis-atlas combination fracture
backfire fracture
banana fracture
Bankart fracture
Barton fracture
Barton-Smith fracture
basal neck fracture
basal skull fracture
baseball finger fracture
basicervical fracture
basilar femoral neck fracture
basilar skull fracture
bayonet position of fracture
beak fracture
bedroom fracture
bend fracture
bending fracture
Bennett basic hand fracture
Bennett comminuted fracture
Berndt-Hardy transchondral fracture
bicolumn fracture
bicondylar T-shaped fracture
bicondylar Y-shaped fracture
bicycle spoke fracture
bilateral condylar fracture
bimalleolar ankle fracture
bipartite fracture
birth fracture
blow-in fracture

blowout fracture
bone fracture
bone shaft fracture
boot-top fracture
Bosworth fracture
both-bone fracture
both-column fracture
bowing fracture
boxer's punch fracture
Boyd type II fracture
Broberg-Morrey fracture
bronchial fracture
bucket-handle fracture
buckle fracture
bumper fracture
bunk bed fracture
burst fracture
bursting fracture
butterfly fracture
buttonhole fracture
calcaneal avulsion fracture
calcaneal displaced fracture
calcaneal stress fracture
calcaneal type I-III fracture
calcaneus tongue fracture
calvarial fracture
Canale-Kelly talar neck fracture
capillary fracture
capitate fracture
capitellar fracture
capitulum fracture
carpal bone fracture
carpal bone stress fracture
carpal navicular fracture
carpal scaphoid bone fracture
carpometacarpal joint fracture
4th carpometacarpal joint fracture
cartwheel fracture
Cedell fracture
cementum fracture
central fracture
cephalomedullary nail fracture
cerebral palsy pathological fracture

cervical fracture
cervical trochanteric displaced fracture
cervicotrochanteric displaced fracture
chalk-stick fracture
Chance vertebral fracture
Chaput fracture
Charcot fracture
chauffeur's fracture
chevron fracture
childhood fracture
chip fracture
chisel fracture
chondral fracture
Chopart fracture
circumferential fracture
clavicular fracture
clay shoveler's fracture
cleavage fracture
closed ankle fracture
closed break fracture
closed fracture
closed indirect fracture
closed reduction of fracture
closed skull fracture
coccygeal fracture
coccyx fracture
Colles fracture
collicular fracture
Coltart fracture
combined fracture
combined radial-ulnar-humeral fracture
comminuted bursting fracture
comminuted intraarticular fracture
comminuted orbital fracture
comminuted skull fracture
comminuted teardrop fracture
complete fracture
complex fracture
complex simple fracture
complicated fracture
composite fracture
compound comminuted fracture
compound complex fracture

compound multiple fractures
compound skull fracture
compressed fracture
compression fracture
condylar compression fracture
condylar process fracture
condylar split fracture
congenital fracture
contrecoup fracture
controlled comminuted fracture
coracoid fracture
corner fracture
coronal split fracture
coronoid process fracture
cortical fracture
Cotton ankle fracture
cough fracture
crack fracture
cranial fracture
craniofacial dysjunction fracture
craniofacial fracture
cribriform fracture
crown fracture
crown-root fracture
crush fracture
crushed eggshell fracture
cuboid fracture
cuneiform fracture
dancer's fracture
Danis-Weber fracture
Darrach-Hughston-Milch fracture
dashboard fracture
de Quervain fracture
Denis Browne spinal fracture
Denis spinal fracture
dens fracture
dentate fracture
dentoalveolar fracture
depressed fracture
depressed skull fracture
depression fracture
depression-type intraarticular fracture
derby hat fracture
Desault fracture

Descot fracture
diacondylar fracture
diametric pelvic fracture
diaphysial fracture
diastatic skull fracture
dicondylar fracture
die punch fracture
direct fracture
direct orbital floor fracture
dishpan fracture
dislocation fracture
displaced intraarticular fracture
displaced malar fracture
displaced pilon fracture
displaced zygomatic fracture
distal femoral epiphysial fracture
distal humeral fracture
distal radial fracture
distraction of fracture
dog-leg fracture
dome fracture
dorsal rim distal radial fracture
dorsal wing fracture
double fracture
double-rib fracture
drill bit fracture
Dupuytren fracture
Duverney fracture
dye punch fracture
dyscrasic fracture
edentulous mandibular fracture
eggshell fracture
elbow fracture
elementary fracture
elephant foot fracture
enamel fracture
endocrine fracture
epicondylar avulsion fracture
epiphysial growth plate fracture
epiphysial plate fracture
epiphysial slip fracture
epiphysial tibial fracture
Essex-Lopresti joint depression fracture
explosion fracture

expressed skull fracture
extension teardrop fracture
external orbital fracture
extraarticular fracture
extracapsular fracture
extraoctave fracture
facial fracture
fat fracture
fatigue fracture
femoral diaphysial fracture
femoral intertrochanteric fracture
femoral neck fracture
femoral shaft fracture
femoral supracondylar fracture
fender fracture
fetal bone fracture
fibular diaphysial fracture
fibular shaft fracture
Fielding-Magliato subtrochanteric
   fracture
fighter's fracture
finger fracture
first carpometacarpal joint fracture
fishmouth fracture
fissure fracture
flake hamate fracture
Fleck fracture
flexion teardrop fracture
flexion-burst fracture
flexion-compression fracture
flexion-distraction fracture
floating arch fracture
floor fracture
folding fracture
foot fracture
forceps fracture
forearm fracture
frontal orbital nasoethmoidal fracture
frontal sinus fracture
Frykman hand fracture
fulcrum fracture
Gaenslen fracture
Galeazzi radical fracture
Garden femoral neck fracture

Gartland humeral supracondylar
   fracture
glabellar fracture
glenoid rim fracture
Gosselin fracture
graft fracture
Grantham femoral fracture
greater trochanteric femoral fracture
greater tuberosity fracture
greenstick fracture
greenstick Le Fort fracture
grenade thrower's fracture
gross fracture
growing skull fracture
growth plate fracture
Guérin fracture
gunshot fracture
Gustilo open fracture scoring
Gustilo tibial fracture
Gustilo-Anderson open clavicular
   fracture
gutter fracture
Hahn-Steinthal fracture
hairline fracture
hamate body fracture
hamate hook fracture
hamate tail fracture
hand fracture
hangman's fracture
Hansen fracture
Hawkins talar fracture
Hawkins talus fracture
head fracture
head-splitting humeral fracture
heat fracture
hemicondylar fracture
hemitransverse fracture
Henderson fracture
Herbert scaphoid bone fracture
Hermodsson fracture
hickory-stick fracture
high-energy fracture
Hill-Sachs posterolateral compression
   fracture

hindfoot fracture
hip avulsion fracture
hockey-stick fracture
Hoffa fracture
Holstein-Lewis fracture
hoop stress fracture
horizontal maxillary fracture
horizontal oblique fracture
humeral condylar fracture
humeral head-splitting fracture
humeral shaft fracture
humeral supracondylar fracture
Hunt and Hess hand fracture
Hutchinson fracture
hyoid bone fracture
hyperextension teardrop fracture
hyperflexion teardrop fracture
ice skater's fracture
idiopathic fracture
impacted articular fracture
impacted subcapital fracture
impacted valgus fracture
impaction fracture
implant fracture
impression fracture
impure blowout fracture
incomplete compound fracture
incomplete vertical root fracture
indented fracture
indirect orbital floor fracture
inflammatory fracture
infraction fracture
infraorbital fracture
Ingram-Bachynski hip fracture
insufficiency fracture
interarticular fracture
intercondylar femoral fracture
intercondylar humeral fracture
intercondylar tibial fracture
internal fixation fracture
internally fixed fracture
interperiosteal fracture
intertrochanteric femoral fracture
intertrochanteric 4-part fracture

intertrochanteric hip fracture
intraarticular calcaneal fracture
intraarticular proximal tibial fracture
intracapsular femoral neck fracture
intraoperative fracture
intraorbital fracture
intraperiosteal fracture
intrauterine fracture
inverted-Y fracture
ipsilateral acetabular fracture
ipsilateral femoral neck fracture
ipsilateral femoral shaft fracture
ipsilateral pelvic fracture
ipsilateral tibial fracture
irreducible fracture
ischioacetabular fracture
isolated hook fracture
Jefferson cervical burst fracture
Jefferson radial fracture
Jeffery radial fracture
joint depression fracture
Jones diaphysial fracture
Jones stress fracture
Judet epiphysial fracture
junctional fracture
juvenile Tillaux fracture
juxtaarticular fracture
juxtacortical fracture
Kapandji radical fracture
Key-Conwell pelvic fracture
Kilfoyle humeral medial condylar
    fracture
Knight and North malar fracture
Kocher fracture
Kocher-Lorenz fracture
Köhler fracture
labral and anterior inferior glenoid rim
    fracture
LaGrange humeral supracondylar
    fracture
laminar fracture
lap seatbelt fracture
laryngeal cartilage fracture
laryngeal fracture

lateral column calcaneal fracture
lateral condylar fracture
lateral condylar humeral fracture
lateral humeral condyle fracture
lateral malleolus fracture
lateral mass fracture
lateral talar process fracture
lateral tibial plateau fracture
lateral wedge fracture
laterally displaced fracture
Lauge-Hansen ankle fracture
Lauge-Hansen stage II supination-
  eversion fracture
Laugier fracture
Le Fort I-III fracture
Le Fort mandibular fracture
Le Fort-Wagstaffe fracture
lead pipe fracture
lesser trochanter fracture
linear skull fracture
Lisfranc fracture
Lloyd-Roberts fracture
local compression fracture
local decompression fracture
long bone fracture
long oblique fracture
longitudinal tibial fatigue fracture
loose fracture
Looser zone in insufficiency fracture
lorry driver's fracture
low lumbar spine fracture
low T humerus fracture
low-energy fracture
lower extremity fracture
lower frontal bone fracture
lumbar spine burst fracture
lumbosacral junction fracture
lunate fracture
Maisonneuve fibular fracture
malar complex fracture
malar fracture
Malgaigne pelvic fracture
malleolar chip fracture
mallet fracture

malunited calcaneus fracture
malunited forearm fracture
malunited radial fracture
mandibular body fracture
mandibular condyle fracture
mandibular ramus fracture
mandibular symphysis fracture
march fracture
marginal ridge fracture
Marmor-Lynn fracture
Mason fracture
mastoid bone fracture
maternal fracture
Mathews olecranon fracture
maxillary fracture
maxillofacial fracture
medial column calcaneal fracture
medial epicondyle humeral fracture
medial malleolar fracture
medial orbital wall fracture
mesiodistal fracture
metacarpal head fracture
metacarpal neck fracture
metacarpal shaft fracture
metaphysial tibial fracture
5th metatarsal base fracture
metatarsal stress fracture
Meyers-McKeever tibial fracture
micronized purified flavonoid fracture
middle tibial shaft fracture
midface fracture
midfoot fracture
midnight fracture
midshaft fracture
midwaist scaphoid fracture
Milch humeral fracture
milkman's fracture
minimally displaced fracture
mini-pilon fracture
missed fracture
Moberg-Gedda fracture
molar tooth fracture
monomalleolar ankle fracture
Monteggia forearm fracture

Montercaux fracture
Moore fracture
Mouchet fracture
multangular ridge fracture
multilevel fracture
multipartite fracture
multiple fractures
multiray fracture
nasal fracture
nasal septal fracture
nasoethmoidal fracture
nasomaxillary fracture
nasoorbital fracture
navicular body fracture
navicular dorsal lip fracture
navicular hand fracture
navicular tuberosity fracture
naviculocapitate fracture
neck fracture
Neer type I-III shoulder fracture
neoplastic fracture
neural arch fracture
neurogenic fracture
neuropathic fracture
neurotrophic fracture
Newman radial neck and head fracture
nightstick fracture
night-walker fracture
nonaccidental spiral tibial fracture
nonarticular distal radial fracture
nonarticular radial head fracture
noncomminuted fracture
noncontiguous fracture
nondepressed skull fracture
nondisplaced fracture
nonpathologic fracture
nonphyseal fracture
nonrotational burst fracture
nonunion fracture
nonunion horse-hoof fracture
nonunion torsion wedge fracture
nutcracker fracture
oblique fracture

oblique spiral fracture
O'Brien radial fracture
obturator avulsion fracture
occipital condyle fracture
occult osseous fracture
occult scaphoid fracture
odontoid condyle fracture
odontoid neck fracture
Ogden epiphysial fracture
olecranon tip fracture
open book fracture
open break fracture
open fracture
open reduction of fracture
open skull fracture
orbital blow-in fracture
orbital blowout fracture
orbital floor fracture
orbital rim fracture
orbital roof fracture
orbital wall fracture
os trigonum fracture
ossification-associated fracture
osteochondral slice fracture
osteoporotic compression fracture
outlet strut fracture
Ovadia-Beals tibial plafond fracture
overlapping fracture
pacemaker lead fracture
Pais fracture
palatal alveolar fracture
palate fracture
Palmer primary fracture
Palmer trapezial ridge fracture
pancraniomaxillofacial fracture
panfacial fracture
Papavasiliou olecranon fracture
parasymphysis fracture
paratrooper's fracture
parry fracture
pars interarticularis fracture
1-part fracture
2-part fracture

3-part fracture
4-part fracture
patellar sleeve fracture
pathologic fracture
Pauwel femoral neck fracture
pedicle fracture
pelvic avulsion fracture
pelvic insufficiency fracture
pelvic rim fracture
pelvic ring fracture
pelvic straddle fracture
pelvis fracture
penetrating fracture
penis fracture
perforating fracture
periarticular fracture
perinatal clavicle fracture
perinatal humerus fracture
peripheral fracture
periprosthetic fracture
peritrochanteric fracture
PER-IV fracture
pertrochanteric fracture
petrous pyramid fracture
phalangeal diaphysial fracture
physeal plate fracture
physis fracture
Piedmont fracture
pillar fracture
pillow fracture
pilon ankle fracture
ping-pong fracture
Pipkin femoral fracture
pisiform fracture
plafond fracture
plaque fracture
plastic bowing fracture
plastic deformation fracture
plate fracture
plateau fracture
plateau tibia fracture
Poland epiphysial fracture
pond fracture

porcelain fracture
Posada fracture
posterior arch fracture
posterior column fracture
posterior element fracture
posterior fracture
posterior process fracture
posterior rib fracture
posterior ring fracture
posterior talar process fracture
posterior wall fracture
postirradiation fracture
postmortem fracture
postoperative fracture
Pott ankle fracture
Pouteau fracture
pressure fracture
profundus artery fracture
pronation-abduction fracture
pronation-eversion fracture
pronation-eversion/external rotation
    fracture
prosthetic fracture
proximal end tibia fracture
proximal femoral fracture
proximal humeral fracture
proximal humeral stress fracture
proximal tibial metaphysial fracture
pseudo-Jefferson fracture
pseudo-Jones fracture
pubic ramus stress fracture
puncture fracture
pure blowout fracture
pyramidal fracture
Quervain fracture
Quinby pelvic fracture
radial head fracture
radial neck fracture
radial styloid fracture
radiographically occult fracture
ramus fracture
resecting fracture
retrodisplaced fracture

reverse Barton fracture
reverse Bennett fracture
reverse Colles fracture
reverse Monteggia fracture
reverse obliquity fracture
reverse Segond fracture
rib fracture
ring fracture
ring-disrupting fracture
Riseborough-Radin intercondylar
     fracture
Rockwood clavicular fracture
Rolando fracture
Rolando-type fracture
roof fracture
root fracture
rotation fracture
rotational burst fracture
Ruedi fracture
Ruedi-Allgower tibial plafond fracture
Russe scaphoid fracture
sacral fracture
sacral insufficiency fracture
sacroiliac fracture
sacrum fracture
sagittal slice fracture
sagittal splitting fracture
Sakellarides calcaneal fracture
Salter I-VI fracture
Salter-Harris epiphysial fracture
sandbagging long bone fracture
Sanders fracture
Sangeorzan navicular fracture
scaphoid fracture
scapular fracture
scotty dog fracture
seatbelt fracture
secondary fracture
segmental fracture
Segond tibial avulsion fracture
Seinsheimer femoral fracture
senile subcapital fracture
sentinel spinous process fracture

septal fracture
SER-IV fracture
sesamoid fracture
shaft fracture
shear fracture
shearing fracture
Shepherd fracture
short oblique fracture
sideswipe elbow fracture
silver fork fracture
simple fracture
simple skull fracture
single fracture
single-column fracture
skier's fracture
Skillern fracture
skull fracture
sleeve fracture
slice fracture
slot fracture
small fracture
Smith ankle fracture
Sneppen talar fracture
snowboarder's fracture
Sorbie calcaneal fracture
sphenoid bone fracture
spinal compression fracture
spine fracture
spinous process fracture
spiral oblique fracture
spiral tibial fracture
splintered fracture
split compression fracture
split-heel fracture
splitting fracture
spontaneous fracture
sprain fracture
Springer fracture
sprinter's fracture
stairstep fracture
Steele intraarticular fracture
stellate skull fracture
stellate undepressed fracture

sternal fracture
sternum fracture
Stieda fracture
straddle fracture
strain fracture
stress fracture
strut fracture
styloid fracture
subcapital fracture
subcapital hip fracture
subchondral fracture
subcondylar fracture
subcutaneous fracture
subperiosteal fracture
subtrochanteric femoral fracture
subtrochanteric fracture
supination external rotation fracture
supination-adduction fracture
supination-eversion fracture
supination-external rotation fracture
supracondylar femoral fracture
supracondylar fracture
supracondylar humeral fracture
supracondylar Y-shaped fracture
supraorbital fracture
suprasyndesmotic fracture
surgical neck fracture
sustentaculum tali fracture
symphysial fracture
synchondritic fracture
T condylar fracture
T fracture
talar avulsion fracture
talar dome fracture
talar neck fracture
talar osteochondral fracture
talus body fracture
tarsal bone fracture
teacup fracture
teardrop burst fracture
teardrop-shaped flexion-compression
  fracture
telescoping septal fracture

temporal bone fracture
tennis fracture
tension fracture
testis fracture
thalamic fracture
Thompson-Epstein femoral fracture
thoracic spine fracture
thoracolumbar burst fracture
thoracolumbar junction fracture
thoracolumbar spine fracture
threatened pathologic fracture
through-and-through fracture
thrower's fracture
Thurston Holland fracture
tibial bending fracture
tibial condyle fracture
tibial diaphysial fracture
tibial open fracture
tibial pilon fracture
tibial plafond fracture
tibial plateau fracture
tibial shaft fracture
tibial stress fracture
tibial triplane fracture
tibial tuberosity fracture
tibiofibular fracture
Tillaux fracture
Tillaux-Chaput fracture
Tillaux-Kleiger fracture
toddler's fracture
tongue fracture
tongue-type intraarticular fracture
tooth fracture
Torg fracture
torsion fracture
torsional fracture
torus fracture
total condylar depression fracture
total fracture
total talus fracture
trabecular bone fracture
tracheal fracture
traction fracture

trampoline fracture
transcaphoid fracture
transcapitate fracture
transcervical femoral fracture
transchondral talar fracture
transcondylar fracture
transhamate fracture
transiliac fracture
translational fracture
transsacral fracture
transscaphoid dislocation fracture
transtriquetral fracture
transverse comminuted fracture
transverse facial fracture
transverse maxillary fracture
transverse process fracture
transversely oriented endplate
   compression fracture
trapezial ridge fracture
trapezium fracture
traumatic fracture
traversing the fracture
trimalar fracture
trimalleolar ankle fracture
triplane fracture
triplane tibial fracture
tripod fracture
triquetral fracture
Tronzo intertrochanteric fracture
trophic fracture
T-shaped fracture
tuberosity avulsion fracture
tuberosity fracture
tuft fracture
ulnar styloid fracture
unciform fracture
uncinate process fracture
undepressed skull fracture
undisplaced fracture
unicondylar fracture
unilateral condylar fracture
unimalleolar fracture
unstable fracture

unstable zygomatic complex fracture
upper thoracic spine fracture
vertebra plana fracture
vertebral body fracture
vertebral compression fracture
vertebral stable burst fracture
vertebral wedge compression
   fracture
vertical oblique pattern fracture
vertical shear fracture
vertical tooth fracture
volar rim distal radial fracture
volar shear fracture
Volkmann fracture
Vostal radial fracture
V-shaped fracture
wagon wheel fracture
Wagstaffe fracture
waist fracture
Walther fracture
Watson-Jones navicular fracture
Watson-Jones tibial tubercle avulsion
   fracture
Weber B fracture
Weber C fracture
wedge compression fracture
wedge flexion-compression fracture
wedge-shaped uncomminuted tibial
   plateau fracture
Wilkins radial fracture
willow fracture
Wilson fracture
Winquist-Hansen femoral fracture
Y fracture
Y-shaped fracture
Y-T fracture
Zickel fracture
zygoma fracture
zygomatic arch fracture
zygomatic body fracture
zygomatic maxillary complex fracture
zygomaticomalar complex fracture
zygomaticomaxillary fracture

Sutures

absorbable suture
adjustable suture
already-threaded suture
alternating suture
aluminum-bronze wire suture
anastomotic suture
anchor suture
anchoring suture
angled suture
antibody-coated suture
antitorque suture
apical suture
arterial silk suture
atraumatic braided silk suture
atraumatic chromic suture
autoplastic suture
back wall suture
basting suture
bioabsorbable Dexon suture
BioSorb suture
Biosyn synthetic monofilament suture
biparietal suture
black braided nylon suture
black braided silk suture
black silk sling suture
black silk suture
black twisted suture
blanket suture
blue twisted cotton suture
blue-black monofilament suture
bolster suture
Bondek absorbable suture
bone wax suture
braided Ethibond suture
braided Mersilene suture
braided Nurolon suture
braided nylon suture
braided polyamide suture
braided polyester suture
braided silk suture
braided suture

braided Vicryl suture
braided wire suture
Bralon suture
bridge suture
bridle suture
bronze wire suture
Bunnell crisscross suture
Bunnell figure-of-8 suture
Bunnell wire pullout suture
buried suture
button suture
cable wire suture
cardinal suture
Cardionyl suture
cardiovascular Prolene suture
cardiovascular silk suture
catgut suture
celluloid linen suture
chain suture
chromic blue-dyed suture
chromic catgut suture
chromic collagen suture
chromic gut suture
chromicized catgut suture
cinch suture
circular suture
circumcisional suture
clove-hitch suture
coated polyester suture
coated Vicryl Rapide suture
coated Vicryl suture
collagen absorbable suture
continuous over-and-over suture
continuous running monofilament
  suture
continuous running suture
continuous sling suture
corner suture
cotton Deknatel suture
cotton nonabsorbable suture
cotton suture

cottony Dacron suture
Dacron bolstered suture
Dacron traction suture
Dafilon nonabsorbable suture
Dagrofil suture
deep dermal suture
deep suspension suture
Deklene II cardiovascular suture
Deklene polypropylene suture
Deknatel silk suture
dermal suture
Dermalon cuticular suture
Dexon absorbable synthetic
    polyglycolic acid suture
Dexon II suture
Dexon Plus suture
double right-angle suture
double-armed suture
double-armed wire suture
double-running penetrating keratoplasty
    suture
dural tack-up suture
elastic suture
Endoloop suture
end-to-end suture
end-to-side suture
epineurial suture
epitenon suture
EPTFE vascular suture
Ethibond extra polyester suture
Ethibond polyester suture
Ethibond suture
Ethicon Mersilk suture
Ethicon silk suture
Ethilon nylon suture
everting mattress suture
everting suture
expanded polytetrafluoroethylene suture
extrachromic suture
eyelid crease suture
Faden suture
false suture
fascial suture

fetal Y suture
figure-of-8 suture
filament suture
fine chromic suture
fine silk suture
fingertrap suture
fishmouth end-to-end suture
fixation suture
flat suture
formaldehyde catgut suture
frontal suture
gastrointestinal surgical gut suture
gastrointestinal surgical linen suture
gastrointestinal surgical silk suture
general closure suture
GI popoff silk suture
glue-in suture
Gore-Tex nonabsorbable suture
gossamer silk suture
grasping suture
green braided suture
green Mersilene suture
green monofilament polyglyconate
    suture
groove suture
gut suture
half-buried mattress suture
Halsted interrupted mattress suture
Halsted interrupted quilt suture
harelip suture
Heaney suture
heavy monofilament suture
heavy retention suture
heavy silk retention suture
heavy silk suture
heavy wire suture
heavy-gauge suture
helical suture
hemostatic suture
horizontal mattress suture
incisive suture
India rubber suture
interfascicular guide suture

internal suture
interrupted loop mattress suture
interrupted manual mucomucosal
    absorbable suture
interrupted nylon suture
interrupted pledgeted suture
interrupted seromuscular suture
interrupted suture
intracameral suture
intracuticular running suture
intracuticular suture
intradermal continuous suture
intradermal suture
intrafascicular suture
intraluminal suture
inverted subcuticular suture
inverting suture
Investa suture
iodine catgut suture
iodized surgical gut suture
iodochromic catgut suture
iris suture
kangaroo tendon suture
Kessler grasping suture
Kessler suture
Kessler-Kleinert suture
Kessler-Tajima suture
Kirschner suture
Krackow suture
Küstner suture
L-25 absorbable surgical suture
LAPRA-TY suture
large-caliber nonabsorbable suture
lashing suture
lateral trap suture
lead suture
lead-shot tie suture
Lembert inverting seromuscular suture
Lembert running suture
Lembert suture
lens suture
limbal suture
limbous suture

Linatrix nonabsorbable suture
Lindner corneoscleral suture
linen suture
locking horizontal mattress suture
locking suture
lock-stitch suture
longitudinal suture
loop suture
lumbar suture
Marlex suture
Mason-Allen suture
mattress suture
Maxon absorbable suture
Maxon delayed-absorbable suture
Maxon suture
Mayo linen suture
McCannel suture
Mersilene braided nonabsorbable suture
mesh suture
metal band suture
metallic suture
Micrins microsurgical suture
Micro-Glide corneal suture
micropoint suture
middle palatine suture
mild chromic suture
Millipore suture
Miralene suture
modified Bunnell suture
modified Frost suture
modified Kessler suture
modified Kessler-Tajima suture
Monocryl poliglecaprone suture
monofilament absorbable suture
monofilament clear suture
monofilament green suture
monofilament nylon suture
monofilament polypropylene suture
monofilament skin suture
monofilament steel suture
monofilament suture
monofilament wire suture
Monosof suture

multifilament steel suture
multistrand suture
muscle-to-bone suture
Mustardé suture
natural suture
nerve suture
neurosurgical suture
nonabsorbable mattress suture
nonabsorbable surgical suture
nonabsorbable suture
nonresorbable suture
Novafil suture
Nurolon suture
nylon 66 suture
nylon monofilament suture
nylon retention suture
nylon suture
oiled silk suture
opaque wire suture
over-and-over suture
overlapping suture
Panacryl suture
Panalok absorbable suture
Pancoast suture
Parker-Kerr basting suture
passing suture
PDS II Endoloop suture
PDS suture
PDS Vicryl suture
Pearsall Chinese twisted suture
Pearsall silk suture
periareolar pursestring suture
pericostal suture
perineurial suture
PERMA-HAND braided silk suture
PERMA-HAND silk suture
permanent mattress suture
pink twisted cotton suture
plain catgut suture
plain collagen suture
plain gut suture
plastic suture
pledgeted Ethibond suture

pledgeted mattress suture
plicating suture
poliglecaprone 25 suture
poliglecaprone suture
polyamide suture
polybutester suture
Polydek suture
polydioxanone suture
polyester fiber suture
polyethylene suture
polyfilament suture
polyglycolate interrupted suture
polyglycolic acid suture
polyglyconate suture
polypropylene button suture
polypropylene suture
Polysorb suture
popoff suture
posterior fixation suture
postplaced suture
PremiCron nonabsorbable suture
Premilene nonabsorbable suture
preplaced suture
primary suture
Prolene polypropylene suture
PRONOVA suture
PROXI-STRIP suture
pullout suture
pursestring suture
quilted suture
Rankin suture
rapid gut suture
Rapide wound suture
reabsorbable suture
reinforcing suture
relaxation suture
releasable suture
retention suture
retracting suture
rhabdoid suture
ribbon gut suture
rip-cord suture
rubber suture

running intradermal suture
running nylon suture
running suture
Sabreloc suture
Safil synthetic absorbable surgical
   suture
scleral flap suture
secondary suture
self-anchoring suture
seromuscular Lembert suture
SERRALNYL suture
SERRALSILK suture
serrated suture
setback suture
seton suture
shoelace suture
shotted suture
silicone-treated surgical silk suture
silk braided suture
silk Mersilene suture
silk nonabsorbable suture
silk popoff suture
silk stay suture
silk suture
silk traction suture
silkworm gut suture
silver suture
silver wire suture
silverized catgut suture
simple flaring suture
simple running suture
simple suture
Sims suture
single running suture
single-armed suture
skin suture
sling suture
Snellen suture
Sofsilk coated and braided suture
Sofsilk nonabsorbable silk suture
Softgut surgical chromic catgut suture
stainless steel wire suture
standard Bunnell suture

staple suture
stay suture
steel mesh suture
sternal suture
Stylus cardiovascular suture
subcutaneous suture
subcuticular continuous suture
subcuticular suture
superficial suture
Supramid bridle collagen suture
Supramid lens implant suture
surgical chromic suture
surgical gut suture
surgical linen suture
surgical silk suture
surgical steel suture
Surgidac suture
Surgidev suture
Surgigut suture
Surgilar suture
Surgilene blue monofilament
   polypropylene suture
Surgiloid suture
Surgilon braided nylon suture
Surgilon monofilament polypropylene
   suture
Surgipro suture
suspending suture
SUTUPAK precut suture
swaged suture
swaged-on suture
synthetic absorbable suture
Synthofil nonabsorbable suture
tacking suture
tag suture
Tajima modified Kessler suture
Teflon pledgeted suture
Teflon-coated Dacron suture
tendon suture
tension suture
tension-requiring suture
Tevdek pledgeted suture
Tevdek suture

through-and-through continuous
  suture
through-and-through reabsorbable
  suture
through-the-wall mattress suture
Ti-Cron suture
tiger gut suture
Tinel suture
traction suture
transdomal suture
transfixation suture
transfixion suture
transition suture
true suture
twisted cotton suture
twisted dermal suture

twisted linen suture
twisted silk suture
twisted virgin silk suture
umbilical tape suture
undyed suture
vascular silk suture
vascular suture
vertical mattress suture
vertical plication suture
Vicryl popoff suture
Vicryl Rapide suture
virgin silk suture
wedge-and-groove suture
white braided silk suture
white nylon suture
white twisted suture

Appendix 6
Poisonous and Hazardous Organisms and Their Antidotes

Organism

Antidote/Treatment

Snakes

Organism	Antidote/Treatment
Central American pit viper	Crotalidae antivenin
copperhead	Crotalidae antivenin
North American rattlesnake	Crotalidae antivenin
Eastern coral snake	Elapidae antivenin
South American pit viper	Crotalidae antivenin
Texas coral snake	Elapidae antivenin
water moccasin	Crotalidae antivenin

Spiders

Organism	Antidote/Treatment
black widow spider	Calcium gluconate / Lactrodectus antivenin
brown recluse spider	No antivenin—treat with pain medications
scorpion	No antivenin—treat with acetaminophen and Benadryl

Marine Animals

Organism	Antidote/Treatment
jellyfish	No antivenin—remove remaining tentacles, apply topical hydrocortisone cream, acetaminophen or ibuprofen for pain
sculpin	No antivenin—immerse the stung extremity in water that is as hot as can be tolerated without producing a burn, for 60 to 90 minutes
stingray	No antivenin—immerse the stung extremity in water that is as hot as can be tolerated without producing a burn, for 60 to 90 minutes

Common Poisonings and Their Antidotes

Poison by Category	Antidote
acetaminophen	acetylcysteine (Mucomyst)
alcohols	
ethylene glycol, methanol, folinic acid	ethanol, folic acid (Folvite)
anticholinergics	
diphenhydramine, benztropine	physostigmine (Antilirium)
anticoagulants	
coumarin derivatives	vitamin K1 (AquaMEPHYTON, Mephyton)
heparin	protamine
benzodiazepines	flumazenil (Romazicon)
botulism	botulinum antitoxin
carbon monoxide	oxygen
carbon tetrachloride	acetylcysteine (Mucomyst)
cardiac medications	
beta-adrenergic blockers	glucagon
calcium channel blockers	calcium chloride
digoxin	digoxin immune fab (Digibind)
chelating agents	
cholinergics	
organophosphates, carbamates	atropine, pralidoxime
cyanide	amyl nitrate, sodium nitrite, sodium thiosulfate, methylene blue, hydroxocobalamin
hydrofluoric acid	calcium gluconate
iron	deferoxamine mesylate (Desferal)
isoniazid	pyridoxine (Aminoxin)
lead	edetate calcium disodium (calcium disodium versenate)
opioids	naloxone (Narcan), nalmefene (Revex), naltrexone (ReVia)
organophosphates, anticholinesterases	atropine, pralidoxime (2-PAM, Protopam)
salicylates	sodium bicarbonate (Neut)
tricyclic antidepressants	sodium bicarbonate (Neut)

Appendix 8
Poisonous Mushrooms and Symptomatology

Type of Mushroom	Symptoms
cyclopeptide	Sharp abdominal pains, violent vomiting, persistent diarrhea that can contain blood and mucus
ibotenic acid-muscimol	Confusion, muscle spasms, delirium, visual disturbances
monomethylhydrazine	Fullness in the stomach, vomiting, watery diarrhea, headache, fatigue, cramps, intense pain in liver and stomach regions, seizures in severe cases
muscarine-histamine	Sweating, drooling, diarrhea, watery eyes, blurred vision, pinpoint pupils, decreased heart rate, decreased blood pressure, asthmatic breathing
psilocybin-psilocin	Intoxicated or hallucinogenic condition, mood may be apprehensive or pleasant, can include compulsive movements and uncontrolled laughter

Appendix 9
Chemical Warfare Agents and Their Antidotes

Warfare Agent	Antidote
anthrax	ciprofloxacin (Cipro)
botulism	trivalent equine antitoxin
brucellosis	doxycycline, ofloxacin
nerve agents	
sarin	atropine, pralidoxime chloride (Protopam)
VX gas	atropine, pralidoxime chloride (Protopam)
hydrogen cyanide	amyl nitrate, sodium nitrate, sodium thiosulfate, vitamin B12
plague	streptomycin, chloramphenicol, gentamicin, doxycycline
Q fever	tetracycline, erythromycin, azithromycin (Zithromax)
ricin-inhaled toxin	no antidote—supportive therapy, gastric lavage, activated charcoal
smallpox	cidofovir (Vistide)
tear gas	no antidote—treatment consists of thorough flushing of eyes, bronchodilators, assisted ventilation, oxygen when necessary, soothing lotions and blister care for skin
tularemia	streptomycin, gentamicin
vesicants	
sulfur mustard	no antidote—treatment consists of supportive care and keeping damaged organs free from infection
lewisite	British anti-lewisite, dimercaprol (BAL in Oil)

Electrocardiogram Leads

Lead	Wall of Heart Viewed
I	lateral wall
II	inferior wall
III	inferior wall
aVF	inferior wall
aVL	lateral wall
aVR	no specific view
V1	anteroseptal wall
V2	anteroseptal wall
V3	anterior and anteroseptal walls
V4	anterior wall
V5	lateral wall
V6	lateral wall

Appendix 11
Spinal Cord Injuries

Type	Symptoms
complete transsection	loss of motor function (quadriplegia with cervical cord transsection, paraplegia with thoracic cord transsection)
	muscle flaccidity
	loss of all reflexes, sensory function below level of injury
	bladder and bowel atony
	paralytic ileus
	loss of perspiration below level of injury
	respiratory impairment
incomplete transsection (central cord)	motor deficits greater in upper than lower extremities
	bladder dysfunction, varying in degree
incomplete transsection (anterior cord)	motor function loss below level of injury
	sensation loss to pain and temperature below level of injury
	touch, pressure, position, vibration senses remain intact
incomplete transsection	ipsilateral paralysis or paresis below level of injury
(Brown-Séquard syndrome)	ipsilateral loss of touch, pressure, vibration, position sense below level of injury
	contralateral loss of pain and temperature sensations below level of injury

Appendix 12
Reed Classification of Level of Consciousness

Stage	Conscious Level	Pain Response	Reflex Response	Respiration	Circulation
0	asleep	arouses	intact	normal	normal
I	comatose	withdrawal	intact	normal	normal
II	comatose	none	intact	normal	normal
III	comatose	none	absent	normal	normal
IV	comatose	none	absent	cyanosis	shock

Appendix 13
Glasgow Coma Scale

Test	Score	Patient Response
Eye opening		
spontaneously	4	spontaneous
to speech	3	opens to verbal command
to pain	2	opens only to painful stimulus
none	1	does not open
Motor response		
obeys	6	correctly shows 2 fingers when asked
localizes	5	reaches toward painful stimulus to remove it
withdraws	4	moves away from painful stimulus
abnormal flexion	3	displays decorticate posturing
abnormal extension	2	displays decerebrate posturing
none	1	lies flaccid with no response
Verbal response (Responding to question of current year)		
oriented	5	correct year given
confused	4	incorrect year given
inappropriate words	3	replies but with inappropriate words
incomprehensible	2	moans or screams to stimuli
no response	1	no response given

Appendix 14
Sample Reports

EMERGENCY ROOM TREATMENT FOR MOTOR VEHICLE ACCIDENT

HISTORY OF PRESENT ILLNESS: The patient is a 17-year-old black female who was brought into the trauma center by helicopter as a priority code yellow trauma following a serious motor vehicle accident. Reportedly, she was the belted passenger of a car involved in a head-on collision with another vehicle at high speed. According to witnesses, there was major damage to both cars. It is not clear if she suffered a brief loss of consciousness on impact, but she was found by the emergency medical services personnel with no clear recall of the events, although awake and alert. She was complaining of severe pain in the chest, the abdomen, the pelvis, and the left thigh. A significant major left thigh deformity was noted, consistent with a fracture. Of note, the patient received 15 mg of morphine sulfate en route to the hospital in the helicopter.

PAST MEDICAL HISTORY: Essentially negative, as she denied current active medical problems. She reported being gravida 0, para 0, with no suspicion of pregnancy.

ALLERGIES: She denied allergies.

MEDICATIONS: She denied medications.

HABITS: She denied alcohol abuse and illicit drug abuse.

PHYSICAL EXAMINATION: She arrived in the trauma bay with a respiratory rate of 20, oxygen saturation of over 98% on oxygen, heart rate 75 to 80, and blood pressure 97/61. Glasgow coma scale 15, moving all extremities except, of course, the left lower extremity where an obvious fracture of the left thigh was noted. The examination of the head showed no evidence of gross injuries. There were no scalp or facial lacerations. The pupils were equal and reactive, and full extraocular movements were noted. There was no abnormal drainage from the ENT orifices. There was no clinical evidence of facial fractures, and normal dental occlusion was noted. The neck was in a collar and showed no JVD, no subcutaneous emphysema, and no localized tenderness on palpation of the spinous processes. The trachea was midline. The chest appeared symmetrical, but there was exquisite tenderness on palpation of the anterior chest wall, particularly over the sternal region. No crepitus was appreciated. The lungs were clear to auscultation. The heart rhythm was regular. The abdomen was soft but tender on palpation, particularly on the left side. There was no guarding or rebound, but there was obvious tenderness. The pelvis was stable on palpation, and the perineum within normal limits. The examination of the back and the extremities was mostly remarkable for an acute angulation deformity of the left thigh, consistent with a closed fracture of the left femoral shaft. No open wounds were noted in the thigh. Of note, the left dorsalis pedis pulse was absent when the patient arrived to the hospital. It was subsequently restored after adequate reduction in traction of the left lower extremity. The examination of the other extremities was unremarkable with no evidence of ecchymosis, swelling, or deformities. Distal pulses were all equal and symmetrical. The neurological examination was also grossly intact, including the peripheral sensorimotor evaluation.

TRAUMA MANAGEMENT: As soon as the patient arrived in the trauma bay, where I was physically present, a full ATLS protocol was maintained. Concomitant with the initial assessment and the physical examination, a large-bore IV line was started and blood was drawn for routine trauma laboratory evaluation. The patient was also connected to an oxygen source and to a monitor for continuous recording of the vital signs. The ultrasound machine was immediately brought into the trauma bay for a focused trauma ultrasonographic examination of the lower chest, abdomen, and pelvis, in an effort to rule out immediately the possibility of life-threatening intrathoracic or intraabdominal hemorrhage. The study was essentially negative, showing no evidence of active bleeding into the chest and the abdomen, and was dictated as a separate report. As she remained hemodynamically stable, additional analgesia was achieved with intravenous fentanyl. Then attention was immediately directed toward the left lower extremity, which showed an acute femoral angulation, and the fracture was adequately reduced. The patient was also placed in traction after verifying her return of the distal pedal pulses. Then multiple x-rays were ordered and obtained.

First, a crosstable lateral cervical spine film showed a normal alignment of C1 through T1 with no evidence of fractures or dislocations. Additional views of the cervical spine were also negative for acute injuries. An anteroposterior view of the pelvis showed no fractures or dislocations.

A supine chest x-ray raised the suspicion of a possible widened mediastinum with aortic injury, but otherwise the lungs appeared fully expanded and clear. There was no evidence of pneumothorax or hemothorax. The diaphragmatic contours appeared normal on both sides.

X-rays of the left femur and the left knee were obtained and confirmed the presence of a displaced left femoral shaft fracture, with no evidence of knee injuries.

At this point, the patient was taken to the computerized tomography suite, where a CT scan of the head, the upper neck, the chest, the abdomen, and pelvis was obtained. The head CT showed no evidence of intracranial injuries or skull fractures. The cervical spine CT appeared within normal limits. The CT scan of the chest was highly suspicious for a mediastinal-aortic injury. The decision was made to immediately obtain an aortogram, and a call was placed to the interventional radiologist on call. CT scan of the abdomen revealed no solid organ injuries, but a small amount of free fluid was noted in the right paracolic gutter. This was thought to be associated with either a mesenteric contusion-laceration or a small bowel injury not immediately appreciated on CT scan.

LABORATORY DATA: A review of the available laboratory data was done at this point showing a WBC of 20.7, hemoglobin 12.3, hematocrit 36.8, and platelet count 277,000. PT 13.0, PTT 22.4. Type and screen O positive. Sodium 136, potassium 3.2, chloride 101, CO_2 25.3, glucose 119, creatinine 0.7, BUN 8, calcium 8.3, phosphorus 4.0, total bilirubin 0.7, alkaline phosphatase 45, total protein 6.3, albumin 3.6, and amylase 149. Beta hCG was negative. Alcohol level was negative.

SECONDARY TRAUMA MANAGEMENT: Under very close monitoring, the patient was taken to the angiography suite, where an aortogram was performed by the interventional radiologist. There was no evidence of aortic injury. A review of the CT scan findings with the radiologist concluded that the images as seen on CT were probably due to motion artifact. The patient was taken back to the emergency room's observation area, where she remained in traction of the left lower extremity and close monitoring. Repeat examination of the abdomen showed continued minimal tenderness, particularly in the left quadrant, somewhat improved by the administration of an analgesic. Again there was no guarding and no rebound suggestive of peritonitis. I made the decision at this point to observe the patient closely on the surgical trauma service with serial abdominal examination every 6 hours in an effort to avoid an unnecessary laparotomy. A call was placed also to the orthopaedic surgeon on call for evaluation of the left femoral fracture and preparation for ORIF in the ensuing 24 hours.

CLINICAL ASSESSMENT
1. Probable closed head injury with concussion.
2. Closed fracture of the left femoral shaft.
3. Severe blunt torso trauma with multiple contusions, probable nondisplaced sternal fracture, and probable mesentery contusions-lacerations.
4. Status post motor vehicle accident as a passenger.

DISPOSITION: The patient was kept in the emergency room's observation area for approximately 2 hours, during which she remained hemodynamically stable. Repeat physical examination again showed no additional findings. A repeat CBC showed a stable hematocrit at 37. As stated above, she was subsequently admitted to the surgical trauma service.

EMERGENCY ROOM TREATMENT FOR SEPTIC SHOCK

HISTORY OF PRESENT ILLNESS: The patient is a 90-year-old male with type 2 diabetes mellitus, brought to the emergency room by EMS status post pulseless electrical activity and intubated secondary to unresponsiveness. The patient's daughter states he vomited several times last night and had chills. This morning he complained of thirst, was given water, and then a short time later was found to be unresponsive. The daughter called EMS, and the patient was intubated and found to be in pulseless electrical activity, treated with epinephrine and atropine.

Per family, the patient denies any other complaints and denies shortness of breath, chest pain, urinary symptoms or fever. He does have severe osteoarthritis of the hips and has been bed bound.

PAST SURGICAL HISTORY: Cholecystectomy.

MEDICATIONS: Include aspirin and dobutamine.

SOCIAL HISTORY: Lives with a daughter.

PHYSICAL EXAMINATION: Vital signs: Systolic blood pressure 80 on Levophed, pulse 107, temperature 95. HEENT: Negative, although pupils were fixed and dilated. Lungs: Clear to auscultation and percussion with scattered rhonchi. Heart: Irregularly irregular. Extremities: Without cyanosis, clubbing, or edema. Neurological: Unresponsive; pupils fixed and dilated.

LABORATORY DATA: White count 48,000 and hemoglobin 4. Lactic acid 28.1, sodium 154, BUN 35, and creatinine 2.2. Urinalysis shows too numerous to count white blood cells. Chest x-ray is without infiltrates. The arterial blood gas on arrival in the ER revealed pH 6.79, pCO_2 21, and pO_2 395.

IMPRESSION: Severe septic shock with multiorgan failure, status post arrest at home with unresponsiveness.

RECOMMENDATIONS: Gatifloxacin in renal doses. Continuous vigorous hydration, fluid resuscitation, and pressors to support blood pressure. Increased BUN and creatinine; follow closely for signs of oliguria and renal failure. Monitor electrolytes. Deep venous thrombosis prophylaxis, nutrition, and hydration.

PROGNOSIS: Extremely poor.

EMERGENCY ROOM VISIT FOR TRANSIENT ISCHEMIC ATTACK

HISTORY OF PRESENT ILLNESS: This 79-year-old female has a past medical history significant for multiple TIAs and hypertension and mild dementia.

Patient is brought in with a sister who says that this morning she was having some speech difficulties. She says occasionally she gets some confusion and feels that the confusion and the trouble speaking both might be TIAs. She is denying having any chest pain, any choking, or dysphagia. She has no numbness or tingling of arms or legs or any focal weakness. No headache. Her difficulty is more of a Broca aphasia, which is improving now and she is able to speak just fine.

ALLERGIES: She has no known allergies.

CURRENT MEDICATIONS: Current medications are lithium, clonazepam, Plavix, and Lopressor. Dose is unknown on the Lopressor. Records show she takes 50 mg once a day.

SOCIAL HISTORY: She lives alone. She does not smoke or drink.

PHYSICAL EXAMINATION: She is in no acute distress. Temperature is 97.8, pulse 76, respiratory rate 16, and blood pressure 187/94. Pupils are equal, round, and react to light and accommodation. Extraocular movements are intact. Mouth and pharynx are clear. Tongue: Slight deviation to the left. She also has a very slight left facial droop. Neck is supple. There is no bruit. Chest is clear. Heart: S1, S2, is regular. There is no murmur or gallops. Abdomen is soft and nontender. Neurologically, cranial nerves are as above. Grip strength is equal bilaterally. Leg strength: Right leg is actually slightly weaker than the left.

STUDIES: CT scan of the head shows chronic vascular changes in deep white matter and old small infarct, anterior internal capsule. Carotid duplex Doppler showed no significant stenosis.

ASSESSMENT: Patient with a transient ischemic attack, which is resolving.

PLAN: I did discuss with the family and the patient the option of perhaps moving to Coumadin; they are very reluctant to do that. I also feel that she needs to be on an antiplatelet medication. We will get her blood pressure controlled and keep her on the Plavix and set her up for outpatient speech therapy. Family is agreeable to that. She does not wish to have any further kind of evaluation. I will get her an appointment with a primary physician in the next week.

EMERGENCY ROOM VISIT FOR VERTIGO

HISTORY OF PRESENT ILLNESS: Patient states she has had intermittent episodes of vertigo over the past 4 days. She called her primary physician today and cannot get in to see her primary physician until Thursday, so she decided to come to the emergency department. She states she is having great deal of difficulty walking, even when she gets up. She describes the dizziness as vertiginous. Denies any light-headedness. Denies prior history of similar problems. She has had no tinnitus. No nausea or vomiting. Has noted no visual changes. Family has noticed her hearing to be somewhat diminished over he past 2 weeks. There has been no fever, chills, nasal congestion, stuffiness, or sore throat. No injuries. Has noted no discomfort, fullness, or pain in her ears. The patient does have history of hypothyroidism, glaucoma, herniated disk in the low back, and history of hypertension.

PHYSICAL EXAMINATION: Patient is quite pleasant, very talkative. Ocular motion does reveal nystagmus on lateral gaze to the right. Ears: Tympanic membranes are pearly with good light reflex. Neck is supple and nontender. Blood pressure is 171/81. Respirations 18. Pulse is 84 and regular. Temperature is 97.4 degrees Fahrenheit. CT scan of the head was unremarkable.

ASSESSMENT: Vertigo, etiology unknown at this time, possible allergic reaction.

PLAN: Patient placed on Nasacort nasal spray 2 sprays in each nostril once a day, meclozine 25 mg p.o. q.8 h. as needed for the vertigo and will complete her followup with her primary physician.

EMERGENCY ROOM VISIT FOR THUMB LACERATION

HISTORY OF PRESENT ILLNESS: This 21-year-old white female accidentally lacerated her left thumb with a knife at home. No other injuries or complaints.

PAST MEDICAL HISTORY: She has no significant past medical problems.

ALLERGIES: No allergies.

MEDICATIONS: Her only routine medication is birth control pills.

SOCIAL HISTORY: No cigarette or drug use. She drinks alcohol about 2 times per week.

PHYSICAL EXAMINATION: Patient is in no distress. Left thumb: There is a 0.5-cm laceration at the radial aspect of the IP joint area. Neurovascularly intact distally.

No active bleeding. It is superficial but gaping. The laceration is anesthetized with 1 mL of 1% Xylocaine without epinephrine, cleansed thoroughly, and sutured with 5–0 Ethilon by our technician with my direct supervision.

ASSESSMENT: Thumb laceration.

PLAN: Stitches out in 7 days. A wound care instruction sheet was given. She is to return for any signs of infection.

EMERGENCY ROOM VISIT FOR NONCARDIAC CHEST PAIN

HISTORY OF PRESENT ILLNESS: This patient comes to emergency because of an episode of wavelike pain or pulsating discomfort, throbbing across the upper sternal and clavicular area, radiating to the arms. This started while he was showering this morning and feels very different from the radiating burning pains that he usually gets from GERD. He typically has burning pains in the epigastrium radiating to the chest, which mainly occur at night and particularly after greasy food. The patient became short of breath with his discomfort this morning. He cannot cause this type of pain with exertion, and he feels that his exercise tolerance has been good; his job involves walking, but no heavy lifting and no rapid walking. He works in a prison.

After today's chest pain, the type of which he has never felt before, the patient asked to see his physician. He was evaluated, EKG taken; labs were drawn, and then referred to emergency for further evaluation. Initial workup was ordered.

PAST MEDICAL HISTORY: GERD treated with Protonix. Patient's GERD has caused precancerous cells in the esophagus. He has also had heartbeat irregularities, hypertension, and some generalized arthritis.

SOCIAL HISTORY: Despite the patient's GERD trouble, he continues to chew tobacco. He drinks 2 to 3 beers per day. He has decreased his caffeine to only a couple of cups on the weekend.

FAMILY HISTORY: Father died of aortic aneurysm. Mother died of cancer.

PHYSICAL EXAMINATION: On examination, the patient appears awake, alert, in no apparent distress. There is no unusual pallor. No respiratory distress. His vital signs are almost normal, blood pressure measured 155/90; see the written record. Pulse oximetry 97% on room air at rest. The pulse is irregularly irregular. Ears, nose, and throat: Normal. Neck: Supple. No adenopathy. There is no jaundice of the eyes. No unusual conjunctival injection. Lungs: Clear to P&A. No rales, no rhonchi, no wheezes. Heart exam: S1, S2 normal. No murmurs; heart tones are somewhat soft. They are also irregularly irregular. Abdomen: Obese. Estimated body weight about 300 pounds. No organomegaly, tenderness, or mass. No chest wall tenderness. Patient cannot reproduce chest pains with motions of the chest or deep breath. Extremities show no cyanosis, mottling, or edema. Vascular: Pulses present in all 4 extremities. No abdominal bruit.

LABORATORY DATA AND STUDIES: EKG shows atrial fibrillation, otherwise unremarkable.

INR on Coumadin is 1.8. PTT is normal. CBC normal with hemoglobin 15.2 and white count 7.15. The chemistry profile shows borderline bilirubin at 1.2. Other liver function tests are normal, as are renal function and electrolytes and others. CPK total 160 with MB 5.6, borderline. Troponin measures normal at 0.01. These tests were taken about 9 hours after his episode of chest pain.

Exercise stress echocardiogram showed very poor exercise tolerance. The patient reached near his predicted peak heart rate at 90 seconds of exercise, even though the treadmill rate was slowed down for him.

ASSESSMENT: Chest pain, suspect noncardiac in origin.

PLAN: The patient has never suffered exertion-related chest pain, and he was not exerting when he had today's episode. Even though it feels different from prior reflux, it seems likely that the pain did come from reflux. I think that his previous pains were surface irritation from acid burn, and today's pain was more likely esophageal spasm. In any case, I feel it is safe for the patient to be at home unless he develops an exertion-related pattern of chest pain. If that develops, he will return to this emergency right away. If he has random episodes of chest pain and if they are not severe, he should try antacid to see if that makes him better. If he has severe pain in the chest of any cause or character, he should return to this emergency; he states understanding. No new medications were prescribed. I did recommend that he stop tobacco and alcohol, but I do not feel that he will comply. He should also try to exercise to increase his tolerance to exercise and lose some weight, but he also is not motivated to follow that instruction.

EMERGENCY ROOM VISIT FOR GASTRITIS

HISTORY OF PRESENT ILLNESS: Patient complaining of abdominal pain for the past month. Has had similar type of abdominal pain in the past. She had endoscopy approximately 3 years ago. She has been on Prevacid and Prilosec in the past for same type of problems, but she states it is currently not helping. She had some blood tests done last week and sonogram of the gallbladder, all of which were normal. She states that she gets early sensation of fullness and bloating sensation of the upper abdomen within 5 to 10 minutes of eating. She has noted this especially with cereal milk. She has noted no other particular foods giving her problems. She has had occasional loose stool with this. The patient does have trouble sleeping. She does take trazodone each night for this and does smoke. Used cocaine approximately 5 years ago, but quit.

PHYSICAL EXAMINATION: The patient appears in no acute distress. Abdomen is soft and nontender; bowel sounds are active. No guarding, no rigidity. Inguinal areas are nontender.

LABORATORY DATA: Laboratory work was reviewed, as well as the sonogram of the abdomen, which was negative for any biliary disease.

ASSESSMENT: Gastritis.

PLAN: Patient was given gastritis instructions and gastritis diet. Placed on Aciphex 20 mg p.o. nightly, Reglan 10 mg p.o. 30 minutes before meals and nightly, and Vicodin 1 or 2 tablets p.o. q.6 h. as needed for pain. She does have an appointment coming up to see the gastroenterologist and was encouraged to keep that appointment.

EMERGENCY ROOM REPAIR OF FINGER LACERATION

PREOPERATIVE DIAGNOSIS: Right index fingertip cut off in a slicer, approximately 1.5 x 1.5 cm.

POSTOPERATIVE DIAGNOSIS: Right index fingertip cut off in a slicer, approximately 1.5 x 1.5 cm.

OPERATION: Full-thickness skin graft to right index fingertip.

ANESTHESIA: Local.

INDICATIONS OF PROCEDURE: The patient is a 20-year-old female who cut off the right index finger at tip in a food slicer. The sliced area measured approximately 1.5 x 1.5 cm. The patient has the fingertip skin with her and reports no other finger injuries, paresthesias, or fractures.

The patient takes no medications and has no allergies to medications.

Past medical and past surgical history is unremarkable.

The social history, family history, and review of systems are also unremarkable.

On physical exam the patient has a 1.5-cm pulp loss off the tip of her right index finger. This goes down to the level of the finger pulp and not to the distal phalanx. The patient has the lacerated piece with her, and the piece is clean and has been kept in a moist sponge.

DESCRIPTION OF PROCEDURE: The patient's finger was blocked using 1% lidocaine without epinephrine, approximately 7 mL. The right index finger tip skin piece was débrided of all devitalized pulp tissue on the dermal side and was sewn back in place using 5–0 Vicryl. A tie-over bolster stent was made of Xeroform and 5–0 nylon sutures, and was applied over the wound. The finger was then splinted and a dry sterile dressing was applied.

FOLLOWUP PLAN: The patient will follow up in about 5 days for stent removal.

EMERGENCY ROOM REPAIR OF KNEE LACERATION

PREOPERATIVE DIAGNOSIS: A 45-cm complex knee laceration with a degloving injury of the patella and patellar tendon.

POSTOPERATIVE DIAGNOSIS: A 45-cm complex knee laceration with a degloving injury of the patella and patellar tendon.

OPERATION: Débridement and 4-layer closure of left knee 45-cm complex laceration with degloving injury of the knee.

ANESTHESIA: Local.

INDICATIONS FOR PROCEDURE: The patient is a 65-year-old female status post fall with a resulting left 45-cm complex laceration which completely degloved the left knee. The patient has a large skin flap that has devitalized a distal portion. The patient has been on steroids, resulting in poor quality of the dermis.

The patient takes asthma medications and has no known drug allergies.

The patient's medical history is significant for asthma. The patient has no significant past surgical history.

The social history, family history, and review of systems are unremarkable.

On physical exam, the patient has a complete degloved left knee with a resulting 45-cm, U-shaped laceration, which goes down to the level of the proximal tibia. The knee is degloved all the way up to the patella with no involvement of the knee joint. This is an extremely large laceration down to the level of the muscle. The distal part of the flap is devitalized, but it is difficult to tell whether this will survive. This distal flap will be débrided, but the patient may need further débridement in the future.

DESCRIPTION OF PROCEDURE: The wound was first infiltrated with 27 cc of 1% lidocaine with epinephrine. The wound was then closed in 4 layers with 3–0 Vicryl for the deep subcutaneous tissue layer to secure the flap all the way back at the level of the patella and the patellar tendon. The sutures were to keep the flap down and reduce dead space. Next the subcutaneous tissue layer was closed using 4–0 Vicryl sutures in interrupted buried fashion. Next, the deep dermis was closed using 5–0 Vicryl sutures, again in deep buried interrupted sutures. Next, the skin was closed using 4–0 nylon suture interrupted in simple and horizontal mattress sutures.

The knee was then dressed in a dry sterile dressing, an Ace wrap, and a knee immobilizer. The patient will follow up in 5 days for a wound check.

PLAN: The sutures will remain in place for 2 weeks. The patient will remain in a knee immobilizer, and the patient will most likely need to have further revision surgery if the distal flap does not survive.

Appendix 15
Common Terms by Procedure

EMERGENCY ROOM TREATMENT FOR MOTOR VEHICLE ACCIDENT

active bleeding
acute angulation deformity
advanced trauma life support (ATLS)
albumin
alkaline phosphatase
amylase
anterior chest wall
anteroposterior view of the pelvis
aortogram
ATLS protocol
beta hCG
blood urea nitrogen (BUN)
blunt torso trauma
brief loss of consciousness
calcium
carbon dioxide (CO2)
chloride
code yellow trauma
complete blood count (CBC)
computerized tomography (CT)
creatinine
crepitus
crosstable lateral cervical spine film
CT scan
diaphragmatic contour
displaced left femoral shaft fracture
distal pedal pulse
dorsalis pedis pulse
ecchymosis, swelling, or deformity
emergency medical services
    personnel
equal and symmetrical
exquisite tenderness on palpation
facial laceration
femoral angulation
femoral shaft

focused trauma ultrasonographic
    examination
free fluid
full extraocular movements
hemodynamically stable
Glasgow coma scale
glucose
gravida 0
grossly intact
guarding or rebound
head-on collision
hematocrit
hemodynamically stable
hemoglobin
illicit drug abuse
interventional radiologist
intraabdominal hemorrhage
intracranial injury
intrathoracic hemorrhage
laparotomy
large-bore IV line
localized tenderness
loss of consciousness
mediastinal-aortic injury
mesenteric contusion-laceration
morphine sulfate
motion artifact
motor vehicle accident
no evidence of fracture or dislocation
nondisplaced sternal fracture
normal alignment of C1 through T1
normal dental occlusion
obvious tenderness
open reduction internal fixation (ORIF)
O positive
oxygen saturation
para 0
paracolic gutter
peripheral sensorimotor evaluation

peritonitis
phosphorous
platelet count
potassium
prothrombin time (PT)
partial thromboplastin time (PTT)
pupils were equal and reactive
serial abdominal examination
skull fracture
small bowel injury
sodium
soft but tender on palpation
solid organ injury
spinous process
stable on palpation
sternal region
subcutaneous emphysema
surgical trauma service
tender on palpation
total bilirubin
total protein
trauma bay
white blood count (WBC)
widened mediastinum
within normal limits

EMERGENCY ROOM TREATMENT FOR SEPTIC SHOCK

arterial blood gas
atropine
bed bound
blood urea nitrogen (BUN)
chest pain
cholecystectomy
clear to auscultation and percussion
creatinine
cyanosis, clubbing, or edema
deep venous thrombosis prophylaxis
diabetes mellitus
dobutamine
emergency medical services (EMS)
epinephrine

fixed and dilated
fluid resuscitation
gatifloxacin
head, eyes, ears, nose, and throat
(HEENT)
hydration
intubated
irregularly irregular
lactic acid
Levophed
multiorgan failure
oliguria
osteoarthritis
pCO2
pH
pO2
pressor
pulseless electrical activity
pupils fixed and dilated
renal failure
scattered rhonchi
septic shock
shortness of breath
sodium
systolic blood pressure
type 2 diabetes mellitus
unresponsiveness
urinary symptom
vigorous hydration
white count

EMERGENCY ROOM VISIT FOR TRANSIENT ISCHEMIC ATTACK

Broca aphasia
bruit
carotid duplex Doppler
clonazepam
chronic vascular change
Coumadin
dementia
dysphagia
extraocular movement

facial droop
focal weakness
grip strength
hypertension
lithium
Lopressor
murmur or gallop
old small infarct
Plavix
transient ischemic attack (TIA)
vascular change
white matter

EMERGENCY ROOM VISIT FOR VERTIGO

glaucoma
good light reflex
herniated disk
hypothyroidism
lightheadedness
meclozine
Nasacort nasal spray
nasal congestion
nausea or vomiting
nystagmus
tinnitus
tympanic membrane
vertiginous
vertigo

EMERGENCY ROOM VISIT FOR THUMB LACERATION

5–0 Ethilon
interphalangeal (IP)
IP joint area
lacerated
neurovascularly intact
thumb laceration
wound care instruction sheet
1% Xylocaine without epinephrine

EMERGENCY ROOM VISIT FOR NONCARDIAC CHEST PAIN

abdominal bruit
acid burn
aortic aneurysm
atrial fibrillation
chemistry profile
chest wall tenderness
cyanosis, mottling, or edema
ears, nose, and throat
electrocardiogram (EKG)
epigastrium
esophageal spasm
exertion-related chest pain
exercise stress echocardiogram
exercise tolerance
gastroesophageal reflux disease (GERD)
heartbeat irregularity
heavy lifting
irregularly irregular
liver function test
noncardiac in origin
no rales, no rhonchi, no wheezes
organomegaly
percussion and auscultation (P&A)
precancerous cell
predicted peak heart rate
Protonix
pulse oximetry
radiating burning pain
reflux
respiratory distress
short of breath
troponin
wavelike pain

EMERGENCY ROOM VISIT FOR GASTRITIS

abdominal pain
Aciphex

biliary disease
bloating sensation
bowel sounds are active
endoscopy
gastritis
gastroenterologist
inguinal area
loose stool
no guarding, no rigidity
Prevacid
Prilosec
Reglan
sensation of fullness
sonogram of the gallbladder
trazodone
Vicodin

EMERGENCY ROOM REPAIR OF FINGER LACERATION

débrided
dermal side
devitalized pulp tissue
distal phalanx
dry sterile dressing
finger pulp
full-thickness skin graft
1% lidocaine without epinephrine
5–0 nylon suture
paresthesia
pulp loss
pulp tissue
splinted

tie-over bolster stent
5–0 Vicryl
Xeroform

EMERGENCY ROOM REPAIR OF KNEE LACERATION

Ace wrap
complex knee laceration
dead space
débridement
deep subcutaneous tissue
degloving injury
deep buried interrupted suture
deep dermis
devitalized
distal flap
dry sterile dressing
interrupted buried fashion
knee immobilizer
knee joint
4-layer closure
1% lidocaine with epinephrine
patellar tendon
proximal tibia
revision surgery
simple and horizontal mattress suture
skin flap
U-shaped laceration
3–0 Vicryl suture
4–0 Vicryl suture
5–0 Vicryl suture
wound check

Appendix 16
Emergency Medicine Abbreviations

Abbreviation	Expansion
AAA	abdominal aortic aneurysm
ABCs	airway, breathing, circulation
ABG	arterial blood gas
ABW	adjusted body weight
ACLS	advanced cardiac life support
AEIOU TIPS	mnemonic for altered mental status check
ALS	advanced life support
AMA	against medical advice
amp	ampule
AO ×3	alert and oriented × 3
ATLS	advanced trauma life support
BF	black female
BLS	basic life support
BM	black male
BMI	body mass index
BSA	body surface area
BVM	bag-valve-mask
CAD	coronary artery disease
CAPD	continuous ambulatory peritoneal dialysis
CCU	coronary care unit
CHF	congestive heart failure
CID	cervical immobilization device
COAD	chronic obstructive airways disease
COPD	chronic obstructive pulmonary disease
CPR	cardiopulmonary resuscitation
CS	cervical spine
CVA	cardiovascular accident
D5 or D5W	dextrose in a 5% normal saline solution
DB	dead body
DIC	death is coming
DNI	do not intubate
DNR	do not resuscitate
DOA	dead on arrival
DVT	deep venous thrombosis
ECC	emergency cardiac care
EMS	emergency medical service
EMT	emergency medical technician
epi	epinephrine
ESR	erythrocyte sedimentation rate

ETA	estimated time of arrival
FACEP	Fellow of the American College of Emergency Physicians
FDIU	fetal death in utero
FHT	fetal heart tone
FOOSH	fall onto outstretched hand
GCS	Glasgow coma scale
GSW	gunshot wound
HF	Hispanic female
HM	Hispanic male
IABP	intraaortic balloon pump
IBW	ideal body weight
ICU	intensive care unit
IM	intramuscular
IO	intraosseous
IUP	intrauterine pregnancy
IV	intravenous
IVDA	intravenous drug abuser
IVP	intravenous push
JONES	mnemonic for assessment of rheumatic fever
lac	laceration
LMA	laryngeal mask airway
LOC	loss of consciousness
LR	lactated Ringer
LS	lumbar spine
MCA	multiple casualty accident
MCI	multiple casualty incident
mg	milligram
MI	myocardial infarction
M&M	morbidity and mortality
MVA	motor vehicle accident
NG	nasogastric (tube)
NICU	neonatal intensive care unit
NS	normal saline
NSR	normal sinus rhythm
OD	overdose
OPQRST	mnemonic for pain scale
PACU	postanesthesia care unit
PALS	pediatric advanced life support
PCU	progressive care unit
PFT	pulmonary function test
PICU	pediatric intensive care unit
p.o.	per os (by mouth)

PQRST	mnemonic to quickly evaluate chest pain
PVC	paroxysmal ventricular contraction
RRR	regular rate and rhythm
SICU	surgical intensive care unit
STD	sexually transmitted disease
STI	sexually transmitted infection
TS	thoracic spine
TTP	trauma transport protocol
UA	urinalysis
URI	upper respiratory infection
UTI	urinary tract infection
Vfib/V-fib	ventricular fibrillation
vitamin H	ER short form for Haldol
Vtach/V-tach	ventricular tachycardia
WD	withdrawal
WF	white female
WM	white male
WNL	within normal limits
WNR	within normal range
WO	weeks old
w/o	without
WOB	work of breathing
WX	wound of exit
XKO	not knocked out
XRT	radiation therapy
Y/N	yes/no
YO	years old

Emergency Medicine Slang

Slang	Meaning
ambo	transporting ambulance
Ambu	ambu Bag
avpu	mnemonic for assessing level of consciousness
bagging	ventilation patient
bag/banana bag	liter of IV fluids given to alcoholic intoxications; named because of its yellow color, and contains multivitamins, folate, thiamine, and sugar. Its goal is to provide hydration as well as depleted nutrients, the absence of which can cause complications in alcoholics.
banger/gang banger	ER patient, often referred to as being in the ER due to traumatic injury, involved in gang activities, specifically violent acts
BIBA	brought in by ambulance
Binky test	ability of an infant to evidence basic stability and an interest in "the important things in life" by placidly sucking on a pacifier
bleed	routine lingo for a hemorrhage (can be used in many phrases, such as arterial bleed, GI bleed, head bleed, venous bleed)
blue bloater/pink puffer	stereotypical description of bodily appearance of COPD patients with chronic bronchitis and emphysema
body packer	drug courier who swallows bags/condoms of drugs
bounce back	patient who returns to ER with same complaint shortly after being released
bus	sometimes used to describe a transporting ambulance
catcher's mask	device used for patients with bleeding varices in throat to stop bleeding
chandelier sign	intense amount of physical response, including near levitation from the bed to the chandelier on the ceiling, induced by examining for cervical motion tenderness in cases of pelvic inflammatory disease
chapter	usually refers to a delusional or hallucinatory patient (from legalese Chapter 51, etc.)

champagne tap	clear tap; no blood
chicken spray	nickname for ethyl chloride spray, liquid used for transiently numbing injection sites
circling the drain	patient's future prospects of life are dim; rapid deterioration
code call	urgent medical emergency
code brown	incontinent patient
code green	ambulatory injury; walking wounded
code yellow	urgent trauma
code red	critical patient
code black	deceased patient
coke	street name for cocaine
crack	street name for a particularly potent crystalline solid form of cocaine
crank	mixture of crack cocaine and another stimulant, such as amphetamine
crasher	someone who passes out in ER (usually family member)
crispy critter	severely burned patient
crock	patient whose physical complaints are without organic or discernible basis or frankly bogus
D&D	"death and donuts"—slang for morbidity/mortality conference
dead shovel	obese male patient who dies while shoveling snow
Demerol sponge	great capacity, tolerance to, and desire for high doses of narcotics by patients with chronic pain management problems
diffusely positive review of systems	patient who reports findings or complaints broadly through each system of the body during the history interview of formal examination
DFO	"done fell out"—dialectical expression of syncope
dope addict	patient addicted to (illicit) substances, usually cocaine or heroin
DRT	"dead right there"—patient has been deceased long enough to greatly decrease the probability of resuscitation
duck	slang for a male urinal from its typical white enamelware construction and its similar silhouette to the bird
the dwindles	slow, vague failure to thrive or senile physical deterioration

dumbbels	mnemonic for cholinergic overdose (diarrhea, urination, miosis/muscle weakness, bronchorrea. bradycardia, emesis, lacrimation, salivation/sweating)
epi sick	pale, green, nauseous, chest-pounding, tachycardiac appearance of patient who has received aggressive subcutaneous epinephrine therapy in anaphylaxis or status asthmaticus
face plant	victim fell forward injuring face against floor or other object
fame	mnemonic for assessment of endocarditis
FLB	"funny-looking beat"—indeterminate or chaotic aberrance on the cardiac monitor that is not well described or not well seen as the tracing went by
floater	patient who has drowned and been in water for some time
FOF	found on floor
FOS	full of stool—clinical or radiographic determination that the patient's intestinal tract is full of stool
	found on sidewalk
four H's	hypoxemia, hypoglycemia, hypovolemia, and high bladder
FTD	fixing to die—patient's future prospects of life are dim; rapid deterioration
frequent flyer	patient who overuses ER
FUBAR'ed	fouled up beyond all recognition—used to describe either the severely traumatized individual or an intoxicated state so profound as to alter the patient's ability to be recognized as himself
GGF1	grandpa's got a fever—battery of tests for elderly with fever of unknown origin
GI cocktail	donnatal, viscous lidocaine, and Mylanta
glove up and dig in	bowel impaction
golden hour/golden window	1st hour after myocardial infarction
gomer	get out of my emergency room—term for elderly patients with multiple complicated medical complaints
gorked	obtunded or not alert, either acutely or chronically
HOD	heroin overdose
JIC tube	just in case—when drawing blood for lab studies, JIC tube is drawn just in case the doctor adds more to the lab order later on

jumper	patient who commits suicide by jumping from a structure
jump start	cardiac defibrillation
junky	patient addicted to illicit substances, usually cocaine or heroin
knife and gun club	used to describe potential patients who could come into the ER by virtue of either form of penetrating traumatic injury, i.e., the traumatic epidemiology from weapons that contributes to the case load of an ER
landmark walking	practice of the ataxic, infirm, seasick, drunk, and others of unconfident stability and gait, of walking from one object to another to steady oneself or rest before moving on to the next
LWBS	"left without being seen"—abbreviation placed upon charts to account for patients who no longer can be accounted for
lytes	electrolytes
meat wagon	transporting ambulance
mud pies	mnemonic for anion gap acidosis
perfed appy	ruptured appendix
perineal towel sign	refers to panty liner, sanitary napkin, tissues, incontinence diapers, washcloths, or towels worn in underwear of elderly women with urinary incontinence which, in the context of otherwise unexplained illness or early urosepsis
popper	a drug abuser who self-injects subcutaneously, usually because the drug habit has sclerosed all peripheral IV sites of access, leaving no other way for injection
pothole sign	method to gauge sufferers of an acute appendicitis attack
preemie	premature infant
pumper	bleeding vessel seen during examination of or repair of a wound
rally pack	combination of sodium chloride, folic acid, thiamine, and multivitamins frequently given to malnourished patients
retic count	reticulocyte blood count test
rig	transporting ambulance
roofie	barbiturate which can be slipped into a drink for abuse, often Rohypnol

rule of 9's	for assessing percentage of body surface area in burns
sad persons	mnemonic for suicide risk factors
scanning a patient	used to describe ordering or performing an imaging study of the patient in the form of CT scan or ultrasound nuclear medicine scan
sed rate	sedimentation rate blood test
sludge	mnemonic for cholinergic overdose
scoop and run	in the event that no treatment is possible at accident scene, patient is urgently transported to ER
shoot and boot	medicate and discharge
shooter	user of injected illicit drugs; perpetrator who actually commits the act of firing on a victim with a firearm
skin popping	used to describe self-injection of drugs subcutaneously, usually because the drug habit has sclerosed all peripheral IV sites of access
stepdown unit	a monitored setting not as intense as any type of ICU
sundowner/sundown syndrome	well-known tendency for senile or demented patients to have a nocturnal worsening of their mental status and confusion
thump	vigorous thrust to the chest in order to try to stimulate heart
triple A	abdominal aortic aneurysm
trumpet	nasopharyngeal airway, said to be so named due to the flared end that keeps the tube from slipping backwards
tweak score	scale for assessing alcoholism dependence
unit	transporting ambulance
the vapors	vague somatization and physical complaints
walking wounded	injured, not critical
wheezer	asthmatic patient